PATHOLOGY OF THE EAR AND TEMPORAL BONE

George T. Nager, M.D., F.A.C.S., (Hon.) F.R.C.S.I.
Andelot Professor and Chairman Emeritus
Department of Otolaryngology–Head and Neck Surgery
The Johns Hopkins University School of Medicine
Otolaryngologist-in-Chief Emeritus
The Johns Hopkins Hospital
Professor Emeritus, Department of Health Services Administration
The Johns Hopkins University School of Hygiene and Public Health
Baltimore, Maryland

With a contribution from
Vincent J. Hyams, M.D.
Professor and Chairman Emeritus
Distinguished Scientist
Department of Otolaryngic Pathology
Armed Forces Institute of Pathology
Washington, DC
Professor Emeritus
Department of Pathology
Uniformed Services University of Health Sciences
Bethesda, Maryland

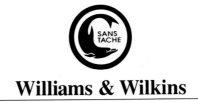

Williams & Wilkins

BALTIMORE • PHILADELPHIA • HONG KONG
LONDON • MUNICH • SYDNEY • TOKYO

A WAVERLY COMPANY

Editor: Charles W. Mitchell
Project Manager: Victoria Rybicki Vaughn
Copy Editor: Bill Cady
Designer: Wilma Rosenberger
Illustration Planner: Wayne Hubbel

Copyright © 1993
Williams & Wilkins
428 East Preston Street
Baltimore, Maryland 21202 USA

Accurate indications, adverse reactions, and dosage schedules for drugs are provided in this book, but it is possible that they may change. The reader is urged to review the package information data of the manufacturers of the medications mentioned.

Printed in the United States of America

Library of Congress Cataloging-in-Publication Data

Nager, George T. (George Theodore), 1917–
    Pathology of the ear and temporal bone   /   George T. Nager, with
contributions by Vincent J. Hyams.
       p.   cm.
    Includes bibliographical reference and index.
    ISBN (invalid) 068363049
    1. Ear—Diseases—Pathogenesis. 2. Ear—Abnormalities. 3. Ear—Histopathology.
4. Ear—Cytopathology. I. Hyams, Vincent J. II. Title.
    [DNLM: 1. Ear Diseases—pathology. 2. Temporal Bone—pathology. 3. Ear—anatomy & histology.   WV 200 N148p 1993]
RF121.N34   1993
616.8′071—dc20
DNLM/DLC
for Library of Congress   93-27739
                                                                                CIP

93 94 95 96 97 98
1 2 3 4 5 6 7 8 9 10

This work is dedicated to my Lord and my Creator, who allowed me to grow up in a family with high standards and a strong academic and rare cultural background, with respect for human dignity and charity toward the poor and the sick. In His infinite generosity and compassion He provided the opportunity for excellent training in various medical disciplines—contacts with remarkable men in outstanding medical institutions that left indelible marks and instilled in me a sense of obligation and commitment. This atmosphere ultimately led to an academic career. One of the great benefits has been the chance to help cultivate, in my own small way, the development of one of the leading departments of otolaryngology– head and neck surgery in one of the finest medical institutions in the world.

Preface

Knowledge of pathology will always be a prerequisite for understanding the pathogenesis, biology, and behavior of a disease process, and it provides a foundation for good patient care. A residency in pathology and three years in medicine, surgery, neurology, neuro-otology, and radiology prior to a residency in otolaryngology–head and neck surgery (ORL-HNS) provided me with a solid base. A year of research on the anatomy and pathology of the ear, following ORL-HNS residency, enabled me to establish my own laboratory and to embark on a lifelong study of diseases affecting the ear and their effect on hearing and equilibrium.

An extensive clinical and surgical practice in one of the largest and foremost medical institutions provided vast and unique clinical material with a broad spectrum of disease entities. These patients have been evaluated by expert clinicians, and their diseases have been thoroughly documented by sophisticated diagnostic tests. Their pathologic changes have been identified by the latest computed tomography and advanced magnetic resonance imaging techniques. The microscopic examination of the serially sectioned temporal bones from many of these and other patients with carefully selected diseases supplied the histopathologic information. Subsequent attempts to correlate the clinical observations and data with the findings during surgical procedures and the morphologic changes observed with the light microscope have provided much valuable new information and clearer insight into a variety of diseases and their effects on hearing and equilibrium. In several instances this has resulted in selection of a better treatment modality for patients, in the technical improvement of surgical procedures, and in the updated training of residents, fellows, and medical students.

In recent years, organizing this type of otologic research, in addition to maintaining a busy surgical practice, directing a residency training program, teaching, and managing a large department in a university setting, has become a progressively more difficult task. Evenings, weekends, and vacations have provided the majority of research time. Collection of valuable anatomical material, rising laboratory expenses, and increasing competition for private and government support have made this work more difficult. Having had the privilege of continuous support from the National Institutes of Health during three decades, I have felt a strong obligation as well as a need to assemble the acquired clinical and pathologic information into a single text and atlas.

The decision to write this book was not undertaken lightly and was actually influenced by John Gardner at Williams & Wilkins. The need for an authoritative text in otologic pathology was obvious. I realized that writing a comprehensive treatise of that kind would require the inclusion of the pertinent clinical information and the latest data on these diseases from the most sophisticated diagnostic, neurologic, and imaging techniques, in addition to their histopathologic documentation and interpretation. Since otolaryngology and, especially, neuro-otology are practiced today in teams and in close collaboration with neuroradiologists, neuro-ophthalmologists, neurosurgeons, neurologists, and pathologists, such a text would also have to consider their interests and be of equal value to them. Therefore, this book has been written primarily for otologists in training, private practice, and academic institutions and for our colleagues in these specialties who daily are intimately concerned with otology and neuro-otology. It will also appeal to senior medical students and postdoctoral fellows who decide to spend elective time or a year of research in this specialty.

The material is organized into 56 chapters according to the different disease processes, neoplasms, injuries, etc. Each chapter was written with the intention of providing the reader with essential clinical information in addition to a comprehensive description and interpretation of the histopathology. Certain topics, i.e., some of the bone dysplasias, were intentionally treated in greater detail in order to provide the reader, especially the otologist, with a better insight and all the important data that are scattered throughout the medical literature and are usually not readily available.

The book begins with a chapter on the gross and microscopic anatomy of the temporal bone based on serial sections in the conventional vertical and horizontal planes. The fact that these planes are identical with the coronal and axial planes used by neuroradiologists in their evaluation of the temporal bone and skull base will make this and many other chapters especially attractive to them.

Dr. Vince Hyams has coauthored Chapters 15–21 of Section III on benign and malignant neoplasms and other lesions involving the external ear, middle ear, and temporal bone. His vast experience and great expertise are clearly reflected in his valuable contributions.

Special attention has also been given to the chapter on fractures and ballistic injuries (Chapter 55), conditions that are still being overlooked but are of great significance with respect to their immediate and long-term effects on cochlear, vestibular, and facial nerve function. The content of this chapter will be of great value to the general radiologist, neurosurgeon, emergency room physician, and forensic pathologist. In only very few instances have I been able to resist including some of the more interesting rare lesions I have come across.

A relatively large number of illustrations in color, halftone, and pen and ink, some of them original, and photomicrographs, many of them original, have been selected to portray the gross and microscopic features of the various diseases.

References at the end of each chapter include original articles, considered to be classical contributions, and more recent information. It is not possible to give bibliographic note to all who have contributed to our knowledge of a given topic, for there are too many. For obvious oversights I ask the reader's indulgence.

The writing of a text like this will continue to remain an imperfect art because of the volume of available knowledge accumulating in seemingly exponential proportions. Thus this book could not include all the disease processes involving the temporal bone.

G.T.N.

Contents

Section IV. Tumors of the Nerve Sheath, Meninges, Brain, and Other Space-occupying Lesions of the Temporal Bone

Section V. Cystic Diseases of the Temporal Bone

Section VI. Bone Dysplasias

SECTION VII. OTHER DISORDERS INVOLVING THE EAR AND TEMPORAL BONE

SECTION I

ANATOMY

1/ Anatomy of the Membranous Cochlea and Vestibular Labyrinth

The inner ear, which comprises the cochlea and the vestibular labyrinth, is situated within the petrous portion of the temporal bone (Fig. 1.1). It consists of an osseous portion, the cochlear and the vestibular capsule, and a membranous portion, enclosed in the former (Figs. 1.2 and 1.3).

The principal components of the membranous or endolymphatic portion include the cochlear duct, the saccule, the utricle, the ductus reuniens, a narrow channel connecting the cochlear duct with the saccule, the three semicircular ducts with their ampullae, and the endolymphatic duct and sac (Figs. 1.4 and 1.5). Utricle and saccule communicate with the sinus of the endolymphatic duct via the utricular and saccular ducts. The opening of the slit-like utricular duct is controlled by the utriculoendolymphatic valve (Fig. 1.6). The membranous cochlea and vestibular labyrinth represent a system of the epithelium-lined tubes and compartments filled with a clear fluid, the endolymph. This endolymphatic system is surrounded by perilymphatic compartments supported by connective tissue containing clear perilymph. These two separate fluid systems together are enclosed in their respective bony capsules.

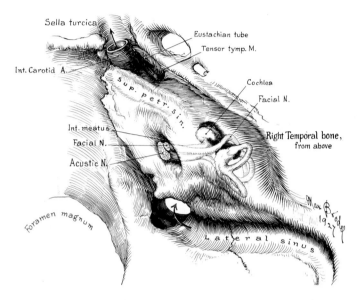

Figure 1.1. Schematic drawing of location of membranous cochlea and vestibular labyrinth within right temporal bone.

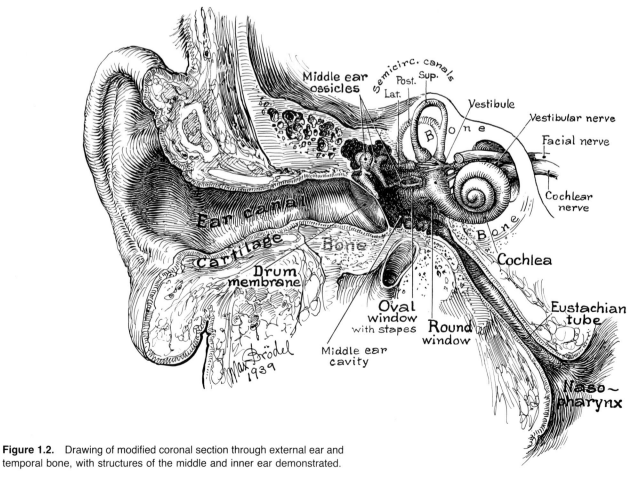

Figure 1.2. Drawing of modified coronal section through external ear and temporal bone, with structures of the middle and inner ear demonstrated.

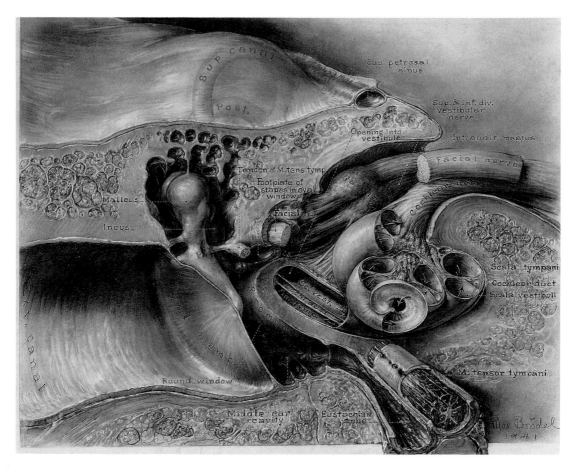

Figure 1.3. Drawing of modified coronal section of right temporal bone, with midmodiolar section through cochlea demonstrating the scala media, scala vestibuli, and scala tympani in each cochlear turn and the seventh and eighth cranial nerves within internal auditory canal.

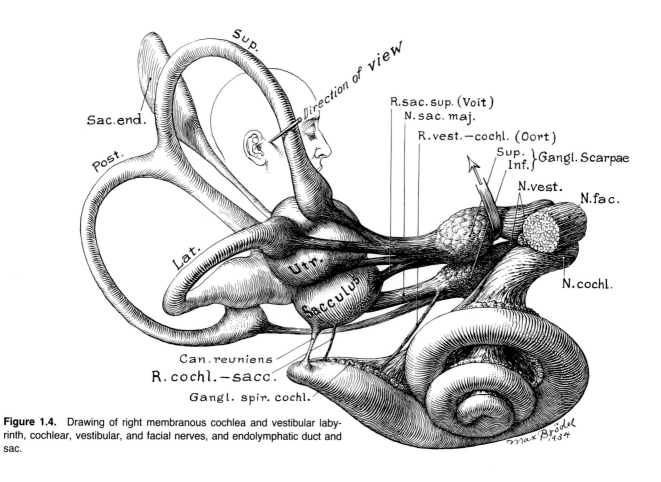

Figure 1.4. Drawing of right membranous cochlea and vestibular labyrinth, cochlear, vestibular, and facial nerves, and endolymphatic duct and sac.

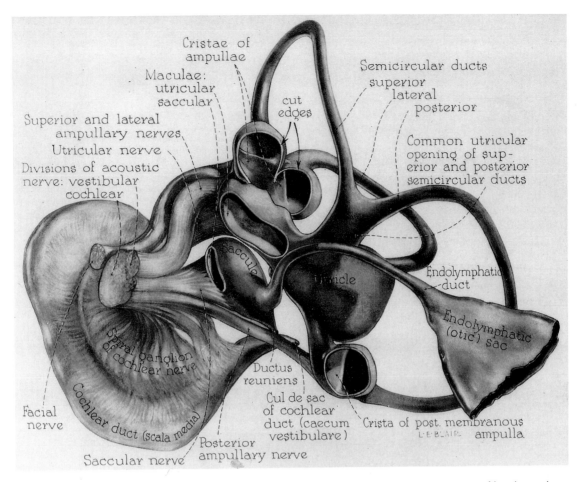

Figure 1.5. Drawing of right eighth cranial (cochlear and vestibular) nerve and sensory organs of hearing and equilibrium that are thereby innervated.

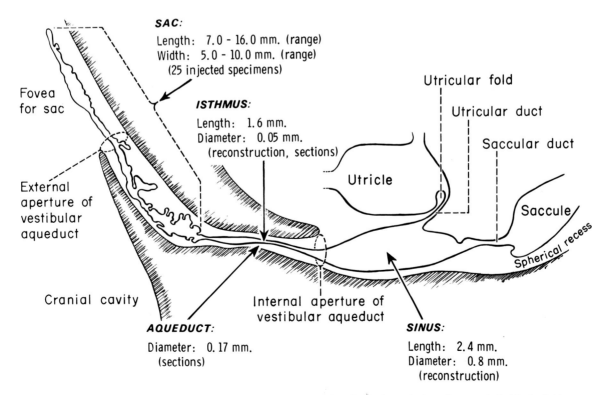

Figure 1.6. Schematic drawing of left utricle, saccule, endolymphatic sinus, duct, and sac and of utricular fold (utriculoendolymphatic valve).

MEMBRANOUS COCHLEA

The membranous cochlea or cochlear duct is a cone-shaped spirally oriented, membranous tube between the osseous spiral lamina and the outer osseous wall of the cochlea to which it is attached. On cross-section, this epithelium-lined tube displays a trigonal configuration (Figs. 1.3, 1.4, and 1.7). The stria vascularis with the underlying spiral ligament represents the height; the basilar membrane, the base; and Reissner's membrane, the hypotenuse of this right-angle triangle (Fig. 1.8). The inferior end of the cochlear duct terminates in a blind pouch, the vestibular cecum (Figs. 1.4 and 1.5). It occupies the cochlear recess of the vestibule and communicates with the saccule through a narrow channel, the ductus reuniens (Figs. 1.4 and 1.5). As the cochlear duct continues its ascending spiral path, it creates the

basal, the middle, and an incomplete apical turn. The apical turn also terminates blindly in the cupular cecum situated just above the hamulus of the osseous spiral lamina (Figs. 1.2–1.4 and 1.7). The cochlear duct contains the spiral organ of Corti. This peripheral sense organ of hearing rests on the basilar membrane (Figs. 1.7–1.9).

The cochlear duct with the basilar and Reissner's membrane divides the osseous cochlear canal into an upper spiral perilymphatic compartment, the scala vestibuli, and a lower spiral perilymphatic compartment, the scala tympani (Figs. 1.3, 1.7, and 1.8). These two scalae communicate apically at the helicotrema above the cupular cecum (Figs. 1.3 and 1.7). Whereas the scala tympani terminates blindly at the round window membrane, the scala vestibuli opens up at that level into the perilymphatic space of the vestibulum.

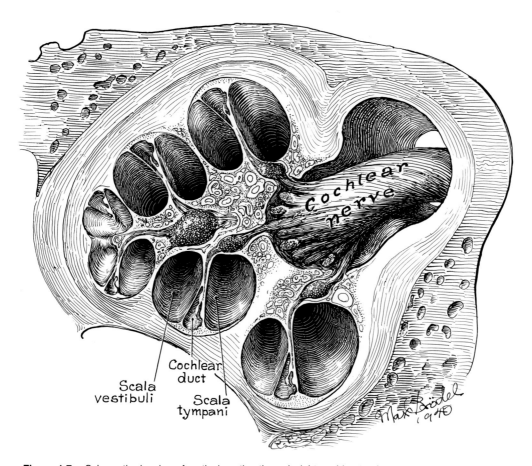

Figure 1.7. Schematic drawing of vertical section through right cochlea to show anatomy of cochlear duct, spiral ligament, and cochlear nerve.

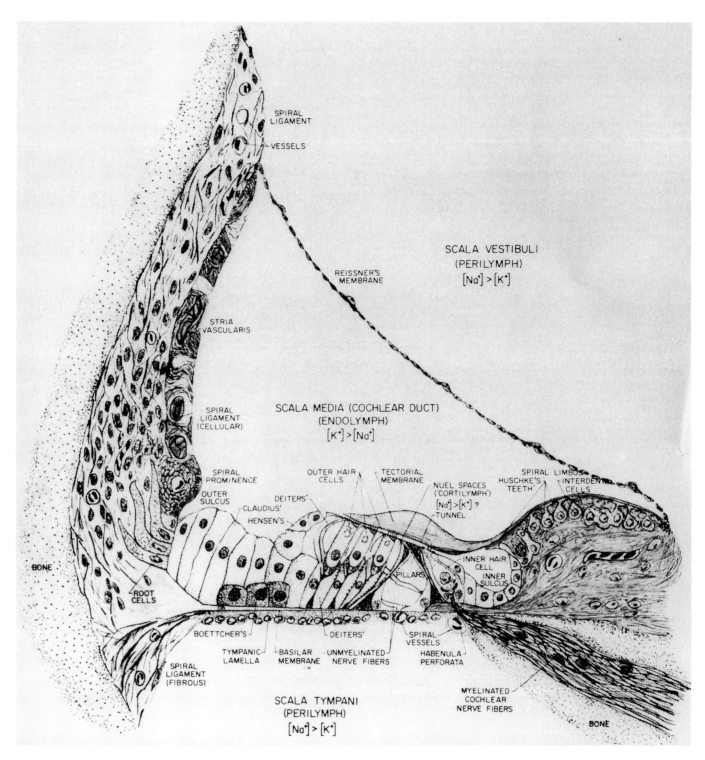

Figure 1.8. Schematic drawing of radial section through cochlear duct, with spiral ligament, Reissner's and basilar membrane, and organ of Corti demonstrated.

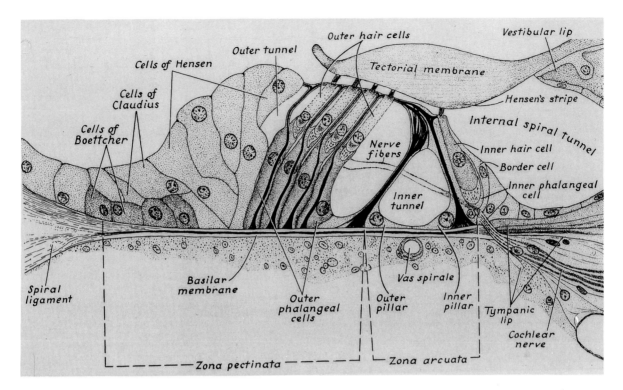

Figure 1.9. Drawing of radial section of organ of Corti from basal turn of human cochlea. The spiral organ extends throughout the length of the cochlea. It is composed of one inner and four outer hair cells, the receptor cells for perception of auditory stimuli, and other cells of various forms that serve to support these sensory elements. The supporting cells include: *(a)* the inner and outer pillar cells, *(b)* the inner and outer phalangeal cells, and *(c)* the cells of Hensen.

COCHLEAR NERVE

The signals from the receptor cells of the spiral end organ of Corti are transmitted to the auditory cortex by the afferent acoustic nerve fibers. The terminal, unmyelinated nerve fibers embrace the lower pole of the hair cells with their synaptic endings in a chalice-like arrangement (Figs. 1.9 and 1.10). They traverse the inner tunnel of Corti, enter the nerve channels of the osseous spiral lamina at the habenula perforata (Figs. 1.8, 1.9, 1.11, and 1.12), and, on reaching the cochlear modiolus, become myelinated. After a short course in the modiolus, these peripheral dendrites join their cell bodies in the spiral ganglion (Figs. 1.4, 1.7, 1.11, and 1.12). The spiral ganglion represents the first of four neurons between the auditory end organ and the auditory cortex. The spiral ganglion is situated in Rosenthal's canal that follows a spiral course to the apex. The central fibers or axons of these bipolar neurons unite to nerve bundles and pass from the cochlear modiolus through nerve channels in the osseous spiral foraminous tract into the internal auditory canal (IAC), where they form the cochlear nerve (Figs. 1.3, 1.4, 1.7, 1.11, and 1.12). In the IAC the cochlear nerve resembles, in structure, a telephone cable made up of numerous wires that has been slightly rotated counterclockwise, as viewed from the porus acusticus (Figs. 1.3, 1.4, and 1.7). This means that the nerve fibers from the third or apical turn of the cochlea run in the center of the nerve and are surrounded by an intermediate layer of nerve fibers from the second or middle turn of the cochlea but that the fibers from the first or basal cochlear turn form the outermost layer of cochlear nerve fibers, with all following a slightly counterclockwise spiral rotation (Figs. 1.3, 1.4, and 1.7). Accordingly, the fiber bundles that transmit the high-frequency responses perceived in the basal turn represent the outer zone of the cochlear nerve.

Within the IAC the cochlear nerve is joined by the vestibular nerve and accompanied by the facial nerve (Figs. 1.1–1.5). Together, the three nerves enter the posterior cranial fossa, traverse the cerebellopontine cistern, and enter the brain stem at the posterior lower lateral aspect of the pons. The intracerebral or central auditory pathways consist of three additional neurons that form numerous connections with nuclei throughout the central nervous system as part of a complex auditory reflex system, as they reach the auditory cortex in the anterior transverse gyrus (Heschl) of the superior temporal lobe (1).

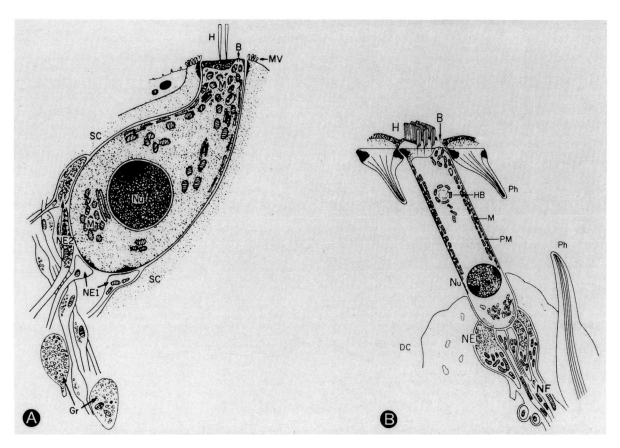

Figure 1.10.   Schematic drawing of cochlear hair cells as visualized with electron microscope. **A.** Inner hair cell. **B.** Outer hair cell. *B,* basal body of kinocilium; *H,* stereocilia; *M,* mitochondrion; *MV,* microvilli on supporting cell; *NE,* nerve ending; *NE1,* afferent nerve ending (agranulated); *NE2,* efferent nerve ending (granulated); and *Ph,* phalangeal process.

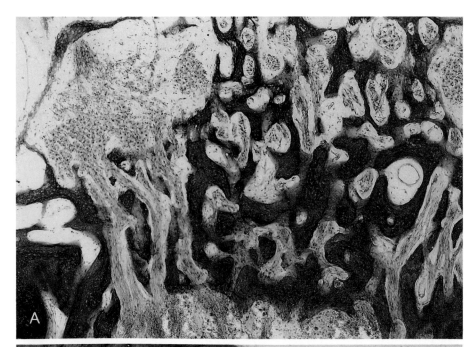

Figure 1.11. A. Vertical section through left cochlear modiolus at fundus of internal auditory canal of a 65-year-old man who died from cerebellar hemorrhage. The cochlear nerve fibers enter the modiolus through short osseous channels in the spiral foraminous tract. (Hematoxylin and eosin, × 65.)

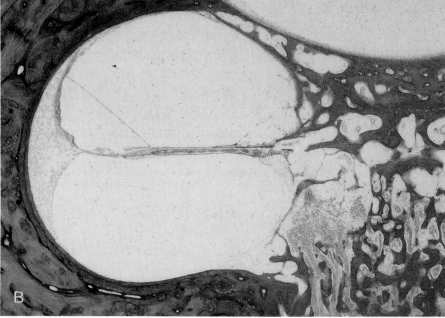

Figure 1.11. B. Cross-section through left upper basal cochlear turn. The cochlear nerve fibers join the bipolar spiral ganglion located adjacent to the medial wall of the scala tympani. (×35.)

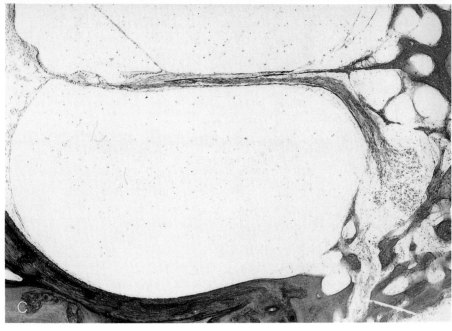

Figure 1.11. C. From the spiral ganglion the peripheral nerve fibers (dendrites) traverse the neural canals in the osseous spiral lamina, leaving them again at the habenula perforata for their final destination. (×65.)

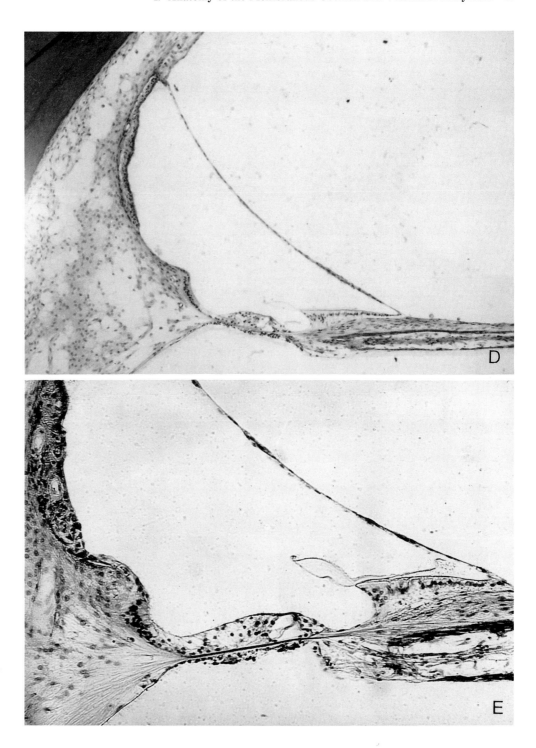

Figure 1.11. **D** and **E.** Cross-sections through organ of Corti in upper basal turn. The inner and outer hair cells are recognized among other cellular structures. ($\times$300 and $\times$500, respectively.)

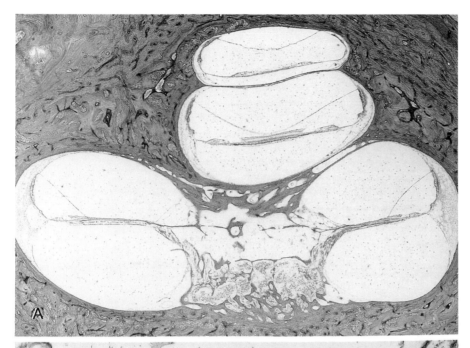

Figure 1.12. A. Vertical paramodiolar section through right cochlea at center of spiral ganglion in a 64-year-old man who died from cardiovascular disease. (Hematoxylin and eosin, ×18.)

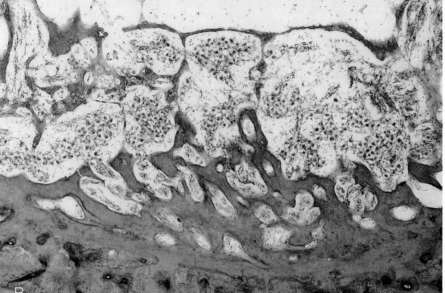

Figure 1.12. B. In its arrangement the spiral ganglion resembles the beads in a string of pearls as it approaches the apex of the cochlea in an ascending concentric spiral pathway. (×70.)

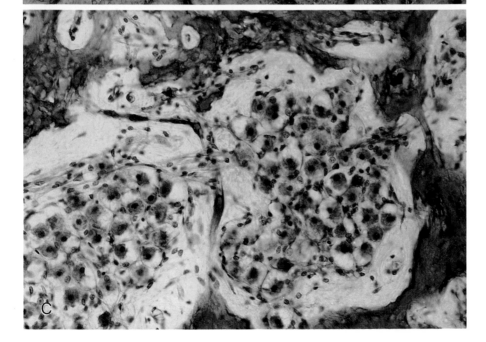

Figure 1.12. C. The individual bipolar ganglion cells are grouped together in separate, communicating osseous compartments. (×260.)

EFFERENT COCHLEAR INNERVATION

The efferent cochlear neurons arise in several areas of the auditory cortex and accompany the ascending auditory pathways. They connect the cortical region with the lower auditory centers and the cochlear end organ. Two systems are distinguished, with one ending in the dorsal cochlear nucleus and the other terminating as the olivocochlear bundle on the hair cells of the organ of Corti (Figs. 1.13–1.15).

Most efferent fibers (75%) of the olivocochlear bundle originate in the contralateral accessory superior olivary nucleus. The remaining fibers arise in the homolateral superior portion of the main olivary nucleus. The efferent fibers leave the brain stem, accompanying the vestibular nerve to the IAC, where they leave the inferior division of that nerve at the saccular ganglion as the vestibulocochlear anastomosis (bundle of Oort) to enter the lower basal turn of the cochlea and become the intraganglionic spiral bundle of Rasmussen (2–6). This bundle continues its spiral

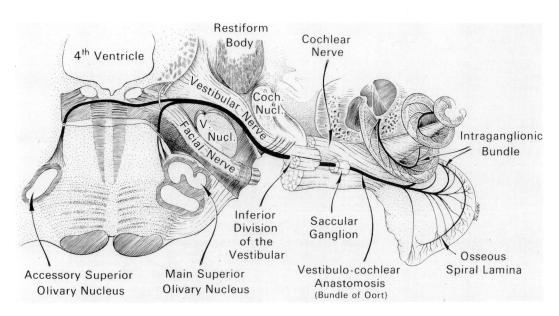

Figure 1.13. Drawing demonstrating origin and course of efferent auditory nerve fibers.

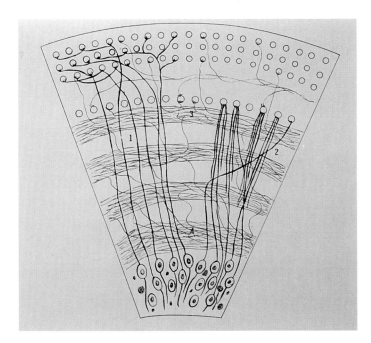

Figure 1.14. Schematic drawing of basilar membrane, demonstrating afferent and efferent innervation of organ of Corti. *1,* afferent nerve fibers to outer hair cells (black); *2,* radial afferent fibers to inner hair cells (black); *3,* interganglionic efferent nerve fibers of Rasmussen (red); and *4,* outer, efferent spiral bundle (red).

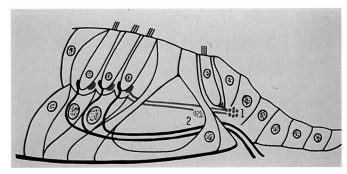

Figure 1.15. Schematic drawing of innervation of outer and inner cochlear hair cells. *1,* inner spiral bundle (red); and *2,* tunnel spiral bundle (black).

pathway upward to the apex of the cochlea as well as in the opposite direction to the round window (Figs. 1.13–1.19). It is most noticeable in the upper basal cochlear turn (Figs. 1.18 and 1.19). The intraganglionic spiral bundle at short intervals gives off between three and six radial nerve fibers, which unite, pass through the osseous spinal lamina, and form two spiral bundles. They form the inner spiral bundle (Figs. 1.13–1.15, 1.18, and 1.19) beneath the inner hair cells, with many of its fibers terminating on the inner hair cells or their afferent nerve fibers (Fig. 1.15). Other radial nerve fibers either extend directly to the outer hair cells or unite to form the delicate midtunnel spiral bundle from where they innervate primarily the outer hair cells or their afferent nerve fibers (Figs. 1.14 and 1.15). These fibers to the outer hair cells form the medial fibers within the tunnel of Corti.

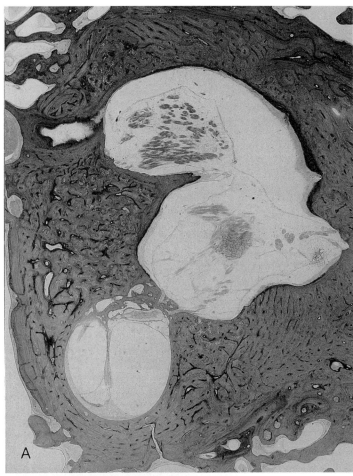

Figure 1.16. **A.** Vertical section through right petrous pyramid near center of IAC and lower basal turn of cochlea. The branch that leaves the inferior vestibular nerve just below the saccular ganglion to join the basal turn of the cochlea is recognized in a series of cross-sections. It represents the vestibulocochlear anastomoses of Oort or the efferent olivocochlear bundle. (Hematoxylin and eosin, ×18.)

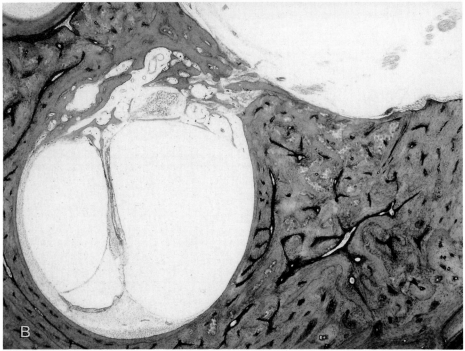

Figure 1.16. **B.** The olivocochlear bundle passes through short channels in the osseous foraminous tract to join the spiral ganglion, where it forms the ascending and descending intraganglionic spiral bundle. (×30.)

Thus, each hair cell is innervated by an efferent fiber, whereby the outer hair cells exhibit a predominantly radial innervation and the inner hair cell exhibits a primarily spiral innervation. In contrast to the afferent cochlear fibers, the efferent fibers display abundant ramifications (Fig. 1.14). The approximately 500 fibers that constitute the vestibulocochlear anastomosis eventually subdivide below the inner and outer hair cells into about 40,000 nerve fibers with their synapses on the lower pole of the hair cells or on their afferent fibers (2).

Close (synaptic) contacts presumably exist between afferent and efferent innervation at the base of the outer hair cells, in the outer and the inner spiral bundle, and in the intraganglionic spiral bundle. It is conceivable that similar contacts may exist in the intraganglionic spiral bundle between efferent and adrenogenic nerve fibers (2, 6).

The efferent or descending nerve fibers have, in general, an inhibitory effect on the ascending afferent fibers and in their function represent to some degree a self-regulating mechanism of the auditory system. That each relay unit along the auditory pathway is considered to have a dual innervation enables incoming signals to be attenuated, modified, or inhibited (5).

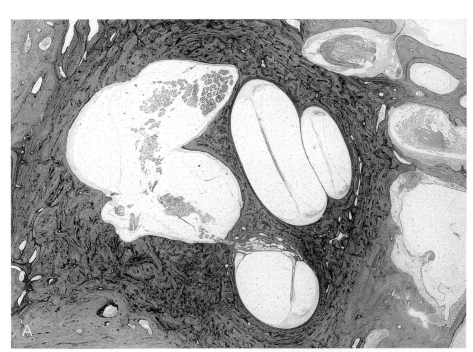

Figure 1.17. A. Vertical paramodiolar section through left IAC and basal cochlear turn of a 56-year-old man who died from cardiovascular disease. The vestibulocochlear anastomosis is seen leaving the inferior vestibular nerve. (Hematoxylin and eosin, ×10.)

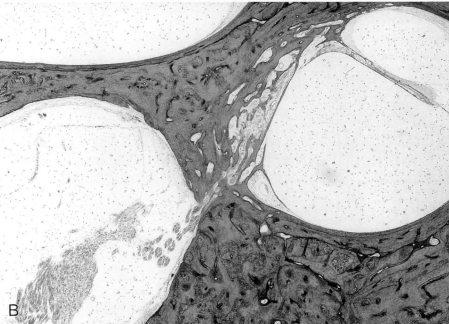

Figure 1.17. B. The vestibulocochlear anastomosis is seen as it joins the spiral ganglion of the lower basal turn of the cochlea. (×25.)

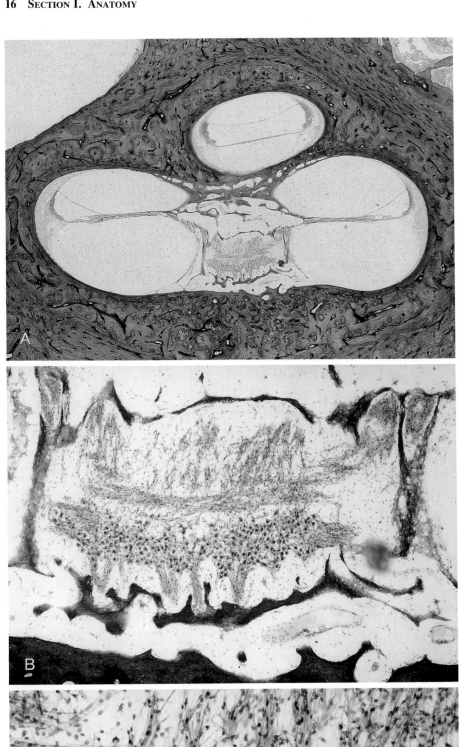

Figure 1.18. A. Vertical paramodiolar section through right cochlea at level of spiral ganglion of a 41-year-old man who died from endotheliomatous meningioma of the right sphenoid wing. (Hematoxylin and eosin, ×16.)

Figure 1.18. B. Dendrites, cell bodies, and axons of the bipolar ganglion cells and the intraganglionic spiral bundle. (×65.)

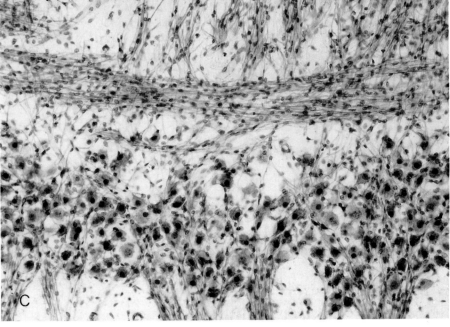

Figure 1.18. C. The longitudinal intraganglionic efferent spiral bundle periodically gives off groups of three to six efferent radial fibers to the organ of Corti. These radial fibers, in turn, give rise to the outer efferent spiral bundle beneath the inner hair cells and to the more lateral efferent, mid-tunnel spiral bundle for the majority of outer hair cells (see Fig. 1.15). (×205.)

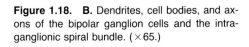

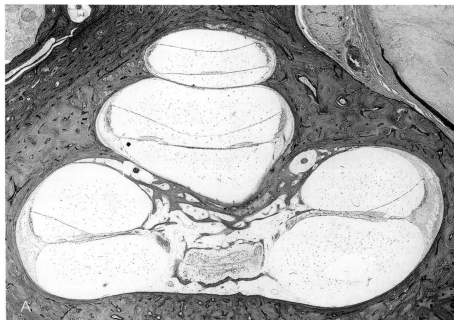

Figure 1.19.   A. Vertical paramodiolar section through left cochlea at level of spiral ganglion in a 78-year-old man who died from generalized arteriosclerosis. (Hematoxylin and eosin, ×27.)

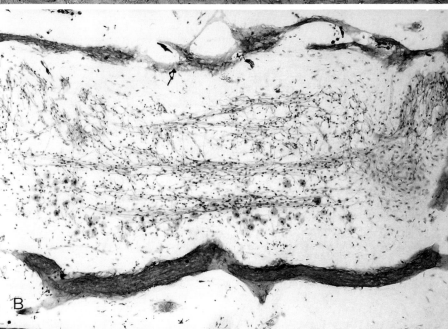

Figure 1.19.   B. Same section of efferent intraganglionic spiral bundle as it continues its spiral course toward the apex (×110.)

AUTONOMOUS INNERVATION OF THE COCHLEA

A long-assumed autonomous innervation of the cochlea has been confirmed by the evidence of adrenergic nerve fibers in the cochlea (2, 6). Two types of fibers may be distinguished: *(a)* a perivascular plexus consisting of a dense network of adrenergic fibers, presumably originating in the pericarotid nervous plexus, that surrounds the basilar artery, the anterior inferior cerebellar artery (AICA), and the labyrinthine artery and whose major branches terminate in the cochlear modiolus; and *(b)* a nerve plexus in the lamina spiralis ossea. This nerve plexus is located distal from the habenula perforata of the spiral osseous lamina. It is independent of the regional blood vessels and has its origin in the superior cervical ganglion. It reaches the inner ear via the tympani plexus, the superficial petrosal nerve, and the facial nerve or via the auricular branch of the vagus nerve, the facial nerve, and the IAC (2).

MEMBRANOUS VESTIBULAR LABYRINTH

The utricle has the form of an irregular, ovoid, somewhat flattened sac. Its position is superior and posterior to the saccule (Figs. 1.4, 1.5, and 1.20). It occupies the elliptical recess in the posterosuperior wall of the vestibule, where it is firmly attached by connective tissue and the penetrating nerve bundles from the utricular division of the superior vestibular nerve. The macula of the utricle is located in the utricular recess, which corresponds to the distended anterior portion of the utricle. It has an oval shape, lies in a horizontal plane, and represents the utricular sensory receptor organ (Figs. 1.4, 1.5, and 1.20). The utricle communicates with the semicircular ducts through openings in its superior and posterior wall. The superior and posterior semicircular ducts form a common crus before joining the utricle (Figs. 1.4, 1.5, and 1.20). The utricular duct originates from the posteroinferior wall of the utricule, passes through the utriculoendolymphatic valve, and opens into the sinus of the endolymphatic duct (Figs. 1.6 and 1.20).

The saccule resembles an irregular-shaped, ovoid sac. It is smaller than the utricle. It is situated anterior and inferior to the utricle and occupies the spherical recess of the medial wall of the vestibule (Figs. 1.4, 1.5, 1.20, and 1.30). It is joined to the anterior wall of the vestibule by fibrous tissue and the entering nerve bundles of the saccular branch of the vestibular nerve. Most nerve fibers are derived from the inferior division, with only a small portion derived from the superior division of the vestibule nerve (Fig. 1.25). The posterosuperior wall of the saccule is firmly attached to the adjacent utricle. The macula sacculi has the shape of a hook and lies in a vertical plane (Figs. 1.4, 1.5, and 1.20). The saccule communicates with the lower basal turn of the cochlea via the narrow ductus reuniens (Figs. 1.4 and 1.5) and through the saccular duct with the sinus of the endolymphatic duct (Fig. 1.6) (1).

VESTIBULAR NERVE

The vestibule nerve originates from bipolar cells of the superior and the inferior division of the vestibular or Scarpa's ganglion inside the IAC (Figs. 1.3, 1.4, and 1.24). The superior division receives afferent fibers from the cristae of the superior and lateral semicircular ducts and from the macula of the utricle and receives a small portion of nerve fibers from the macula of the saccule (Figs. 1.4, 1.5, and 1.25). The inferior division receives the major portion of afferent fibers from the macula of the saccule (Figs. 1.4 and 1.5) and, by its posterior branch or singular nerve afferent fibers, from the crista of the posterior semicircular duct (Figs. 1.4, 1.5, and 1.20) (7–11). The central axons from the bipolar cells of Scarpa's ganglion form the main trunk of the vestibular nerve, which, on entering the medulla, divides into an ascending and a descending root. Branches from the ascending root continue to the superior, medial, and lateral vestibular nuclei, with a few extending to the inferior peduncle of the cerebellum, to the vermis, and to the nucleus fastigii. The fibers from the cristae of the semicircular canals end in the superior and rostral part of the medial nucleus, whereas the ones from the maculae of the utricle and saccule are directed to the lateral and the caudal part of the medial nucleus. The fibers that form the descending (spinal) root of the vestibular nerve terminate in the inferior (spinal) vestibular nucleus (8).

INNERVATION OF THE UTRICLE AND SACCULE

Whereas the macula of the utricle is innervated exclusively by the superior vestibular nerve, the saccular macula is supplied by all three divisions of the eighth cranial nerve. These three branches are: *(a)* the ramus saccularis superior (Voit (12)), a branch from the superior vestibular nerve (Fig. 1.25); *(b)* the ramus saccularis major, the largest branch of the inferior vestibular nerve (Fig. 1.27); and *(c)* the ramus cochleosaccularis (Hardy (13)), a branch of the cochlear nerve (Fig. 1.28). The ramus saccularis superior, initially described for mammals in 1907 (12), is a constant finding in the adult. With thick nerve fibers it innervates the anterior saccular macula (Figs. 1.29 and 1.30). The ramus saccularis major supplies the main posterior portion of the saccular macula with medium-sized nerve fibers (Figs. 1.29 and 1.30). The cochleosaccular nerve is the smallest of the three nerves. It is usually present but frequently missed because of its small size (13). It originates as a tiny nerve bundle from the spiral ganglion near its basal end. It courses generally in the vertical plane of the section through tiny bony channels of about 1-mm in length medial and upward in the bony ridge between the cochlea and the spherical recess to the undersurface of the posterior end of the saccular macula (Fig. 1.28). The canalis reuniens lies on the surface of the bony ridge above and slightly posterior to the delicate cochleosaccular nerve bundle made up of the smallest caliber of nerve fibers (Fig. 1.30). These nerve fibers mingle with those from the ramus saccularis major under the posterior tip of the saccular macula. The cochleosaccular nerve is considered to be a true branch of the cochlear nerve. It is quite distinct from the vestibulocochlear anastomosis (Oort (14)). As there is some intermingling of the three calibers of nerve fibers, the boundaries of the innervated macular areas are not clearly defined (Fig. 1.30). In general, however, the thick nerve fibers innervate the anterior end, the medium nerve fibers innervate the main part of the posterior end, and the thin nerve fibers innervate the posterior end and the superior margin of the saccular macula (15–17). Autogenetically and phylogenetically, the sacculus is the primary structure; the utricle and semicircular canals develop later and only indirectly become connected (13).

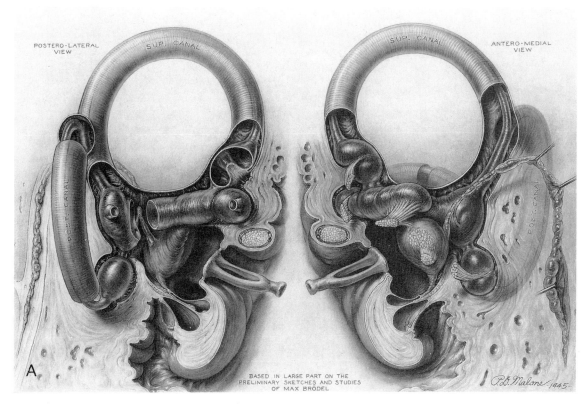

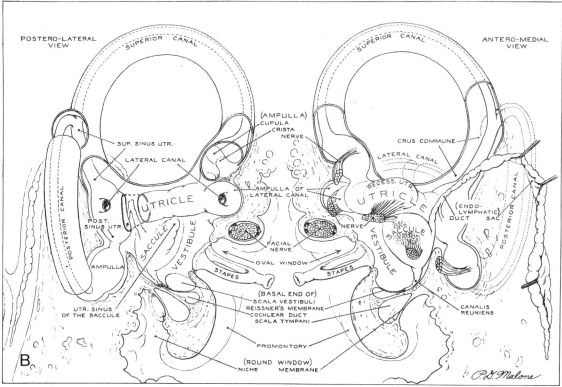

Figure 1.20.   Drawing of vertical section through right vestibular labyrinth at level of oval and round windows, with branches of vestibular nerve, endolymphatic duct, and sac demonstrated.

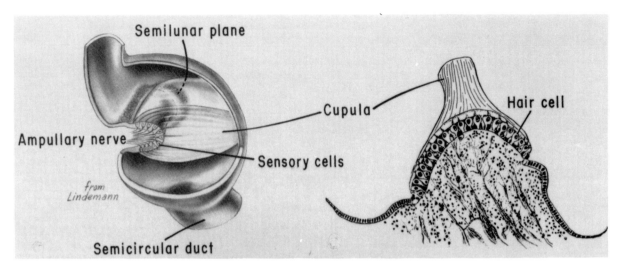

Figure 1.21. Semischematic drawing of architecture of cupula. The crista, crossing the ampullary expansion of the semicircular duct, is invested by sensory epithelium. The hairs of the sensory cells protrude into the cupula, which extends from the surface of the epithelium of the roof of the ampulla and outward to the planum semilunare on the side of the ampulla. The transitional epithelium is located at the base of the crista.

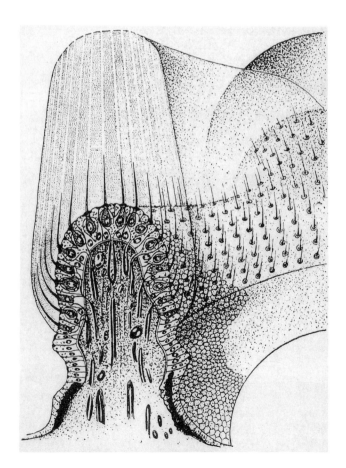

Figure 1.22. Schematic representation of section through ridge of crista ampullaris. It shows the organization of the hair cells along the surface of the crista and the insertion of the cilia into the cupula.

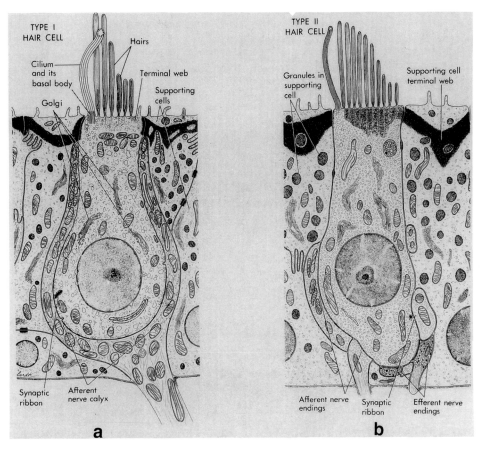

Figure 1.23. Schematic representation of ultrastructure of vestibular hair cells. It shows the principal features of the vestibular type I and type II hair cells and their supporting cells.

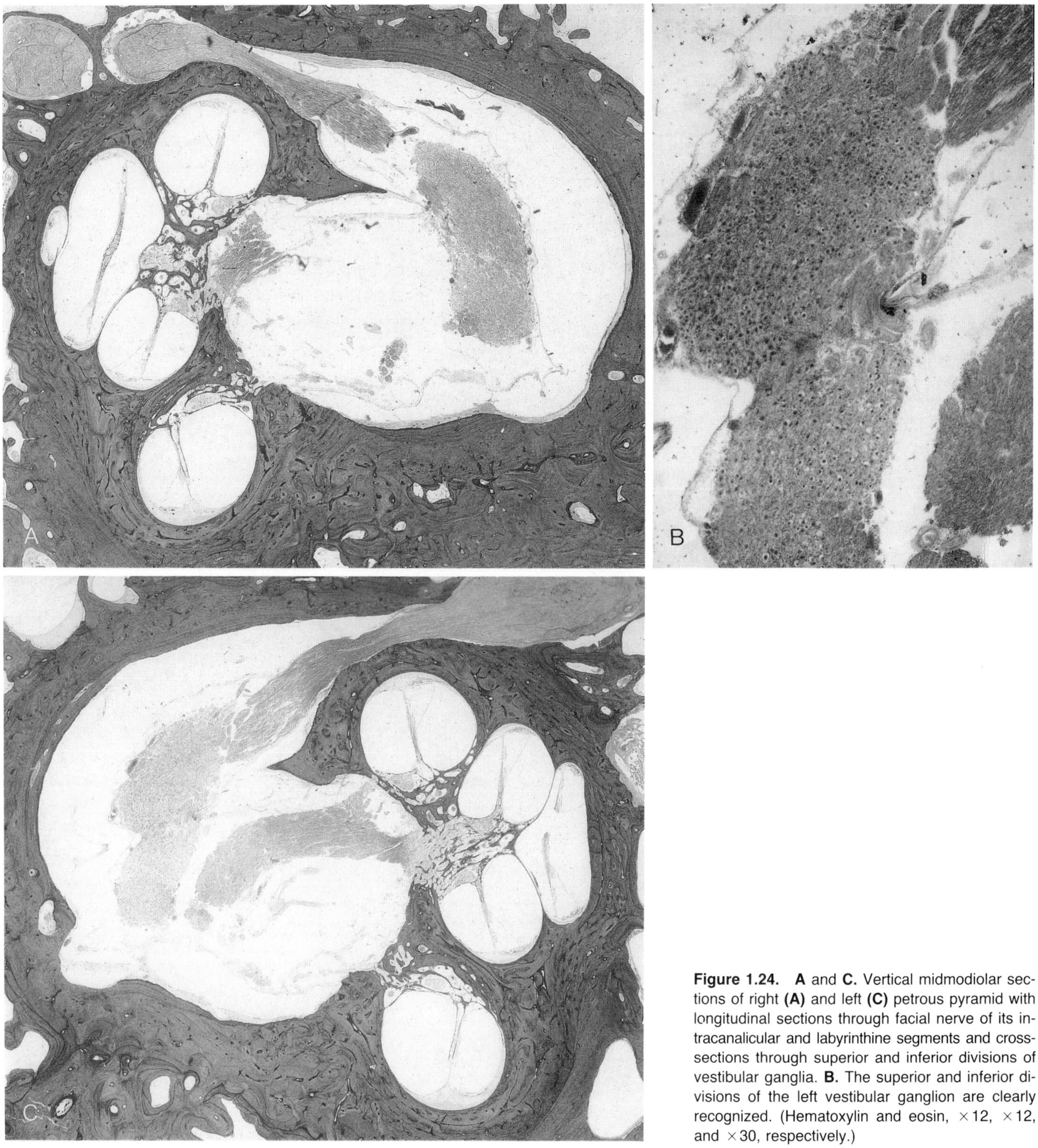

Figure 1.24. A and **C.** Vertical midmodiolar sections of right **(A)** and left **(C)** petrous pyramid with longitudinal sections through facial nerve of its intracanalicular and labyrinthine segments and cross-sections through superior and inferior divisions of vestibular ganglia. **B.** The superior and inferior divisions of the left vestibular ganglion are clearly recognized. (Hematoxylin and eosin, ×12, ×12, and ×30, respectively.)

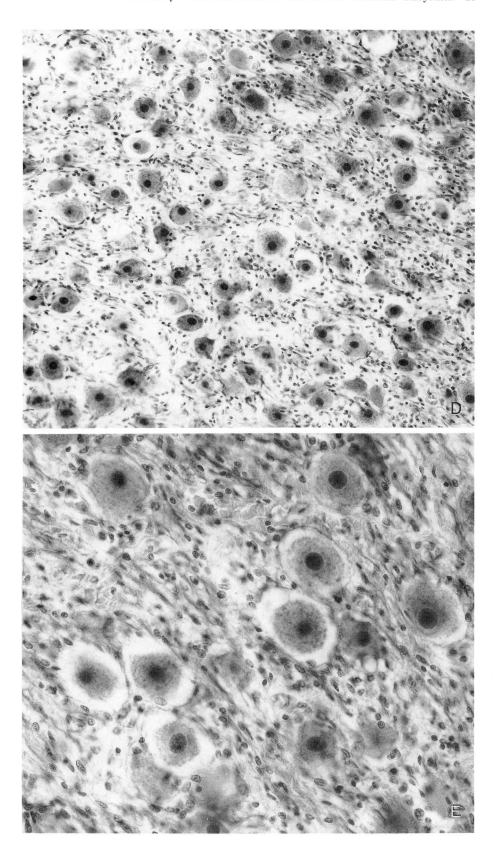

Figure 1.24. D and **E.** The bipolar vestibular ganglion cells with their peripheral dendrites and central axons represent the first of several neural units that constitute the vestibular pathways. ($\times 70$ and $\times 440$, respectively.)

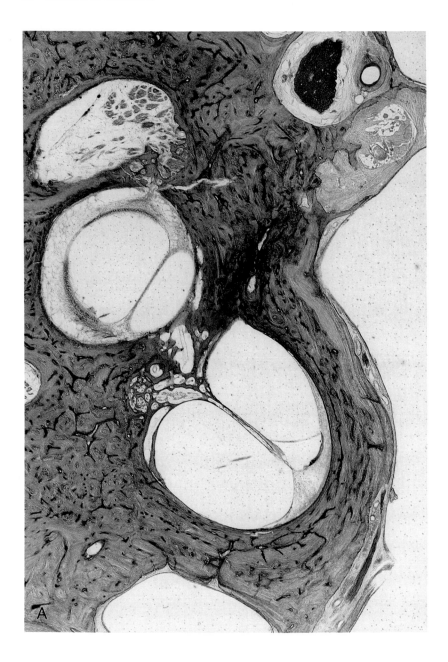

Figure 1.25.   A. Vertical section through left pyramid at level of macula sacculi in 56-year-old man who died from chronic pyelonephritis and generalized arteriosclerosis. (Hematoxylin and eosin, ×18.)

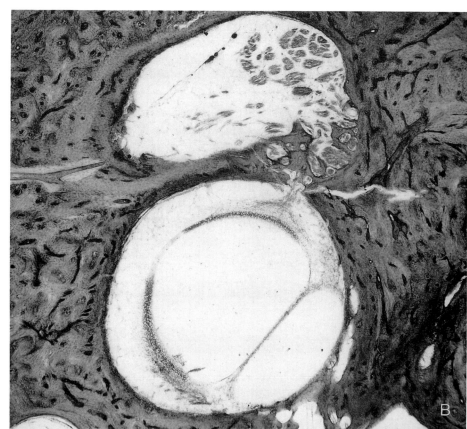

Figure 1.25. B. A branch from the superior division of the vestibular nerve is leaving the IAC and entering the spherical recess of the vestibule to supply a small portion of the macula sacculi. (×30.)

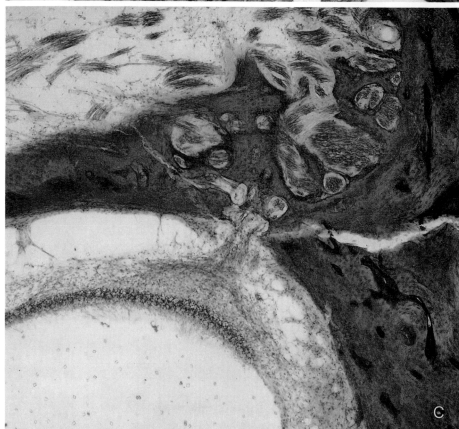

Figure 1.25. C. The saccular branch of the superior vestibular nerve forms a delicate network beneath the neurosensory epithelium of the adjacent macula sacculi. (×70.)

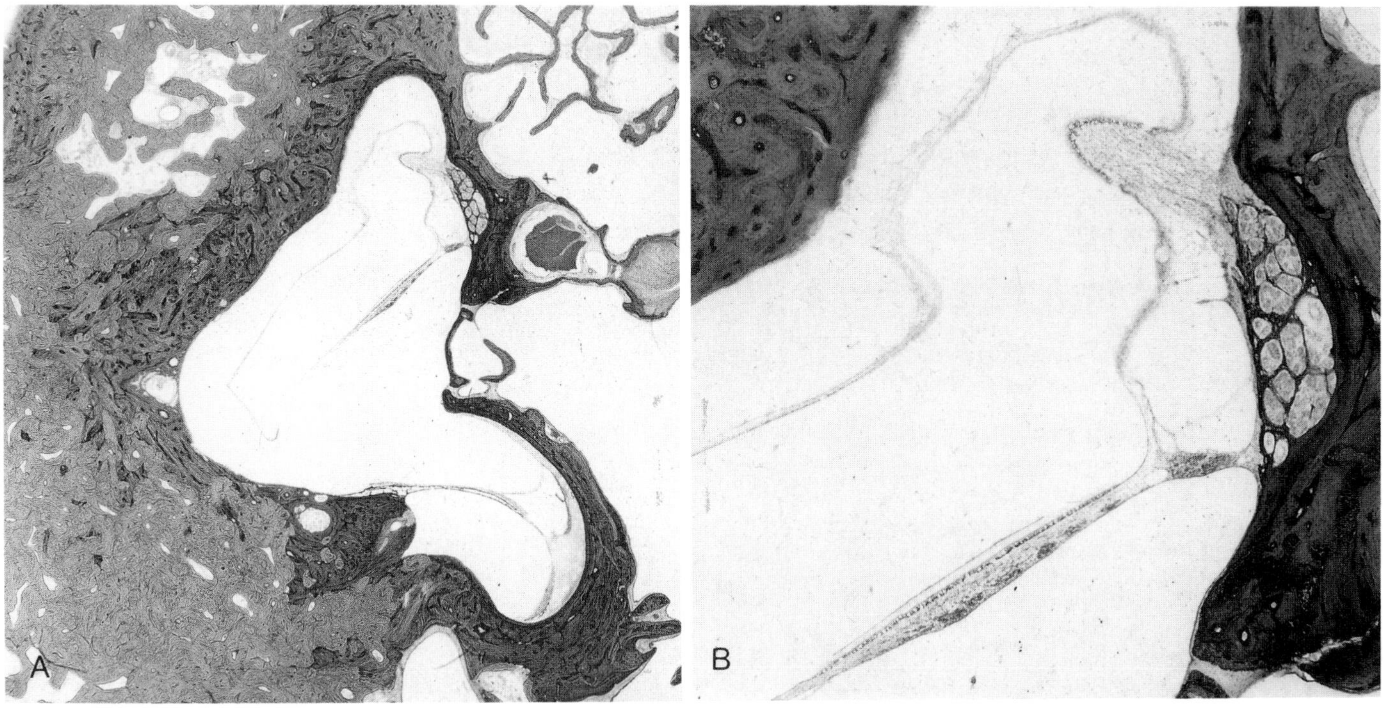

Figure 1.26. **A.** Vertical section through left petrous pyramid at level of oval window in a 65-year-old man. It shows the utricle and the ampulla of the superior semicircular canal. **B.** Branches from the superior division of the vestibular nerve are innervating the crista of the superior semicircular canal and the macula of the utricle. (Hematoxylin and eosin, ×9 and ×30, respectively.)

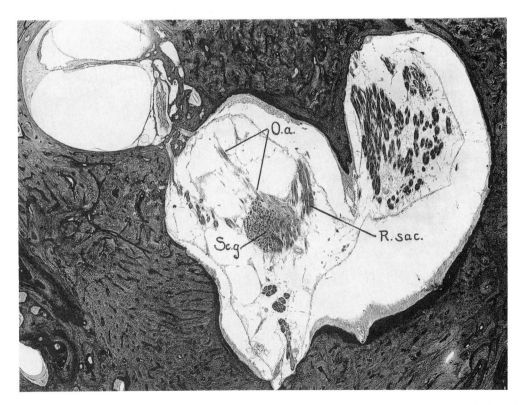

Figure 1.27. Vertical section through right petrous pyramid and posterior part of fundus of IAC. It shows the vestibulocochlear anastomosis (Oort (14)) *(O. a.)* as it passes from the inferior division of Scarpa's ganglion *(Sc. g.)* to join the spiral ganglion of the lower basal cochlear turn. The ramus saccularis *(R. sac.)* of the inferior division of the vestibular nerve and the superior division of this nerve are clearly recognized. (Hematoxylin and eosin, ×15.)

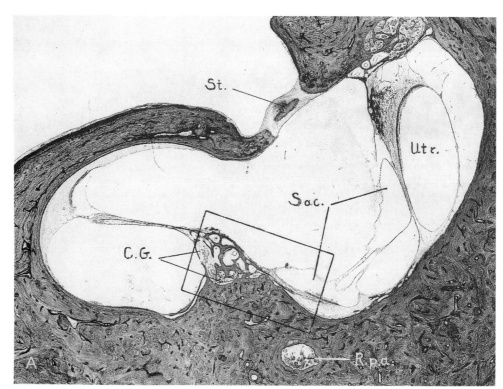

Figure 1.28. A. Vertical section through right petrous pyramid *(R. p. a.)* at level of anterior oval window margin. It shows the relation of the cochleosaccular nerve (Hardy) to the lower basal turn of the cochlea and the spherical recess in the anterior wall of the vestibule. (Hematoxylin and eosin, ×15.)

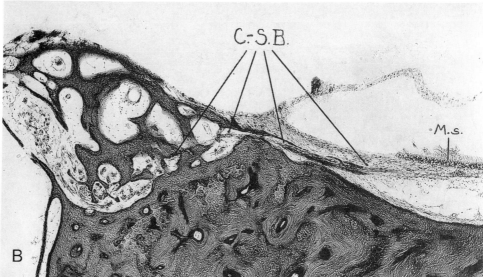

Figure 1.28. B. The cochleosaccular nerve bundle *(C.-S. B.)*, seen in a longitudinal section in its entire length, leaves the spiral ganglion to join the posterior tip of the saccular macula *(M. s.)*. (×44).

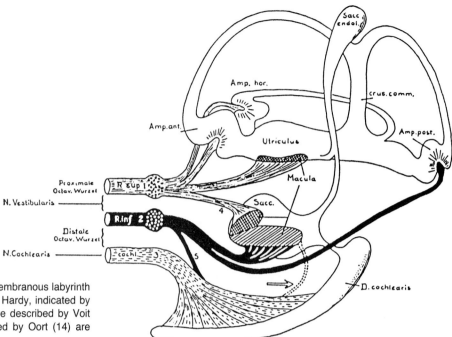

Figure 1.29. De Burlet's schema of innervation of membranous labyrinth with addition of third nerve (cochleosaccular nerve of Hardy, indicated by *arrow*) to macula sacculi. The superior saccular nerve described by Voit (12) and the vestibulocochlear anastomosis described by Oort (14) are labeled *4* and *5*, respectively.

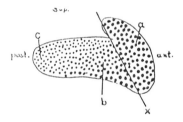

Figure 1.30. Lorente de No's schema of distribution of nerve fibers of various sizes in macula sacculi. *a*, thick fibers; *b*, medium fibers; and *c*, thin fibers.

EFFERENT VESTIBULAR INNERVATION

The efferent vestibular fibers originate ventromedially to the ventral portion of the lateral vestibular nucleus. They follow the efferent cochlear nerve fibers in the vestibular nerve to the level of the vestibular ganglion (Scarpa), where they part and join the individual vestibular nerve branches to the cristae of the semicircular canals and maculae of the utricle and saccule to terminate on their respective neuroepithelial structures (2).

AUTONOMOUS INNERVATION OF THE VESTIBULAR LABYRINTH

Two adrenergic systems are recognized in the vestibular labyrinth: *(a)* the perivascular nervous plexus from the basilar artery, extending along the labyrinth artery and its major branches, possibly innervating the blood vessels of the vestibular ganglion; and *(b)* a separate adrenergic nervous plexus, independent from the local blood vessels, that exists in the vestibular ganglion and beneath the vestibular sensory receptor cells. Contacts between the autonomous and the efferent nervous system apparently have so far not been identified (2).

NEURAL COMPARTMENT OF THE JUGULAR FORAMEN

The jugular foramen is a large aperture posterior to the carotid canal, formed by the petrous portion of the temporal bone and the lateral portion of the occipital bone. It is generally larger on the right side. It may be subdivided into three compartments. The anterior compartment transmits the inferior petrosal sinus. The intermediate or neural compartment represents the conduit for the passage of the glossopharyngeal, vagus, and spinal accessory nerves (Fig. 1.31). The posterior compartment includes the sigmoid portion of the transverse sinus and some meningeal branches from the ascending pharyngeal and occipital arteries. The glossopharyngeal nerve traverses the jugular foramen slightly anterior and superior to the 10th and 11th cranial nerves (Fig. 1.31). It is separated from them by a sheet of dura and forms the small superior ganglion within the jugular canal (Fig. 1.31) and, immediately on exiting it, the larger elongated petrosal ganglion. Occasionally, both ganglia are fused into one. The vagus and accessory nerves traverse the jugular canal together within an extension of the dura and arachnoid and are thereby clearly separated from the glossopharyngeal nerve (Fig. 1.31). Within the jugular canal the vagus nerve forms the jugular ganglion and immediately thereafter receives the internal branch of the spinal accessory nerve and then increases in size to give rise to the elongated spindle-shaped ganglion nodosum. These two ganglia are structurally similar to the spinal ganglia and represent the original neurons of the sensory fibers of the nerve. The motor fibers of the vagus bypass the ganglion. Smaller ganglion cells may frequently be encountered along the nerve and its branches. The spinal accessory nerve arises from the combination of the superior and the inferior root of the nerve. It joins the vagus nerve at its passage through the neural (intermediate) compartment of the jugular foramen, which it traverses in a laterally downward, arch-shaped direction. On exiting the jugular foramen it divides into an internal and an external branch.

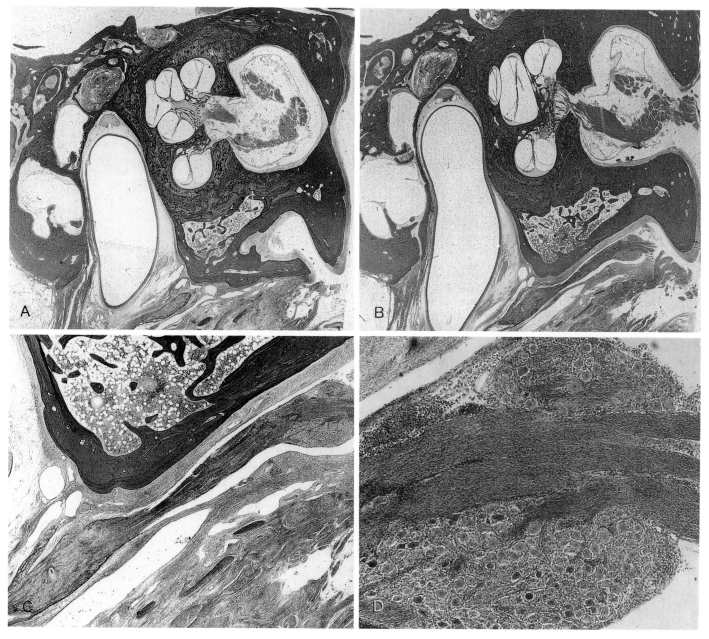

Figure 1.31.   A. Vertical section through right temporal bone with mid-modiolar section of cochlea, cross-section through neural (intermediate) compartment of jugular foramen, and cross-section through external aperture of cochlear canaliculus. **B.** Vertical section through right temporal bone with anterior paramodiolar section through cochlea. The glossopharyngeal nerve, seen in longitudinal section with its two ganglia, occupies the upper portion of the neural compartment; the vagus nerve occupies the middle portion; and the spinal accessory nerve occupies the lower portion. **C.** Vertical section through right temporal bone with anterior paramodiolar section of cochlea. Cranial nerves IX, X, and XI (from *top* to *bottom*) traverse the jugular foramen (canal). **D.** Vertical section through right temporal bone with paramodiolar section through cochlea. Longitudinal section of right glossopharyngeal nerve and its superior ganglion on its entrance into jugular canal (foramen). (Hematoxylin and eosin, × 5½, × 5½, × 15, and × 65, respectively.)

ENDOLYMPHATIC DUCT AND SAC

The endolymphatic duct traverses the medial portion of the petrous pyramid in its own bony canal, the vestibular aqueduct (Fig. 1.6). On its route it is accompanied by the vein of the vestibular aqueduct. The vestibular aperture is part of the perilymphatic vestibular compartment. It represents the Y-shaped junction of the utricular and saccular ducts. The common channel opens up into the distended segment of the endolymphatic duct, known as the sinus (Fig. 1.6). The next intermediate segment of the duct is narrow, hence is referred to as the isthmus.

Thereafter, the endolymphatic duct widens again to become the endolymphatic sac. The greater part of this sac is located within the funnel-shaped cranial aperture of the cochlear aqueduct. It lies within a duplication of the posterior fossa dura and is partially covered medially by a thin bony shelf, the operculum (Figs. 1.6 and 1.32A). Two portions of the endolymphatic sac are distinguished: *(a)* a proximal rugose portion with an irregular lumen caused by the numerous folds of the epithelial lining; and *(b)* a distal portion with a smooth cuboidal epithelial lining (Figs. 1.6 and 1.27). The location of the endolymphatic sac shows considerable variation.

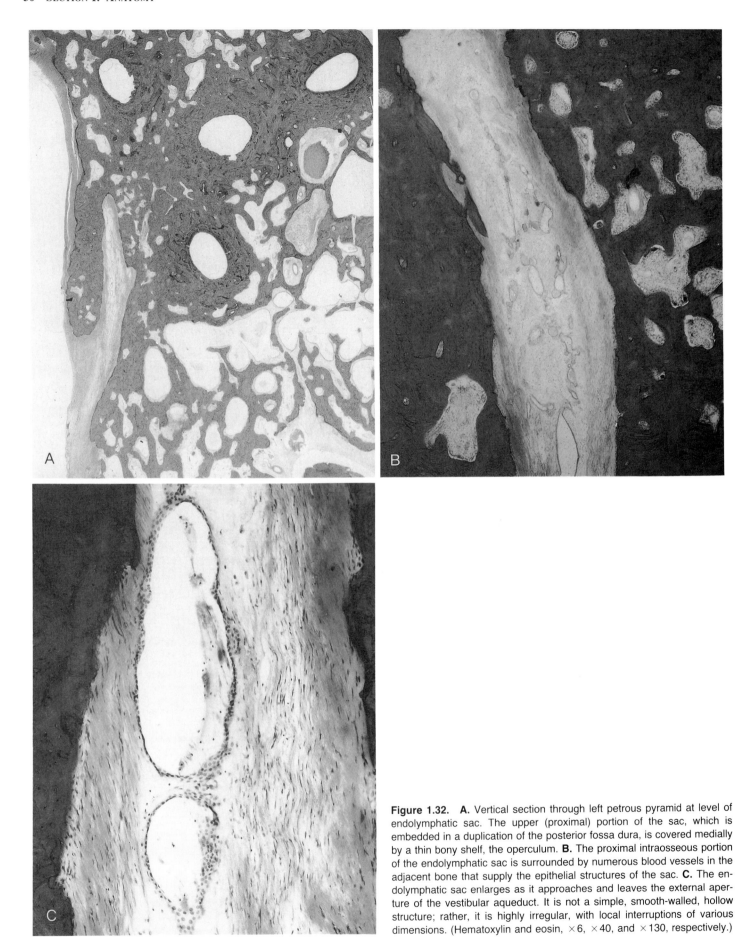

Figure 1.32. **A.** Vertical section through left petrous pyramid at level of endolymphatic sac. The upper (proximal) portion of the sac, which is embedded in a duplication of the posterior fossa dura, is covered medially by a thin bony shelf, the operculum. **B.** The proximal intraosseous portion of the endolymphatic sac is surrounded by numerous blood vessels in the adjacent bone that supply the epithelial structures of the sac. **C.** The endolymphatic sac enlarges as it approaches and leaves the external aperture of the vestibular aqueduct. It is not a simple, smooth-walled, hollow structure; rather, it is highly irregular, with local interruptions of various dimensions. (Hematoxylin and eosin, $\times 6$, $\times 40$, and $\times 130$, respectively.)

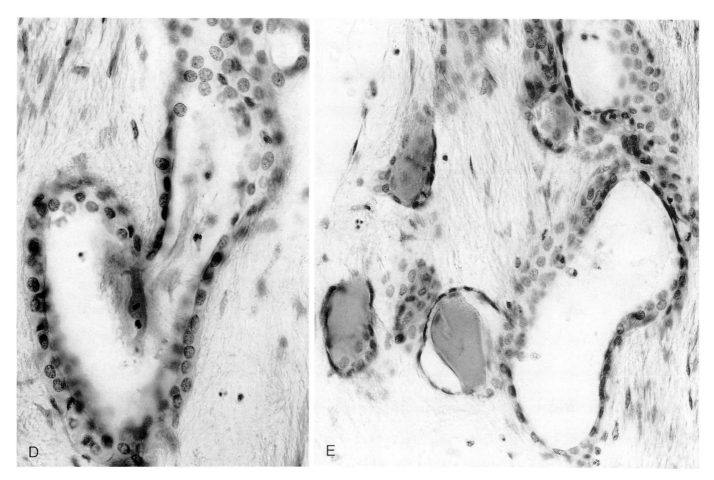

Figure 1.32.   D. The distal, rugose portion of the endolymphatic sac is lined by a cuboidal endothelium. **E.** In the more peripheral portion of the endolymphatic sac, the lumen frequently contains an eosinophilic, homo-geneous, viscous fluid, some erythrocytes, and cellular debris. (×400 and ×350, respectively.)

MICROSCOPIC ANATOMY OF THE TEMPORAL BONE

The photomicrographs in this chapter are from histologic sections of human temporal bones sectioned serially in the vertical or coronal (Figs. 1.33–1.58) and horizontal or axial (Figs. 1.59–1.76) planes. These specimens were removed at autopsy and prepared in the usual manner for examination with the compound microscope. Each section was cut at a thickness of 20 μm. In the vertical series the sections begin in the region of the petrous apex and continue toward the mastoid antrum in an anterior-to-posterior direction. In the horizontal series the sections start at the arcuate eminence and proceed toward the jugular bulb in a superior-to-inferior direction. The initial effort for the investigator is to develop a clear three-dimensional concept from these two-dimensional sections of a given anatomical region or structure within these temporal bones. To achieve this it is necessary to look at these serial sections sequentially, forward and backward, to become familiar with the anatomical relationship. As these planes correspond with the two planes commonly used in computed tomography scanning of the temporal bone, the knowledge thus acquired greatly facilitates the otologist's ability to recognize normal and abnormal anatomy and pathology involving the temporal bone (Fig. 1.77).

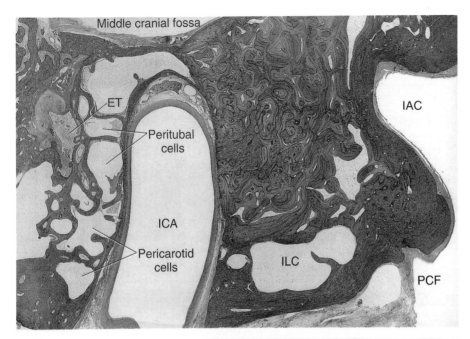

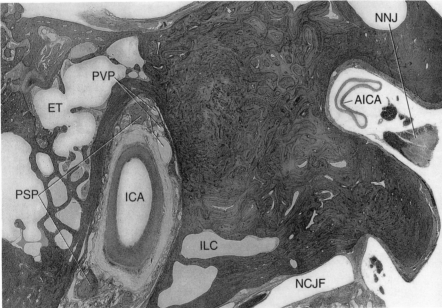

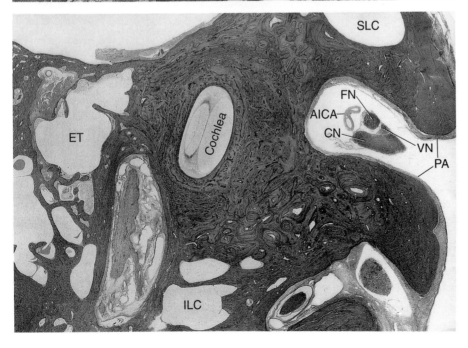

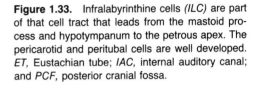

Figure 1.33. Infralabyrinthine cells *(ILC)* are part of that cell tract that leads from the mastoid process and hypotympanum to the petrous apex. The pericarotid and peritubal cells are well developed. *ET,* Eustachian tube; *IAC,* internal auditory canal; and *PCF,* posterior cranial fossa.

Figure 1.34. The IAC opens into the posterior cranial fossa. It contains a loop of the AICA and the cranial nerves VII and VIII. The neuroglial-neurolemmal junction *(NNJ)* of the cochlear and the vestibular nerve is usually located inside the canal near the porus. *ET,* Eustachian tube; *ICA,* internal carotid artery; *ILC,* infralabyrinthine cells; *NCJF,* neural compartment jugular foramen; *PSP,* pericarotid sympathetic plexus; and *PVP,* pericarotid venous plexus.

Figure 1.35. The Eustachian tube *(ET)* widens as it approaches the middle ear. The pericarotid sympathetic and the venous plexus are embedded in the loose connective tissue that ensheathes the internal carotid artery. As the vagus nerve passes through the neural compartment of the jugular foramen, it forms first the smaller jugular ganglion. After receiving the internal branch from the accompanying accessory nerve, it gives rise to the considerably larger, spindle-shaped ganglion nodosum. *CN,* cochlear nerve; *FN,* facial nerve; *ILC,* infralabyrinthine cells; *PA,* porus acusticus; *SLC,* supralabyrinthine cells; and *VN,* vestibular nerve.

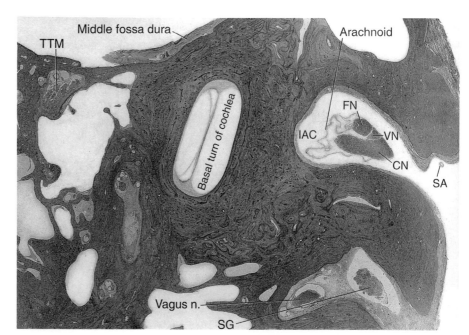

Figure 1.36. The tympanic branch of cranial nerve IX or the nerve of Jacobson courses toward the promontory in the tympanic canaliculus. It is accompanied by the inferior tympanic artery and vein. The subarachnoid space surrounds cranial nerves VII and VIII and extends to the fundus of the IAC. *CN*, cochlear nerve; *FN*, facial nerve; *SA*, subarcuate artery; *SG*, superior ganglion; and *TTM*, tensor tympani muscle.

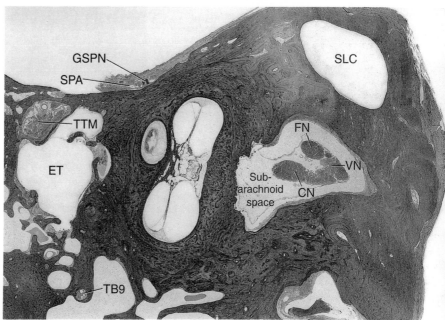

Figure 1.37. An anterior tangential cross-section through its basal and second turn marks the appearance of the cochlea. The large air space above the IAC represents a supralabyrinthine air cell. It is part of the supralabyrinthine cell tract that extends from the mastoid toward the petrous apex. *CN*, cochlear nerve; *ET*, Eustachian tube; *FN*, facial nerve; *GSPN*, greater superficial petrosal nerve; *SLC*, supralabyrinthine cells; *SPA*, superficial petrosal artery; *TB9*, tympanic branch of cranial nerve IX; *TTM*, tensor tympani muscle; and *VN*, vestibular nerve.

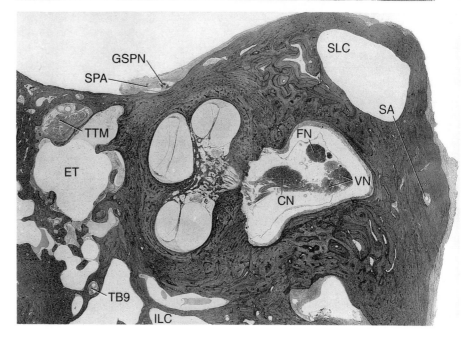

Figure 1.38. The anterior paramodiolar cross-section through the cochlea displays the architecture of the modiolus and membranous cochlea. It shows the passage of the cochlear nerve bundles through the spiral foraminous tract and the arrangement of the spiral ganglion. *CN*, cochlear nerve; *ET*, Eustachian tube; *FN*, facial nerve; *GSPN*, greater superficial petrosal nerve; *ILC*, infralabyrinthine cells; *SA*, subarcuate artery; *SLC*, supralabyrinthine cells; *SPA*, superficial petrosal artery; *TB9*, tympanic branch of cranial nerve IX; *TTM*, tensor tympani muscle; and *VN*, vestibular nerve.

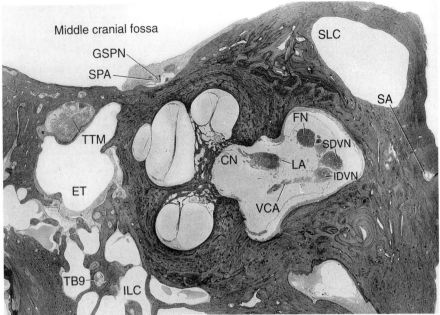

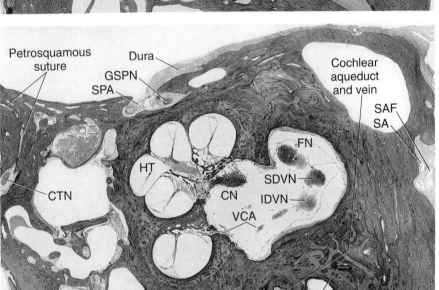

Figure 1.39. The petrosquamous suture marks the junction of the petrous and squamous portion of the temporal bone. The tensor tympani muscle *(TTM)* runs in a semicanal along the roof of the Eustachian tube *(ET)*. The inferior aperture of the cochlear aqueduct is about to form. *CN*, cochlear nerve; *FN*, facial nerve; *GSPN*, greater superficial petrosal nerve; *IDVN*, inferior division of vestibular nerve; *ILC*, infralabyrinthine cells; *LA*, labyrinthine artery; *SA*, subarcuate artery; *SDVN*, superior division of vestibular nerve; *SLC*, supralabyrinthine cells; *SPA*, superficial petrosal artery; *TB9*, tympanic branch of cranial nerve IX; and *VCA*, vestibulocochlear anastomosis.

Figure 1.40. The facial nerve *(FN)* is about to enter the labyrinthine segment of the Fallopian canal. The hiatus of the facial nerve is located above the second turn of the cochlea. It contains the greater superficial petrosal nerve *(GSPN)* and the superficial petrosal artery *(SPA)*. The cochlea is seen in its midmodiolar plane. The vestibulocochlear anastomosis *(VCA)* (Oort) enters the basal turn of the cochlea. It is part of the olivocochlear bundle (Rasmussen) (4) that carries efferent nerve fibers to the cochlea. *CN*, cochlear nerve; *CTN*, chorda tympani nerve; *HT*, helicotrema; *IDVN*, inferior division of vestibular nerve; *SA*, subarcuate artery; *SAF*, subarcuate fossa; and *SDVN*, superior division of vestibular nerve.

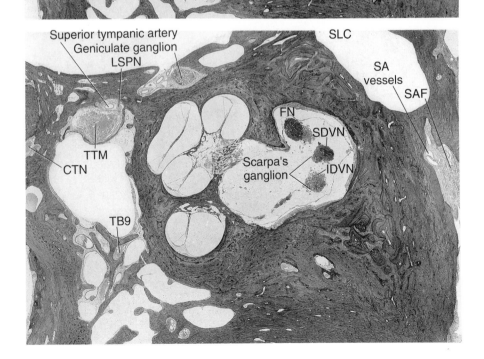

Figure 1.41. An invagination of the posterior fossa dura marks the subarcuate fossa *(SAF)* and the entrance of the subarcuate artery *(SA)*. The artery is accompanied by two veins. The cochlear aqueduct and the accompanying vein of the cochlear aqueduct are seen in separate channels midway between the posterior fossa and scala tympani of the basal turn of the cochlea. *CTN*, chorda tympani nerve; *FN*, facial nerve; *IDVN*, inferior division of vestibular nerve; *LSPN*, lesser superficial petrosal nerve; *SDVN*, superior division of vestibular nerve; *SLC*, supralabyrinthine cells; *TB9*, tympanic branch of cranial nerve IX; and *TTM*, tensor tympani muscle.

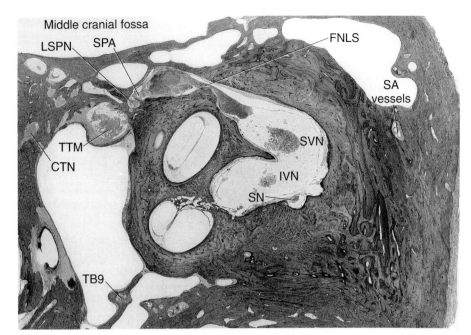

Figure 1.42. The geniculate ganglion is located at the lateral opening of the labyrinthine segment of the Fallopian canal. It represents the sensory ganglion of the nerve. The central processes of its ganglion cells reach the brain stem through the nervus intermedius. The saccular nerve is about to enter its separate canal. *CTN,* chorda tympani nerve; *FNLS,* facial nerve labyrinthine segment; *IVN,* inferior vestibular nerve; *LSPN,* lesser superficial petrosal nerve; *SA,* subarcuate artery; *SN,* singular nerve; *SPA,* superficial petrosal artery; *SVN,* superior vestibular nerve; *TB9,* tympanic branch of cranial nerve IX; and *TTM,* tensor tympani nerve.

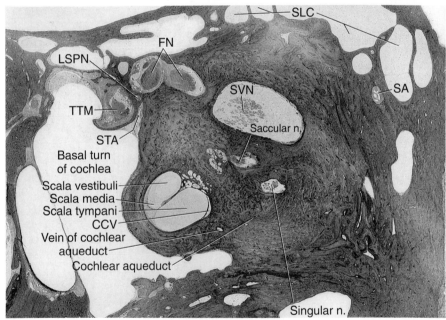

Figure 1.43. The saccular nerve is about to pass through the inferior cribriform vestibular area to join the macula of the saccule. The two collecting veins from the scala vestibuli and scala tympani have joined to form the common modiolar vein. The cross-section of this vein is seen at the inferior medial angle of the scala tympani. *CCV,* common cochlear vein; *FN,* facial nerve; *LSPN,* lesser superficial petrosal nerve; *SA,* subarcuate artery; *SLC,* supralabyrinthine cells; *STA,* superior tympanic artery; and *SVN,* superior vestibular nerve.

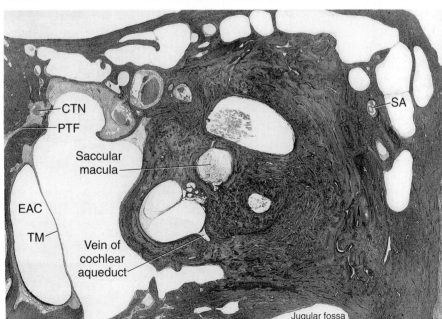

Figure 1.44. Before reaching the round window, the common modiolar vein confluates with the vestibulocochlear vein to form the vein of the cochlear aqueduct, seen here as it leaves the scala tympani. The macula of the saccule occupies the spherical recess of the vestibule. *CTN,* chorda tympani nerve; *EAC,* external auditory canal; *PTF,* petrotympanic fissure; *SA,* subarcuate artery; and TM, tympanic membrane.

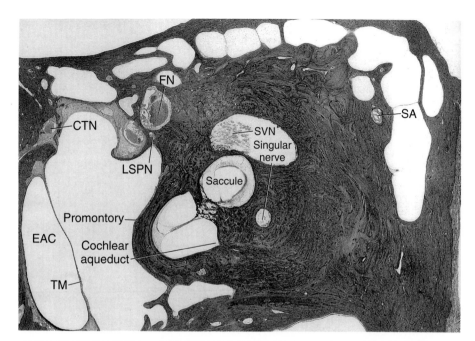

Figure 1.45. The nerve of Jacobson is passing over the promontory in front of the oval window. The cochlear aqueduct is about to open up into the scala tympani. The tympanic membrane, external auditory canal *(EAC)* and jugular bulb have come into view. *CTN,* chorda tympani nerve; *FN,* facial nerve; *LSPN,* lesser superficial petrosal nerve; *SA,* subarcuate artery; *SVN,* superior vestibular nerve; and *TM,* tympanic membrane.

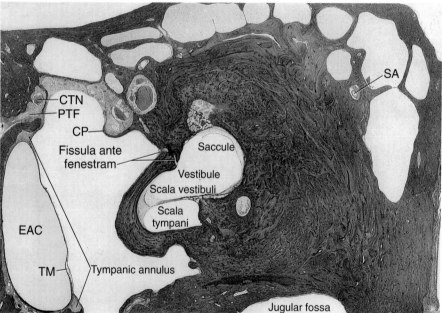

Figure 1.46. The aperture of the cochlear aqueduct and the fissula ante fenestram are recognized. The chorda tympani nerve *(CTN)* appears in the lateral wall of the epitympanum after its passage through the petrotympanic fissure *(PTF). CP,* cochleariform process; *EAC,* external auditory canal; and *TM,* tympanic membrane.

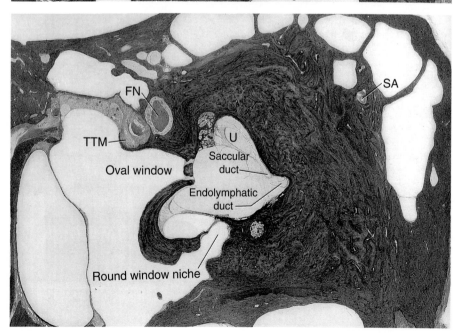

Figure 1.47. Within the vestibule the saccular and utricular duct are about to unite to give rise to the endolymphatic duct. A part of the macula of the utricle *(U)* occupies the elliptical recess that represents a depression in the posterosuperior aspect of the medial wall of the vestibule. All the perilabyrinthine cells are well pneumatized. *FN,* facial nerve; *SA,* subarcuate artery; and *TTM,* tensor tympani membrane.

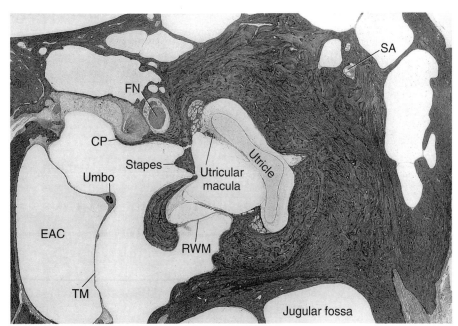

Figure 1.48. The niche to the round window and the round window membrane *(RWM)* covering the cochlear fenestra are seen. *CP,* cochleariform process; *EAC,* external auditory canal; *FN,* facial nerve; *SA,* subarcuate artery; and *TM,* tympanic membrane.

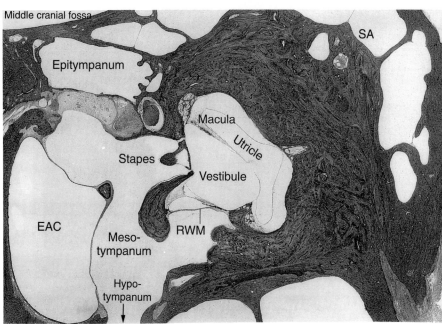

Figure 1.49. The cross-section through the oval window displays the attachment of the anterior crus of the stapes to the footplate. *EAC,* external auditory canal; *RWM,* round window membrane; and *SA,* subarcuate artery.

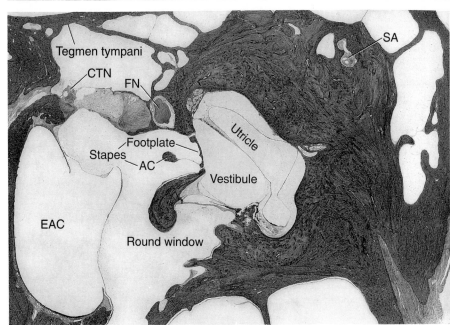

Figure 1.50. The vein of the vestibular aqueduct collects the blood from the membranous ducts of the semicircular canals. It is seen here as it joins the vestibular aqueduct, which it accompanies in a common or separate canaliculus. It drains into the lateral sinus. The macula of the utricle is much closer to the superior than the inferior portion of the stapes footplate. *AC,* anterior crus; *CTN,* chorda tympani nerve; *EAC,* external auditory canal; *FN,* facial nerve; and *SA,* subarcuate artery.

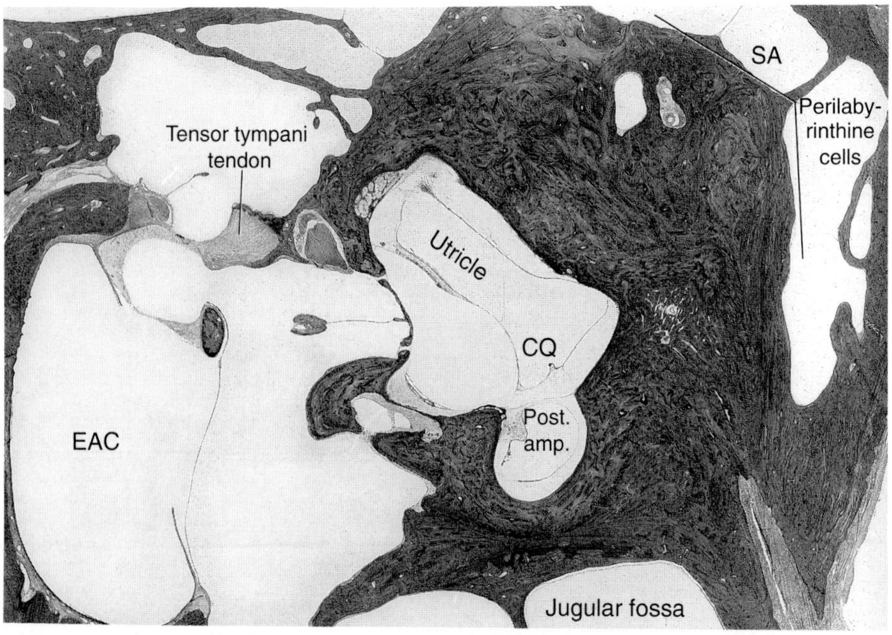

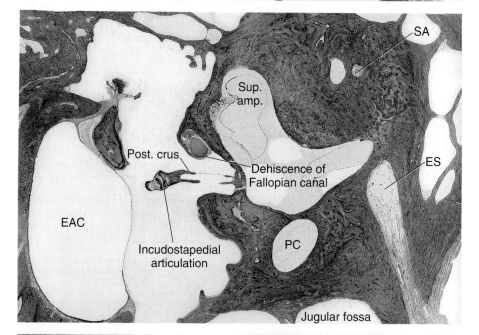

Figure 1.51. The ampulla and crista of the posterior semicircular canal and the crista quarta *(CQ)* of the utricle are demonstrated. *EAC,* external auditory canal; and *SA,* subarcuate artery.

Figure 1.52. The posterior crus of the stapes displays its characteristic centrally concave, excavated structure. The ampulla and crista of the superior semicircular canal have come into view. *EAC,* external auditory canal; *ES,* endolymphatic sac; *PC,* posterior canal; and *SA,* subarcuate artery.

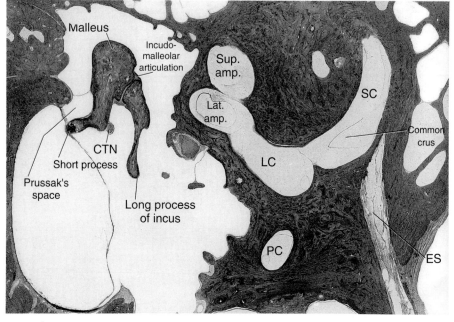

Figure 1.53. Malleus and incus, with the chorda tympani nerve *(CTN)* between them, and the ampulla and crista of the lateral semicircular canal have made their appearance. The endolymphatic sac *(ES)* is embedded in a duplication of the posterior fossa dura and is partially protected medially by the operculum, a bony shelf. *LC,* lateral canal; *PC,* posterior canal; and *SC,* superior canal.

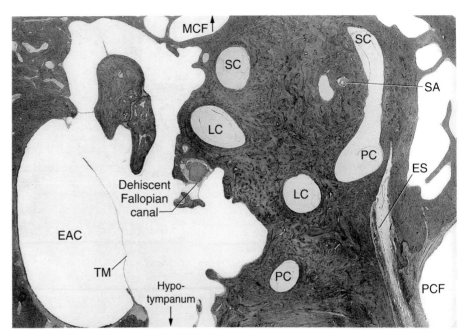

Figure 1.54. The nonampullated segment of the superior semicircular canal joins the common crus. A dehiscence in the floor of the Fallopian canal with exposure of the nerve is a frequent observation in that region. *EAC,* external auditory canal; *ES,* endolymphatic sac; *LC,* lateral canal; *MCF,* middle cranial fossa; *PC,* posterior canal; *PCF,* posterior cranial fossa; *SA,* subarcuate artery; *SC,* superior canal; and *TM,* tympanic membrane.

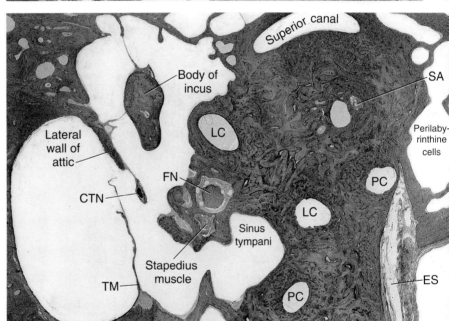

Figure 1.55. The stapedius muscle is recognized anterior to the facial nerve *(FN).* The chorda tympani nerve *(CTN)* is seen as it approaches the Fallopian canal. *ES,* endolymphatic sac; *LC,* lateral canal; *PC,* posterior canal; *SA,* subarcuate artery; and *TM,* tympanic membrane.

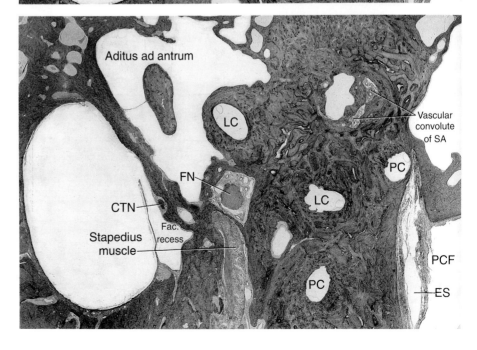

Figure 1.56. At the center of the superior semicircular canal, the subarcuate artery *(SA)* often gives rise to a vascular convolution. The stapedius muscle is seen in a longitudinal section. Irregular punched-out defects in the walls of the semicircular canals are not a rare observation and are of pathologic significance. *CTN,* chorda tympani nerve; *ES,* endolymphatic sac; *FN,* facial nerve; *LC,* lateral canal; *PC,* posterior canal; and *PCF,* posterior cranial fossa.

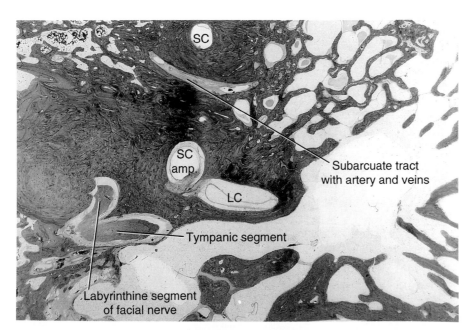

Figure 1.62. The short process of the incus points toward the mastoid antrum. The medial arm of the facial nerve emerges from the labyrinthine segment while the lateral arm enters the tympanic segment of the Fallopian canal. The nearby cross-section of the superior canal *(SC)* displays the ampulla with the crista and the nerve. Adjacent is the ampullated end of the lateral canal *(LC)* and its corresponding nerve. The subarcuate tract that runs through the center of the superior canal contains the subarcuate artery and two veins.

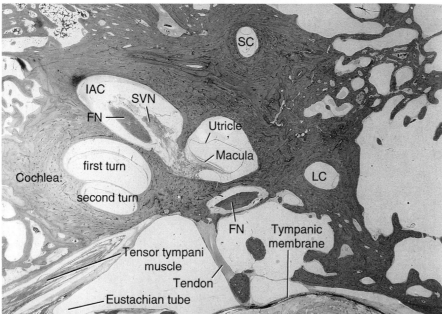

Figure 1.63. The tensor tympani muscle runs parallel to the Eustachian tube within its mediosuperior wall; its tendon attaches to the neck of the malleus. The facial nerve *(FN)* is seen passing above the oval window. A tangential section through the cochlea reveals the first and second turn. In the IAC the facial nerve is entering the labyrinthine segment of the Fallopian canal. The superior vestibular nerve *(SVN)* is recognized. A cross-section through the vestibule displays the superior portion of the utricle with the macula and nerve. *LC,* lateral canal; and *SC,* superior canal.

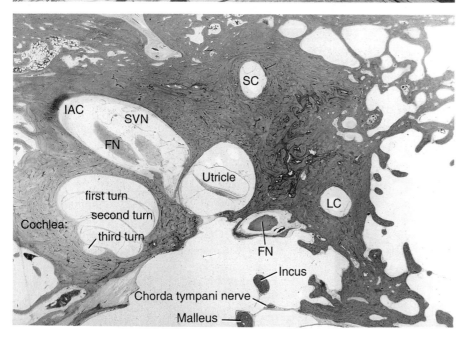

Figure 1.64. The subarcuate fossa is seen as an invagination of the posterior fossa dura. It continues as the subarcuate tract, which runs superiorly and laterally through the center of the superior canal *(SC)* toward the mastoid antrum. The third turn of the cochlea is coming into view. *FN,* facial nerve; *LC,* lateral canal; and *SVN,* superior vestibular nerve.

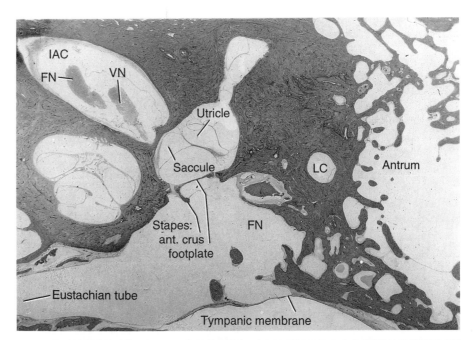

Figure 1.65. The openings of the periantral cells are all oriented toward the center of the mastoid antrum. The common crus, resulting from the junction of the nonampullated segments of the superior and posterior canals, approaches the utricle. The location of the facial nerve *(FN)* is at the junction of the tympanic and the mastoid segment of the Fallopian canal. The tympanic membrane and its relation to the manubrium of the malleus are recognized. *LC,* lateral canal; and *VN,* vestibular nerve.

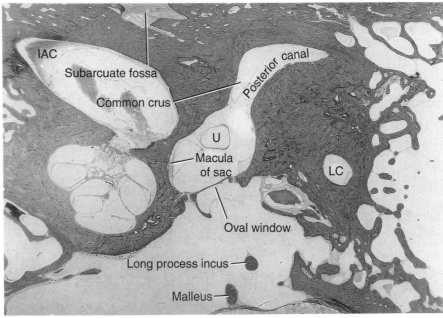

Figure 1.66. The posterior canal is emerging from the common crus. The saccule has come into view. Its mascula occupies the spherical recess, a depression in the anteroinferior wall of the vestibule. The stapedial footplate with the base of the anterior crus covers the oval (vestibular) window. The architecture of the cochlea is displayed in a midmodiolar cross-section. *LC,* lateral canal; and *U,* utricle.

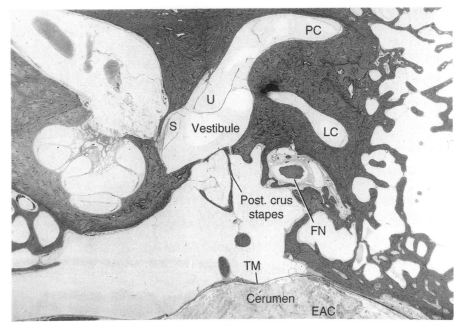

Figure 1.67. The membranous duct of the posterior canal *(PC)* has joined the utricle *(U).* The nonampullated end of the lateral canal *(LC)* is approaching the vestibule. The attachment of the posterior crus of the stapes to the footplate is seen. *EAC,* external auditory canal; *FN,* facial nerve; *S,* saccule; and *TM,* tympanic membrane.

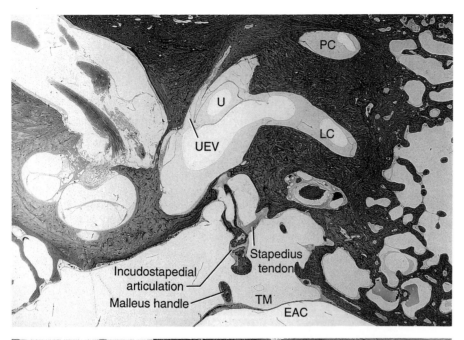

Figure 1.68. The tendon of the stapedius muscle emerges from the pyramidal process and attaches to the capitulum of the stapes below its articulation with the incus. The vestibular aperture and sinus of the endolymphatic duct and the utriculoendolymphatic valve *(UEV)* are recognized. *EAC,* external auditory canal; *LC,* lateral canal; *PC,* posterior canal; *TM,* tympanic membrane; and *U,* utricle.

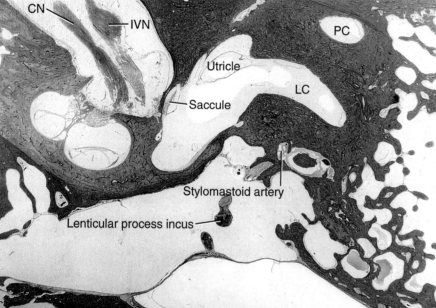

Figure 1.69. The stylomastoid artery that accompanies the facial nerve is about to enter its separate bony canal, whereas the facial vein continues inside the Fallopian canal. The proximal part of the endolymphatic sac is recognized. *CN,* cochlear nerve; *IVN,* inferior vestibular nerve; *LC,* lateral canal; and *PC,* posterior canal.

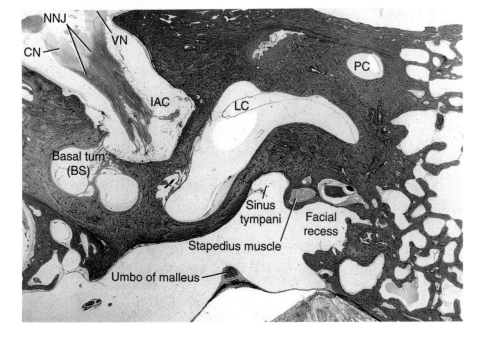

Figure 1.70. The membranous duct of the lateral semicircular canal has made connection with the utricle. The neuroglial-neurolemmal junction *(NNJ)* of the cochlear nerve *(CN)* and vestibular nerve *(VN)* lies within the IAC near its aperture. *BS,* basal turn; *LC,* lateral canal; and *PC,* posterior canal.

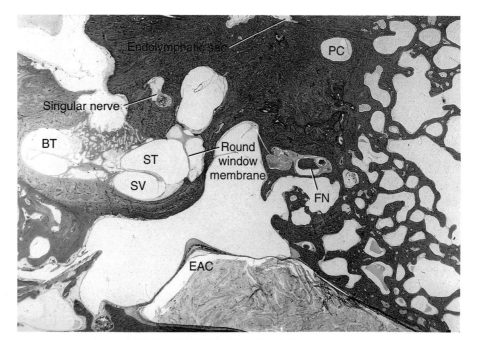

Figure 1.71. The separate bony canal for the singular nerve is localized between the IAC and the inferior extension of the vestibule. It houses the branch from the inferior vestibular nerve for the posterior ampulla. The niche to the round window and round window membrane covering the cochlea fenestra are recognized. The tympanic membrane is attached to the wall of the tympanic sulcus by the tympanic annulus in a circumferential fashion. *BT,* basal turn; *EAC,* external auditory canal; *FN,* facial nerve; *PC,* posterior canal; *ST,* scala tympani; and *SV,* scala vestibuli.

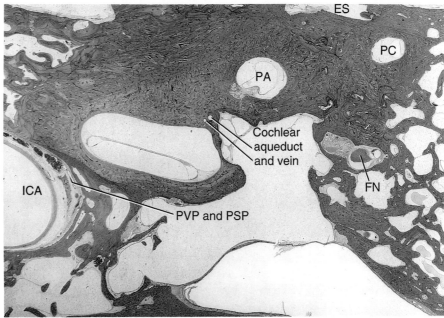

Figure 1.72. The larger of the two cross-sections through the posterior canal *(PC)* exhibits the ampulla and crista and the nerve that supplies it. The cochlear duct and its accompanying vein have already left the scala tympani of the basal turn of the cochlea. Within its bony canal the internal carotid artery *(ICA)* is surrounded by a sheath of loose connective tissue that includes the pericarotid venous plexus *(PVP)* and the pericarotid sympathetic nerve plexus *(PSP). ES,* endolymphatic sac; *FN,* facial nerve; and *PA,* posterior ampulla.

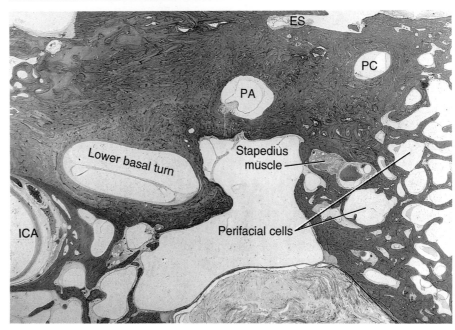

Figure 1.73. The endolymphatic sac *(ES)* extends into a duplication of the posterior fossa dura. It is partially covered by a bony shelf, the operculum. The external auditory canal is filled with cerumen. *ICA,* internal carotid artery; *PA,* posterior ampulla; and *PC,* posterior canal.

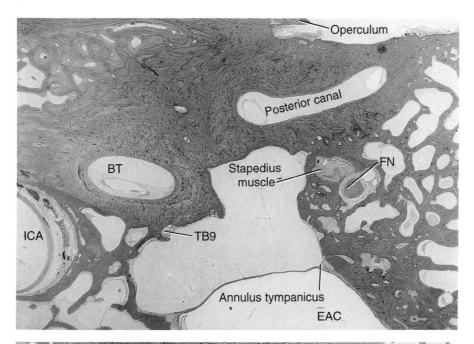

Figure 1.74. The two segments of the posterior canal have joined. The inferiormost extension of the lower basal turn *(BT)* is viewed in a tangential cut. *EAC,* external auditory canal; *FN,* facial nerve; *ICA,* internal carotid artery; and *TB9,* tympanic branch of cranial nerve IX.

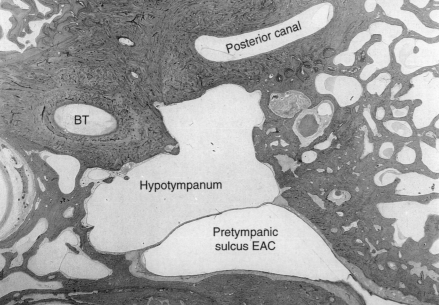

Figure 1.75. The pretympanic sulcus seen here corresponds to a depression in the most medial part of the floor of the external auditory canal *(EAC)*. *BT,* basal turn.

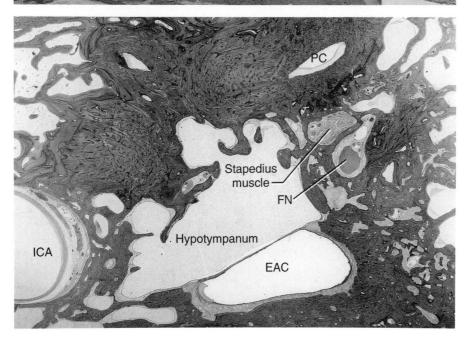

Figure 1.76. Cell tracts from the hypotympanum extend to the petrous apex around the internal carotid artery *(ICA)* and around the Fallopian canal to the lower portion of the mastoid process. *EAC,* external auditory canal; *FN,* facial nerve; and *PC,* posterior canal.

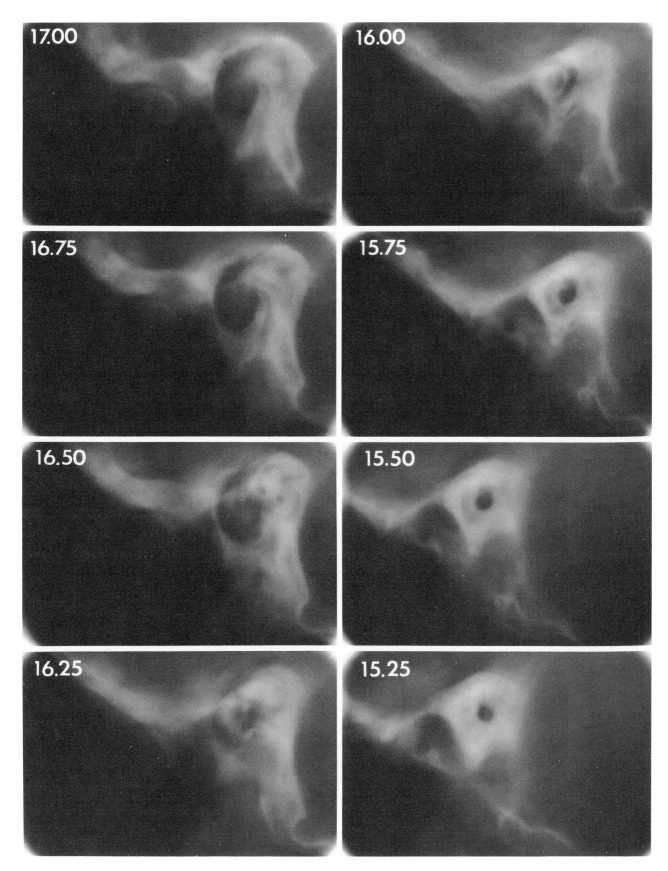

Figure 1.77.   Serial lateral multidirectional tomograms of left temporal bone of adult, to show normal radiologic anatomy. *Sections 17.00* and *16.75* show the lateral semicircular canal and the mastoid segment of the Fallopian canal. *Sections 16.50* and *16.25* show the superior and posterior semicircular canals. *Sections 16.00* and *15.75* show the cochlea. *Sections 15.50* and *15.25* show the IAC, the jugular bulb, and the internal carotid artery.

References

1. Celesia GG, Puletti F. Organization of auditory cortical areas in man. Brain 1976;99:403.
2. Beck CHL. Anatomie und Histologie des Ohres. In: Berendes J, Link R, Zöllner F, eds. Hals-Nasen-Ohrenheilkunde in Praxis und Klinik, 2: Aufl, Ohr I. Stuttgart: Georg Thieme, Chap 2 1979;5:1–60.
3. Rasmussen GL. An efferent cochlear bundle. Anat Rec 1942;82:441.
4. Rasmussen GL. Efferent fibers of the cochlear nerve and cochlear nucleus. In: Rasmussen GJ, Windle W, eds. Neural mechanisms of the auditory and vestibular systems. Springfield, Illinois: Charles C Thomas, 1960.
5. Hawkins JE Jr. Hearing anatomy and acoustics. In: Best CH, Taylor NE, eds. The physiological basis of medical practice. 8th ed. Baltimore: Williams & Wilkins, 1966.
6. Spoendlin H. The innervation of the organ of Corti. Laryngol 1967;81:717.
7. Anson BJ, McVay X. Surgical anatomy. 5th ed. Philadelphia: WB Saunders, 1971.
8. Donaldson JA, Miller JM. Anatomy of the ear. In: Paparella M, Shumrick DA, eds. Otolaryngology. 2nd ed. Philadelphia: WB Saunders, 1980;I:26–62.
9. Anson BJ, Donaldson JA. Surgical anatomy of the temporal bone. 3rd ed. Philadelphia: WB Saunders, 1981.
10. Blum W, Fawcett DW. A textbook of histology. 9th ed. Philadelphia: WB Saunders, 1968.
11. Wersall J, Lundquist PG. Morphological polarization of the mechanoreceptors of the vestibular and acoustic system. In: Graybiel A, ed. Second symposium on the role of the vestibular organs in space exploration. NASA publication no SP-115. Washington, DC: National Aeronautics and Space Administration, 1966.
12. Voit M. Zur Frage der Verästelung des Nervus acusticus bei den Säugetieren. Anat Anz 1907;31:635–640.
13. Hardy M. Observations on the innervation of the macula sacculi in man. Anat Rec 1934;59(4):403–418.
14. Oort H. Über die Verästelung des Nervus octavus bei Säugetieren. Anat Anz 1918;51:272–280.
15. Poliak S. Über die Doppelte Innervation der Macula Sacculi und über das cochleo-vestibuläre Bundel bei den Säugetieren. Gesamte Anat Abt 1927;84:145–152.
16. Lorente de No R. Études sur l'anatomie et la physiologie du labyrinthe de l'oreille et du VIII 'nerv. Trav Lab Rech Biol Madrid 1916;24:53–153.
17. de Burlet HM. Zur Innervation der Macula Sacculi bei Säugetieren. Anat Anz 1924;84:26–32.

2/ Ossification of the Cochlear and Vestibular Capsule

Around the seventh week of fetal life the mesenchyme surrounding the developing otic vesicle is transformed into precartilage and, after another week, undergoes modification to true hyaline cartilage (1). During the next 2 months the cartilaginous capsule increases in size to allow the cochlea to grow. Around the 16th week the membranous cochlea has reached adult size and differentiation. At this stage the cartilaginous capsule undergoes a gradual conversion to bone. Ossification begins from 14 ossification centers that develop in succession. By the 20th week they will have fused to form the bony capsule. Conversion to bone is therefore accomplished over a period of about 4–6 weeks. At that time the ossification centers display a three-layer structure with an outer and an inner periosteal layer and an intermediate endochondral bony layer (Fig. 2.1B and C). This structural pattern persists throughout adult life. These three layers develop according to independent timetables and follow individual principles of histologic differentiation (2).

The outer periosteal layer is formed by periosteum surrounding the cartilaginous capsule. It is made up of lamellar bone and provides growth and mass to the otic capsule (Fig. 2.1C and D). The inner periosteal layer immediately encloses the perilymphatic and endolymphatic labyrinthine compartments. It is derived from the inner periosteum and consists of lamellar bone including remnants of cartilage cells. It is thin and dense and remains practically inactive. It is also known as the endosteal layer of the capsule (Fig. 2.1D).

The middle layer of the otic capsule consists of a framework of irregular islands of intrachondral and endochondral bone, embedded in primitive bone marrow (Fig. 2.1C and E). The intrachondral tissue is composed of heteromorphous areas of calcified hyaline cartilage that contains true bone within the original framework of cartilage cells or lacunae. These areas form the scaffold on which the endochondral bone is gradually being deposited (Fig. 2.1E and F). The ossification process develops in the following manner: Around the 17th week the hyaline cartilage cells begin to enlarge and become partially calcified. At the same time the matrix undergoes mineralization and takes on a darker hue. The cartilage cells then are being eroded, opened, and invaded by osteoblasts that deposit new bone within their lacunae in the form of small osseous globules known as "globuli ossei" (Fig. 2.1F) (3). This process is recognized as intrachondral ossification (1). Osteoblasts from the surrounding marrow spaces subsequently deposit endochondral bone on the outer surface of these areas or islands of partially ossified cartilage cells or lacunae, a process recognized as endochondral ossification (Fig. 2.1F) (3). Continuous deposition of endochondral bone gradually reduces the once capacious marrow spaces to relatively small vascular channels. As a result the bone of the middle layer develops a compact, firm, and petrous structure.

The extracapsular regions of the petrous pyramid—the petrous apex and the region of the antrum—develop as extensions from the outer periosteal layer. They remain cancellous and subsequently become pneumatized. Pneumatization develops from the Eustachian tube and middle ear cavity and extends into the periosteal bony layer and from there into the adjacent endochondral bony layer.

Ossification advances more rapidly in the cochlear capsule than in the vestibular capsule. The cartilaginous vestibular capsule at first becomes more loose and spongy to accommodate the continuing expansion of the semicircular ducts. Even about the 24th week it shows no sign of conversion to bone. Ossification of its endochondral layer becomes complete only during the early weeks of postnatal life.

The features that make the development of the inner ear capsule unique within the skeletal system are: *(a)* it maintains its fetal bone structure throughout adult life; *(b)* it reaches adult dimensions around the 21st week of embryonic life; *(c)* it develops from 14 ossification centers without an intermediate zone of epiphyseal growth; and *(d)* each of these centers and, consequently, the entire capsule display a trilaminar structure with an independent timetable of growth and a separate process of histologic differentiation for each capsule layer (4).

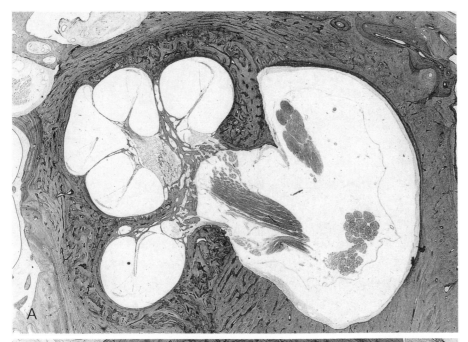

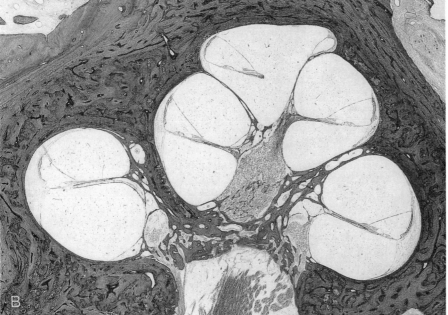

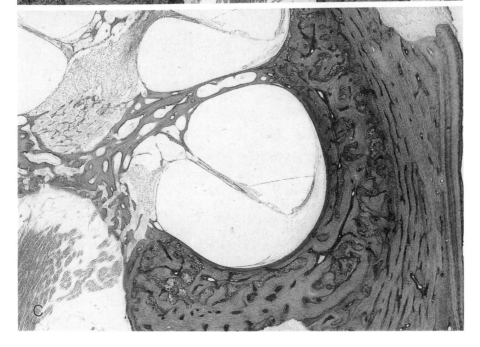

Figure 2.1. A. Vertical midmodiolar section of right temporal bone of a 35-year-old woman. It shows the usual bony architecture of the otic capsule. (Hematoxylin and eosin, ×10½.)

Figure 2.1. B. The cochlear capsule displays the characteristic trilaminar structure. (×16.)

Figure 2.1. C. Cross-section through upper basal turn of cochlea, demonstrating three layers of adult cochlear capsule. (×35.)

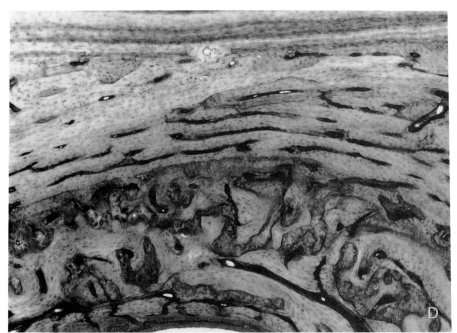

Figure 2.1. **D.** Cross-section through cochlear capsule surrounding upper basal turn. The outer periosteal layer, recognized in the upper half of the section, is made up of lamellar bone with lamellae in parallel arrangement. (×55.)

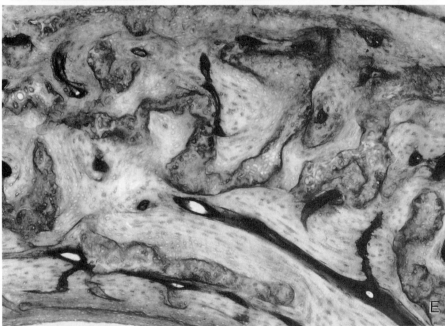

Figure 2.1. **E.** The middle, intermediate, or endochondral layer occupies most of the lower half of the section. It consists of numerous irregular islands of partially calcified cartilage cells. The inner periosteal layer is recognized near the lower left corner of the section as a small, dense band of lamellar bone with the lamellae arranged in a straight parallel fashion. The islands of partially calcified cells are surrounded by lamellar endochondral bone that has been deposited on their surface in an irregular manner. (×110.)

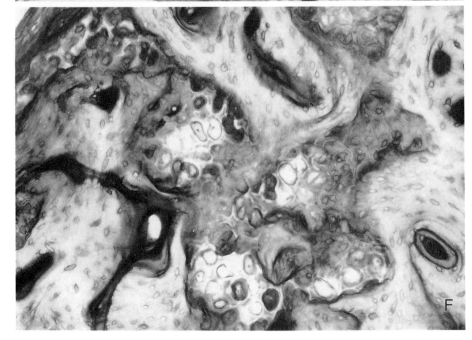

Figure 2.1. **F.** In these irregular islands of residual cartilage there are: *(a)* cartilage cells that are enlarged, calcified, and empty; *(b)* cartilage cells that have been eroded and occupied by osteoblasts that have deposited into these empty lacunae new bone in the form of spherical globules referred to as "globuli ossei"; and *(c)* cartilage cells that are in the process of being eroded and ossified. (×195.)

References

1. Bast TH, Anson BJ. The temporal bone and the ear. Springfield, Illinois: Charles C Thomas, 1949.
2. Anson BJ, Donaldson JA. Surgical anatomy of the temporal bone. 3rd ed. Philadelphia: WB Saunders, 1981.
3. Manasse P. Über knorpelhaltige Interglobularräume in der menschlichen Labyrinthkapsel. Z Ohrenheilkd 1987;341:1–10.
4. Goycoolea MV. Otosclerosis. In: Paparella MM, Shumrick DA, Gluckman JL, Meyerhoff WL, eds. Otolaryngology, Vol II: Otology and neuro-otology. 3rd ed. Philadelphia: WB Saunders, 1991.

3/ Pneumatization of the Temporal Bone

During the third week of fetal life, while the auditory vesicle is being formed, an outpocketing develops from the foregut to become the first pharyngeal pouch. The dorsal end of this pouch, through gradual expansion, becomes in succession the Eustachian tube, the tympanic cavity, and the extensions of the latter, namely, the epitympanic and hypotympanic recess, antrum, and mastoid air cells. Between the fourth and the sixth week, the lower part of the tympanic cavity begins to develop while the upper part is still occupied by embryonic connective tissue that originally filled the entire middle ear space. During the 23rd week, the epitympanum begins to form, and by the 30th week, the middle ear cavity is almost completely developed (1). As the mesenchyme gradually disappears, the walls and contents of the middle ear cavity become lined by endodermal epithelium from the tubotympanic recess.

In the newborn the rudimentary mastoid bone contains only a single air space, the antrum, which is surrounded by diploic bone containing hematopoietic marrow. As the mastoid process develops, the marrow spaces gradually become hollowed out. The mesenchyme originally occupying that space is being resorbed, and the developing air-containing cells become outlined by the advancing endodermal epithelium. The newly formed periantral air cells communicate with each other and become part of the steadily expanding air cell system of the temporal bone.

Pneumatization of the petrous pyramid generally does not begin until after the third year of life (1). It proceeds from the middle ear and antrum through recognized expanding air cell tracts (2). These include: *(a)* a posteromedial tract extending from the antrum along the posterior wall of the pyramid through the roof of the internal auditory canal toward the apex (Figs. 3.2, 3.3, and 3.6); *(b)* a superior tract extending from the epitympanum along the floor of the middle cranial fossa over the superior semicircular canal toward the apex (Figs. 3.2, 3.3, and 3.6); *(c)* a subarcuate cell tract extending from the antrum through the center of the superior canal toward the apex following the subarcuate canal (Fig. 3.6); *(d)* an inferior tract extending from the hypotympanum underneath the cochlea toward the apex (Figs. 3.2, 3.3, 3.5, and 3.6); and *(e)* an anterolateral tract that includes the peritubal and pericarotid cells on its course toward the apex (Fig. 3.3). Pneumatization of the petrous pyramid is observed in about 30% of temporal bones. It is encountered most frequently in the perilabyrinthine areas (Figs. 3.2, 3.3, 3.5, and 3.6) and somewhat less often in the petrous apex (Figs. 3.1 and 3.4). It tends to be symmetrical, but in about 25% of specimens

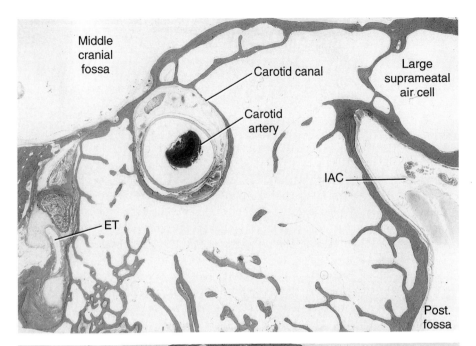

Figure 3.1. Vertical section through right petrous pyramid in anterior portion of internal auditory canal *(IAC)*. The petrous apex is unusually well pneumatized and osteoporotic, so that the bony canal of the internal carotid artery appears almost hanging in the air. *ET,* Eustachian tube. (Hematoxylin and eosin, ×7.5.)

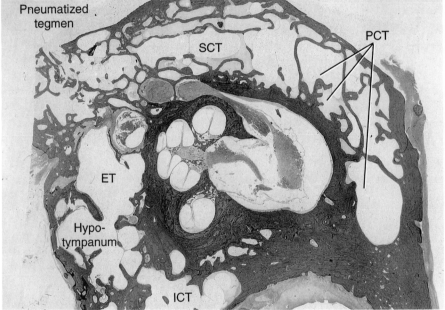

Figure 3.2. Vertical midmodiolar section through right temporal bone of a 52-year-old man. The petrous pyramid is so well pneumatized that the different cell tracts are easily recognized. Note the extensive pneumatization of the tegmen. *ET,* Eustachian tube; *ICT,* inferior cell tract; *PCT,* posteromedial cell tract; and *SCT,* superior cell tract. (Hematoxylin and eosin, ×4.5.)

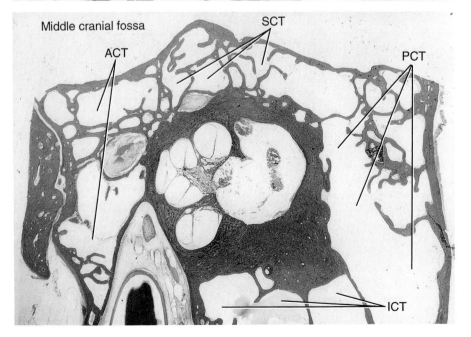

Figure 3.3. Vertical midmodiolar section through unusually well pneumatized right petrous pyramid of a 17-year-old black man. The posteromedial, the superior, the inferior, and the anterolateral cell tracts are recognized. *ACT,* anterolateral cell tract; *ICT,* inferior cell tract; *PCT,* posteromedial cell tract; and *SCT,* superior cell tract. (Hematoxylin and eosin, ×5.)

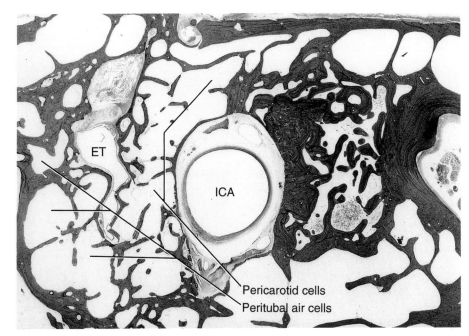

Figure 3.4. Vertical section through right petrous pyramid near anterior wall of internal auditory canal. The peritubal and periocarotid air cells are well developed. *ET,* Eustachian tube; and *ICA,* internal carotid artery. (Hematoxylin and eosin, × 7.)

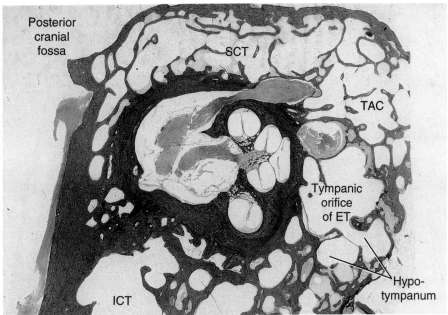

Figure 3.5. Vertical midmodiolar section of unusually well pneumatized left petrous pyramid of a 52-year-old white woman. The superior cell tract *(SCT)* and the tegmental air cells *(TAC)* are clearly recognized. *ET,* Eustachian tube; and *ICT,* inferior cell tract. (Hematoxylin and eosin, ×5.)

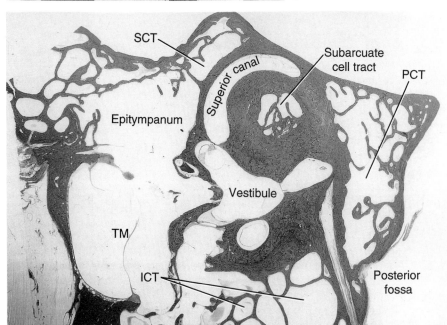

Figure 3.6. Vertical section through right temporal bone at level of oval and round windows of a 16-year-old black man. The subarcuate cell tract passes through the center of the superior semicircular canal. *ICT,* inferior cell tract; *PCT,* posteromedial cell tract; *SCT,* superior cell tract; and *TM,* tympanic membrane. (Hematoxylin and eosin, ×4.5.)

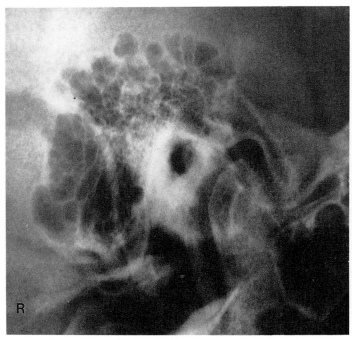
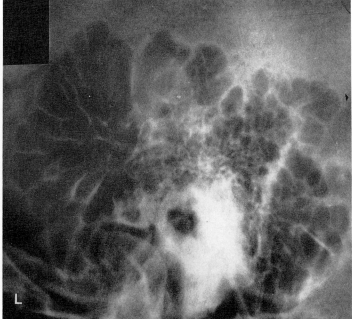

Figure 3.7. Lateral (Schüller) projection of well-developed temporal bones of a 31-year-old woman, to show occasional observation of asymmetrical pneumatization. The unusually extensive cellular development on the left involves the squama and the root of the zygoma.

the extent of cellular development varies between the two sides (Fig. 3.7).

Cellular architecture and the extent of pneumatization show considerable variation (Fig. 3.7). They are influenced by infection (Fig. 3.8) and environmental, nutritional, and genetic factors and are dependent on Eustachian tubal function (3–7). The observation of very similar cellular patterns in the majority of identical twins and the occasional familiar occurrence of hypocellular pneumatization support the likelihood of a contributing genetic influence. If pneumatization fails, the bone remains diploic and may develop into compact bone, and the mastoid process may become hypocellular or acellular (Figs. 3.9–3.12).

Inflammatory involvement of a previously pneumatized mastoid process may result in destruction of the original bone and replacement by sclerotic bone. This can be recognized histologically, in that the original bone displays a regular lamellar structure, whereas the sclerotic bone shows an irregular arrangement of cement lines.

Depending on location, pneumatized cell groups may be divided according to different regions and areas in these regions. This is primarily of surgical importance. In the middle ear region, air cells are located in the epitympanum, mesotympanum,

and hypotympanum (Figs. 3.2 and 3.3–3.5). In the mastoid region, cell groups are recognized in the periantral, tegmental, sinodural, perifacial, and tip areas and adjacent to the sigmoid sinus. In the perilabyrinthine region, supralabyrinthine and infralabyrinthine cells are encountered (Figs. 3.2, 3.3, 3.5, and 3.6). In the apical region, the cells surrounding the Eustachian tube and the internal carotid artery are of significance (Fig. 3.4). The significance of these cell tracts is that they can serve as an avenue for extension of a neoplastic lesion or an inflammatory process from the middle ear cleft to a remote area in the petrous pyramid, where they can give rise to serious secondary infections involving the endocranium, adjacent soft tissues in the neck, and major venous vessels.

In some instances, pneumatization can be so extensive that cell complexes extend into the temporal and occipital squama, route of the zygoma, base of the styloid process, and adjacent sphenoid bone (Figs. 3.7, 3.13, and 3.14). In such situations, the dense vestibular and otic capsule gives the radiologic appearance of being suspended within the petrous pyramid by a delicate trabecular network created by the intercellular partitions (Figs. 3.5, 3.13, and 3.14).

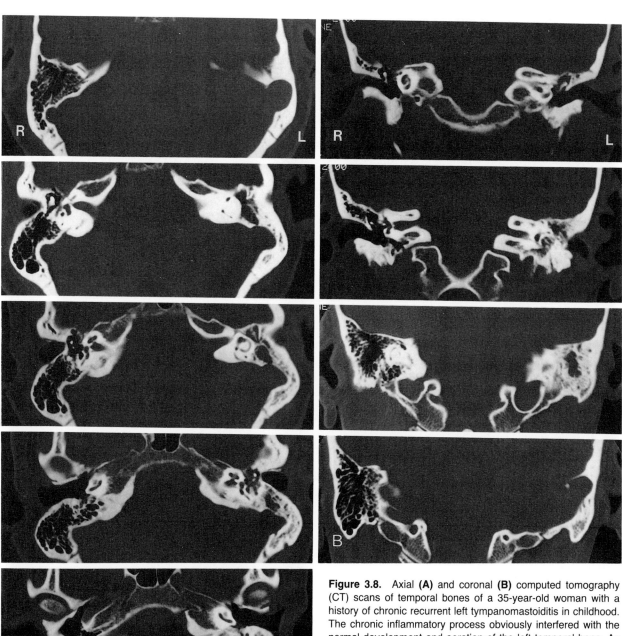

Figure 3.8. Axial **(A)** and coronal **(B)** computed tomography (CT) scans of temporal bones of a 35-year-old woman with a history of chronic recurrent left tympanomastoiditis in childhood. The chronic inflammatory process obviously interfered with the normal development and aeration of the left temporal bone. As a result, the left mastoid process remained underdeveloped, poorly pneumatized, and sclerotic.

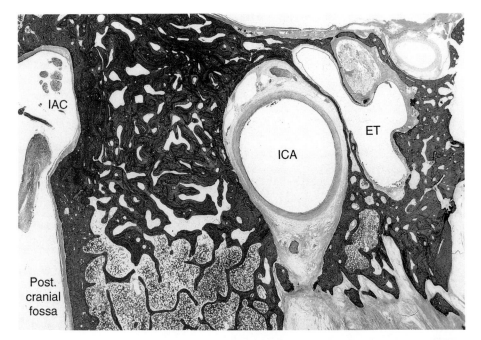

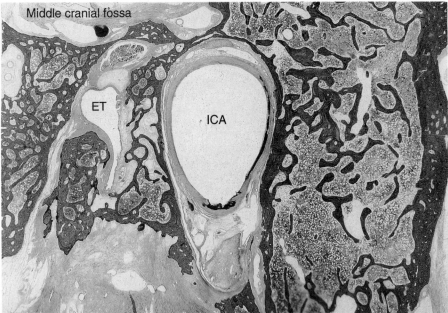

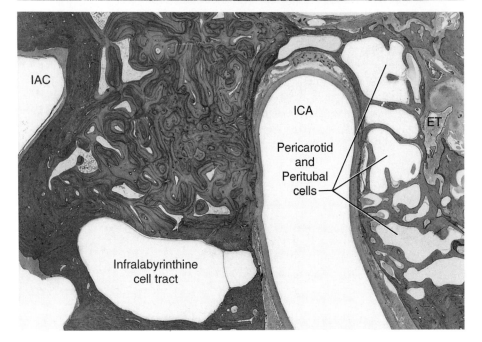

Figure 3.9. Vertical section through left petrous pyramid at level of anterior wall of internal auditory canal *(IAC)* in a 64-year-old white man. The acellular petrous apex consists of compact and cancellous bone with hematopoietic marrow. *ET,* Eustachian tube; and *ICA,* internal carotid artery. (Hematoxylin and eosin, ×7.)

Figure 3.10. Vertical section through left petrous pyramid anterior to internal auditory canal of a 51-year-old white man. The acellular petrous apex consists exclusively of cancellous bone with hematopoietic marrow. *ET,* Eustachian tube; and *ICA,* internal carotid artery. (Hematoxylin and eosin, ×6.5.)

Figure 3.11. Vertical section through left petrous pyramid near anterior wall of internal auditory canal *(IAC)* in a middle-aged white man. A large single inferior labyrinthine air cell is seen beneath the otherwise acellular compact bone of the petrous apex. The peritubal and pericarotid air cells are well developed. *ET,* Eustachian tube; and *ICA,* internal carotid artery. (Hematoxylin and eosin, ×7.)

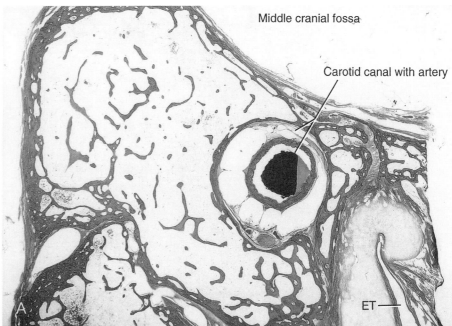

Middle cranial fossa

Carotid canal with artery

ET

Figure 3.12. A. Vertical section through left petrous pyramid anterior to internal auditory canal of a 52-year-old white man. The originally well developed but clearly osteoporotic acellular petrous apex consists of cancellous bone with fat marrow. *ET,* Eustachian tube. (Hematoxylin and eosin, ×7.)

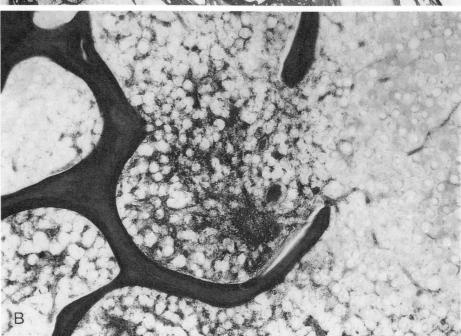

Figure 3.12. B. Few marrow spaces contain residues of hematopoietic tissue. (×50.)

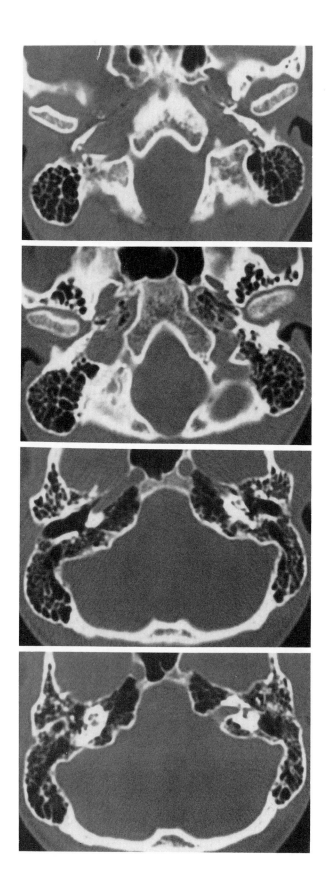

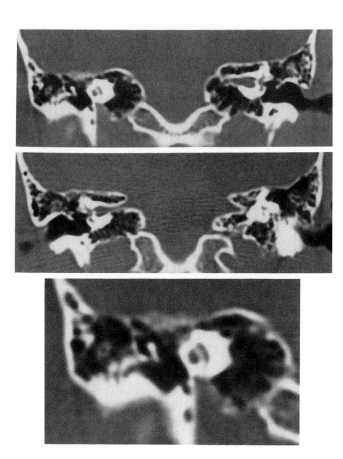

Figure 3.13. Axial *(left)* and coronal *(right)* CT scans of temporal bones of a 17-year-old black man with extensive pneumatization. The cellular development is especially noticeable in the regions of the squama, root of the zygoma, and the petrous apex. The dense cochlear and vestibular capsule gives the impression of being suspended in the surrounding network of air cells of the petrous pyramid.

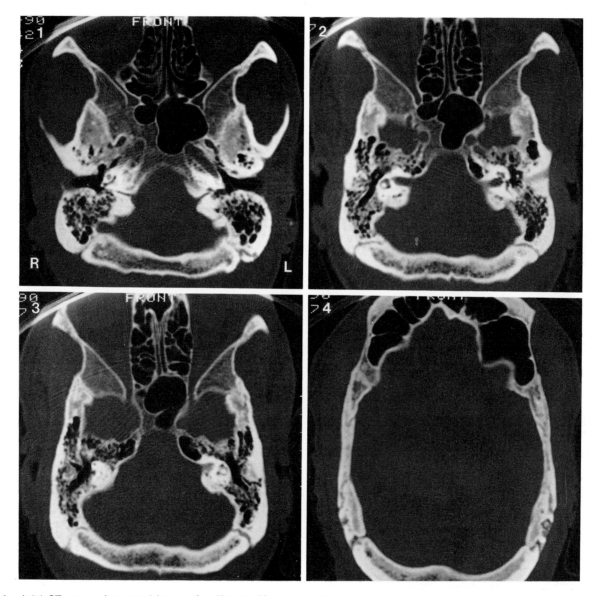

Figure 3.14. Axial CT scans of temporal bones of a 43-year-old man with extensive, symmetrical pneumatization of mastoid process, petrous pyramid, squamous portion, and root of the zygoma. Both petrous pyra-mids are very well pneumatized with large single apical air cells bilaterally. The internal and external tables of the calvaria are unusually sclerotic.

References

1. Donaldson JA. Surgical anatomy of the temporal bone. 3rd ed. Philadelphia: WB Saunders, 1981.
2. Beck CHL. Anatomie und Histologie des Ohres. In: Berendes J, Link R, Zöllner F, eds. Hals-Nasen-Ohrenheilkunde, Ohr I. Stuttgart: Georg Thieme, Chap 2, 1979;5:27–60.
3. Tumarkin A. On the nature and significance of hypocellularity of the mastoid. J Laryngol 1959;73:34.
4. Rotermundt F. Die Beeinflussung der Pneumatisation des Felsenbeins durch die Otitis des Säuglings. Z Laryngol Rhinol 1969;48:925.
5. Lesoine W. Die Mittelohrentzündung und die Pneumatisationhemmung des Warzenfortsatzes. Monatsschr Ohrenheilkd 1970;104:388.
6. Schwartz M. Schleimhaut und Pneumatisation. Arch Ohren Nasen Kehlkopfheilkd 1958;173:116–27.
7. Diamant M. The ''pathologic size'' of the mastoid air cell system. Acta Otolaryngol (Stockh) 1965;60:1.

4/ Blood Supply to the Temporal Bone and Membranous Labyrinth

The arteries that supply the different constituents of the temporal bone—the bony structure, the middle ear, and the membranous cochlea and labyrinth—are branches from the external and internal carotid and vertebral arteries.

The bony structure of the temporal bone receives its blood supply from branches of the external carotid artery, namely, from the occipital, retroauricular, maxillary, and ascending pharyngeal branches, from a meningeal branch of the vertebral artery, and from the subarcuate artery (SA). The SA is a branch of the anterior inferior cerebellar artery (AICA). These vessels with their ramifications form the vascular network in the periosteum that covers the entire surface of the temporal bone. Smaller branches from that periosteal network supply the adjacent bone, the marrow spaces in the bone, and the mucoperiosteum lining the air cell system. These vessels also provide larger penetrating branches to various more deeply located areas within its bony structure. Although each of these vessels supply primarily a certain area, they anastomose among one another, and several join to form the vascular network in the bony capsule of the cochlea and labyrinth.

The middle ear or, more specifically, the vascular network in the mucoperiosteum lining the walls of the middle ear cavity receives its blood supply from the same branches of the external carotid artery and from one or two of the caroticotympanic arteries, a small branch or branches of the internal carotid artery. This mucoperiosteal network supplies the adjacent bone, marrow spaces, and air cells and contributes significantly to the vascular network of the cochlear and labyrinthine capsule (Figs. 4.1 and 4.2).

The membranous cochlea and the vestibular labyrinth are exclusively supplied by the labyrinthine artery that arises from the AICA.

BLOOD SUPPLY OF THE MIDDLE EAR

The description of the blood supply of the middle ear, which follows, is based on earlier observations gained from tracing individual blood vessels through serial histologic sections of the temporal bone, via a compound microscope (1). This method, although tedious and time-consuming, proved to be more accurate than the technique of vascular injection used by previous investigators.

The arteries that participate in the blood supply of the middle ear are: *(a)* the caroticotympanic, *(b)* the inferior tympanic, *(c)* the stylomastoid, *(d)* the superficial petrosal, *(e)* the superior tympanic, *(f)* the subarcuate, *(g)* the anterior tympanic, *(h)* the deep auricular, and *(i)* the artery, whatever its origin, that courses along the Eustachian tube from its nasopharyngeal end.

The arteries anastomose extensively with each other, both by continuity of their main stem and via the mucosal networks

to which they contribute. It has been possible, in the sections examined, not only to trace each artery from its entrance into the temporal bone to its junction with the main stem of another artery but also to trace each branch to its finest ramifications in the mucosa or adjacent structures (bone, muscle, nerve). Often, in tracing branches of an artery into a mucosal network of vessels, a branch of somewhat larger caliber than the others is found to be continuous with a branch of similar caliber that has arisen from a neighboring stem artery. The presence of such connections between stem arteries is the basis for the statements about anastomosis via the mucosal network of a specific region. If the intervascular connections potentially present by way of the smaller vessels of the mucosal networks were included, then each artery to the middle ear would have to be described as anastomosing with each of the others.

The first six and the last of the arteries listed above are portrayed in Figure 4.3; the anterior tympanic artery is shown in Figures 4.4 and 4.5. It has not been practicable to show the finer ramifications, or most of the anastomotic possibilities via the networks, in the drawings. In these drawings the region of the junction between two main stems is portrayed as determined by comparing the diameters of the two vessels; of course, it is the region of the smallest caliber, from which the vascular lumen increases in size in either direction. Thus, for instance, it was found that the junction between the stylomastoid and the superficial petrosal artery usually occurs in the upper third of the descending portion of the Fallopian canal rather than at the level of the geniculate ganglion, which is stated in most textbooks.

The vascular mucosal network is denser in some areas than in others; the denser networks are in the floor, over the promontory, and over the lower portions of the anterior and posterior walls of the tympanic cavity. Blood to certain regions of the middle ear appears to be supplied mainly via one of these denser networks rather than a single artery. Thus, the lower third of the inner aspect of the tympanic membrane and the corresponding segment of the inner peripheral vascular ring get their main supply from the vascular network of the floor, and the region of the round window is supplied with blood from the network over the promontory.

The *caroticotympanic artery* (arteria caroticotympanica), usually stated to be a single vessel, in the material examined is often represented by two small arteries. These arteries arise as separate branches of the internal carotid artery (in its course through the vertical part of the carotid canal, a region included in the sections studied) and pass through separate channels in the bony partition between the carotid canal and the lower part of the anterior wall of the middle ear. If two vessels are present, one is superior to the other as they enter the middle ear and as they course across the promontory in its mucosa to join the stem of the inferior tympanic artery in the same way as does the ves-

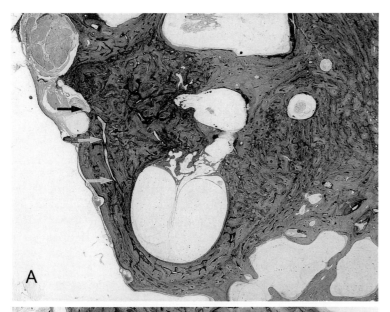

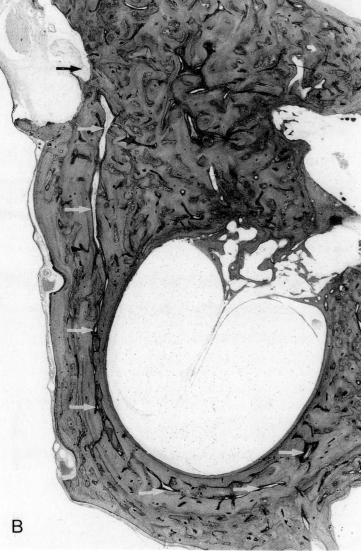

Figure 4.1. **A.** Vertical section through right temporal bone of an adult, just anterior to oval and round windows. A branch from the superior tympanic artery in the promontorial mucosa is seen entering the bony capsule of the lower basal cochlear turn below the facial canal *(arrows).* (Hematoxylin and eosin, ×12.)

Figure 4.1. **B.** The artery supplies the radial and circumferential intraosseous vascular network of the cochlea *(arrows).* (×25.)

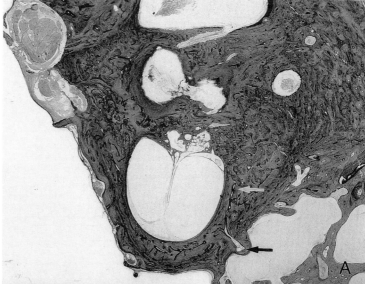

Figure 4.2. A. Section of same temporal bone as shown in Figure 4.1, 10 sections closer to oval and round windows. A branch from the inferior tympanic artery in the middle ear mucosa is seen as it enters the osseous capsule of the lower basal turn of the cochlea *(arrow).* (Hematoxylin and eosin, ×12.)

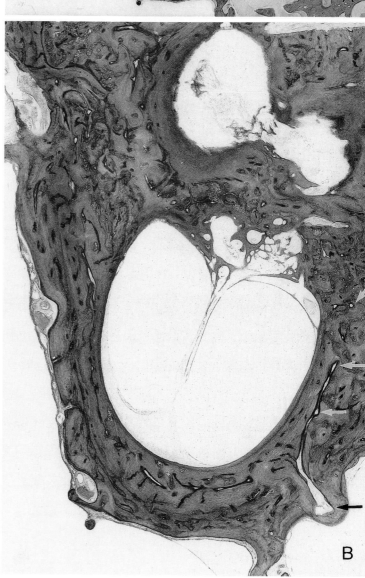

Figure 4.2. B. This artery is one of the several contributing vessels to the radial and circumferential intraosseous vascular cochlear network *(arrows).* (×25.)

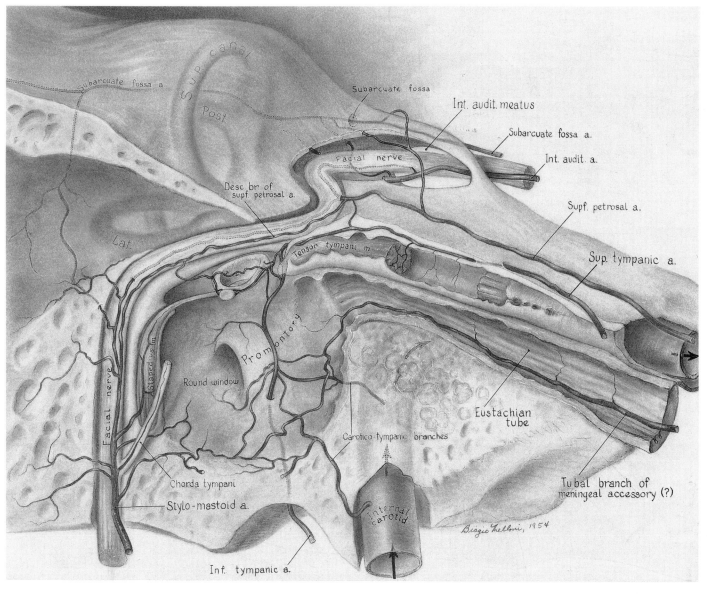

Figure 4.3. Illustration of arteries that supply the middle ear and mastoid, except for occipital, deep auricular, and anterior tympanic arteries.

sel when single. The region of the middle ear supplied from the internal carotid artery is the same whether one or two caroticotympanic branches are present; the branches extend to the anterior wall and the anterior part of the medial wall of the middle ear, from the tubal orifice to the floor.

The *inferior tympanic artery* (arteria tympanica inferior), a branch of the ascending pharyngeal artery, enters the anterior part of the floor of the middle ear, accompanied by the nerve of Jacobson, by passing through the inferior tympanic canaliculus from the jugular fossa (Fig. 4.3). The artery then ascends over the promontory, anterior to the round window region, usually in a bony groove but occasionally in a bony canal. In the promontorial part of its course the vessel is joined by the caroticotympanic artery or arteries. Still in close relationship with the tympanic branch of the ninth nerve, it unites with the superior tympanic artery in front of the oval window or somewhat below that level. Its branches supply primarily the dense vascular networks in the floor and over the promontory; this artery also contributes to the mucosal networks around the tympanic orifice of the Eustachian tube and over the lower anterior wall of the tym-

panic cavity and supplies the adjacent nerve of Jacobson. The main stem gives rise also to a small artery that supplies the anterior part of the stapes (Figs. 4.3 and 4.5).

The *stylomastoid artery* (arteria stylomastoidea), a branch of the posterior auricular artery, enters the facial canal through the stylomastoid foramen and courses upward in the canal alongside the facial nerve to terminate by joining branches of the superficial petrosal artery. In the lower third of the vertical portion of the facial canal, this vessel gives off branches posteriorly to bone and mucosa of the mastoid region, medially to the bone between the nonampullated end of the lateral and the ampullated end of the posterior semicircular canals (sometimes, these branches can be traced as far as the bone at the center of the posterior semicircular canal), and anteriorly to the mucosal vascular networks in the floor and over the lower posterior wall of the tympanic cavity. Lateral branches of the stylomastoid artery anastomose also at this level with the posterior branches of the deep auricular artery in the posterior wall and in the floor of the external auditory meatus (not shown in the drawings). Small vessels originating from the posterior meningeal artery, accompany-

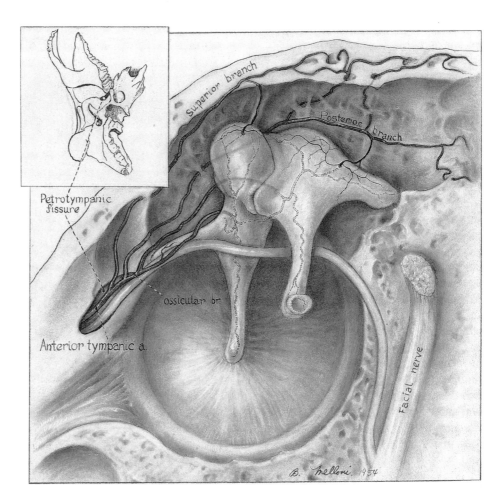

Figure 4.4. Somewhat schematic illustration of branching of anterior tympanic artery and of relationship of branches to other structures. The ossicular branch is the principal source of blood to the malleus and incus. The *insert* shows, at a much reduced scale, the location of the outer end of the petrotympanic (Glaserian) fissure through which the anterior tympanic artery enters the middle ear.

ing the nerve of Arnold, anastomose with branches from the stylomastoid artery in the region where the nerve of Arnold crosses the seventh nerve, within or near the Fallopian canal. In the lower third of the facial canal a branch of the stylomastoid artery occasionally enters the facial nerve. This vessel ascends within the trunk and may give rise to a smaller branch that descends toward the stylomastoid foramen. These branches supply the nerve fibers and soon terminate between them. One or more small branches are also given off to the chorda tympani nerve; this is the posterior tympanic artery (arteria tympanica posterior) of some textbooks. It has a much smaller caliber than the other tympanic arteries and follows the chorda only to the tympanic orifice of the canaliculus chordae tympani. There it supplies mainly the posterior part of the inner peripheral vascular ring of the tympanic membrane. In a few instances a very tiny vessel accompanies the chorda farther through the middle ear cavity to an anastomosis with a tiny terminal vessel from the anterior tympanic artery.

The largest branch of the stylomastoid artery is given off anteriorly at the level of the lower end of the stapedius muscle, which it supplies. In the middle third of the descending facial canal, branches are also sent posteriorly and medially; some of them, within the bone of the region, unite with branches from the subarcuate artery (Fig. 4.3). The stem of the stylomastoid artery, whose caliber is considerably diminished beyond the origin of the branch to the stapedius muscle, then anastomoses with the descending main branch of the superficial petrosal artery, which courses in the facial canal between its wall and the trunk of the facial nerve. Moreover, it may anastomose with that

descending branch of the superficial petrosal artery that courses peripherally within the substance of the facial nerve. This vessel usually terminates within the nerve trunk but exceptionally may continue and leave it, to join the stem of the stylomastoid artery (Fig. 4.3). Both anastomoses are usually near the junction of the middle and the upper third of the vertical portion of the facial canal. At this level, small arteries are also given off posteriorly and laterally to the mastoid region, to the medial half of the floor of the aditus, and to the posterosuperior segment of the inner peripheral tympanic vascular ring, which in this region may have anastomotic connections with the outer peripheral vascular ring. From this part of the inner vascular ring a vessel passes, in a mucosal fold near the lower border of the posterior plica of the tympanic membrane, to the medial surface of the neck of the malleus to join a vessel from the posterior branch of the anterior tympanic artery. Together they form the descending artery in the mucosal membrane over the medial aspect of the handle of the malleus; the branches of this vessel, together with those from the inner peripheral vascular ring, supply the mucosal surface of the tympanic membrane.

The *superficial petrosal artery* (ramus petrosus superficialis arteriae meningeae mediae) arises from the meningeal artery just above the foramen spinosum and runs posteriorly and laterally, in the floor of the middle cranial fossa, with the greater superficial petrosal nerve in a groove (sulcus nervi petrosi superficialis majoris) to the hiatus of the facial canal (Fig. 4.3). In the sulcus, several small vessels are given off to the adjacent dura, and one larger vessel frequently branches off and crosses over the petrous crest, in front of the superior semicircular canal, to

and 4.5). For this branch, which seems previously not to have been recognized, the name of "ossicular artery" is proposed later in this chapter.

The *deep auricular artery* (arteria auricularis profunda), a branch from the mandibular portion of the internal maxillary artery, enters the temporal bone at the inferior aspect of the osseous portion of the external auditory canal. In the bony floor of the canal it usually divides into two major branches, an anterior and a posterior branch and several smaller ramifications. The posterior branch largely supplies the bony structures and the overlying integument of the posterior half of the canal wall, anastomoses medially and posteriorly with branches from the stylomastoid artery, and supplies vessels to the posteroinferior segment of the outer peripheral vascular ring of the tympanic membrane. It then ascends superficial to or, sometimes, within the posterior bony canal wall to the posterosuperior segment of the outer vascular ring and, at this higher level, frequently anastomoses again with branches from the stylomastoid artery. The posterior branch then approaches the tympanic membrane and descends between the epidermis and the layer of radial fibers, passing at first behind the manubrium of the malleus and then superficial to it, in its lower half. Branches from this descending vessel follow the direction of the radial fibers to the periphery. In some instances the artery divides near the distal end of the manubrium into two branches that form an elliptical loop around the umbo and send vessels radially to the inferior part of the pars tensa. In other instances the same artery simply ramifies radially at the umbo.

The anterior branch of the deep auricular artery supplies the bone and overlying integument of the anterior half of the external auditory canal wall and sends vessels to the anteroinferior segment of the outer peripheral vascular ring. It also, via branches that pass through the bone beneath the tympanic sulcus, contributes to the mucosal vascular network of the floor of the middle ear and by this route may anastomose with the other vessels that contribute to this network. The stem of the anterior branch ascends in the anterior canal wall, where it gives a few small branches that anastomose in the bone with ones from the posterior branch of the anterior tympanic artery, and terminates by entering the anterosuperior segment of the outer peripheral vascular ring of the tympanic membrane.

The artery, whatever its origin, that courses in the wall of the Eustachian tube not only supplies the walls of the tympanic part of the tube but also participates in the blood supply of the middle ear. It sends branches to the mucosal networks of the anterior wall and of the promontory and anastomoses with the caroticotympanic artery. In the drawing (Fig. 4.3), this artery is labeled with a *question mark* as being from the meningeal accessory artery, because this appears to have been its origin in the only case in which it could be traced, in the histologic sections, to a source that can be identified with reasonable certainly. In this specimen, the origin is from a small artery that runs near the middle meningeal artery beneath the foramen spinosum; the internal maxillary artery, however, was not included in the block of tissue sectioned. The artery along the upper part of the tube may, of course, arise from any of the several arteries that are known to send branches to the nasopharyngeal end of the Eustachian tube or from the anastomotic network there formed by these branches.

The blood supply of the posterior part of the mastoid region could not be determined from the histologic material ex-amined, because this part of the temporal bone had usually not been included in the blocks of tissue sectioned. The observations made on this point give no reason to doubt the customary statement in textbooks that the mastoid branch of the occipital artery supplies this part of the middle ear.

BLOOD SUPPLY OF THE MALLEUS AND THE INCUS

Early in the course of our efforts to trace the vessels supplying the malleus and incus, it became apparent that in our material the major vessel to the outer ossicles was a branch of the anterior tympanic artery, not the middle meningeal artery, as stated earlier, and that it entered the middle ear through or near the petrotympanic (Glaserian) fissure, not along the tendon of the tensor tympani muscle. For this branch of the anterior tympanic artery, which seems previously not to have been recognized, we propose the name, ossicular artery. This vessel, the major one to the outer ossicles, branches from its parent artery in the upper part of the petrotympanic fissure. It enters the middle ear either by accompanying the chorda tympanic nerve through the fibrous tissue of the fissure or by passing through a small osseous canal in one or the other of the bones that border the fissure. The ossicular artery usually divides into two branches, one for the malleus and one for the incus, within the petrotympanic fissure or soon after entering the middle ear (Figs. 4.4 and 4.5). In two instances the division occurred near the malleus, which the ossicular artery reached by the route usual for its malleolar branch.

The branch to the malleus or the *malleolar artery* enters the middle ear near the anterior part of the attachment of the lateral malleolar ligament and courses in the mucosa on the upper surface of the anterior edge of the ligament. Near the attachment of this ligament to the malleus, the artery enters the bone through a niche or a "nutrient foramen," at the anterolateral aspect of the neck, or of the lower part of the head of the malleus (Figs. 4.4–4.6). Usually inside the niche, but occasionally just before reaching it, the malleolar artery sends a branch to the root of the short process and may receive an anastomosis from the incudal artery. This anastomosis, which is not always present, runs in the mucosa over the joint capsule and unites the malleolar and incudal arteries before they penetrate the respective ossicles; its location is shown in Figure 4.5.

The course of the branch to the incus or the *incudal artery* varies more than does that of the malleolar artery. As stated earlier, the ossicular artery usually gives off the incudal branch soon after or even before it enters the middle ear. In these typical cases, the incudal artery either traverses for a short distance the lower part of the bony lateral wall of the attic or courses in the mucosa of the wall, then passes across the lateral part of the epitympanum in a mucosal fold. In this mucosal fold the incudal artery usually extends directly to the lateral part of the body of the incus, but it may extend to the region of the neck of the malleus and then run in the mucosa over the joint capsule to reach the incus. In the latter cases it is slightly above the lateral malleolar ligament. In the two instances in which the ossicular artery did not divide until near the neck of the malleus, the incudal artery passed from its origin to the incus by running in the mucosa over the lateral part of the incudomalleolar articulation.

In contrast to the malleolar artery, which always enters the same part of the bone it supplies, the incudal artery varies considerably. It may enter the lateral (Fig. 4.7) or, less frequently, the medial aspect of the body of the incus in close proximity to the joint capsule, or it may enter the incus at the anterolateral surface of the root of the long crus (Fig. 4.5). Not infrequently, the main stem of the incudal artery enters the bone in one of these areas, and a small branch continues in the mucosa to enter

the bone at one of the other two areas or at the lower end of the long crus. In those cases in which the incudal artery enters the root of the long crus or the medial aspect of the body of the incus, its course from the lateral wall of the attic is to the region of the neck of the malleus and then across the incudomalleolar articulation. If it is to enter the root of the long crus, the incudal

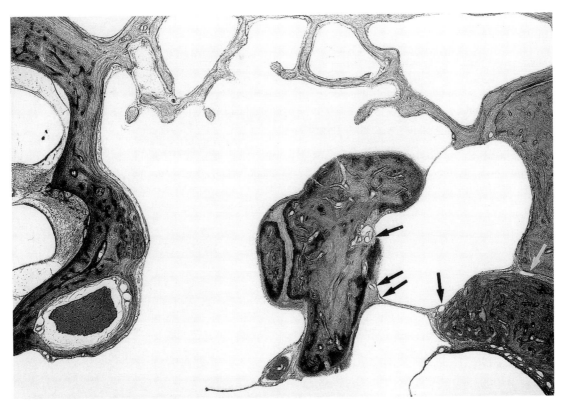

Figure 4.6. Vertical section through left epitympanic region. The malleolar artery has been cut in five places *(arrows)* along its course from the tympanic end of the petrotympanic fissure (on right) across the anterior lateral malleolar ligament to its entrance into the malleus. (Hematoxylin and eosin, ×20.)

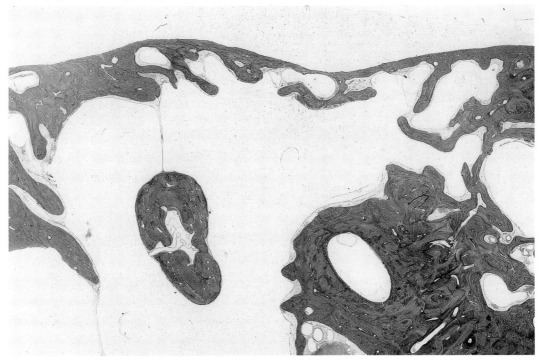

Figure 4.7. Vertical section through right epitympanic region at level of incus. It shows the entrance of the incudal artery into the lateral side of the body of the incus. Sections anterior to the one photographed show that in this one the incudal artery reaches the ossicle in a mucosal fold by passing directly across the lateral epitympanic space. The small vessel in the mucosal fold from the tegmen to the incus is a tributary, from the posterior branch of the anterior tympanic artery to the vascular network in the mucosa of the incus. (Hematoxylin and eosin, ×18.)

artery passes only across the lateroinferior portion of the joint capsule; if it is to enter the medial aspect of the body of the incus, the artery continues across the capsule, between the long crus of the incus and the manubrium of the malleus. Often, as noted above, the incudal artery receives an anastomotic branch from the malleolar artery before it enters the incus.

The malleolar artery, after reaching the marrow space of the malleus, which may even extend into the upper part of its head, forms an irregular vascular convolute, often extremely complex in arrangement, and divides into several branches. One of the branches can be traced into the short process, two or more can be traced into the bone of the head, and another can be followed down toward the tip of the manubrium.

The anterior process of the malleus (processus gracilis or processus Folii), which extends as a delicate spicule into the dense fibrous tissue of the petrotympanic fissure, receives one or two tiny branches from the ossicular artery or from its malleolar branch. The exact source depends on the level at which the branching occurs.

Inside the body of the incus, the incudal artery forms a vascular convolute (Fig. 4.8) similar to that in the malleus. This artery gives rise to branches that pass within the bone to the short and the long process.

The mucous membrane of the outer ossicles contains a dense vascular network. Over the head and the neck of the malleus this network is supplied by small vessels that pass in mucosal folds from the tegmen tympani and from the lateral wall of the attic to the head of the malleus. These vessels arise from the superior branch and the posterior branch of the anterior tympanic artery, the same vessel that gives origin to the ossicular artery (Figs. 4.4 and 4.5). Most of the ramifications of these vessels remain in the mucosa, but a few penetrate the substance of the malleus and join the convolute inside the marrow space. Thus, to a limited degree, the mucosal vessels provide a collateral circulation for the malleus and the incus, in spite of the fact that they and the ossicular artery arise from a common source, the anterior tympanic artery.

The vascular network in the mucosa over the manubrium is supplied by branches from three arteries, the anterior tympanic, the stylomastoid, and the deep auricular. Only rarely does a vessel from this network penetrate the bone to unite with the branch of the malleolar artery inside the manubrium.

The mucosal network over the incus and the incudostapedial articulation is supplied by vessels that arise from the posterior branch of the anterior tympanic artery. Most of them pass in mucosal folds from the lateral wall of the attic to the lateral aspect of the body of the incus, but occasionally such vessels pass from the tegmen to the superior surface of the incus. From this network a few tiny branches pass through the cortical layer of the incus and join the vascular convolute inside the marrow space. From the mucosal network over the long process of the incus, vessels seldom pass into the bone.

BLOOD SUPPLY OF THE STAPES

Blood vessels within the osseous tissue of the stapes are present only in the thickened margin of the footplate and in the neck and the head of the bone; the crura and the thin central part of the footplate seem normally to be nourished entirely by diffusion from the mucosal network of vessels. That this is the case

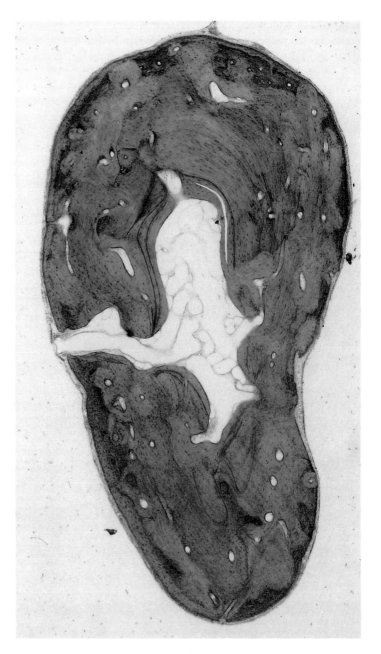

Figure 4.8. Higher magnification of part of incus shown in Figure 4.7, to demonstrate complexity of arterial vascular convolute in marrow space. (Hematoxylin and eosin, ×165.)

is not surprising when the thickness of a normal stapedial crus (measured from the outer to the inner face of the U-shaped section of the structure) is compared with the thickness of a Haversian lamellar system in other bones. The mucosal networks of the two surfaces of a stapedial crus are seldom separated from each other by more than three or four lamellae of osseous tissue. The distance to be traversed by diffusion through the canaliculi of the bone is, therefore, often much less than is the case in a typical Haversian system, between the vessel in the Haversian canal and the outer lamellae of the system.

Other than in definitely pathologic specimens, blood vessels in the crura or in the central part of the footplate have been found only twice in all the material examined. The two exceptions are the stapes of a 53-year-old man in whom an arrest of development of this ossicle appears to have occurred. The appearance of each stapedial crus of this man is normal for the embryonic stage before resorption of the bone of the primitive rod has been completed (5, 6). A section through the anterior crus of the left stapes of this man is shown in Figure 4.9.

The vessels within the substance of the normal stapes, in the thickened margin of the footplate and in the neck and head, are branches from the vessels of the mucosal network. The usual tributaries to the mucosal vascular network over the stapes are shown in Figures 4.3 and 4.5.

It should be noted that the vascular supply of the stapedial region, as traced in sections, differs considerably from that found by the injection technique (7, 8). Two small arteries can be traced to the mucosa of the region of the anterior crus; one is from the superior tympanic artery, while the other branches from the inferior tympanic artery near the anastomotic junction of the parent vessels. The vessel from the superior tympanic artery either comes off well above the oval window, even near the geniculate ganglion, and descends for some distance or comes off in front of the oval window as a shorter branch. Both of the possible sources are shown in Figure 4.3; only the former is included in Figure 4.5. The two small arteries contribute to the vascular network around the anterior crus and, after giving off one or two tiny

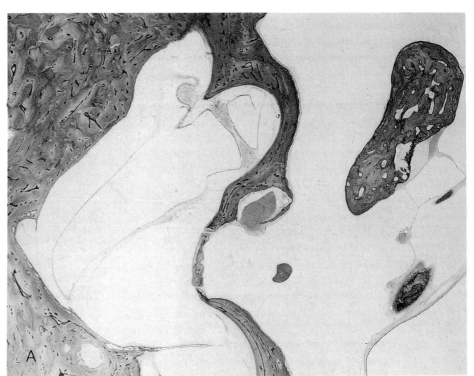

Figure 4.9. A. Vertical section through left temporal bone near center of oval window in a 53-year-old man with abnormal stapes in which blood vessels are present in the crura and in the central part of the footplate. (Hematoxylin and eosin, ×25.)

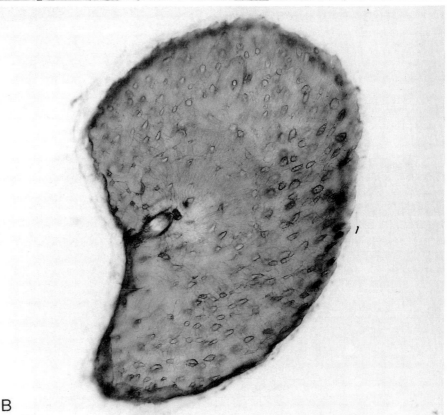

Figure 4.9. B. At higher power, the anomalous crus that includes a blood vessel near the center can be seen. (×230.)

vessels that pass, at the base of the crus, into the thickened bone of the margin of the footplate, join each other and course along the convex aspect of the anterior crus. This vessel terminates by supplying the dense vascular network over the incudostapedial articulation and by a branch that enters the bone of the neck and head of the stapes. Before uniting and passing along the shaft of the anterior crus, the two vessels receive anastomoses from the vessels in the region of the posterior crus (Fig. 4.5).

The principal supply to the region of the posterior crus is a small artery that emerges from the facial canal above the posterior margin of the annular ligament; this vessel arises from that descending main branch of the superficial petrosal artery that courses in the facial canal between its wall and the trunk of the facial nerve (Fig. 4.3). (For the source and course of the parent vessel, see the account of the blood supply of the entire middle ear.) The small artery, after emerging from the facial canal, passes in the mucosa across the annular ligament, supplies the vascular network over the posterior crus and the posterior part of the stapedial footplate, gives rise to one or two tiny branches that enter the posterior part of the thickened osseous rim of the footplate, and then passes along the convex surface of the posterior crus to contribute to the vascular network over the incudostapedial articulation and to send a branch into the bone of the neck and head of the stapes (Fig. 4.5). Additional contributions to the vascular network over the incudostapedial articulation along the stapedius tendon (not shown) may originate in the adjacent facial canal and the overlying mucoperiosteum.

The anastomotic connections between the vessels that supply the region of the anterior crus and those of the region of the posterior crus are usually three in number: (a) the tiny vessels in the bone of the rim of the footplate, from the two sources, communicate with each other; (b) a vessel of a size larger than those of the general mucosal network courses in the mucosa of the footplate or, occasionally, in a mucosal fold from one crus to the other, as illustrated in Figure 4.5; and (c) a similar-sized vessel often but not always courses in the mucosa near the inferior margin of the oval window (Fig. 4.5).

In perhaps a fifth of the material a vessel could be traced from the region of the facial canal above the oval window downward to the mucosal network of the promontory. In some instances this vessel in crossing the oval window niche passes between the stapedial crura (i.e., through the obturator foramen) in a mucosal fold; in other instances it passes downward in front of the anterior crus or behind the posterior crus or by the neck of the stapes. Its course in all the positions is approximately perpendicular to the plane of the stapedial arch. In a few instances this vessel arises within the facial canal directly from the descending main branch of the superficial petrosal artery that gives origin to the artery to the posterior crus of the stapes; in other instances it appears to arise indirectly from the same source as a branch from the mucosal network of vessels over the facial canal. Because this vessel in any of its variant relationships occurs in only a small proportion of the material studied, it has been omitted from the illustrations (Figs. 4.3 and 4.5) of the normal vascular pattern of the stapedial region; it may, however, eventually prove to be of interest to the embryologist.

To establish a relationship between the stapedial artery of embryonic life and any of the small arteries we have observed in the stapedial region of the adult, it would be necessary to make an intensive study of all the intermediate stages from less than 40 mm in length to that in the adult. Merely because an artery in the adult has a similar position with respect to the stapes that an embryonic vessel had to the developing ossicles does not warrant the conclusion that the embryonic artery persisted and directly participated in the formation of the adult artery. Most investigators of blood vessels of the stapedial region in human embryos, in fact, reported inability to identify the remnants of the stapedial artery, near the stapes, beyond the third month (5, 9). Only two authors concluded otherwise (7, 8).

Comments

Our method of studying the vascular patterns within the tympanic membrane as part of the middle ear has not added much to the findings of earlier investigators. Good descriptions and illustrations of these vascular networks can be found in their publications (10–14). A drawing to show these patterns is therefore superfluous. In our description, emphasis has been placed only on where the respective tributaries enter the inner and outer vascular rings.

Tracing vessels and their branches through serial histologic sections reveals that anastomotic connections between the arteries of the middle ear are even more plentiful than was hitherto recognized from studies based on injection and dissection techniques. Tracing clearly demonstrates the blood supply to the middle ear ossicles, identifies the ossicular artery as the principal source of the malleus and incus, and establishes the avascular nature of the crura of the stapes.

BLOOD SUPPLY TO THE INTERNAL AUDITORY CANAL, MEMBRANOUS COCHLEA, VESTIBULAR LABYRINTH, AND SURROUNDING BONE

The labyrinthine artery (internal auditory artery) supplies the dura and arachnoid within the internal auditory canal, the cranial nerves VII and VIII, and the membranous cochlea and labyrinth. It also contributes significantly to the vascular network of the surrounding bony capsule. The origin of this artery and its distribution had been examined earlier by several investigators using dissection and vascular injection techniques (2, 15–19). In the early 1950s, Smith (20–22) demonstrated the capillary areas in the cochlea and labyrinth of the guinea pig, cat, and human, and in the late 1960s, Axelsson (23) published an excellent treatise on the vascular anatomy of the cochlea in the guinea pig and human. Two decades ago, Mazzoni (3, 24, 25) in several studies examined the origin and course of the labyrinthine and SA in humans. The following account attempts to summarize the essential observations of these investigators.

The *labyrinthine artery (LA)* arises regularly from an arterial (cerebellar) loop that either extends into the internal auditory canal (40%), lies at the porus (27%), or lies in close proximity to it (33%) (Fig. 4.10). This loop represents the main trunk or a collateral branch of the anterior inferior cerebellar artery (AICA) in about 80%, an accessory AICA in about 17%, and the posterior inferior cerebellar artery (PICA) in about 3% (24). The AICA originates from the basilar artery and supplies the anterior inferior surface of the cerebellum. The collateral branch of the AICA arises from that artery near the entrance to the auditory canal. The accessory AICA originates from the basilar artery just anterior to the AICA. The PICA arises from the vertebral artery, supplies the posterior inferior surface of the cere-

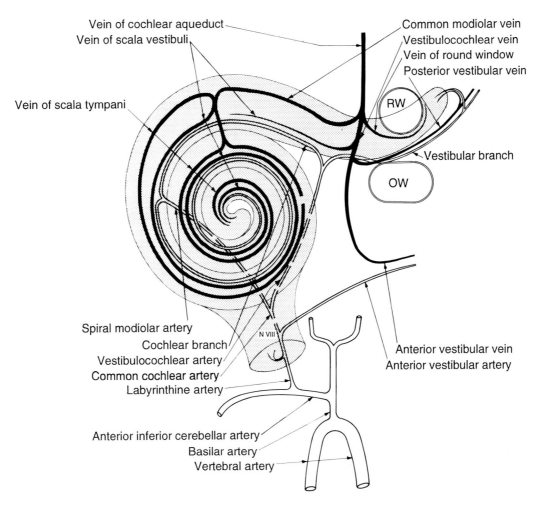

Figure 4.10. Schematic drawing of arterial supply and venous draining of cochlea. The labyrinthine artery arises as a branch of the AICA and gives rise to the anterior vestibular and common cochlear arteries. The common cochlear artery divides into the vestibulocochlear artery and the spiral modiolar artery. The vestibulocochlear artery subdivides into the cochlear and vestibular branches. The vestibular branch supplies the terminal section of the lower basal turn of the cochlea. The cochlear branch runs in the opposite direction toward the apex to anastomose with one or two descending branches of the spiral modiolar artery. It supplies the lower half or the entire length of the lower basal turn of the cochlea. The spiral modiolar artery follows the cochlear duct to the apex and, except for the initial segment of the lower basal turn, supplies the entire cochlea.

Two independent venous systems, one from the scala vestibuli and the other from the scala tympani, provide venous drainage for the cochlea. The two collecting veins, the vein of the scala vestibuli and vein of the scala tympani, join to form the common modiolar vein. The common modiolar vein unites with the vestibulocochlear vein to form the vein of cochlear aqueduct that drains into the lateral sinus. *OW*, oval window; and *RW*, round window.

bellum, and anastomoses with the AICA. The (cerebellar) arterial loop, the parent vessel of the LA, varies considerably in size and relation to the seventh and eighth cranial nerves. In the 67 of 100 specimens in which the arterial loop had a close relation to the canal and porus, it was passing between the nerves in 52%, inferiorly in 27%, anteriorly in 12%, posteriorly in 7.5%, and superiorly in 1.5%. In two-thirds its course was in a horizontal plane, and in one-third its course was either in an oblique or a vertical plane. In the 33 specimens in which the arterial loop had no close relation to the canal, it was inferior to the nerves in 76%, intermediate and posterolateral in 9% each, and anteromedial in 6% (24).

The LA was represented by a single vessel in about half, by two vessels in nearly half of the specimens, and as three vessels in only a few instances. As the LA enters the canal, it passes over the inferior border of the porus and runs between the seventh and eighth nerves along the anterior superior or posterior inferior surface of the latter. In the presence of two LAs, one courses anterior while the other courses posterior along the eighth nerve. The larger one usually represents the main artery, eventually dividing into its three terminal branches, whereas the smaller one may terminate within the canal or, in one-fourth of cases, becomes the vestibulocochlear artery or supplies the saccule. Within the canal the LA supplies branches to the seventh and eighth cranial nerves, arachnoid, outlining dura, and adjacent bone (25). Whereas smaller branches from the dural vascular network supply the adjacent bone, larger branches traverse the dura to enter the deeper regions of the osseous canal wall. The LA gives off a branch to the superior vestibular ganglion, where it may form a vascular convolution (25). This branch also supplies the vascular networks in the superior and inferior vestibular ganglia. From the superior ganglion a vascular branch joins the dura of the adjacent posterior canal wall and, after giving off a few tributaries to the dural network, enters the bone between the posterior canal wall and the medial wall of the vestibule and semicircular canals to supply the regional bony structures (25). Other branches mainly from the main stem of the LA supply the superior, anterior, and inferior osseous canal wall. The LA then

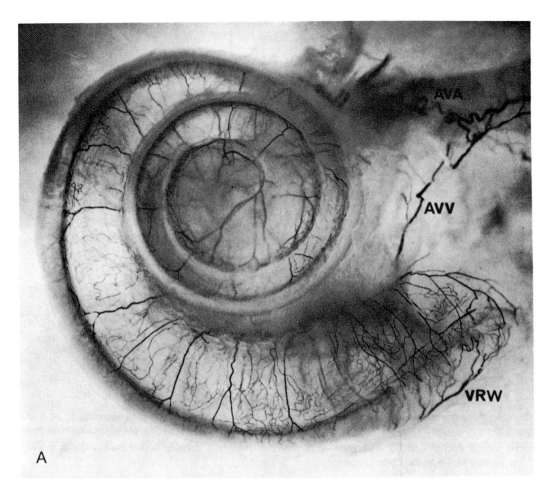

Figure 4.16. A. Blood supply of cochlea, demonstrated in injected temporal bones. Vascular patterns in the vestibular scala and spiral lamina are revealed. *AVA,* anterior vestibular artery; *AVV,* anterior vestibular vein; and *VRW,* vein of the cochlear fenestra.

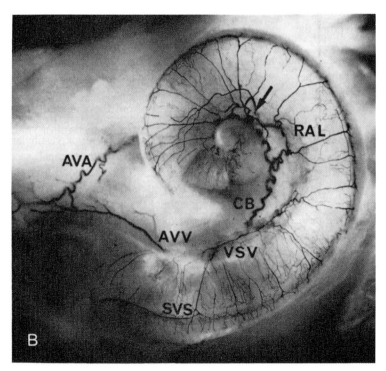

Figure 4.16. B. Two of the three sources of arterial supply to the basal turn of the cochlea are demonstrated: *(a)* the cochlear branch of the vestibulocochlear artery, and *(b)* the spiral modiolar artery. *AVA,* anterior vestibular artery; *AVV,* anterior vestibular vein; *CB,* cochlear branch of the vestibulocochlear artery; *RAL,* radiating arterioles; *SVS,* vessels of the stria vascularis; *VRW,* vein of the cochlear fenestra; and *VSV,* vein of the scala vestibuli.

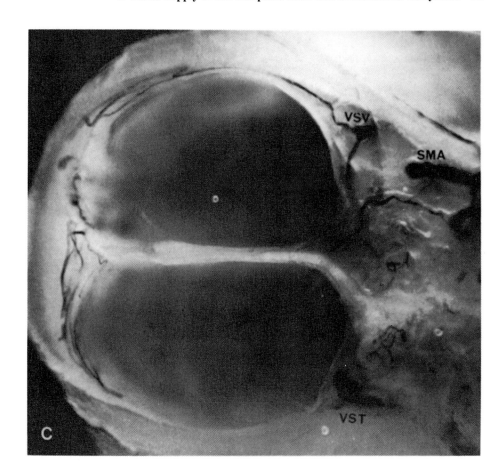

Figure 4.16. C. The spiral modiolar artery seen here supplies the apical half of the lower basal turn as well as the second and third turns of the cochlea. *SMA,* spiral modiolar artery; *VST,* vein of the scala tympani; and *VSV,* vein of the scala vestibuli.

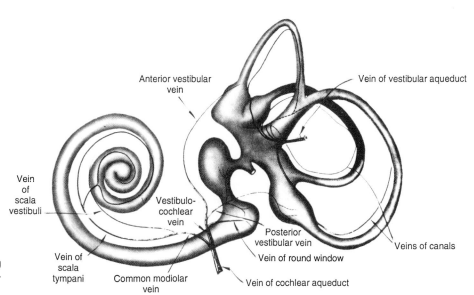

Figure 4.17. Schematic drawing demonstrating venous drainage of cochlea and vestibular labyrinth.

References

1. Nager GT, Nager M. The arteries of the human middle ear, with particular regard to the blood supply of the auditory ossicles. Ann Otol Rhinol Laryngol 1953;62:923–950.

2. Siebermann F. Die Blutgefässe im Labyrinth des menschlichen Ohres. Wiesbaden: J Bergmann, 1894.

3. Mazzoni A. The subarcuate artery in man. Laryngoscope 1970;80:69–79.

4. Nager GT. Origins and relations of the internal auditory artery and the subarcuate artery. Ann Otol Rhinol Laryngol 1954;63:51–62.

5. Broman I. Die Entwicklungsgeschichte der Gehörknöchelchen beim Menschen. Anat Hefte Abt 1898;11:507–668.

6. Bast TH, Anson BJ. The temporal bone and the ear. Springfield, Illinois: Charles C Thomas, 1949.

7. Nabeya D. The blood vessels of the middle ear, in relation to the development of the small ear bones and their muscles (a preliminary report). Okajimas Folia Anat Jpn 1923;1:243–245.

8. Adachi B. Das Arteriensystem der Japaner, Bd. 1:99–103, Kyoto, 1928.

9. Tandler, J. Zur Entwicklungsgeschichte der Kopfarterien bei den Mammalia. Gegenbaurs Morphol Jahrb 1902;30(1–2):275–373.

10. Prussak A. Zur Physiologie und Anatomie des Blutstromes in der Trommelhöhle. Berichte über die Verhandlungen der Königlich Sächsischen Gesellschaft der Wissenschaften zu Leipzig, Mathematisch-Physische Classe 1868;20:101–118.

11. Popper M. Die Gefässe und Nerven des Trommelfells. Monatsschr Ohrenheilkd 1869;3:79–86.

12. Burnett IM. Über das Vorkommen von Gefässchlingen im Trommelfell einiger niedrigen Tiere. Monatschr Ohrenheilkd 1876;10:74.

13. Moos S. Untersuchungen über das Verhalten der Blutgefässe und des Blutgefässkreislaufs des Trommelfells und Hammergriffes. Arch Augen-Ohrenheilkd Ohrenärztlicher Teil 1877;6:475–495.

14. Gerlach W. Microscopische Studien aus dem Gebiete der menschlichen Morphologie. Erlangen, 1858.

15. Shambaugh GE. Blood vessels in the labyrinth of the ear. Vol X, Dicentennial Publication. Chicago: University of Chicago Press, 1903.

16. Shambaugh GE. The distribution of blood vessels in the labyrinth of the ear of the sheep and calf. Arch Otol 1905;34:71.

17. Asai K. Die Blutgefässe des häutigen Labyrinthes der Ratte. Anat Hefte 1908;36:711.

18. Asai K. Die Blutgefässe im häutigen Labyrinth des Hundes. Anat Hefte 1908;36:369.

19. Nabeya D. A study in the comparative anatomy of the blood vascular system of the internal ear in mammalia and in homo [Japanese]. Acta Sch Med 1923;6:1–132.

20. Smith CA. Capillary areas of the cochlea in the guinea pig. Laryngoscope 1951;61:1073–1095.

21. Smith CA. The capillaries of the vestibular membranous labyrinth in the guinea pig. Laryngoscope 1953;63:87–104.

22. Smith CA. Capillary areas of the membranous labyrinth. Ann Otol Rhinol Laryngol 1954;63:435–474.

23. Axelsson A. The vascular anatomy of the cochlea in the guinea pig and in man. Acta Otolaryngol Suppl (Stockh) 1968;243:1–134.

24. Mazzoni A. Internal auditory canal arterial relations at the porus acusticus. Ann Otol Rhinol Laryngol 1969;78:797–814.

25. Mazzoni A. Internal auditory artery supply to the petrous bone. Ann Otol Rhinol Laryngol 1972;81:13–21.

26. Schuknecht HF, Gulya AJ. Anatomy of the temporal bone with surgical implications. Philadelphia: Lea & Febiger, 1986.

5/ Dysplasia of the External and Middle Ear

Congenital aural atresia is a relatively common unilateral or bilateral malformation that is usually associated with a deformity of the auricle and regularly accompanied by a developmental anomaly of the middle ear. A combination with an abnormality of the inner ear is observed in approximately 10% of cases (1–4).

Moderate and severe forms of congenital aural atresia are encountered in about 1 in 10,000 to 1 in 20,000 individuals (5, 6). It occurs more commonly in the male, is observed much more often unilaterally, and for reasons still unknown affects the right ear more frequently than the left (7, 8).

At one time, congenital aural atresia was considered a well defined and independent entity. However, our observations have shown that this malformation often represents only one of several malformations involving the derivatives of the posterior segments of the first and second branchial arches (9, 10). Aural atresia may also be associated with abnormalities affecting other organ systems as the result of single-gene disorders, chromosomal abnormalities, or environmental teratogens.

EMBRYOLOGY

A brief review of the normal development of the ear is given here to facilitate comprehension of the problems encountered in congenital aural atresia. The inner ear and the middle and outer ear develop independently. Differentiation of the inner ear begins early in the third week of intrauterine development with the appearance of the ectodermal auditory placode at the level of the myelencephalon. The auditory placode invaginates during the fourth week to form the auditory pit, which later becomes the auditory vesicle. Around the 31st day, the labyrinthine recess develops from the dorsal end of the auditory vesicle. This recess gives rise to the endolymphatic duct and sac. During the fifth week, a superior dorsal and an inferior ventral compartment develop from the auditory vesicle. The superior compartment differentiates into the semicircular canals and the antrum, which, in turn, develop into the utricle and saccule. The lower compartment, through evagination and involution, becomes the cochlear duct. During the 7th week, the cochlear duct completes 1 turn; during the 8th week, it completes 1½ turns; and during the 10th week, it completes 2½ turns. At about the 12th week, the endolymphatic labyrinth is fully differentiated except for part of the organ of Corti in the apical turn (11).

In the 2.7-mm-long embryo a conglomeration of ganglion cells appears adjacent to the anterior wall of the auditory vesicle and gradually advances toward its medial wall. This represents the acousticofacial ganglion. The origin of this ganglion is not uniform. The acoustic ganglion originates from cells of the rostral wall of the auditory vesicle. The facial ganglion originates mainly from the ganglion crest and, to a lesser extent, from cells of the first epibranchial placode. While the facial ganglion separates from the original acousticofacial ganglion during the third week, the acoustic ganglion maintains its close relationship to the developing auditory vesicle. The acoustic ganglion divides (at the same time as the auditory vesicle) into a superior and an inferior portion. The superior portion sends nerve fibers to the utricle and to the superior and the lateral ampulla. The inferior portion sends nerve fibers to the saccule and to the posterior ampulla. The remaining part of the inferior portion of the acoustic ganglion later becomes the spiral ganglion situated at the concave side of the cochlear duct. The close relationship of this ganglion to the developing cochlear duct leads to its typical spiral arrangement. At about the same time, the facial nerve comes into view. Nerve fibers grow from the neural tube into the mesenchyme of the second branchial arch. The chorda tympani nerve arises from peripheral nerve fibers of the geniculate (formerly facial) ganglion. The chorda tympani joins the developing facial nerve for a short distance and, by the fifth week, unites with the third branch of the trigeminal nerve (7).

While the membranous labyrinth is taking shape, a gradual concentration of mesenchyme takes place around it (fourth week). This surrounding mesenchyme is transformed into cartilage after the seventh week and, subsequently, is converted into bone to form the inner ear capsule. Ossification of the labyrinthine capsule begins at about the 16th week, as the endolymphatic labyrinth reaches adult form, and develops from 14 centers. Ossification begins near the round window and ends in the area of the oval window and fissula ante fenestram. It is generally completed by the 23rd week (12).

During the third week of fetal development, while the auditory vesicle is being formed, an outpocketing develops from the foregut and becomes the first pharyngeal pouch. The dorsal end of this first pharyngeal pouch, through gradual expansion, becomes in succession the Eustachian tube, tympanic cavity, and extensions of the latter, namely, the epitympanic recess, antrum, and mastoid air cells. Between the fourth and sixth weeks, the lower portion of the tympanic cavity begins to form. In the eighth week, the upper portion is still occupied by mesenchyme. During the 23rd week, the upper portion of the cavity begins to develop, and in the 30th week, the middle ear cavity is almost completely formed. Subsequently, the mesenchyme gradually disappears from the middle ear cavity and the walls, and contents become lined by endodermal epithelium of the tubotympanic recess.

The malleus and incus are derived from the first and second branchial arches. The first branchial arch forms the head of the malleus and the body and short process of the incus. The second branchial arch forms the short process and handle of the malleus, long process of the incus, and stapes, with the exception of the vestibular portion of the footplate. The vestibular portion of the stapedial footplate is a derivative of the otic capsule. The head of the malleus, body of the incus, and cartilaginous mandible are initially continuous as Meckel's cartilage of the first branchial arch. The styloid process, hyoid bone, stapedial arch and tympanic portion of the footplate, long crus of the incus, and malleus handle are initially continuous as Reichert's cartilage of the second branchial arch. Subsequently, the ossicles separate from their parent cartilages and begin an independent growth. Interference with their later differentiation may give rise to malformations occasionally encountered during explorations of the middle ear.

Shortly after the appearance of the primordium of the stapes (sixth week), a condensation of the mesenchyme signifies the beginning development of malleus and incus. The incudomalleolar and incudostapedial articulations are already established during the eighth week when chondrification begins. Ossification of malleus and incus begins during the 16th week and is largely completed by the 30th week (12).

A spherical condensation of mesenchyme during the fourth week marks the beginning of the development of the stapes. This mesenchymal mass is perforated by the stapedial artery during the fifth week, assumes a ring-like form during the sixth week, approaches the periotic mesenchyme during the seventh week, and fuses with that portion of the periotic mesenchyme that forms the stapedial lamina. Chondrification of the stapes begins during the 8th week, and ossification begins around the 18th week. Originating in the center of the tympanic portion of the footplate, ossification spreads along the crura and reaches the capitulum by the 21st week (12), by which time the stapes has reached its ultimate dimensions. At this stage, the crura are bony cylinders, with a thin cortical layer of bone and a central marrow space. The footplate consists of an inner and an outer layer of bone, a small central marrow space, and an inner layer of cartilage that covers the vestibular and articular surface. After the 24th week, an excavation process transforms the cylindrical crura into inward-concave semicanals, transforms the capitulum into an empty cylinder open toward the footplate, and removes the outer, tympanic osseous layer of the footplate (11). This final remodeling process of the stapes is completed by the 38th week.

The annular ligament of the oval window develops between the 10th and 13th week by dedifferentiation of the cartilaginous stapedial lamina of the otic capsule into mesenchyme, with subsequent differentiation into fibrous tissue. The annular ligament is fully developed by the 16th week.

The round window area is recognized during the 11th week as a condensation of embryonic connective tissue between the scala tympani and the fossula of the cochlear fenestra, which itself is filled with mesenchyme. At this stage, the round window extends directly to a portion of the wall of the periotic duct. Subsequent differentiation of the respective areas into cartilage, bone, and fibrous connective tissue results in the formation of the round window niche and round window membrane by the 26th week.

The tensor tympanic muscle and tendon are derivatives of the first branchial arch; their development begins between the 8th and the 11th week. The stapedius muscle begins to develop at 8½ weeks from a group of mesenchymal cells located adjacent to the interhyal. The stapedius tendon, in turn, develops from mesenchymal cells in close proximity to the head of the stapes. The pyramidal process and the anterior wall of the Fallopian canal are formed by fusion of the laterohyal capsule with the otic capsule. The laterohyal and tympanohyal capsules both participate in the formation of the descending portion of the Fallopian canal. As a result of their malformation, the facial nerve may take an abnormal course and leave the middle ear in a more anterior and lateral direction (7).

As the inner ear is being developed, the middle and the outer ear are also taking shape. On the outside of the embryonic head, between the first and second branchial arches, branchial groove develops opposite a corresponding outpocketing of the pharynx (Fig. 5.1). The epithelium at the medial end of the groove is, for a time, in contact with the entoderm of the first pharyngeal pouch. Later, during the enlargement of the head, mesoderm grows between and separates these two epithelial layers. Near the close of the second fetal month, the branchial groove deepens again into a funnel-shaped tube. This tube, which subsequently becomes supported by the cartilages of the outer ear, represents the outer one-third of the external acoustic meatus. The medial extremity of this funnel then produces a solid core of epithelial cells that grows inward to meet the outer epithelium of the pharyngeal pouch again until only a thin seam of connective tissue remains to separate the two epithelial layers. This seam of connective tissue, which is derived from the mesenchyme, becomes the tunica propria of the tympanic membrane.

The core of epithelial cells remains solid until near the end of fetal life. Meanwhile, the connective tissue around the margin of the tympanic membrane begins to ossify at about the third month. It gives rise to the tympanic ring that serves as a support for the tympanic membrane. Finally, in the seventh month of fetal life, when all other structures of the outer, the middle, and the inner ear are well differentiated, the solid core of epithelial cells splits, first in its deepest portion to form the outer surface of the tympanic membrane and then extending and opening outward to join the lumen of the primitive meatus. This tube, with the surrounding connective tissue and expanded bony tympanic annulus, becomes the inner two-thirds of the external acoustic meatus, i.e., the bony external auditory canal. Therefore, congenital atresia of the meatus may occur with a normally differentiated and functioning tympanic membrane and ossicular chain, as well as with various malformations of these structures, depending on the age at which development was delayed or arrested.

The auricle is formed by growth of mesenchymal tissue flanking the first branchial groove. At about the sixth week, six knob-like hillocks appear from the mandibular and hyoid arch tissues (Fig. 5.2). The coalescence of these tubercles, by the third month, and their further development mold the auricle (11). Whereas the tragus derives from the first (mandibular) arch, all the auricle except the tragus develops from the second (hyoid) arch.

Failure in differentiation of the first and second branchial arches may affect the auricle and result in microtia, anotia, or malposition of the pinna, or the middle ear ossicles may be malformed, fused, or aplastic. Malformation of the stapedial footplate, on the other hand, results from total lack of differentiation, incomplete differentiation, or failure of the lamina stapedialis to separate from the otic capsule (13).

Failure of the first branchial groove to develop may result in stenosis or atresia of the external meatus. A disturbance in differentiation of the first pharyngeal pouch will affect the architecture of the Eustachian tube and middle ear, as well as the extent and character of the pneumatization of the mastoid process.

Since the membranous labyrinth derives from the ectodermal otocyst and develops independently from the rest of the ear, which is mainly a derivative of the branchial apparatus, com-

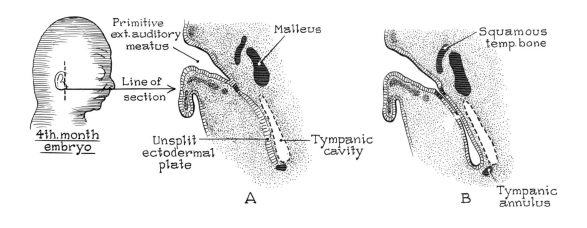

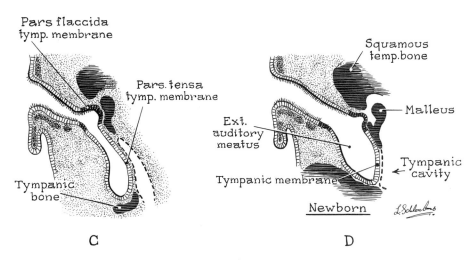

Figure 5.1. Schematic drawing of development of external auditory canal. **A.** About fourth embryonic month. A funnel-shaped tube (first ectodermal branchial groove) represents the future cartilaginous external auditory canal. A cord of epithelial cells has grown from the deep extremity of this funnel medially and downward to meet the outer epithelium of the pharyngeal pouch. This cord later contributes to the formation of the tympanic membrane and osseous external auditory canal. **B.** About seventh embryonic month. The solid cord of epithelial cells splits, beginning in its deepest portion. **C.** About eighth embryonic month. Progressive separation of the epithelial cells leads to an outward opening of the lumen into the primitive meatus. **D.** Newborn.

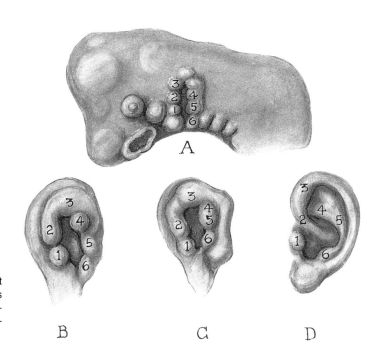

Figure 5.2. Development of auricle. **A.** Primordial elevations on first (mandibular) and second (hyoid) arches in 11-mm embryo. **B–D.** Progress of embryonic fusion of hillocks and adult configuration of auricle (with corresponding numerals *1–6* on derived parts). **B.** 13.5-mm embryo. **C.** 15-mm embryo. **D.** Adult form of auricle with parts identified.

bined malformations of the inner, the middle, and the outer ear should theoretically not be expected to occur frequently; however, a significant number of combined malformations have been documented (3, 7).

PATHOLOGY

The more severe forms of congenital auricular malformation are always associated with meatal atresia, whereas meatal atresia may, in a rare instance, be seen in patients with a normal pinna.

Atresia of the meatus may be membranous or osseous. Membranous atresia is much less common and is characterized by a rudimentary cartilaginous canal, separated from the middle ear by a dense structure of connective tissue. In the osseous form of meatal atresia, the bony portion of the external meatus is absent, and a more or less solid mass of compact bone forms the lateral wall of the middle ear cavity (Fig. 5.3). Osseous atresia is regularly accompanied by a malformation of the cavity and structures of the middle ear. These malformations vary in degree. The origin, formation, and location of the atresia plate and anomalies involving the middle ear are discussed later. It was stated earlier that unilateral atresia is more common than bilateral atresia. In unilateral atresia it is not unusual for the other ear to show a less severe malformation, with a narrow meatus and hypoplastic tympanic membrane or abnormal middle ear ossicles. The mechanisms by which developmental anomalies of the branchial apparatus occur are not clear. Developmental failure in any particular instance depends on which portion of the branchial apparatus was involved and at which embryonic stage normal development was arrested.

An analysis of the case histories of 241 patients with congenital aural atresia seen at Johns Hopkins Hospital between 1955 and 1975 (8) revealed the following:

1. Seventy patients showed bilateral involvement, an incidence of 29% (Fig. 5.4A–F).
2. The deformity occurred more commonly in the male (61%) than in the female and affected the right ear more frequently (57%) than the left ear.
3. A positive family history of a congenital ear deformity affecting either a sibling or another relative was obtained in 14%.
4. Additional malformations were found in 56% of patients. A specific malformation syndrome could be recognized in 35 patients (15%). Fifteen of these patients had mandibulofacial dysostosis (14–16), three had craniofacial dysostosis (17), three exhibited a first and second branchial arch syndrome, three had the rubella syndrome, and two had achondroplasia. Congenital aural atresia was also found associated, in one instance each, with Goldenhar's syndrome, thalidomide embryopathy, Möbius' syndrome, Noonan's syndrome, the otopalatal-digital syndrome, the oral-facial-digital syndrome, the Pierre-Robin anomaly, and von Reckinghausen's neurofibromatosis. However, the association of congenital aural atresia with many of these malformation syndromes may have been fortuitous, and further studies are necessary.
5. In the presence of congenital aural atresia, a careful search for other abnormalities in the head and neck as well as in other organ systems is indicated.
6. Although the degree of the deformity of the external ear is generally proportional to the malformation of the middle ear, no characteristic correlation patterns could be identified radiologically, and each patient has to be evaluated individually.

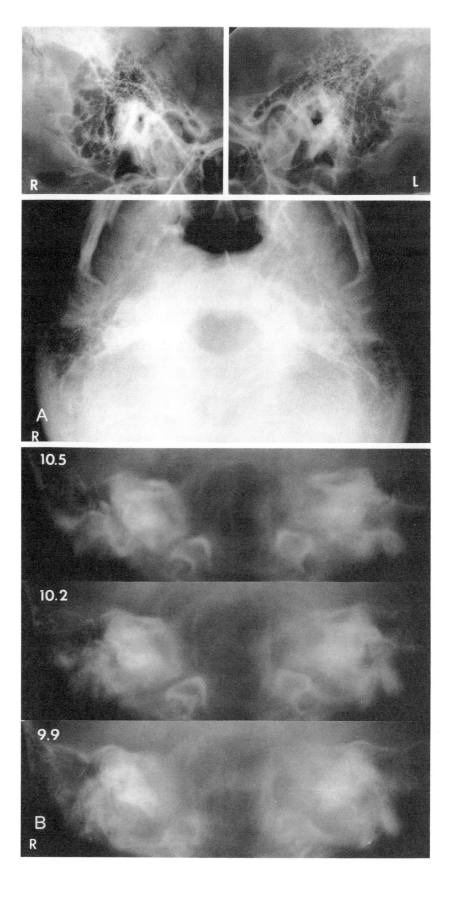

Figure 5.3.   A. Law's view of both temporal bones and submentovertical view of skull of an 18-year-old woman with congenital aural atresia of right ear. The right mastoid process is well pneumatized, but the external auditory canal is absent, and the right condyloid process is in a posterior location and in apposition to the right mastoid process. **B.** Anteroposterior polytomograms reveal an osseous meatal atresia and a moderate reduction of the right middle ear cavity.

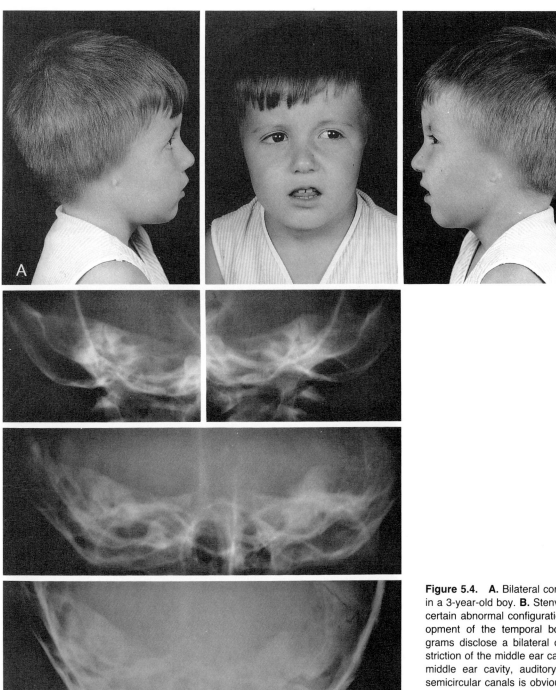

Figure 5.4. **A.** Bilateral congenital aural atresia with anotia in a 3-year-old boy. **B.** Stenvers and occipital views reveal a certain abnormal configuration and very poor cellular development of the temporal bones. **C.** Anteroposterior tomograms disclose a bilateral osseous meatal atresia and restriction of the middle ear cavity. **D** and **E.** Hypoplasia of the middle ear cavity, auditory ossicles, cochlea, and lateral semicircular canals is obvious in the additional anteroposterior polytomograms. **F.** Conglomeration of malleus and incus and underdevelopment of the lateral and posterior semicircular canal are best recognized in the lateral polytomograms of the right temporal bone.

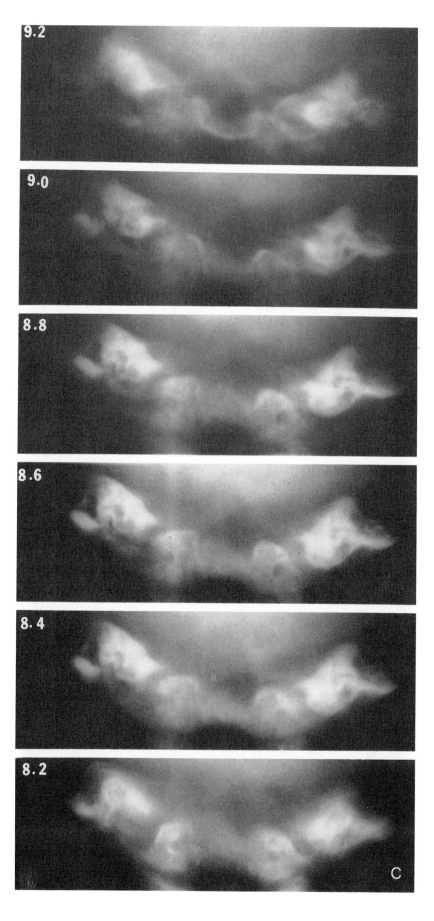

Figure 5.4.   C.

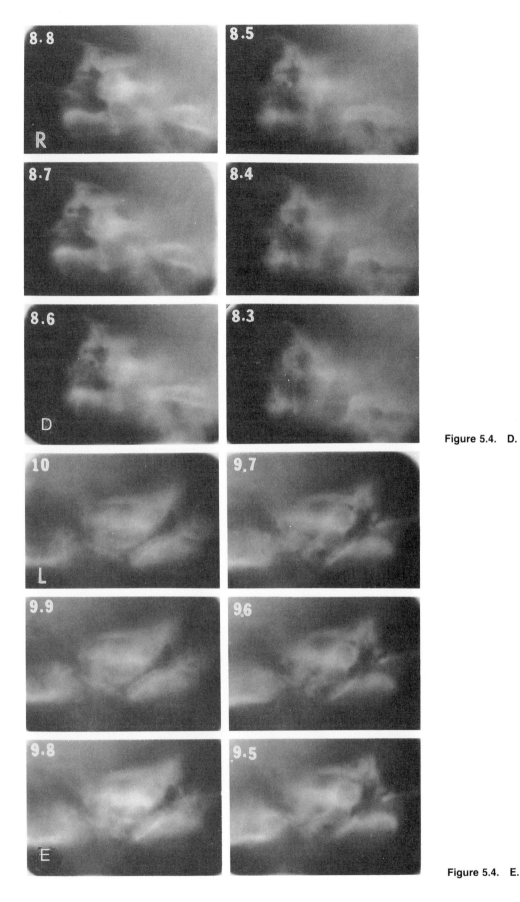

Figure 5.4.   D.

Figure 5.4.   E.

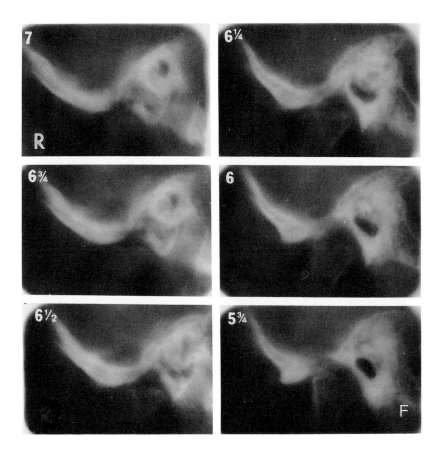

Figure 5.4.   F.

CLASSIFICATION OF EXTERNAL AND MIDDLE EAR MALFORMATIONS

Developmental anomalies of the external and the middle ear may be conveniently classified into the following three groups, depending on the degree of malformation and the structures involved: minor (group I), moderate (group II), and severe (group III) malformation (7).

Minor External and Middle Ear Malformations (Group I)

In group I malformations the auricle can be normal but frequently reveals some intimation of malformation. Whereas the auricle may reveal no abnormalities in overall dimensions and position, it may display minor variations in relief, resembling the later developmental stages of the pinna (Fig. 5.5*B*). Many of these variations show a hereditary tendency. The external auditory canal can also be normal; it is occasionally hypoplastic in its entire length (Fig. 5.6*A* and *B*). In a rare instance it is present only in its medial portion. The tympanic membrane can be normal in the presence of a regular canal. More often it is thickened and appears opaque. A normal tympanic membrane, however, does not preclude the presence of anomalies of the middle ear. Such anomalies can include a hypoplastic middle ear cavity, malformation of the malleus and incus, abnormalities of middle ear muscles and nerves, and agenesis of the oval and round windows. The handle of the malleus is often deformed and in an abnormal position. In a rare instance the inner ear is abnormal. The semicircular canals can be hypoplastic, with the lateral being the most frequently involved (6). Minor external and middle ear malformations are commonly seen in craniofacial dysostosis (17) (see Fig. 5.17).

Moderate External and Middle Ear Malformations (Group II)

Group II malformations encompass the majority of ear deformities. The auricle is rarely normal and is usually represented by a small rudimentary soft tissue structure of variable size, often in an abnormal anterior and inferior position. Anomalies of the auricle have been divided into three types: microtia types I, II, and III (Fig. 5.5) (18). In microtia type I, the different parts of the rudimentary auricle are still recognizable. In microtia type II, the auricle is represented by a vertical, somewhat curving ridge that usually includes some cartilage and resembles a primitive helix. In microtia type III, the rudiment of soft tissue no longer has any resemblance to any portion of the auricle. In a rare instance the auricle may be absent (Fig. 5.5*I*); however, this severest expression of the malformation, known as anotia, is usually found in severe external and middle ear malformations (group III).

The external auditory canal in group II malformations is either hypoplastic or aplastic, or it may end blindly with one fistulous tract or, occasionally, two fistulous tracts leading toward a rudimentary tympanic membrane. If the tympanic bone is absent and if the upper portion of Reichert's cartilage is very hypoplastic, bony processes from the squamous portion of the temporal bone and hypotympanum join in the formation of a lateral osseous wall of the tympanic cavity. In such instances the chorda tympani nerve also courses laterally to the atresia plate. The atresia plate is again medial to where the tympanic membrane would

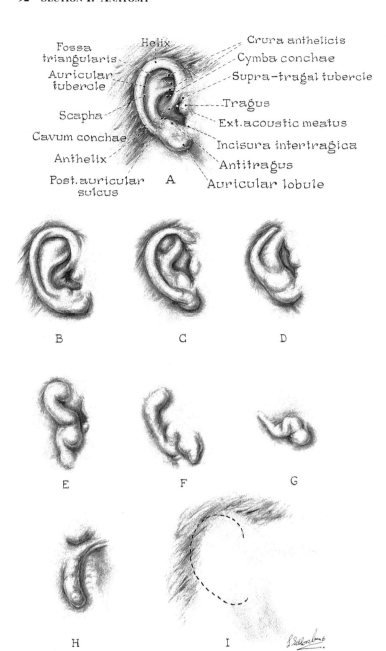

Fossa triangularis
Helix
Crura anthelicis
Cymba conchae
Auricular tubercle
Supra-tragal tubercle
Tragus
Scapha
Ext. acoustic meatus
Cavum conchae
Incisura intertragica
Anthelix
Antitragus
Post. auricular sulcus
A
Auricular lobule

B   C   D

E   F   G

H   I

Figure 5.5. Examples of auricular malformations. **A.** Normal adult pinna. **B.** Example of minor malformation. The pinna reveals regular overall dimensions and position but incomplete differentiation. **C** and **D.** Examples of microtia type I. The auricle is smaller, rudimentary, and often located in an abnormal position. The different parts of the pinna are still discernible. **E** and **F.** Examples of microtia type II. The auricle, in addition to being smaller and often in abnormal position, is represented by a vertical curving ridge resembling a primitive helix. **G** and **H.** Examples of microtia type III. The rudiment of the auricle has no resemblance to any portion of the pinna. **I.** Example of anotia.

normally be encountered but less medial than when formed by Reichert's cartilage (18). The fistulous tract can be associated with an epidermoid inclusion cyst (cholesteatoma).

The tympanic bone can be either present or absent. If present, it is invariably severely malformed and usually represented by an osseous plate whose central portion may consist of connective tissue. This atresia plate forms the lateral wall of the middle ear cavity. If the tympanic bone is absent, the upper portion of Reichert's cartilage may show anomalies in both configuration and position. It can form the principal portion of the atresia plate. In such instances the chorda tympani nerve courses laterally to it (7, 18). The atresia plate, therefore, is medial to the normal location of the tympanic membrane, and the middle ear cavity represents only the medial half of a normal cavum tympani.

The cellular development of the mastoid process varies greatly. It can be normal, limited, or absent. In most instances it is restricted. Differentiation of the antrum and periantral cells is directly related to the degree of pneumatization. Normal pneu-

matization is occasionally associated with fairly good differentiation of middle ear structures.

Ossicular malformations are regularly encountered in group II malformations (Fig. 5.7A–P). In general, they are more frequent and more severe than those in group I. The malleus and incus frequently form a conglomeration or have bony unions with the atresia plate and walls of the epitympanic recess. Infrequently, the incus lacks a connection with the stapes. The stapes may be malformed or even absent. The stapedial arch may be fixed by an osseous connection to the Fallopian canal or the promontory or by a bony structure that takes the place of the stapedius tendon. The stapedial footplate can be fixed as a result of incomplete differentiation of the annular ligament or total lack of it. The middle ear muscles may be anomalous, supernumerary, and malpositioned.

The facial nerve may be hypoplastic or, in a rare instance, absent. Its course from the geniculate ganglion can be straight downward over the promontory. The nerve may course uncovered by bone above or below the oval window or even through

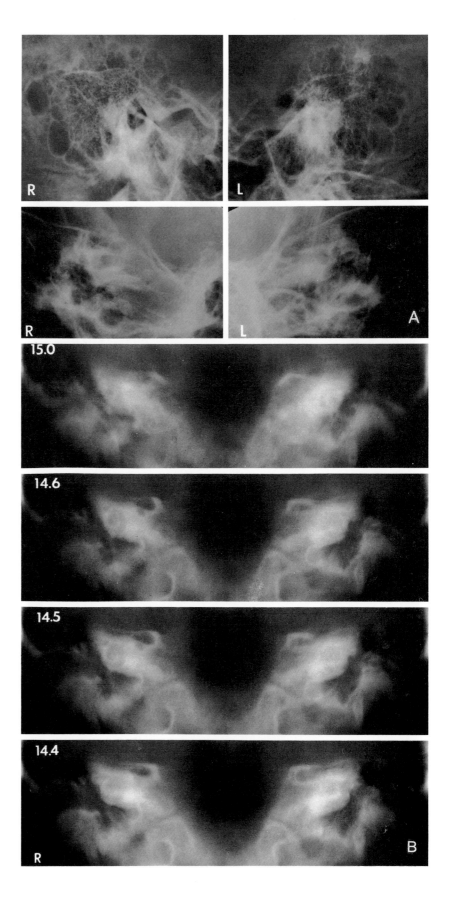

Figure 5.6. Congenital aural atresia of left ear in an 18-year-old man. Both mastoid processes (Schüller view) and petrous pyramids (Stenvers view) display extensive and equal pneumatization **(A)**. Abnormally narrow left external auditory canal is recognized in the anteroposterior polytomograms **(B)**. The middle ear cavities, malleus and incus, and cochlear and labyrinthine capsules appear normal bilaterally.

the stapedial arch. On rare occasions it may bifurcate around the oval window or divide into three portions distal from it. The greater and the lesser superficial petrosal nerves and the chorda tympani nerve can be absent (7).

Severe External and Middle Ear Malformations (Group III)

In group III malformations the auricle is generally severely malformed; it can even be absent (Fig. 5.5*I*). The external auditory canal is aplastic. Strands of connective tissue and epidermis or a fistulous tract is occasionally encountered as a rudiment of an external meatus. Very often the mastoid process is hypoplastic and not pneumatized. The middle ear and antrum may be absent or may be represented by a slit-like lumen (see Fig. 5.15*B* and 5.18–5.20). Such a rudimentary middle ear cleft may contain embryonic mesenchyme, mature connective tissue, or osseous trabeculae. Anomalies of the facial nerve are the rule. The middle ear ossicles are frequently absent. Malformations of the inner ear are most frequently encountered in this group. The inner ear malformations can involve one or several semicircular canals and the vestibule, as well as the cochlea. Severe external and middle ear malformations are often associated with the se-

vere cranial malformations. They are regularly encountered in mandibulofacial dysostosis (Fig. 5.9). They have commonly been observed in thalidomide embryopathy.

ATRESIA IN GENETIC DISORDERS

Despite the frequency of congenital aural atresia, little is known about its genetics as an isolated trait, or in conjunction with abnormalities of the pinna, middle ear, and inner ear, or in association with abnormalities in other organ systems. Family histories have rarely been taken, and the results of complete physical examinations are only occasionally reported. Therefore, it is difficult to delineate more than a few disorders in which a genetic etiology is significant. The paucity of well-documented reports indicates that complete evaluation, including a family history, of all individuals with external ear malformations is necessary to determine the role of heredity in the development of abnormalities of the ear.

Microtia, Meatal Atresia, and Hearing Impairment

Unilateral or bilateral external ear abnormalities including atresia of the external auditory meatus and microtia have been

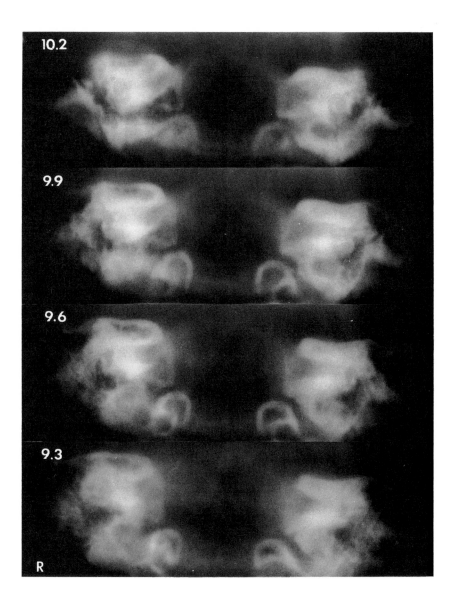

Figure 5.8. Anteroposterior polytomograms of petrous pyramids of a 16-year-old girl with Treacher Collins syndrome. Complete, dense bony plates separate in the middle ear cavity from the region of the outer ear canals. Their absence resulted from aplasia of their lower margins. The left malleus and incus appear cramped into a smaller epitympanic recess. Pneumatization and cochlear and vestibular capsules appear normal.

reported in association with hearing loss as a recessive disorder by Konigsmark and coworkers (19). The pinnae may be almost completely absent (20, 21). Both conductive and sensorineural hearing losses have been noted. Middle ear abnormalities consisting of absence of or malformed ossicles and reduction in size of the middle ear cavity have been described. The oval window, semicircular canals, cochlea, and internal auditory canal are normal (19). Also reported were two sibs (22), one with bilateral aural atresia without microtia and one with both unilateral atresia and microtia; these differences may represent variation in expression of the same disorder. No mention was made of the patients' hearing status or whether the parents were similarly affected, and it is possible that these two patients had the same disorder (19).

Conductive hearing loss, microtia, and meatal atresia have been described in a family in which the inheritance pattern was compatible with a dominant disorder (23). Another case reported involved a father and son with aural atresia and microtia (24). The father had a unilateral mixed hearing loss of unknown degree and had a history of noise exposure; hearing in the other ear was normal. No audiometric studies were performed on the son (25).

Mandibulofacial Dysostosis (Treacher Collins Syndrome)

Mandibulofacial dysostosis (Treacher Collins syndrome) is an autosomal dominant disorder characterized by bilateral and, in most cases, symmetric abnormalities. Distinguishing features include flattening of the frontonasal angle, antimongoloid obliquity of the palpebral fissures, colobomas of the lower eyelids with absence of eyelashes medial to the colobomas, and hypoplasia of the maxillary sinuses and malar bones (Fig. 5.9). Hypoplasia or absence of the zygomatic processes, mandibular hypoplasia, increased mandibular angle, and prominent antegonial notch are common. In some cases, the palate may be cleft, lacrimal puncta and Meibomian glands may be absent, blind fistulae may be present between the ear and oral commissures, and there may be macrostomia (26).

Otologic abnormalities are a prime feature of the disorder and include microtia, external auditory canal atresia, and moderately severe conductive hearing loss (see Fig. 5.8) (27). However, hearing may be normal in some cases (28, 29). The malleus, incus, and stapes have been reported to be malformed (27, 28, 30–35). Inner ear structures have been reported to be present and normal by some investigators (27, 30, 34, 38, 39) and abnormal by others (27, 34, 36, 37, 40, 41). The middle ear cavity is usually hypoplastic or absent (27).

Most patients are of normal intelligence. Those reported to be mentally retarded are probably ''retarded'' secondary to hearing impairment.

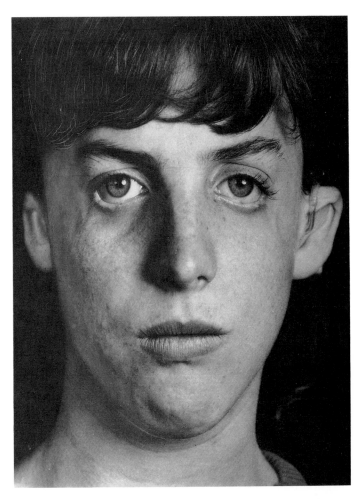

Figure 5.9. Face of patient with mandibulofacial dysostosis (Treacher Collins syndrome). The lower eyelashes are absent medially. There are bilateral depressions in the regions of the malar eminences and zygomatic arches. The ears are malformed.

Variation in expression among affected individuals is marked. That is, both severely and mildly affected individuals may be present in the same family (28, 29, 39, 42–48). The extent of the variation emphasizes the importance of evaluating all relatives of an affected individual for minor stigmata, so that accurate genetic counseling may be provided. Examinations should include a clinical evaluation of the craniofacies, radiographic study of the facial bones and mandible, and audiologic evaluation. Several reports have described affected sibs with this syndrome, although the parents were presumed normal (28, 32–34). However, careful examination of the parents was not performed. The high number of new mutation cases reported may, in reality, reflect inadequate investigation of relatives of affected individuals.

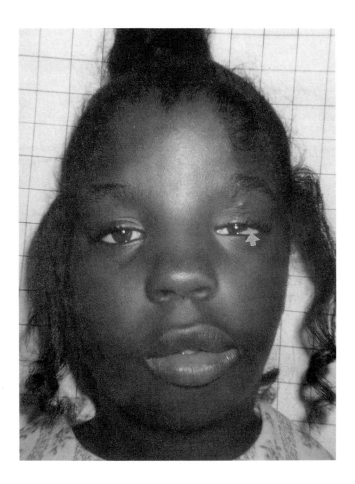

Figure 5.13. Facies of patient with OAVD (Goldenhar's syndrome). The face is asymmetric and an epibulbar dermoid is present on the left eye *(arrow)*.

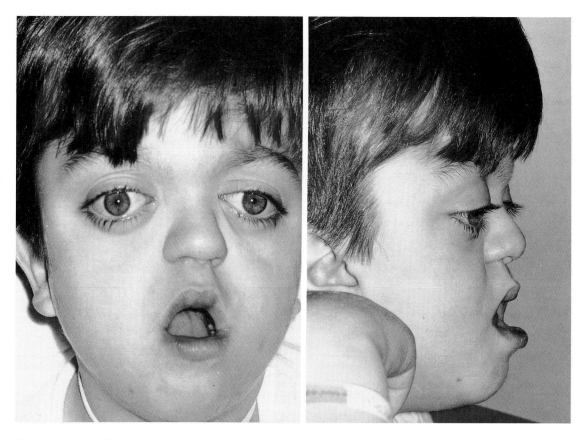

Figure 5.14. Facies of patient with craniofacial dysostosis (Crouzon's disease). There is proptosis, midface hypoplasia, and relative mandibular prognathism, and the nose is bulbous. (Courtesy of Dr. M. Michael Cohen, Jr., Seattle, Washington.)

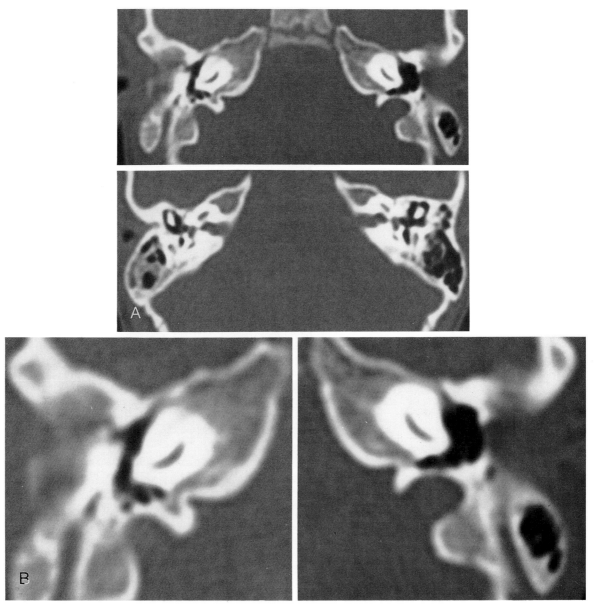

Figure 5.16. Axial computed tomography scans of a 5-year-old girl with bilateral microtia types I and II and atresia of EAC. **A.** The right temporal bone displays a thick, predominantly osseous atresia plate where the tympanic membrane would normally be encountered. The right middle ear cavity is severely hypoplastic, and the right mastoid process is poorly pneumatized and shows a considerable amount of unresorbed mesen-chyme. The left temporal bone demonstrates a much thinner atresia plate that is predominately membranous. The tympanic cavity is much larger, and the mastoid process exhibits a normal age-related size and cellular development. **B.** In the enlargement of scan 1, the difference in size of the two middle ear cavities and the structure of the two atresia plates become even more obvious. (Courtesy of Dr. D. Mattox.)

Craniofacial Dysostosis (Crouzon's Disease)

Patients with distinctive craniofacial deformity have premature fusion of the cranial sutures, ocular hypertelorism and proptosis, midface hypoplasia, and beak-shaped nose (Fig. 5.14) (77, 78). Premature synostosis of the sagittal, lambdoid, and coronal sutures results in brachycephaly and acrocephaly; however, no definitive calvarial form can be said to be diagnostic of craniofacial dysostosis, since head shape is in part related to the sequence in which skull sutures fuse prematurely (79). Nausea, vomiting, and headaches are frequent symptoms. As a result of shallow orbits, proptosis may be severe. There may be divergent strabismus, loss of vision, papilledema, and optic atrophy (80).

A hyperostotic ridge may be palpable in the area of the metopic suture (81), and a bony prominence may be present in the region of the anterior fontanel. The mandible is prognathic relative to the maxilla, there is malocclusion, and the palate is V-shaped.

On radiographs of the skull, premature suture closure, thinning of the skull, and prominent convolutional markings are noted (81–84).

External auditory canal atresia has been reported by several investigators (49, 85–88).

Hearing loss has been noted (68, 81, 85, 87, 88, 89, 90), but formal audiometric studies have not been done in most cases to document the type of hearing impairment accurately.

The absence of hand malformations in craniofacial dysostosis serves to differentiate it *(a)* from acrocephalosyndactyly type I (Apert syndrome) (91), in which premature craniosynostosis is associated with osseous and soft tissue syndactyly of the hands and feet, and *(b)* from acrocephalosyndactyly type V (Pfeiffer's syndrome) (92), in which premature craniosynostosis is associated with brachydactyly, soft tissue syndactyly, and broad thumbs and toes. Other forms of craniosynostosis from which craniofacial dysostosis should be distinguished have been reviewed (77).

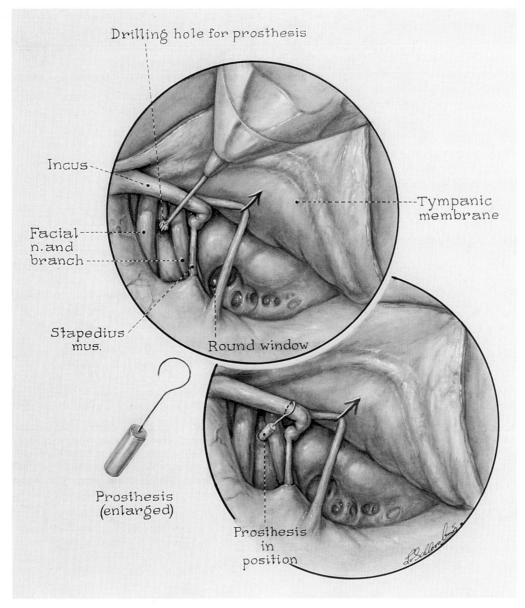

Figure 5.17. Drawing showing creation of vestibular fenestra in congenital absence. The facial nerve forms a bifurcation in the area where normally the right oval window would be encountered. A wire Teflon piston prosthesis was inserted through an opening in the vestibular capsule between the two branches of the seventh nerve instead of the congenitally absent stapes.

Hypertelorism, Microtia, and Clefting

One team of investigators (93) reported two female sibs with mental retardation, microcephaly, short stature, orbital hypertelorism, primary telecanthus, cleft lip and cleft palate, and hypoplasia of thenar eminences. In addition, one patient had a pelvic kidney, while the other had crossed ectopia of the left kidney that was positioned in the right lumbar region.

Abnormalities of the ears in these girls included microtia, atresia of the external auditory canal, and hypoplasia of the auditory ossicles. The vestibule, cochlea, semicircular canals, and internal auditory canals were normal. Hearing loss was noted, but the type and the degree were not specified.

Both sisters had congenital heart disease. However, some of their relatives had congenital heart disease without otologic or facial abnormalities, suggesting that heart disease was segregating independently.

18q Syndrome

Individuals with 18q syndrome have psychomotor retardation, hypotonia, short stature, microcephaly, hypoplastic midface, epicanthus, ophthalmologic abnormalities, cleft palate, congenital heart disease, abnormalities of the genitalia, and tapered fingers with an increased number of whorls (94–96). The external ear canals may be normal, stenotic, or atretic, and the anthelix and antitragus may be prominent. Three of four patients reported by another investigator (97) had bilateral atresia or hypoplasia of the external auditory canal, conductive hearing loss, and normal pinnae. Their middle ears were normal; polytomograms revealed atresia plates in the region of the tympanic membranes. The fourth patient, who had normal ear canals, had normal tomographic studies but had a mixed hearing loss.

Atresia in Embryopathies

During the 1950s and 1960s, it became obvious that a medicament (thalidomide) and the rubella virus may also produce the syndrome of congenital aural atresia.

THALIDOMIDE

Ingestion of the tranquilizer thalidomide (Contergan, in the former West Germany) produced a host of malformations that included deformities of the limbs, malformations of the heart, anomalies of the respiratory, digestive, and urinary systems, clefts of face, lip, and palate, eye anomalies, malformations of the ear, and transient or persistent hemangiomas of the face. Thalidomide embryopathies were observed in West Germany and England between 1959 and 1962. In West Germany during that period, about 7000 children were born with malformations of the limbs (98). If isolated malformations of the hands and fingers are included, the actual number of affected children is closer to 10,000. Since malformations of the limbs are associated with anomalies of the ears in approximately 10% of patients, it can be estimated that about 1000 of these children also had ear deformities (99, 100). In these children, aural atresia occurred with microtia or anotia, with sixth and seventh nerve palsy, and at times with malformations and even agenesis of the inner ear (101).

Ingestion of thalidomide during the 35th and the 36th day and occasionally during the 37th day after the last menstrual period produced anotia, facial nerve palsy, and damage to the eye muscle nuclei (102). Lesser ear deformities occurred after ingestion between the 38th and the 45th day. The infrequent duplication of the thumb was seen following ingestion prior to the 38th day. Partial or total agenesis of both arms corresponded to the period from the 39th to the 44th day. Cardiac malformations, duodenal atresia, and congenital subluxation of the hip occurred with ingestion between the 39th and the 45th day. Ingestion around the 50th day produced lesser thumb malformations, rectal stenosis, and anal atresia. Thus, prolonged ingestion of thalidomide by a pregnant woman obviously can, during sensitive phases of fetal development, affect several organization centers, which, in turn, can lead to a kaleidoscopic combination of developmental defects. Nevertheless, many women in spite of regular thalidomide ingestion gave birth to normal children, suggesting that not all women are sensitive to this teratogenic drug.

MATERNAL RUBELLA

The introduction of polytomography led to a reevaluation and revision of the original concept that malformations of the middle ear were never associated with developmental defects of the inner ear. Radiologic investigation as well as surgical exploration provided evidence that malformations of the middle ear are not infrequently combined with severe anomalies of the labyrinth and cochlea (103, 104). Furthermore, it became evident that in maternal rubella not only the inner ear but also the middle and the outer ear can be affected (105).

Case Reports

The following four cases are examples of dysplasias involving the outer and the middle ear and in three instances explain their management. Case 1 depicts a bilateral malformation of the auricle and external auditory canal (EAC) as visualized in the axial view of serial computed tomography (CT) scans of the petrous pyramid. Case 2 illustrates a malformation of the right oval window in association with a bifurcation of the facial nerve anterior to the vestibular fenestra. Case 3 demonstrates the clinical, anatomical, and pathologic aspect of oculoauriculovertebral dysplasia (OAVD) or Goldenhar's syndrome. Case 4 is an example of a syndrome characterized by the association of dysplasias of the external and the middle ear with developmental anomalies involving the musculoskeletal and urogenital systems.

Case 1. *Bilateral dysplasia of auricle and external auditory canal (EAC). Microtia types I and II. Aplasia of left EAC with partially osseous and membranous atresia plate. Hypoplasia of right EAC with thick, predominantly osseous atresia plate. Epidermoid inclusion cyst (external cholesteatoma) in right pretympanic area. Marked hypoplasia of right tympanic cavity. Bony fusion of malleus and incus with osseous synostosis between malleus and lateral wall of attic. Bilateral conductive hearing loss. Postoperative successful construction of right EAC, tympanic membrane, and mobilization of ossicular chain, resulting in satisfactory improvement of hearing.*

A 5-year-old girl who was first examined at the age of 6 months when she presented with bilateral malformation of the external ears was seen. Her family history was negative for dysplasia and hearing loss. The pregnancy was remarkable only in that the mother had been treated with antibiotics during the fifth month of pregnancy for a severe viral infection that lasted for the remaining 4 months.

Otologic examination showed bilateral microtia types I and II. There was no left EAC. The right EAC was thread-like and blind-ending at the distance of 6–10 mm from the entrance. Cranial nerves

VI and VII were intact. A brain stem evoked response (BSER) indicated a bilateral conductive hearing loss of approximately 60 dB with a bone conduction response at 20 dB.

Radiologic examination. Axial computed tomography (CT) scans of the temporal bones at the age of 4 years disclosed a thread-like cartilaginous ear canal on the right with a thick, predominantly osseous atresia plate and a hypoplastic middle ear cavity. The left EAC was completely atretic, but the atresia plate was much thinner and partially membranous and osseous (Fig. 5.16). Cochlear function studies then showed an average pure tone loss of 60 and 35 dB in the right and the left ear, respectively.

At *operation*, a right external canal was constructed, the ossicular chain was mobilized, and a tympanoplasty was performed. Malleus and incus were found to be fused and firmly attached to the lateral wall of the attic by a bony union. The stapes and oval window were normally differentiated with a mobile footplate. A small epidermoid inclusion cyst (external cholesteatoma) had been removed from the osseous portion of the EAC. Postoperatively, hearing was significantly improved.

Case 2. Bilateral aplasia of oval window with maximal conductive hearing loss. Bifurcation of right facial nerve anterior to right dysplastic vestibular fenestra.

An 18-year-old man who was born with a severe bilateral hearing loss was seen. His family history was negative for dysplasia and hearing improvement.

Otologic examination at the age of 12 years revealed normal auricles, EACs, and tympanic membranes. The audiogram showed a bilateral severe conductive hearing loss with a bilateral speech reception threshold (SRT) of 68 dB and a discrimination score of 100% and 96% for the right and the left ear, respectively.

At *operation,* the right middle ear cavity was of normal size, and the malleus and incus were normal in appearance. Of the stapes, only the capitulum and the stapedius tendon were present, whereas the crural arch and the footplate were nonexisting. The niche to the oval window was only intimated by a horizontal oval depression in the area of the vestibular capsule, where the oval window would normally be encountered. Just anterior to that depression, the exposed facial nerve formed a bifurcation, with the greater portion following the superior and a lesser portion running along the inferior margin of the poorly differentiated oval window niche. An opening was made through the wall of the vestibule between the two branches of the nerve, and a wire Teflon piston prosthesis was used to replace the congenitally absent stapes (Fig. 5.17). This provided the patient with normal hearing, which 5 years later, at the age of 17, still showed an SRT of 8 dB and a discrimination score of 98%.

Case 3. Oculoauriculovertebral dysplasia (OAVD) (Goldenhar's syndrome). Left-sided hemifacial microsomia. Hypoplasia of left mandibular ramus. Anterior and inferior position of left auricle with microtia type I. Bilateral auricular appendices. Complete atresia of left EAC. Dysplasia of middle ear ossicles. Bilateral conductive hearing loss.

A 1-year-old boy born with OAVD was seen.

Otologic examination disclosed a left hemifacial microsomia with mandibular hypoplasia, bilateral microtia type I and auricular appendices, a low-set left ear with total atresia of the left EAC and dysplastic middle ear ossicles (Fig. 5.18). Responses to various acoustic stimuli in free field were noticed between 30 and 40 dB. Bone conduction studies without masking were said to be excellent from 500 to 4000 cycles.

Microscopic examination of the left temporal bone revealed an osseous atresia plate, a reduced middle ear cavity, and dysplasia of all three middle ear ossicles. The stapedial superstructure was represented by a rudimentary arch. The oval window was absent. The round window was fully differentiated, but the niche was filled with mesenchyme and closed to the middle ear cavity that was also totally occupied by mesenchyme (Fig. 5.19). The facial nerve took an abnormal course through the tympanic cavity, and the stylomastoid foramen was in an abnormal lateral position (Fig. 5.20). The membranous cochlea and vestibular labyrinth were unremarkable.

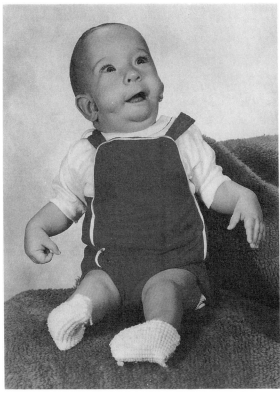
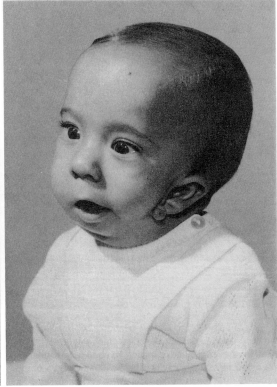

Figure 5.18. Oculoauricular vertebral dysplasia (OVAD) (Goldenhar's syndrome) in a 1-year-old boy. The left hemifacial microsomia, mandibular hypoplasia, anterior and inferior position of the left auricle, and bilateral microtia type I with preauricular appendices are recognizable.

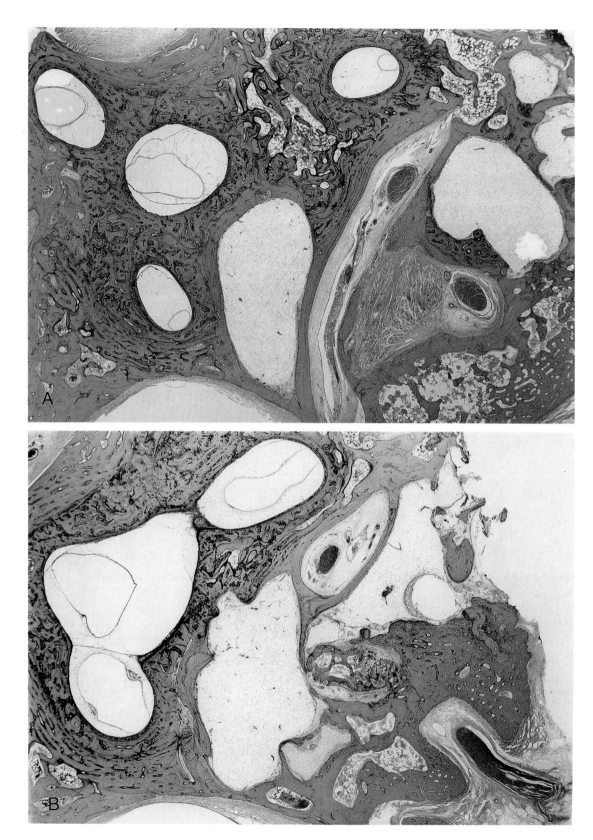

Figure 5.20. Vertical section through left temporal bone (same patient as in Figs. 5.18 and 5.19) at level of descending portion of Fallopian canal **(A)** and stylomastoid foramen **(B).** Note the abnormal course of the facial nerve and the lateral position of the stylomastoid foramen. (Hematoxylin and eosin, ×14 and ×13, respectively.)

Case 4. *Dysplasia of both temporal bones, EACs, middle ear os-sicles, and left oval window. Right hemifacial microsomia, right microtia, and bilateral conductive hearing loss. Short, webbed neck and torticollis. Klippel-Feil deformity, cervical and thoracic sco-liosis, and ocult lumbar spina bifida. Aplasia of left and ptosis of right kidney, aplasia of vagina and uterus—a syndrome (106).*

A 24-year-old woman who was referred for evaluation of bilat-eral conductive hearing loss, torticollis, and genital anomalies was seen. The family history was negative. The patient had two normal younger sibs. The parents were unrelated and were aged 22 and 17 years, respectively, at the time of the patient's birth. Torticollis to the right, webbed neck and right microtia were present at birth. Milestones were normal. Hearing impairment was first noticed at the age of 3 years after an otitis media. She never menstruated. Second-ary sex characteristics developed normally. Aplasia of the uterus was noted during an appendectomy at the age of 13 years.

Otologic examination revealed a mild right hemifacial micro-somia, a short webbed-shaped neck and torticollis to the right, and restricted neck mobility. The sternocleidal muscles were normal. There was an inferior prognathism and a cross-bite. The nuchal hairline was low. The right auricle was low set and trumpet shaped, with a preauricular appendage (Fig. 5.21A–C). The EACs were distorted and assumed, particularly on the right, and were in a downward-slanting direction. The tympanic membranes were normal. The au-diogram disclosed a bilateral conductive hearing loss of 65 and 60 dB and a discrimination score of 92 and 100% for the right and the left ear, respectively.

Radiologic examination disclosed a severe bilateral malformation of the temporal bones with depression of the lateral posterior portion of the middle cranial fossa and downward slanting of both, espe-cially the right EACs. Anteroposterior multidirectional tomograms of the petrous pyramids showed, besides other anomalies, a malfor-mation and fusion of malleus and incus with synostosis to the lateral wall of the attic (Figs. 5.22 and 5.23). There was an upper thoracic scoliosis with a compensatory cervical scoliosis, a possible fusion of the lower fourth and fifth cervical vertebrae (Fig. 5.21D), and an ocult lumbar spina bifida.

Additional abnormalities included an aplasia of the left and ptosis of the right kidney, a surgical correction for an aplastic vagina, and an aplasia of the uterus. There were multiple moles and café-au-lait spots, a cubitus, a genu valga, and a ligamentous hyperlaxity of the fingers. The chromosomal analysis showed a normal female 46, XX karyotype, and her IQ was estimated to be 109.

At *operation,* the malleus and incus were found to be malformed, fused, and firmly attached to the lateral wall of the attic by a bony union. The lenticular process of the incus was absent, but a fibrous band connected the incus with the capitulum of the stapes. The stapes superstructure was dysplastic, and the oval window was poorly dif-ferentiated (Fig. 5.24). The stapedial superstructure was replaced by a wire Teflon piston prosthesis, providing the patient with normal hearing in that ear (Fig. 5.25).

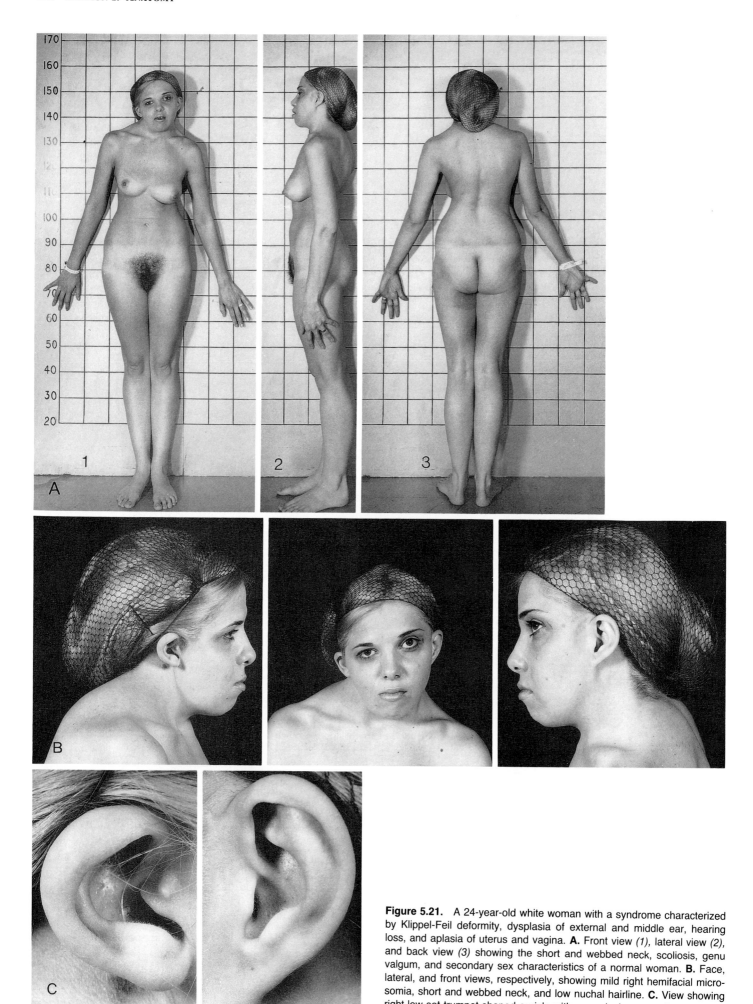

Figure 5.21. A 24-year-old white woman with a syndrome characterized by Klippel-Feil deformity, dysplasia of external and middle ear, hearing loss, and aplasia of uterus and vagina. **A.** Front view *(1)*, lateral view *(2)*, and back view *(3)* showing the short and webbed neck, scoliosis, genu valgum, and secondary sex characteristics of a normal woman. **B.** Face, lateral, and front views, respectively, showing mild right hemifacial microsomia, short and webbed neck, and low nuchal hairline. **C.** View showing right low-set trumpet-shaped auricle with preauricular appendage.

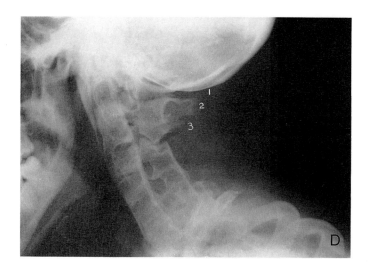

Figure 5.21. D. Lateral view of cervical spine of the same patient as in Figure 5.21*A–C,* with possible fusion of lower cervical vertebrae shown.

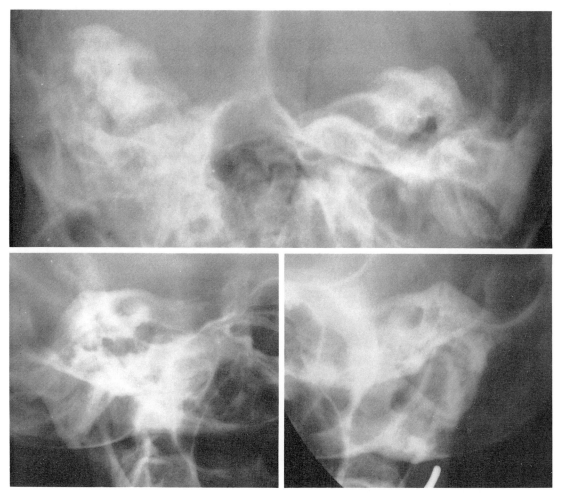

Figure 5.22. Suboccipital and Stenvers views of petrous pyramids, demonstrating depression of lateral posterior portion of middle cranial fossa, which is more marked on the right.

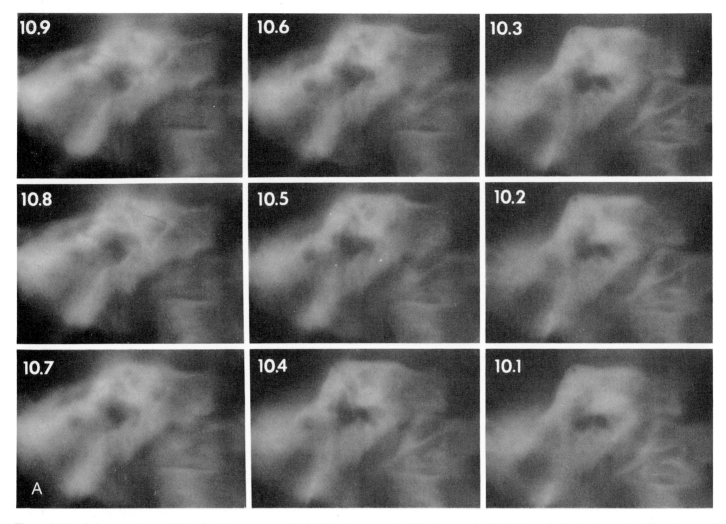

Figure 5.23. Anteroposterior multidirectional tomograms of right **(A)** and left **(B)** temporal bones. The depression of the lateral posterior portion of the middle cranial fossa, the downward slanting of the EACs (more marked on the right than on the left), the ossicular fusion and malformation, and the bony synostosis between the malleus and lateral wall of the attic are well recognized.

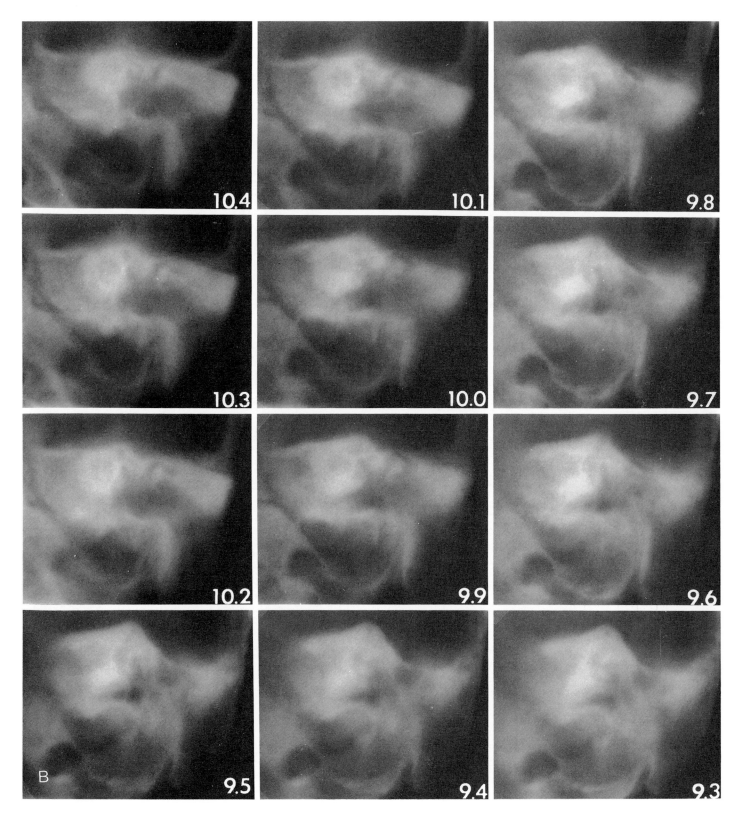

Figure 5.23. B.

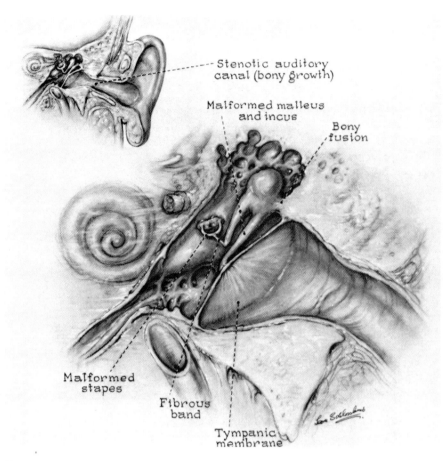

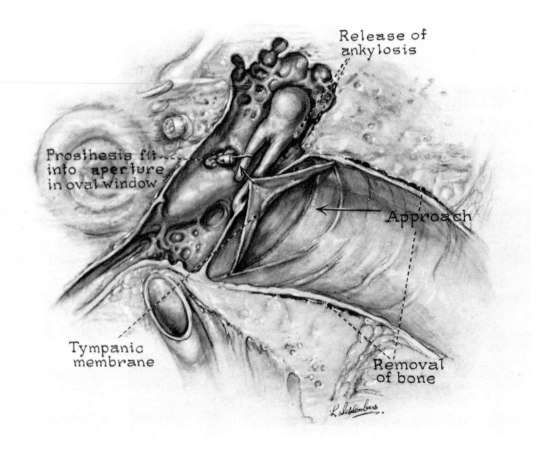

Figure 5.24. Drawing of left middle ear showing anomalies involving auditory ossicles and oval window.

Figure 5.25. Drawing of left middle ear showing surgical correction of malformation. Insertion of a wire Teflon piston prosthesis provided the patient with normal hearing in that ear.

References

1. Altmann F. Problem of so-called congenital atresia of the ear. Histologic report of a new case. Arch Otolaryngol 1949;50:759.
2. Naunton RF, Valvassori GE. Inner ear anomalies: their association with atresia. Laryngoscope 1968;78:1041.
3. Bergstrom LV, Hemenway WG, Downs MP. A high risk registry to find congenital deafness. Otolaryngol Clin North Am. 1971;4(2):369–399.
4. Jahrsdoerfer RA. Congenital atresia of the ear. Laryngoscope 1978;88(Suppl 13):1–48.
5. Bezold F, quoted by Bauer G, Stein C. Konstitutions-pathologie in der Ohrenheilkunde. Berlin: Springer Verlag, 1926.
6. Mündnich K, Terrahe K. Missbildungen des Ohres. In: Berendes J, Link R, Zöllner F, eds. Hals-Nasen-Ohrenheilkunde, Ohr I. Stuttgart: Georg Thieme, Chap 1, 1979;5:1–49.
7. Altmann F. Missbildungen des Ohres. In: Berendes J, Link R, Zöllner F, eds. Hals-Nasen-Ohrenheilkunde, Teil 1. Stuttgart: Georg Thieme, 1966;3:643.
8. Jafek BW, Nager GT, Strife J, Gaylor RW. Congenital aural atresia: an analysis of 311 cases. Trans Am Acad Ophthalmol Otolaryngol 1975;8:588.
9. Thompson A. A description of congenital malformation of the auricle and external meatus of both sides in 3 persons. Proc R Soc Edinb 1845;1:443.
10. Virchow R. Über Missbildungen am Ohr und im Bereiche des ersten Kiemenbogens. Virchows Archiv 1864;30:221.
11. Bast TH, Anson BJ. Embryology of the ear. In: Paparella MM, Shumrick DA, eds. Otolaryngology. Philadelphia, WB Saunders, Chap 1, 1980;1(7):3–25.
12. Richany SF, Bast TH, Anson BJ. The development and adult structures of the malleus, incus and stapes. Ann Otol 1954;63:394.
13. Lindsay JR, Saunders SH, Nager GT. Histopathologic observations in so-called congenital fixation of the stapedial footplate. Laryngoscope 1966;70:1587.
14. Collins ET. Case with symmetrical congenital notches in outer part of each lower lid and defective development of molar bones. Trans Ophthalmol Soc U K 1900;20:190.
15. Franceschetti A, Zwahlen P. Un syndrome nouveau: la dysostose mandibulo-faciale. Bull Schweiz Akad Med Wiss 1944;1:60.
16. Franceschetti A, Klein D. Mandibulo-facial dysostosis. A new hereditary syndrome. Acta Ophthalmol 1949;27:143.
17. Crouzon O. Dysostose cranio-faciale héréditaire. Bull Soc Med Hop (Paris) 1912;33:545.
18. Marx H. Beitrag zur Morphologie und Genese der Mittelohrmissbildungen mit Gehörgangsatresie. Z Hals-Nasen-Ohrenheilkd 1922;2:230.
19. Konigsmark BW, Nager GT, Haskins HW. Recessive meatal atresia and hearing loss. Report of sibship. Arch Otolaryngol 1972;96:105.
20. Ellwood LC, Winter ST, Dar H. Familial microtia with meatal atresia in two sibships. J Med Genet 1968;5:289.
21. Dar H, Winter ST. Letter to the editor. J Med Genet 1973;10:305.
22. Meurmon Y. Congenital microtia and meatal atresia. Observations and aspects of treatment. Arch Otolaryngol 1957;66:443.
23. Kunkel VO. Mikrotie bei Mutter und drei von vier Kindern. HNO 1959;8:80.
24. Balci S. Familial microtia with meatal atresia in father and son. Turk J Pediatr 1974;16:140.
25. Balci S. Personal communication to BW Konigsmark, 1978.
26. Gorlin, RL, Pindborg JJ, Cohen MM Jr. Syndromes of the head and neck. 2nd ed. New York: McGraw-Hill, 1976:453.
27. Hutchinson JC Jr, Caldarelli DD, Valvassori GE, Pruzansky S, Parris PJ. The otologic manifestations of mandibulofacial dysostosis. Trans Am Ophthalmol Otolaryngol 1977;84:520.
28. Axelsson A, Brolin I, Engstrom H, Liden G. Dysostosis mandibulo-facialis. J Laryngol Otol 1963;77:575.
29. Farrar JE. Mandibulo-facial dysostosis (Treacher Collins syndrome). Arch Dis Child 1955;30:391.
30. McKenzie J, Craig J. Mandibulo-facial dysostosis (Treacher Collins syndrome). Arch Dis Child 1955;30:391.
31. Harrison SH. Treacher Collins syndrome. Br J Plast Surg 1950–1951;3:282.
32. Stovin JJ, Lyon JA Jr, Clemens RL. Mandibulo-facial dysostosis. Radiology 1960;74:225.
33. Holobrow CA. Deafness and the Treacher Collins syndrome. J Laryngol Otol 1961;75:978.
34. Herberts G. Otological observations in the ''Treacher Collins syndrome.'' Acta Otolaryngol 1962;54:456.
35. Edwards WG. Congenital middle-ear deafness with abnormalities of the face. J Laryngol Otol 1964;78:152.
36. Sando I, Hemenway WG, Morgan WR. Histopathology of the temporal bones in mandibulo-facial dysostosis. Trans Am Acad Ophthalmol Otolaryngol 1968;72:913.
37. Sugar HS, Berman M. Relationship between the mandibulofacial dysostosis syndrome of Franceschetti and the oculoauriculovertebral dysplasia syndrome of Goldenhar. Am J Ophthalmol 1968;66:510.
38. Böök JA, Traccaro M. Genetical investigations in a North Swedish population of mandibulo-facial dysostosis. Acta Genet (Basel) 1955;5:327.
39. Behrents RG, McNamara JA, Avery JK. Prenatal mandibulo-facial dysostosis (Treacher Collins syndrome). Cleft Palate J 1977;14:13.
40. Mann I, Kilner TP. Deficiency of malar bones with defect of the lower lids. Br J Ophthalmol 1943;27:13.
41. Livingstone G. The establishment of sound conduction of congenital deformities of the external ear. J Laryngol Otol 1959;73:231.
42. Leopold IH, Mahoney JF, Price ML. Symmetric defects in the lower lids associated with abnormalities of the zygomatic process of the temporal bones. Arch Ophthalmol 1945;34:210.
43. Straith CL, Lewis JR. Associated congenital defects of the ears, eyelids and malar bones (Treacher Collins syndrome). Plast Reconstr Surg 1949;4:204.
44. Wildervanck LS. Dysostosis mandibulo-facialis (Franceschetti-Zwahlen) in four generations. Acta Genet Med Gemellol (Roma) 1960;9:447.
45. Maran AGD. The Treacher Collins syndrome. J Laryngol Otol 1964;78:135.
46. Rovin S, Dachi SF, Borenstein DB, Cottler WB. Mandibulofacial dysostosis, a family study of five generations. J Pediatr 1964;65:215.
47. Fazen LE, Elmore J, Nadler HL. Mandibulo-facial dysostosis (Treacher Collins syndrome). Am J Dis Child 1967;113:405.
48. Hall JG. Mandibulofacial dysostosis (Treacher Collins-Franceschetti syndrome). Birth Defects 1969;5(2):215.
49. Nager FR, de Reynier JP. Das Gehörorgan bei den angeborenen Kopfmissbildungen. Pract Otorhinolaryngol (Basel) 1948;10(Suppl 2):1.
50. O'Connor GB, Conway ME. Treacher Collins syndrome (dysostosis mandibulo-facialis). Plast Reconstr Surg 1950;5:419.
51. McNeill KA, Wynter-Wedderburn L. Choanal atresia—a manifestation of the Treacher Collins syndrome. J Laryngol Otol 1953;67:365.
52. Altmann F. Congenital atresia of the ear in man and animals. Ann Otol Rhinol Laryngol 1955;644:824.
53. Brocher JEW, Klein D. Die Dysostosis mandibulofacialis im Roentgenbild. Fortschr Geb Roentgenstr Nuklearmed 1960;93:67.
54. Chou Y-C. Mandibulofacial dysostosis. Chin Med J 1960;80:373.
55. Fernandez AO, Ronis ML. The Treacher Collins syndrome. Arch Otolaryngol 1964;80:505.
56. Marden PM, Smith DW, McDonald MJ. Congenital anomalies in the newborn infant, including minor variations. J Pediatr 1964;64:357.
57. Jones RG. Mandibulofacial dysostosis. Cent Afr J Med 1968;14:193.
58. Genée E. Une Forme extensive de dysostose mandibulofaciale. J Genet Hum 1969;17:45.
59. Pfeiffer RA. Associated deformities of the head and hands. Birth Defects 1969;5(3):18.
60. Neidhart E. Die Dysostosis mandibulo-facialis Franceschetti-Zwahlen-Klein syndrome) in Kombination mit Missbildungen der obern Extremitaten. Thesis, Zürich, 1968; cited in Ref 63.
61. Klein D, Konig H, Tobler R. Sur une forme extensive de dysostose mandibulofaciale (Franceschetti) accompagnée de malformations des extremitées et d'autres anomalies congénitales chez une fille dont le frère ne presente qu'une forme fruste du syndrome (fistula auris congenita retrotragica). Rev Otoneuro-ophthalmol 1973;42:432, cited in Ref 63.
62. Vatre JL. Étude génetique et classifications clinique de 154 cas de dysostose mandibulo-faciale (syndrome de Franceschetti) avec déscription de leurs associations avec malformations. J Genet Hum 1971;19:17, cited in Ref 63.
63. Bowen P, Harley F. Mandibulofacial dysostosis with limb malformations (Nager's acrofacial dysostosis). Birth Defects 1974;10(5):109.
64. Walker FA. Apparent autosomal recessive inheritance of the Treacher Collins syndrome. Birth Defects 1974;10(8):135.
65. Herrmann J, Pallister PD, Kaveggia EG, Opitz JM. Acrofacial dysostosis type Nager. Birth Defects 1975;11(5):341
66. Burton BK, Nadler HL. Nager dysostosis. Report of case. J Pediatr 1977;91:84.
67. Lowry RB. The Nager syndrome (acrofacial dysostosis): evidence for autosomal dominant inheritance. Birth Defects 1977;13(3C):195.

68. Meyerson MD, Jensen KM, Meyers JM, Hall BD. Nager acrofacial dysostosis: early intervention and long-term planning. Cleft Palate J 1977;14:35.

70. Ross RB. Lateral facial dysplasia (first and second branchial arch syndrome, hemifacial microsomia). Birth Defects 1975;11(7):51.

71. Coccaro PJ, Becker MH, Converse JM. Clinical and radiographic variations in hemifacial microsomia. Birth Defects 1975;11(2):314.

72. Gorlin RJ, Pindborg JJ, Cohen MM Jr. Syndromes of the head and neck, 2nd ed. New York: McGraw-Hill, 1976:546.

73. Gorlin RJ, Jue KL, Jacobsen U, Goldschmidt E. Oculoauriculovertebral dysplasia. J Pediatr 1963;63:991.

74. Shokeir MH. The Goldenhar syndrome: a natural history. Birth Defects 1977;13(3C):67.

75. Budden SS, Robinson GC. Oculoauricular vertebral dysplasia. J Dis Child 1973;125:431.

76. Darling DB, Feingold M, Berkman M. The roentgenological aspects of Goldenhar's syndrome (oculoauriculovertebral dysplasia). Radiology 1968;91:254.

77. Cohen MM Jr. An etiologic and nosologic overview of craniosynostosis syndromes. Birth Defects 1975;11(2):137.

78. Gorlin RJ, Pindborg JJ, Cohen MM Jr. Syndromes of the head and neck. 2nd ed. New York: McGraw-Hill, 1976:220.

79. Bertelson TI. The premature synostosis of the cranial suture. Acta Ophthalmol (Suppl) 1958;51:1.

80. Koziak PH. Craniosynostosis: report on 22 cases. Am J Ophthalmol 1954;37:380.

81. Parks MM, Costenbader FD. Craniofacial dysostosis (Crouzon's disease). Am J Ophthalmol 1950;33:77.

82. Arce M, Arce F. Roentgenographic study of craniofacial dysostosis. Report of cases. Nonfamilial and nonhereditary. AJR 1942;47:275.

83. Pinkerton OD, Pinkerton FJ. Hereditary craniofacial dysplasia. Am J Ophthalmol 1952;35:500.

84. Vulliamy DG, Normandale PA. Cranio-facial dysostosis in a Dorset family. Arch Dis Child 1966;41:375.

85. Aubrey M. Examen otologique de 10 cas de dysostosis craniofacialis de Crouzon. Rev Neurol (Paris) 1935;63:302.

86. Wiegand R. Dysostosis craniofacialis (Morbus Crouzon 1912) mit beidseitigen (häutiger) Gehörgangsatrisie. Arch Ohren-Nasen-Kehlkopfheilkd 1954;166:128.

87. Blodi FC. Developmental anomalies of the skull affecting the eye. Arch Ophthalmol 1957;57:593.

88. Baldwin JL. Dysostosis craniofacialis of Crouzon. A summary of recent literature and case reports with emphasis on involvement of the ear. Laryngoscope 1968;78:1600.

89. Boedts D. La surdité dans la dysostose craniofaciale ou maladie de Crouzon. Acta Otorhinolaryngol Belg 1967;21:143.

90. Kreiborg S, Jensen BL. Variable expressivity of Crouzon's syndrome within a family. Scand J Dent Res 1977;85:175.

91. Gorlin RJ, Pindborg JJ, Cohen MM Jr. Syndromes of the head and neck. 2nd ed. New York: McGraw-Hill, 1976:32.

92. Gorlin RJ, Pindborg JJ, Cohen MM Jr. Syndromes of the head and neck. 2nd ed. New York: McGraw-Hill, 1976:609.

93. Bixler D, Christian JC, Gorlin RJ. Hypertelorism, microtia and facial clefting. A newly described inherited syndrome. Am J Dis Child 1969;118:495.

94. deGrouchy J. The 18p-, 18q- and 18r syndrome. Birth Defects 1969;5(5):74.

95. Schnizel A, Hayashi K, Schmid W. Structural aberrations of chromosomes 18. II. The 18q-syndrome. Report of three cases. Hum Genet 1975;26:123.

96. Konigsmark BW, Gorlin RJ. Genetic and metabolic deafness. Philadelphia: WB Saunders, 1976;369.

97. Bergstrom LV, Stewart JM, Kenyon B. External auditory atresia and the deleted chromosome. Laryngoscope 1974;84:1905.

98. Weicker H, Bachmann KD, Pfeiffer RA, Gleiss J. Thalidomid-Embryopathie. Dtsch Med Wochenschr 1962;87:1597.

99. Kleinsasser O, Schlothane R. Die Ohrmissbildungen im Rahmen der Thalidomid-Embryopathie. Z Laryngol Rhinol 1964;43:344.

100. Mündnich K. Höprverbessernde und plastische Operationen bei Ohrmissbildungen. In: Berendes J, Link RL, Zöllner F, eds. Hals-Nasen-Ohrenheilkunde, Teil 1. Stuttgart: Georg Thieme, 1966;3:637.

101. Lenz W, Knapp K. Die Thalidomid Embryopathie. Schweiz Med Wochenschr 1962;87:1232.

102. Lenz W. Das Thalidomid Syndrom. Fortschr Med 1963;81:148.

103. Ombrédanne M. 100 opérations d'aplasie de l'oreille avec imperforation du conduit. Acta Oto-rino-laringol Ibero-Am 1957;8:315.

104. Frey KW, Mündnich K. Schichtaufnahmen des Felsenbeins mit polyzyklischer Verwischung bei angeborenen Ohrmissbildungen. Fortschr Geb Roentgenstr Nuklearmed 1957;87:164.

105. Leicher H. Taubstummheit, Vestibularisschaden und Missbildungen des äusseren Ohres als Symptome der Röteln-Embryopathie. Laryngol Rhinol Otol [Stuttg] 1952;31:128.

106. Nager GT, Chen SCA, Hussels IE. A new syndrome in two unrelated females: Klippel-Feil deformity. Conductive deafness and absent vagina. In: Bergsma D, ed. Clinical delineation of birth defects. Part X. The endocrine system. Baltimore: Williams & Wilkins, 1971;VII(6):311–317.

6/ Dysplasia of the Osseous and Membranous Cochlea and Vestibular Labyrinth

Multiplanar tomography and histologic examination of serially sectioned temporal bones with suspected or documented anomalies of the bony and membranous cochlea and vestibular labyrinth have disclosed in recent decades a number of hitherto unrecognized malformations. This made it necessary to modify the original categorization of anomalies. A more recent and more specific classification takes into account that the superior compartment of the inner ear capsule, which includes the semicircular canals, the utricle, the endolymphatic duct and sac, and the inferior compartment, which includes the cochlea and saccule, may undergo independent or combined anomalous developments (1). This classification divides the anomalies as follows (Fig. 6.1):

Type I: Isolated aplasia or dysplasia of lateral semicircular canal. The lateral canal may be absent, form with the vestibule a plump single cavity, may be represented by a cul-de-sac or a lateral ovoid evagination of the vestibule, or may appear as a plump, thick, rudimentary canal with a smaller diameter. The other semicircular canals and the cochlea are normally configured. Type I represents the most common and the least severe of malformations.

Type II: Aplasia or dysplasia of lateral semicircular canal as described in type I, associated with dysplasia of the cochlea. Dysplasia of the cochlea may be characterized by an elongated evagination of the vestibule that lacks the configuration of a cochlear turn or by a single cochlear turn or 1½ cochlear turns (2).

Type III: Aplasia or dysplasia of lateral semicircular canal as described in type I, associated with an aplasia or a rare club-shaped distension of the vestibule, representing a rudimentary superior or posterior semicircular canal but with a normally configured cochlea. The posterior of the three semicircular canals is the least frequently involved.

Type IV: Aplasia or dysplasia of two or all three semicircular canals as described in types I and III, associated with a severe dysplasia of the cochlea. In the absence of all three semicircular canals, a spherical or ovoid cavity with a finger-like projection resembling a rudimentary common crus portrays a "Labyrinth Anlage" that did not develop beyond the otocystic stage.

Type V: Aplasia of all three semicircular canals, associated with a normally configured cochlea (3, 4).

Type VI: Aplasia of all three semicircular canals, associated with a dysplasia of the cochlea (3).

Type VII: Normally configured vestibular labyrinth associated with an aplasia of the cochlea (5, 6).

Type VIII: Aplasia of vestibular labyrinth and cochlea (7).

This more detailed classification is very helpful in the delineation of aberrations of the bony cochlear and vestibular capsule. However, for evaluating morphologic changes that involve the cochlear modiolus, osseous spiral lamina, and contents of the vestibule and endolymphatic sac and duct as observed in the Mondini type of dysplasia or that involve the cochlear duct and saccule as encountered in Scheibe's dysplasia, it is advantageous to refer to these generally recognized patterns.

The original information on dysplasia of the cochlea and vestibular labyrinth in patients with profound congenital hearing loss is based on the observations of Mondini (8) (1791), Michel (7) (1864), Scheibe (9, 10), and Siebenmann (11) (1907). The pertinent types and observations are here summarized briefly.

TYPES OF DYSPLASIA

Michel Type

Michel (7) described a bilateral aplasia of the cochlear and vestibular capsule and of the eighth nerve. The external and the middle ear were normal, but the stapes, stapedius muscle, and mastoid process were absent. He also reported an instance in which the inner ear components were represented by rudimentary structures in an otocyst-like cavity. In two other instances the petrous pyramids and middle ears were absent (12, 13). In another case a child whose mother had taken thalidomide during the first month of pregnancy was born with an aplasia of the cochlea and vestibular labyrinth on one side and a dysplastic inner ear on the opposite side. The dysplasia was represented by a single cavity surrounded by a bony capsule containing structures resembling rudimentary sense organs (14). Isolated observations of aplasia have since been reported. Because of its rarity this type of developmental anomaly is of relative significance.

Mondini Type

The characteristic feature of the Mondini type of dysplasia is that it may consistently involve anomalies of the cochlear and vestibular capsule and their membranous structures. Mondini (8) provided the initial gross description of a flattened cochlea represented only by a single curved tube in combination with a bony aperture on the posterior aspect of the petrous pyramid housing an enlarged endolymphatic sac. The scalae vestibuli and tympani were present only in the lower 1½ turns of the cochlea, and the regional neural and vascular structures appeared unremarkable. The remaining cochlear turns formed a common cavity. The endolymphatic duct was greatly distended. Alexander (15) described the histopathology of more extensive findings in this form of dysplasia. This dysplasia has subsequently been referred to by Siebenmann as the Mondini type (11, 16, 17). In the Mondini type the dysplasia of the cochlea may vary between a cochlea represented by a single coil and one with a near-normal config-

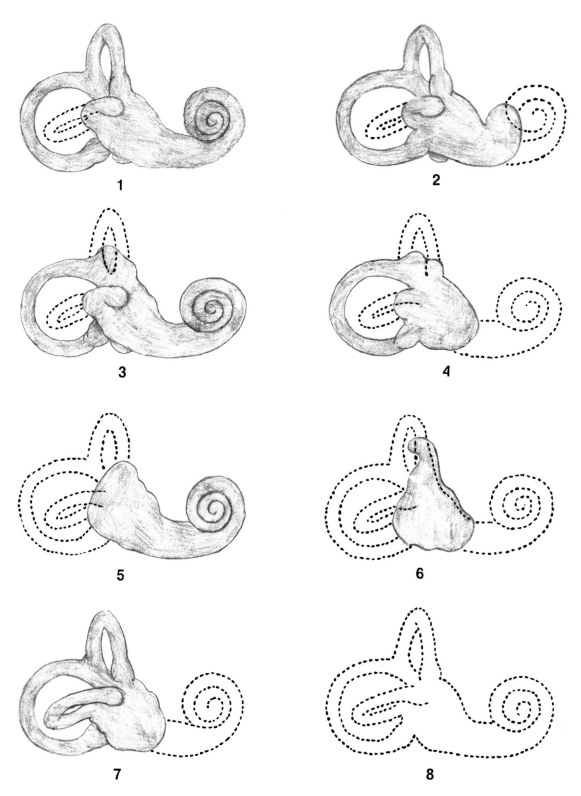

Figure 6.1.   Illustrations of various types of developmental anomalies involving the osseous cochlea and vestibular labyrinth according to a modified classification by K. Mündich and K. Terrahe (1). *1,* dysplasia or aplasia of lateral canal; *2,* dysplasia or aplasia of lateral canal and cochlea; *3,* dysplasia and aplasia of lateral and superior or posterior canal; *4,* dysplasia or aplasia of lateral and superior or posterior canal and cochlea; *5,* dysplasia or aplasia of all three canals; *6,* dysplasia or aplasia of all three canals and cochlea; *7,* dysplasia or aplasia of cochlea; and *8,* aplasia of cochlea and vestibular labyrinth.

uration (see Figs. 6.13–6.15). In general, the cochlea appears flattened with an underdeveloped apex. The cochlear modiolus and osseous spiral lamina are deficient, extend only to the middle turn, and in rare instances may be almost completely absent (Figs. 6.2–6.4) (18). The absence of a bony septum between the second and third cochlear turn creates a common apical space or common scala (Fig. 6.3). The cochlear aqueduct and its medial apertures into the subarchnoid space and the internal auditory canals are often distended. There may be an abnormal additional communication between the subarachnoid space of the internal auditory canal and the perilymphatic space of the lower basal turn of the cochlea and the perilymph cistern of the vestibule. The endolymphatic duct and sac may be distended or dysplastic. The cochlear capsule may display an abnormal development of its trilaminal bony structure. It may be associated with a dysplasia or aplasia of the oval and round windows. A dysplasia of the oval window can be accompanied by a dehiscence in the stapedial footplate.

Children with a dehiscent stapedial footplate have a persistent perilymph fistula and cerebrospinal otorrhea and usually present with a history of recurrent otogenic meningitis. The cochlear duct that may occupy 1, 1½, and sometimes 2 cochlear turns is usually dilated but is sometimes collapsed (Fig. 6.4). The organ of Corti can be missing in some areas, may be severely altered, or may resemble some early stage of development (Fig. 6.3D). The stria vascularis displays various stages of dysplasia and atrophy. Dysplasia of the vestibular labyrinth includes anomalies or absence of all semicircular canals, the vestibule, and the vestibular nerve. The utricle, saccule, and endolymphatic duct and sac are often dilated (Figs. 6.5–6.9). The Mondini type of dysplasia occurs more often bilaterally. It has been observed in genetically determined as well as prenatally acquired forms of profound childhood hearing loss (16, 19). Depending on the extent of morphologic changes encountered in the cochlea and vestibular labyrinth, it can be accompanied by a partial or total loss of cochlear and vestibular function. It includes a broad spectrum of structural abnormalities. It may present as a single malformation, in association with atresia of the middle or outer ear, or in combination with other malformation syndromes.

Scheibe Type

The distinctive feature of the Scheibe type of dysplasia is that the morphologic changes are limited to the membranous cochlea and saccule, the phylogenetically younger structure of the inner ear. The utricle and semicircular canals are not involved. In Scheibe's initial case the nerves supplying the basal turn of the cochlea, the saccule, and the posterior ampulla were described to be atrophic. In Scheibe's second case the atrophy of the nerve to the basal turn was associated with other degenerative changes of the membranous cochlea (9, 10). In one instance of a full-term infant (of deaf-mute parents) with bilateral Scheibe dysplasia who died 10 hours after birth, the stria vascularis formed multiple layers between the spiral ligament and a

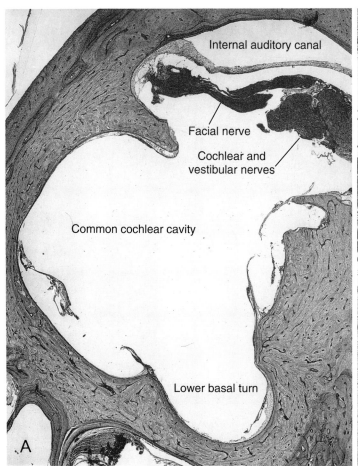

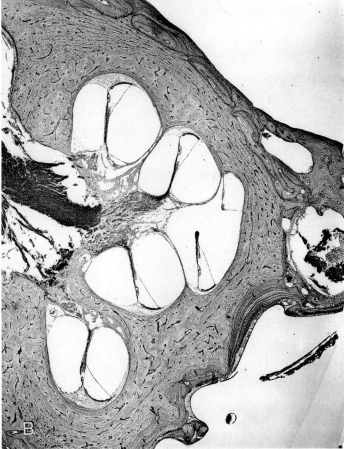

Figure 6.2. Vertical midmodiolar section of right cochlea. The overall dimensions of the right cochlea **(A)** are slightly larger than those of the normal left cochlea **(B)**. The subtotal absence of the modiolus and osseous spiral lamina creates a common cochlear cavity that includes all three turns and communicates widely with the subarachnoid space of the internal auditory canal. (Hematoxylin and eosin, ×20.)

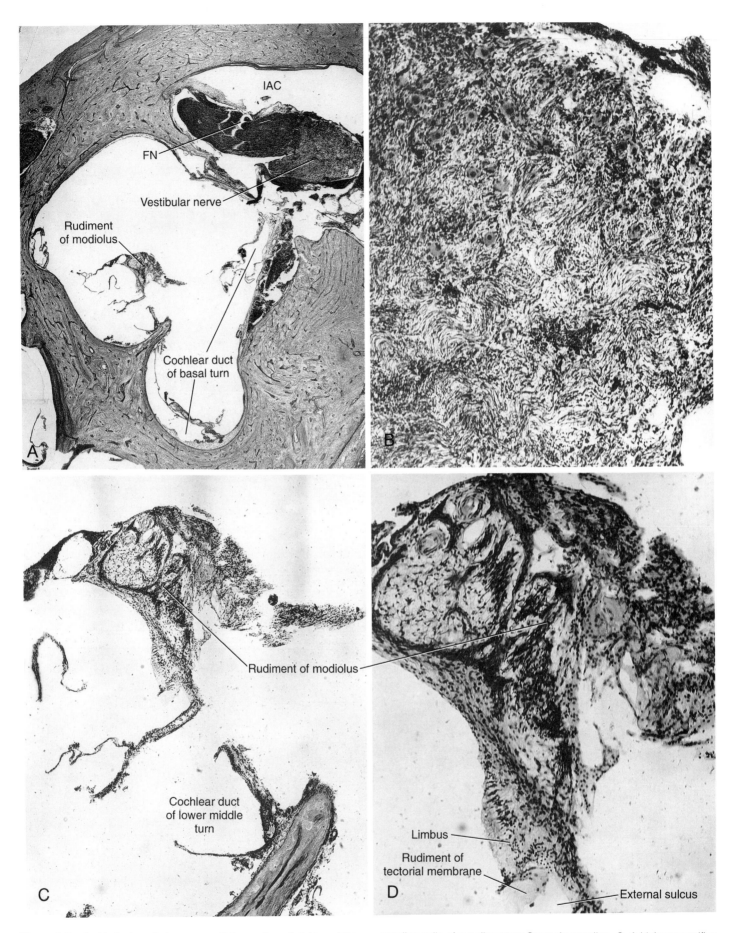

Figure 6.3. **A.** Vertical posterior paramodiolar section of right cochlea and internal auditory canal *(IAC).* Near the center of the cochlear cavity, a cross-section through the rudiment of the modiolus with the adjacent osseous spiral lamina and the torn undifferentiated cochlear duct can be recognized. The IAC contains the facial nerve *(FN)* as it enters the labyrinthine segment of the Fallopian canal and the vestibular and cochlear nerve. **B.** A higher magnification of the vestibular nerve displays some scattered ganglion cells of a rudimentary Scarpa's ganglion. **C.** A higher magnification of the rudimentary modiolus discloses some cochlear nerve fibers. **D.** A still higher magnification of the modiolus shows that the osseous spiral lamina supports an incompletely differentiated limbus with a primitive tectorial membrane lying in the internal sulcus covered by a single layer of endothelial cells. (Hematoxylin and eosin, ×20, ×150, ×67, and ×150, respectively.)

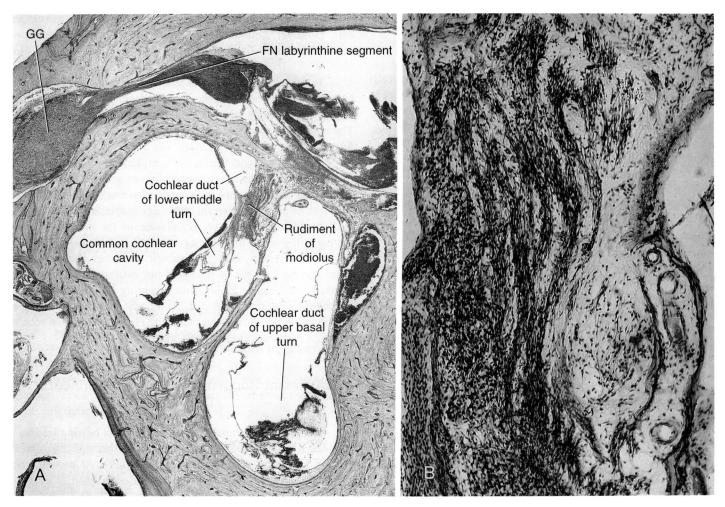

Figure 6.4. **A.** Vertical section through right cochlea near posterior tangent of middle turn. It displays the rudiment of the modiolus with cochlear nerve fibers. At that level, an incomplete interscalar bony septum separates the basal turn from the middle turn. The cochlear duct that extends along 1¼ turns is poorly differentiated. *FN*, facial nerve; and *GG*, geniculate ganglion. **B.** A higher magnification of the modiolus reveals some scattered ganglion cells of the primitive spiral ganglion between the cochlear nerve bundles. (Hematoxylin and eosin, ×20 and ×150, respectively.)

partially collapsed Reissner's membrane in the basal turn but was missing in other areas. The tectorial membrane had a spherical shape and was lying in the internal sulcus. A few hair cells could be identified. The cochlear neuron was normal. The macula of the saccule was aplastic, with the saccular wall collapsed onto the macula (20). In two other patients, ages 10 and 66 years, with profound hearing loss since birth and bilateral Scheibe dysplasia, the severe morphologic alterations involving the cochlear duct and saccule are quite similar. The stria vascularis is atrophic in some and hyperplastic in other areas or may exhibit an irregular mass of strial tissue in the region of the spiral prominence. The organ of Corti is missing in some areas and in other areas or throughout consists of a flattened mound of undifferentiated cells in which remnants of pillar cells may be recognized. The tectorial membrane has a spherical shape and lies in the internal sulcus. Reissner's membrane is depressed onto the stria vascularis, onto the organ of Corti, and onto the limbus so as to obliterate the cochlear duct, and there may be a varying loss of cochlear neurons in the basal turn or in all turns of the cochlea. The utricle and saccule are normal (20). These cases illustrate the structural changes involving the cochlear duct and saccule encountered in the Scheibe dysplasia that may be genetically determined or acquired during fetal life (21).

Siebenmann-Bing Type

In the Siebenmann-Bing type of dysplasia the cochlear capsule displays a normal configuration. The membranous cochlea and vestibular labyrinth can be dysplastic. Siebenmann (11) also described a malformation involving the membranous cochlea and vestibular labyrinth with a dislocation of the organ of Corti. It was in a patient with congenital deafness and retinitis pigmentosa. The organ of Corti was missing in the major portion of the basal turn, but in its upper end, it began to appear as a mound of undifferentiated epithelial cells in an atypical location, laterally from where it would normally be encountered, almost outside the reach of the tectorial membrane. From the middle turn on upward it gradually assumed a more normal position. The spiral ganglion cell population was severely diminished. The maculae and cristae of the vestibular labyrinth disclosed minor atrophic changes, and there was an apparent paucity of blood vessels in the labyrinth, particularly in the cochlea.

Vestibular System

Two of the three patients tested showed a normal response, and one showed a slightly abnormal response.

Radiography

The tomograms of the temporal bones of three patients showed no abnormalities.

Pathology

No histopathologic studies have been presented.

Summary

The characteristic features include: *(a)* autosomal dominant transmission, *(b)* symmetric low-frequency sensorineural hearing loss with slow progression to moderately severe loss involving all frequencies, and *(c)* normal vestibular responses.

Dominant Progressive Middle-Frequency Sensorineural Hearing Loss

Dominant progressive sensorineural hearing loss of the middle frequencies has been studied extensively (27, 43, 44). Most investigators found dominant transmission. Some, however, assume the recessive mode of inheritance.

CLINICAL FINDINGS

Auditory System

This type of hearing loss is characterized audiometrically by a slowly progressive loss in the middle-frequency range, manifested by a shallow saucer-shaped depression with a hearing loss involving 1000–2000 Hz that is most severe in younger persons, with normal thresholds in the low- and high-frequency ranges. In older patients, all frequencies eventually become affected. The degree of hearing loss may vary considerably among the same age group, suggesting a variable expression of the gene. The SISI test is positive, and tone decay tests are negative.

Vestibular System

Vestibular tests are normal.

Pathology

The temporal bones of a woman whose father also had a middle-frequency 55–100-dB sensorineural hearing loss showed a complete absence of the organ of Corti in the basal turn, with clumps of cells remaining in the middle and apical turns. The stria vascularis was atrophic. The spiral ganglion cells were deficient in the basal turn of the cochlea.

Summary

The major characteristic features include: *(a)* autosomal dominant transmission, *(b)* progressive sensorineural hearing loss involving the middle frequencies in childhood and eventually all frequencies, and *(c)* normal caloric responses.

Dominant Progressive High-Frequency Sensorineural Hearing Loss

Dominant progressive high-frequency sensorineural hearing loss was recognized as a possible distinct form of hearing loss in 1934 (45) and was subsequently demonstrated in four generations in 1974 (46).

CLINICAL FINDINGS

Auditory Systems

The audiograms display an abrupt high-tone loss above 2000 Hz, 1000 Hz, and 500 Hz, with progressive involvement of the lower frequencies as age increases. The SISI tests are positive at high frequencies, and speech discrimination is poor.

Vestibular System

No studies have been reported.

Radiography

Tomographic studies were unremarkable.

Pathology

There is a localized atrophy of the organ of Corti in the basal turn that is associated with a corresponding partial atrophy of the cochlear nerve fibers.

Summary

The characteristic features are: *(a)* autosomal dominant inheritance, *(b)* abrupt sensorineural high-tone loss, and *(c)* progressive involvement of the lower frequencies with age.

Otosclerosis

Otosclerosis is one of the major causes of progressive loss of hearing in adults. It is a bone dysplasia involving the temporal bone that is more often present in its histologic form than in its clinically manifest form. Its characteristics include: *(a)* autosomal dominant inheritance with about 40% penetration; *(b)* gradual onset of hearing loss in early decades of life, rarely in childhood or beyond the age of 50 years; *(c)* slowly progressive, predominantly conductive or combined, symmetrical, very rarely purely sensorineural hearing loss leading to a profound deafness or total loss of hearing only in very rare instances; *(d)* normal vestibular responses; and *(e)* occasionally encountered in association with osteogenesis imperfecta in adults. It was first recognized in 1735 (47, 48) and since then has been the subject of over 1000 publications (49). It is discussed in a separate chapter under bone dysplasia involving the temporal bone.

Recessive Congenital Severe Sensorineural Hearing Loss

A high percentage of sporadic, congenital deafness is of recessive origin. Recessive congenital severe sensorineural hearing loss represents an estimated 40%, the largest group, of all forms of profound hearing loss in children (29, 50). The dominant congenital severe sensorineural form accounts for about 10%

(29). It is assumed that about four or five genes are involved (50). Most parents of these children apparently had normal hearing, but the percentage of consanguinity is high. In most instances, both ears are involved.

CLINICAL FINDINGS

Auditory System

The audiogram generally reveals a high-frequency loss, occasionally a profound bilateral loss of 80–100 dB in all frequencies with absent bone conduction. Three subgroups may be distinguished: *(a)* normal hearing in the low and middle frequencies followed by an abrupt drop with no response in the high frequencies; *(b)* a gradually increasing hearing loss beginning in the low frequencies; and *(c)* residual hearing in the low frequencies, in rare instances combined with residual hearing in the middle frequencies (27). The SISI score is positive, but tone decay tests are negative.

Vestibular System

The vestibular responses may be normal, severely impaired, or absent (51).

Radiography

No abnormal radiographic findings have been reported.

Pathology

The histologic examination of these temporal bones in most instances disclosed the Scheibe-type cochleosaccular dysplasia (27), but in one patient a Mondini-type dysplasia with involvement of the labyrinthine capsule was reported (18, 27).

Summary

The characteristic features include: *(a)* autosomal recessive transmission, *(b)* congenital severe sensorineural hearing loss, and *(c)* normal and abnormal vestibular responses.

Recessive Congenital Moderate Sensorineural Hearing Loss

The disorder characterized by congenital moderate nonprogressive sensorineural hearing loss was first recognized in 1970 (52), with additional observations in 1971 (53).

CLINICAL FINDINGS

Auditory System

The hearing loss was first noticed in children. Repeated audiograms in all persons involved over periods up to 16 years showed no progression. In all, the hearing loss was moderately severe with a three-frequency (500, 1000, 2000 Hz) average loss of 30–50 dB. The tracings were flat with a minimal increase in the higher frequencies. SISI scores were positive, and tone decay tests were negative.

Vestibular System

Vestibular responses in five of six affected individuals were normal.

Pathology

No histopathologic studies are available.

Summary

The characteristic features are: *(a)* autosomal recessive transmission, *(b)* congenital symmetric nonprogressive moderate sensorineural hearing loss that is slightly more marked in the higher frequencies, and *(c)* normal vestibular function.

Recessive Early-Onset Sensorineural Hearing Loss

Early onset of severe progressive sensorineural hearing loss in childhood was described in 1964 (54) and in 1967 (55).

CLINICAL FINDINGS

Auditory System

Each of 10 affected individuals in one family had at least some hearing at birth, responded to sounds, and in some instances learned to articulate a few words. Between the ages of 1½ and 6 years, hearing decreased rather rapidly in all to a severe sensorineural hearing loss of 60–100 dB in all frequencies. Only one child was able to attend a public school for a few years before being transferred to a school for the deaf. SISI scores were positive in the two who were tested.

Vestibular System

The vestibular responses were normal.

Radiography

Tomograms of the temporal bones from a member of one family showed no abnormalities.

Pathology

No histologic findings are available.

Summary

The characteristic features include: *(a)* autosomal recessive transmission, *(b)* early-onset severe sensorineural hearing loss with essentially no hearing after 5 or 6 years of age, and *(c)* normal vestibular function.

X-Linked Congenital Recessive Sensorineural Hearing Loss

Sex-linked congenital hearing loss has been identified in several families (56–58). Congenitally deaf males were found in each family in several generations. These males were born to normal-hearing mothers who frequently had deaf brothers.

CLINICAL FINDINGS

Auditory System

The audiograms in all instances showed a 70–100-dB sensorineural hearing loss in all frequencies.

ing at the fundus at internal auditory canal with aplasia of all its peripheral branches.

A 27-year-old woman had been totally deaf in the right ear since early childhood was seen. Her family history was negative for any form of hearing impairment, maternal illness during pregnancy, or complications in the perinatal period.

Five months prior to admission, the patient had several fleeting episodes of lightheadedness and giddiness, lasting a few seconds. Two months later, while getting out of her car, she experienced, without premonitory symptoms, a sudden severe attack of rotatory vertigo with nausea, vomiting, tinnitus in the right ear, loss of balance, and severe bilateral frontal headaches lasting 24 hours, followed by prostration. She subsequently suffered 12 similar episodes, with several accompanied by a spontaneous nystagmus, occurring once or twice a week, steadily increasing in intensity in spite of medication. The diagnosis of Ménière's disease was made, and the patient was referred to a neurosurgeon for right vestibular nerve section.

Otologic examination on admission revealed normally developed auricles and external auditory canals. The tympanic membranes disclosed some myringosclerosis and an atrophic scar of the left pars tensa. Cochlear function studies showed total loss of hearing in the right ear but normal hearing in the left ear. Vestibular responses to caloric stimulation were absent on the right but normal on the left.

Radiologic examination of the temporal bones exhibited somewhat wide but symmetrical, normally configured internal auditory canals and reduced cellular development of both mastoid processes, with a mild sclerosis on the left compatible with a history of recurrent bilateral otitis media in childhood.

At *operation* the seventh and eighth cranial nerves appeared unremarkable, and the right vestibular nerve could be easily divided. Death occurred suddenly from cardiac arrest on the second postoperative day.

The temporal bones were removed 1½ hours after death, processed in our laboratory, and referred to me for final analysis and interpretation.

On *examination of the right temporal bone,* the cochlear capsule appeared slightly larger, compared with the normal one on the left side. Its configuration, thickness, and trilaminar osseous structure were unmarkable. However, the cochlear modiolus and the osseous spiral lamina were almost totally absent except for a small rudiment around the junction of the upper basal turn with the lower middle turn of the cochlea (Figs. 6.2–6.4). Therefore, there was a wide open communication between the common cochlear cavity, which included all three turns, and the subarachnoid space of the internal auditory canal, which appeared slightly widened (Fig. 6.2). The vestibular nerve ended at the partially developed semilunar-shaped membranous bony plate that forms the basis of the modiolus and contains the tractus spiralis foraminosus, the superior and inferior vestibular areas or formina of exit for the two main branches of the vestibular nerve, and the opening of the labyrinth segment of the facial canal (Fig. 6.3). Several cochlear nerve bundles can be followed as they leave the rudiment of the modiolus, where together with a small group of spiral ganglion cells they represent a maldeveloped first cochlear neuron (Fig. 6.4). Their peripheral dendrites terminated at the lateral end of the rudimentary osseous spiral lamina. Within the terminal portion of the vestibular nerve, there was a small group of ganglion cells (Fig. 6.3B). The facial nerve followed its usual course through the petrous pyramid (Figs. 6.4–6.8). In the posterior half of the common cochlear cavity, a maldeveloped osseous interscalar septum partially divided the rudiments of the upper basal turn from the lower middle cochlear turn (Fig. 6.4A). A poorly differentiated cochlear duct extended from the round window for the length of about 1¼ turns (Figs. 6.3 and 6.4). Except for a limited area in the lower middle turn, where a cellular structure resembled

a limbus with an internal sulcus and a very primitive portion of a tectorial membrane, no other structures, such as a spiral ligament, stria vascularis, or organ of Corti, were recognized or even intimated by a corresponding formation of endothelial cells (Fig. 6.3A, C, and D). The lower end of the cochlear duct communicated widely with an enormously distended saccule that extended laterally to the vestibular surface of the stapes footplate and compressed the utricle toward the medial and posterior wall of the vestibule (Figs. 6.5–6.7). Posteriorly, the utricle formed a hemispherical evagination (Fig. 6.8). No neural or macular structures were recognized in either the saccule or the utricle (Figs. 6.5–6.7). All three osseous and membranous semicircular canals were absent (Figs. 6.6–6.8). All branches of the vestibular nerve to the respective vestibular end organs were absent. The endolymphatic duct ended in a somewhat dysplastic endolymphatic sac (Figs. 6.6–6.8). Whereas the vestibular fenestra is normally developed, the cochlear fenestra appears incompletely differentiated (Figs. 6.6–6.7). The middle ear cavity and middle ear structures, as far as they were included in the sections, were normal in appearance.

In summary, the right temporal bone displayed a severe malformation of the osseous and membranous cochlea and vestibular labyrinth. The cochlear malformation was characterized by a near-total absence of the modiolus and osseous spiral lamina and by a dysplastic cochlear duct that extended for 1¼ cochlear turns with an almost complete absence of cochlear nerve fibers and spiral ganglion cells and with total absence of a spiral ligament, stria vascularis, and organ of Corti. The severe malformation of the vestibular labyrinth included an enormous distension of the saccule on account of the utricle, with aplasia of the respective neural structures (maculae and nerve fibers) and aplasia of all three osseous and membranous semicircular canals. These observations represent a very severe form within the broad spectrum of Mondini-type dysplasias. They are consistent with the clinical findings of a complete loss of cochlear and vestibular responses in the right ear.

Examination of the left temporal bone was remarkable only for a localized tympanosclerotic process involving the anterior oval window margin and anterior crus of the stapes without significantly interfering with the mobility of that ossicle (Figs. 6.5B and 6.9B). Air and bone conduction in the left ear were essentially normal in all frequencies.

Comment. In the absence of the sensory epithelia of utricle, saccule, and all three semicircular canals and their vestibular nerve fibers and in the presence of an essentially normal function and morphologic appearance of the cochlea and vestibular labyrinth on the opposite side, the conventional explanation for the etiology of the vertiginous episodes is no longer applicable.

Case 2. *Multiple congenital anomalies involving the ears and other areas.*

Ears: Bilateral deformities of pinna (microtia type I), distortion of external auditory canals, and dysplasia of malleus and incus and stapedial arch; poorly differentiated oval windows associated with abnormal course of exposed facial nerve inferior to vestibular fenestra; aplasia of cochlear fenestra; bilateral congenital severe conductive hearing loss; bilateral aplasia of all three semicircular canals with questionable rudiment of left superior canal; prominent nystagmus to right associated with gaze to the right; definite left-beating nystagmus following cold caloric stimulation of right ear; possible increase in right-beating nystagmus above existing level following cold caloric stimulation of left ear.

Other areas: Mental retardation; truncus arteriosus; midline facial defects (clefting of lip and palate); right microphthalmia and coloboma of right eye and nerve; limitation of flexion of right knee; poor dentition; dysplasia of kidneys with urethral reflux.

A 15-year-old girl with a history of recurrent chronic otitis media with intermittent malodorous discharge from the right ear and bilat-

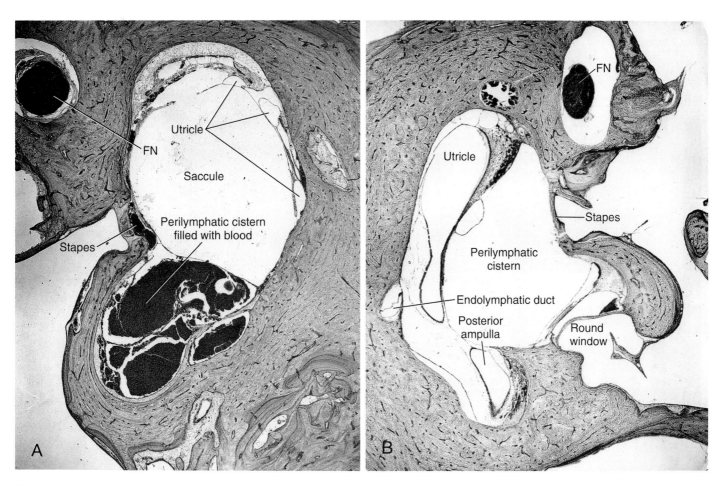

Figure 6.5. Vertical section through right and left vestibule at level of oval and round windows. **A.** The right vestibule displays an enormous distension of the saccule, partially compressing the utricle and almost impinging on the undersurface of the stapes footplate. The perilymphatic cistern is filled with blood. Note the absence of vestibular nerve branches to the right utricle, saccule, and three aplastic semicircular canals. **B.** A tympanosclerotic mass arises in the mucoperiosteum, covering the anterior oval window margin, and surrounds the anterior crus of the stapes without significantly immobilizing it. *FN,* facial nerve. (Hematoxylin and eosin, ×20.)

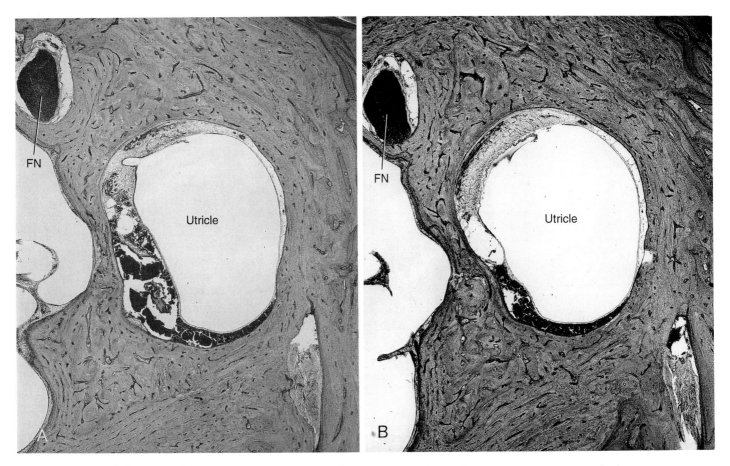

Figure 6.8. **A** and **B.** Continuing vertical sections through posterior portion of right vestibule 10 sections apart. The utricle is dysplastic. Blood occupies most of the perilymphatic cistern. *FN,* facial nerve. (Hematoxylin and eosin, ×20.)

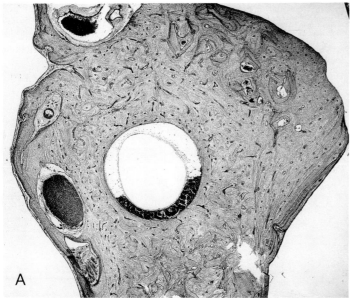

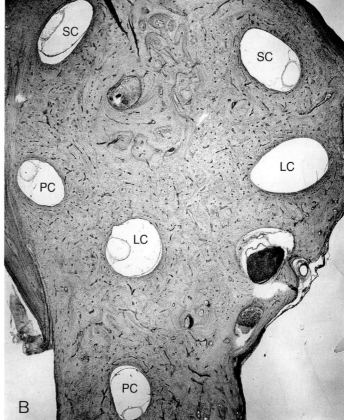

Figure 6.9.   A and **B.** Vertical sections through right and left vestibular labyrinth at corresponding levels. The posterior portion of the right petrous pyramid **(A)** is much smaller in overall dimensions. The right utricle displays a posterior hemispherical evagination. There is an aplasia of all semicircular canals. The left vestibular labyrinth **(B)** reveals normally developed semicircular canals. *LC,* lateral canal; *PC,* posterior canal; and *SC,* superior canal. (Hematoxylin and eosin, ×20.)

eral congenital severe hearing loss was seen. There was no family history of developmental anomalies or hearing loss.

Otologic examination on admission disclosed: *(a)* bilaterally deformed pinnae (microtia type I) and external auditory canals; *(b)* a right attic retraction pocket cholesteatoma; *(c)* a severe bilateral conductive hearing loss according to the (BSER) audiogram that was greater on the left; *(d)* a prominent nystagmus to the right on gaze to the right; a definite left-beating nystagmus after cold caloric stimulation of the right ear; and a possible increase in the right-beating nystagmus above the preexisting level, following cold caloric stimulation of the left ear.

Radiologic examination showed an almost total absence of pneumatization of the mastoid processes (Fig. 6.10) and an aplasia of all three semicircular canals bilaterally with a questionable rudiment of a left superior canal (Figs. 6.11 and 6.12).

At *operation* (a right radical mastoidectomy for removal of cholesteatoma), the malleus, incus, and stapedial arch were found to be dysplastic. The oval window was poorly differentiated, and the facial nerve was exposed and followed an abnormal course along the inferior margin of the vestibular fenestra. There was no evidence of a cochlear fenestra.

Case 3. *Congenital severe progressive bilateral sensorineural hearing loss associated with recurrent episodes of rotatory vertigo, nausea, vomiting, nystagmus, and fluctuating hearing loss. Bilateral Mondini-type dsyplasia involving the cochlear capsule. Family history of temporal headaches, repeated attacks of vertigo and disequilibrium (brother, mother, and maternal grandmother).*

A girl 3 years 7 months old with a progressive bilateral hearing loss suspected to have occurred before the age of 3–4 months was seen. An audiogram by auditory brain response (ABR) at the age of 2½ years showed a threshold of 50 dB on the left and 60 dB on the right. Five months prior to admission, she woke up early one morning vomiting, went back to sleep, and 2 hours later woke up again vomiting, was very dizzy, and was observed to have a spontaneous horizontal and torsional nystagmus lasting 30 seconds. The nystagmus recurred every couple of hours during the next 48 hours. She had had no preceding viral syndrome. Three months later she fell backward and hit her head, did not lose consciousness, but 4 hours later developed vertigo, disequilibrium, and nystagmus lasting 24 hours. The next day the mother noticed that the child was not responding to sound at all in either ear. She was admitted and started on intravenous steroids.

Neuro-otologic examination on admission disclosed no evidence of dysmorphic features. The tympanic membranes were normal in appearance and mobility. No positive fistula test could be elicited. Pregnancy and delivery had been normal. The mother did not take any drugs during pregnancy, and the patient had not received any recognized ototoxic medications.

Cochlear function. No threshold could be obtained by play audiometry. The ABR during natural sleep disclosed no identifiable responses at 90 dB on the right and an equivocal response on the left.

Vestibular function. Evaluation of vestibular function by the neuro-otologist revealed no responses on the right and about normal responses on the left.

Radiologic examination. The axial CT scan of the temporal bones demonstrated a very prominent widening of the medial aperture of both cochlear aqueducts and of the internal auditory canals. The configuration of the cochlear capsule appeared somewhat unusual in that 1½ turns of the cochlea could be identified, compared with 2½ turns usually observed (Fig. 6.13). The neuroradiologist believed that the reduced number of cochlear turns may represent a Mondini type of cochlear malformation.

Operation. A right exploratory tympanotomy was performed for a possible perilymph fistula. The stapes was normally configured and mobile. No dehiscence was noted in the center of the footplate. The round window niche was normally configured. There was no visible leak of perilymph in the central region of the footplate, in the annular ligament, in the round window membrane, and in areas of the fissula ante fenestram and fissula post fenestram on Valsalva maneuver. The oval and round windows were packed with fibrous tissue. Two weeks postoperatively, the patient developed a transient Horner's syndrome on the left side that was considered to represent a form of ophthalmoplegic migraine. There was no return of cochlear function.

Case 4. *Bilateral Mondini-type malformation involving cochlea, lateral semicircular canal, endolymphatic duct and sac, internal auditory canal, and medial aperture of cochlear aqueduct. Perilymph fistula at left fissula ante fenestram. History of severe bilateral sensorineural hearing loss since birth with delayed speech and language development. Sudden onset of fluctuating hearing loss in left ear at age 15 years. Postoperative closure of perilymph fistula with revision 8 months later.*

A 20-year-old man with a history of bilateral moderately severe hearing loss since birth and delayed development of speech and language was seen. At the age of 8, he suffered a dramatic drop of hearing in the left ear and since then has had a continuous fluctuating hearing loss with significant drops and partial return of hearing at ages 10 and 14 years.

Otologic examination at age 15 years revealed normal tympanic membranes. Cochlear function studies disclosed a severe bilateral sloping sensorineural hearing loss with an SRT for the right ear of 85 dB with no measurable discrimination and an SRT for the left ear of 75 dB with 56% discrimination.

Radiologic examination with axial and coronal CT scans of the temporal bones suggested a malformation of the cochlea with 1½ cochlear turns and a common scala for the upper middle and apical turn. Both lateral semicircular canals were slightly hypoplastic with a reduced diameter. Both endolymphatic ducts and endolymphatic sacs were greatly distended. The internal auditory canals were somewhat widened, and the medial aperture of the cochlear aqueducts was visibly enlarged. All of these aberrations were somewhat more pronounced on the left side (Fig. 6.14).

Operations. A left exploratory tympanotomy was performed for closure of a perilymph fistula. Except for an abnormally low and shallow anterior oval window margin, all middle ear structures appeared unremarkable. When the mucoperiosteum was elevated from that area, a brisk accumulation of clear fluid was encountered of what seemed to be the external aperture of the fissula ante fenestram. That area and both windows were packed in the usual fashion. Postoperatively, the patient's hearing remained stable for 8 months, then suddenly dropped again, and the left ear was reexplored. Again, there was a suspicion of a perilymph fistula in the area of the fissula ante fenestram, and the region was repacked. A 6-month postoperative audiogram disclosed the left ear with a stable 60-dB SRT and a discrimination score of 100%.

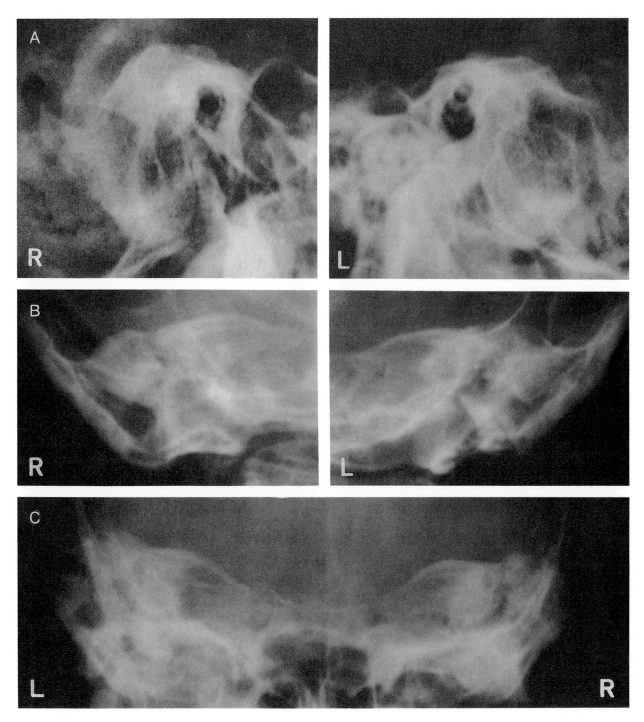

Figure 6.10.   A. The Schüller projection of the temporal bones shows almost no mastoid air cell development on either side. **B.** In the Stenvers view, the cochlear capsule is recognized, but all three semicircular canals are absent bilaterally. **C.** In the occipital view, no semicircular canals can be identified on either side.

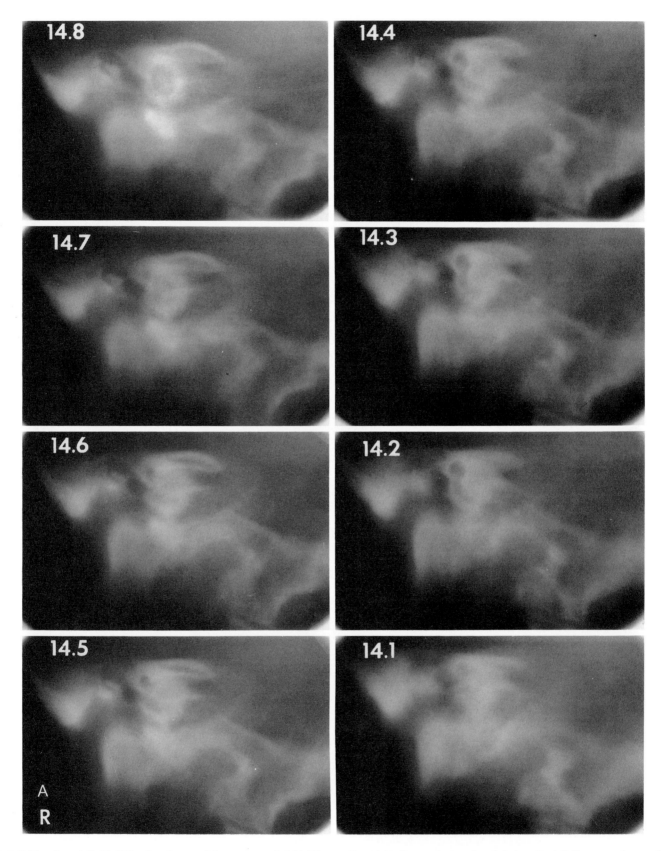

Figure 6.11. A and **B.** Multidirectional coronal tomograms of right **(A)** and left **(B)** temporal bones at corresponding levels. The external auditory canals display an unusual configuration and a certain vertical orientation. Malleus and incus appear dysplastic and are laterally rotated. On the right, all semicircular canals are absent, but on the left, there may be a rudiment of a superior canal. The labyrinthine and the mastoid segment of the Fallopian canal are unremarkable. The osseous structure of the oval window niche seems denser than usual, especially on the left.

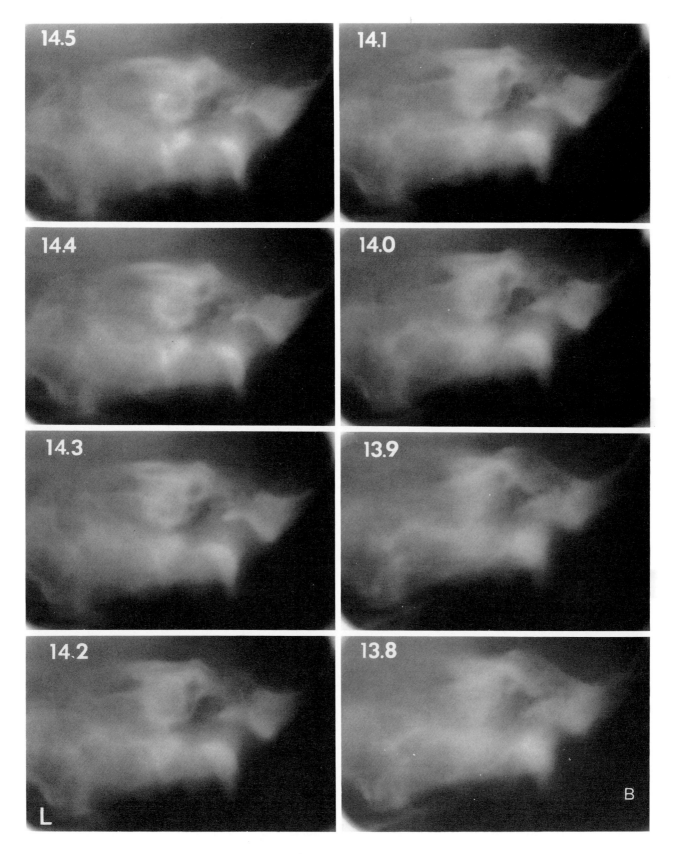

Figure 6.11.   B.

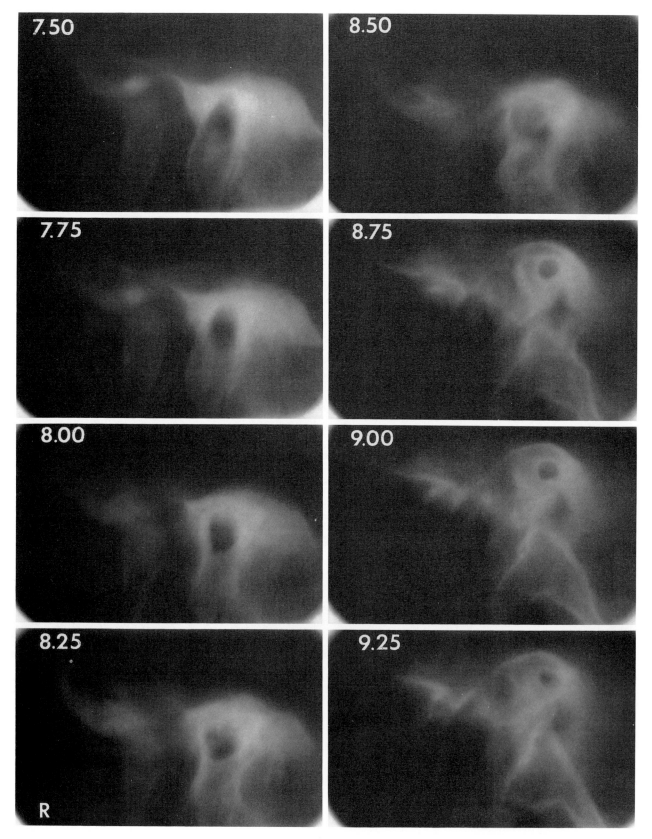

Figure 6.12. Multidirectional lateral tomograms of the right temporal bone display a vestibular space but no semicircular canals.

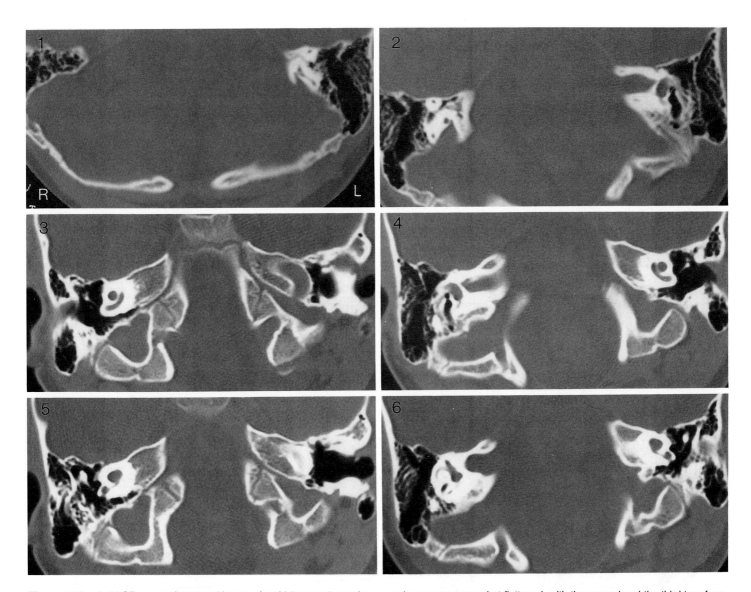

Figure 6.13.   Axial CT scans of temporal bones of a girl 3 years 7 months old with bilateral Mondini-type malformation involving the cochlear capsule, internal auditory canals, and cochlear aqueducts. The cochlear capsule appears somewhat flattened, with the second and the third turn forming a common cavity. The internal auditory canals and the medial apertures of the cochlear aqueduct are distended. (Courtesy of Dr. D. Mattox.)

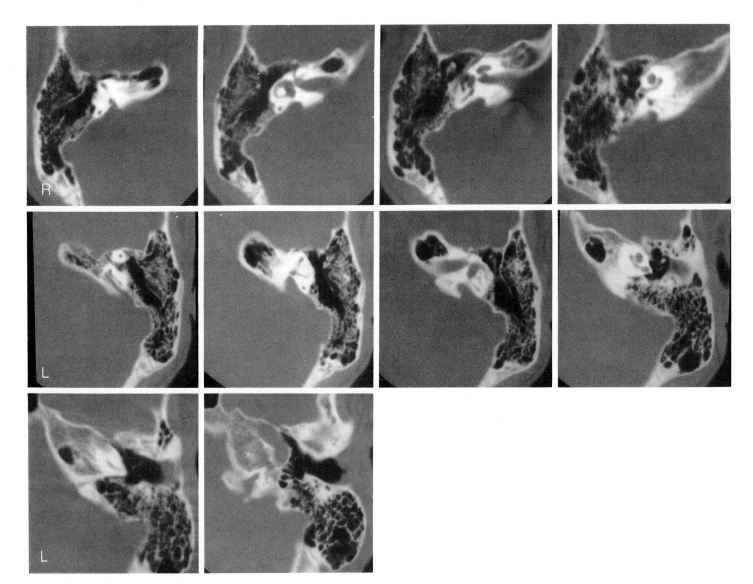

Figure 6.14. Axial CT scans of temporal bones of a 20-year-old man with bilateral Mondini-type malformation. The cochlear capsules appear somewhat flattened, with 1½ turns, with the upper middle and apical turn forming a common cavity. The lateral semicircular canals are slightly hypoplastic with a reduced diameter. The internal auditory canals are widened, and the medial apertures of the cochlear aqueducts are enlarged. (Courtesy of Dr. D. Mattox.)

Case 5. *Bilateral Mondini-type malformation of cochlea associated with 1½ turns and a common scala for the upper middle and apical turn. Surgically documented perilymph fistula at left fistula ante fenestram. Possible additional perilymph fistula in area of left round window niche. Normal speech and language development up to age 2 years. Recurrent episodes of spontaneous left-beating horizontal nystagmus associated with severe disequilibrium (inability to sit, stand, and walk, with nausea and vomiting), lasting between 1 and 3½ days. Noticeable retardation in further speech and language development after last episode of nystagmus and ataxia. Bilateral, moderately severe sensorineural high-tone loss.*

A 3-year-old girl with normal speech and language development during the first 2 years of life was seen. She had had recurrent episodic truncal ataxia associated with left-beating horizontal nystagmus, nausea, and vomiting since the age of 12 months, lasting up to 3½ days. After the most recent, fifth episode at the age of 2 years, which was 7 months prior to admission, she was observed to have made no further progress in her speech and language development.

The family history revealed a maternal grandfather with a hearing loss attributed to noise exposure. The mother has had a history of episodes of vertigo lasting for an entire day that have occurred approximately every other year for 10 years. During these episodes she is completely incapacitated and must remain in bed. However, she has never had any tinnitus or hearing loss. Both parents suffer from migraine headaches. There was no family history of dominant hereditary paroxysmal ataxia, congenital lues, or endolymphatic hydrops.

The patient gave no history of ear infections, head injuries, or exposure to Lyme disease.

Otologic examination at age 2 years 5 months revealed normal tympanic membranes with no discernible fluid in the middle ears. Cochlear function studies showed a bilateral hearing loss of 60–70 dB at 2000–4000 Hz, with an SRT of 40 dB on the right and 50 dB on the left and prolonged latency between wave III and V of her BSER, consistent with a cochlear lesion.

Radiologic examination. Serial, axial and coronal CT scans of the temporal bones disclosed normally configured cochleae with recognizable 1½ turns and a somewhat distended space suggesting the possibility of a common scala of the upper middle and apical turn of the cochlea. The internal auditory canals were enlarged, but the endolymphatic duct and sac and the medial aperture of the cochlear aqueduct were not widened.

Operation. Exploration of the left tympanic cavity disclosed the oval window niche, the intercrural space of the stapes, and the niche of the round window covered by mucosal membranes. After removal of the membrane over the oval window, a definite leakage of clear fluid, which increased during the Valsalva manuever, was discovered at the middle ear aperture of the fissula ante fenestram. After removal of the membrane overlying the round window, it appeared that there possibly was a small leak of clear fluid in the area of that niche. The oval and the round window niche and the fissula ante fenestram were packed in the usual fashion. Postoperatively, the child has had no further episodes of nystagmus and ataxia, and sound field right ear aided testing using play audiometry disclosed what was believed to be a reliable SRT of 20 dB.

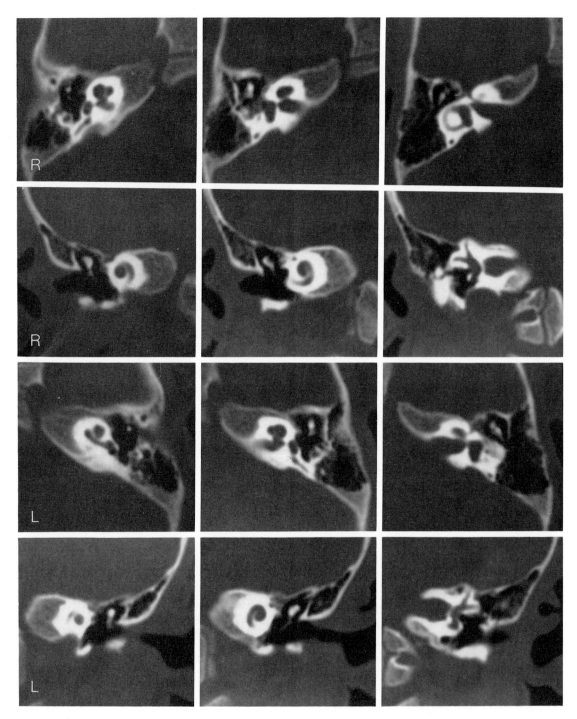

Figure 6.15. Axial and coronal CT scans of temporal bones of a 3-year-old girl with bilateral Mondini-type malformation of cochlea and perilymph fistula at middle ear aperture of left fissula ante fenestram. The cochlea reveals a normal configuration with discernible 1½ turns and a slightly ectatic space, suggesting a common scala of the upper middle and apical turn. The internal acoustic meati are distended, but there is no evidence of an enlargement of the endolymphatic duct, the sac, and the medial orifice of the cochlear aqueduct. (Courtesy of Dr. D. Mattox.)

DISCUSSION

The designation congenital, as applied to deafness, concerns cases in which the developmental anomaly or disease entity is present at or about the time of birth. It comprises the genetically determined diseases and those that result from environmental influences during the prenatal and perinatal period. Differentiation between inherited deafness and deafness acquired during embryonic life becomes a problem in the more common recessive forms in which a positive family history is lacking (67).

The prevailing assumption today is that about 35–50% of profound childhood deafness is determined by Mendelian inheritance of single genes (68). Genetic deafness includes many different entities that vary considerably in distribution and incidence among the various populations. The autosomal recessive forms account for 60–70% of the cases. The autosomal dominant forms account for about 20–30%. The amount of hearing loss varies considerably in individuals that carry the responsible mutant allele (68). A small group of patients, about 2%, with mutant alleles on the X-chromosome account for deafness inherited in a sex-linked fashion (68).

The other 50% of patients with profound childhood deafness owe their hearing loss primarily to acquired causes. Maternal ingestion of ototoxic drugs (thalidomide and chloroquine phosphate), maternal viral infections (prenatal rubella, cytomegalovirus, and herpes virus infections), metabolic diseases, and radiation exposure are such examples.

In the remaining number of cases, a profound childhood deafness may be associated with perinatal problems. These include severe jaundice, birth injuries, hemorrhages, reactions to administration of drugs, hypoxia, and anoxia.

Developmental anomalies of the middle ear accompanied by congenital deafness are often part of a broader malformation syndrome. Although some may be inherited in a simple Mendelian manner, more complex etiologic mechanisms are involved in the majority of congenital malformations (68). The assumption is that such malformations result from interactions between multiple factors, some of which are genetic, while others are of environmental origin. Frequently, one or the other will predominate. The thalidomide and rubella embryopathies are examples of conditions in which environmental factors play a predominant roll (68). The teratogenic effect of thalidomide to some extent depends on the genotype of the mother and the fetus, and in the rubella embryopathy the genome of the virus probably represents an additional factor (68). It is possible that in many instances, multiple genes are involved in profound childhood deafness (68, 69). In situations of polygenic inheritance, the mechanism may involve interaction between several genes, each of which has a small effect but interact synergistically to produce a major developmental aberration (69). In such instances, the morphologic changes often include malformations of the outer, middle, and inner ear. Similar malformations may also be encountered in chromosomal aberrations (trisomies 13–15, 18, and 21), which likewise share a complex genetic origin. By contrast, in the simply inherited profound deafness of childhood, the morphologic changes are limited to the cochlear duct and saccule and reflect a degeneration at a cellular level involving the organ of Corti, stria vascularis, first cochlear neuron, and the configuration and macula of the saccule.

Evaluation and management of profound prelingual deafness involve a team effort that, depending on the nature of the problem, includes the expertise of the pediatrician, otologist, neurologist, audiologist, geneticist, microbiologist, and pathologist of the ear and temporal bone. The continuous accumulation of histopathologic information gained from various carefully documented malformations and degenerative processes will, it is hoped, lead to a better understanding of the pathogenesis of the different forms of profound deafness in children and adults and, ultimately, to control and prevention of some of these conditions and their emotionally heavy burdens.

References

1. Mündnich K, Terrahe K. Missbildungen des Ohres. In: Berendes J, Link R, Zöllner F, eds. Hals-Nasen-Ohren Heilkunde in Praxis und Klinik, Ohr I. Stuttgart: Georg Thieme, Chap 18, 1979;5:1–49.
2. Terrahe K. Missbildungen des Innen- und Mittelohres als Folge der Thalidomidembryopathie. Fortschr Geb Röntgenstr 1965;17:102.
3. Scholtz HJ. Probleme der Vestibularis-Untersuchung bei Ohrmissbildungen mit Fehlen aller Bogengänge. Z Laryngol Rhinol 1967;46:758.
4. Jensen J. Tomography of the inner ear in Waardenburg syndrome. AJR 1967;51:828.
5. Partsch CJ. Angeborene Ohrmissbildungen als Ursache der Taubheit. Ann Univ Sarav Med 1971, cited in Reference 1.
6. Terrahe K. Diagnostik der Missbildungen des Ohres und des Ohrschädels. Arch Ohren Nasen Kehlkopfheilkd 1972;85:202.
7. Donaldson GA, Anson BJ. Surgical anatomy of the facial nerve. Symposium on disease and injury of the facial nerve. Otolaryngol Clin North Am 1974;7(2):289–308.
8. Mondini C. Anatomico surdi nati sectio: De bononsiensi scientiarum et artium instituto atque academia commentarii. Bononiae 1791;7.
9. Scheibe A. Ein Fall von Taubstummheit mit Acusticus-Atrophie und Bildungsanomalien im häutigen Labyrinth beidseits. Z Ohrenheilkd 1892;22:11.
10. Scheibe A. Bildungsanomalien im häutigen Labyrinth bei Taubstummheit. Z Ohrenheilkd 1895;27:93.
11. Siebenmann F, Bing R. Über den Labyrinth und Hirnbefund bei einem an Retinitis pigmentosa erblindeten angeborenen Taubstummen. Z Ohrenheilkd 1907;54:265.
12. Virchow R. Über Missbildungen am Ohr. Virchows Arch Pathol Anat Physiol 1864;30(1):221–239.
13. Marphan A-D. Paralyse faciale congenitale. Soc Med Hop 1901;1007.
14. Jorgensen MB, Kristensen HK, Buch NH. Thalidomide-induced aplasia of the inner ear. J Laryngol 1964;78:1095–1101.
15. Alexander G. Zur Pathologie und pathologischen Anatomie der kongenitalen Taubheit. Arch Ohren Nasen Kehlkopfheilkd 1904;61:183.
16. Siebenmann F. Grundzüge der Anatomie und Pathologie der Taubstummheit. Wiesbaden: JF Bergmann, 1904.
17. Marx H. Die Missbildungen des Ohres. In: Henke F, Lubarsch O, eds. Handbuch der speziellen pathologischen Anatomie und Histologie, Bd XII: Gehörorgan. Berlin: Julius Springer, Chap 7, 1926;XII:609–734.
18. Lange W. Aplasie des Ganglion spirale und des Nervus cochlearis als Ursache angeborener Taubheit. Arch Ohren Nasen Kehlkopfheilkd 1914;93:123–133.
19. Nager FR. Missbildungen der Schnecke und Hörvermogen. Z Hals Nasen Ohrenheilkd 1925;11:149–176.
20. Schuknecht FH. Pathology of the ear. Cambridge, Massachusetts: Harvard University Press, 1974:198.
21. Altmann F. The inner ear in genetically-determined deafness. Acta Otolaryngol (Stockh) 1964; Suppl 187(4):1–39.
22. Bergstrom L, Hemenway WG, Downs MP. A high risk registry to find congenital deafness. Otolaryngol Clin North Am 1971;4:369–399.
23. Konigsmark BW, Gorlin RJ. Genetic and metabolic deafness. Philadelphia: WB Saunders, 1976.
24. Proctor CA, Proctor B. Understanding hereditary nerve deafness. Arch Otolaryngol 1967;85:45–62.
25. Frazer GF. Profound childhood deafness. J Med Genet 1964;1:118–161.
26. Chung CS, Brown KS. Family studies of early childhood deafness ascertained through the Clark School for the Deaf. Am J Hum Genet 1970;22:630–644.

27. Huizing EH. Hereditare Innenohrschwerhörigkeit. In: Berendes J, Link R, Zöllner F, eds. Hals-Nasen-Ohren Heilkunde in Praxis und Klinik. Ohr II. Stuttgart: Georg Thieme, Chap 40, 1980;6:1–26.

28. Fay EA. Marriages of the deaf in America. Washington, DC: Volta Bureau, 1898.

29. Sank D. Genetic aspects of early total deafness. In: Rainer JD, Altschuler K, Kallmann F, eds. Family and mental health problems in a deaf population. Springfield, Illinois: Charles C Thomas, 1963;28–81.

30. Müller E. Vestibularisstörungen bei erblicher Taubheit. Arch Ohren Nasen Kehlkopfheilkd 1936;142:156–163.

31. Altmann F. Histologic pictures of inherited nerve deafness in man and animals. Arch Otolaryngol 1950;51:852–890.

32. Dolowitz DA, Stephens FE. Hereditary nerve deafness. Ann Otol Rhinol Laryngol 1961;70:851–859.

33. Huizing EH, van Bolhuis AH, Odenthal DW. Studies on progressive hereditary perceptive deafness in a family of 355 members. Acta Otolaryngol (Stockh) 1966;61:35–41, 161–167.

34. Huizing EH, Odenthal DW, van Bolhuis AH. Results of further studies on progressive hereditary sensorineural hearing loss. Audiology (Basel) 1972;12:261–263.

35. Teig E. Hereditary progressive perceptive deafness in a family of 72 patients. Acta Otolaryngol (Stockh) 1968;65:365–372.

36. Belluci RJ. Congenital aural malformations, diagnoses and treatment. Otolaryngol Clin North Am 1981;14(1):95–124.

37. Smith AB. Unilateral hereditary deafness. Lancet 1939;2:1172–1173.

38. Everberg G. Unilateral anacusis. Clinical, radiological and genetic investigations. Acta Otolaryngol (Stockh) 1960; Suppl 158:366–374.

39. Everberg G. Etiology of unilateral total deafness. Ann Otol Rhinol Laryngol 1906;69:711–721.

40. Everborg G. Further studies on hereditary unilateral deafness. Acta Otolaryngol (Stockh) 1960;51:615–635.

41. Vanderbilt University Hereditary Deafness Study Group. Dominantly inherited low-frequency hearing loss. Arch Otolaryngol 1968;88:242–250.

42. Konigsmark BW, Mengel MC, Berlin CI. Familial low-frequency hearing loss. Laryngoscope 1971;81:759–771.

43. Konigsmark BW, Salman S, Haskins H, Mengel MC. Dominant mid-frequency hearing loss. Ann Otol Rhinol Laryngol 1970;79:42–54.

44. Paprella MM, Sugiura S, Hoshino T. Familial progressive sensorineural deafness. Arch Otolaryngol 1969;90:44–51.

45. Crowe SJ, Guild SR, Polvogt LM. Observations on the pathology of high-tone deafness. Bull Johns Hopkins Hosp 1934;54:315–380.

46. Nance WE, McConnell FE. Status and progress of research in hereditary deafness. Adv Hum Genet 1974;4:173–250.

47. Valsalva AM. Valsalvae opera et Morgagni epistolae. Venetiis, 1741.

48. Valsalva AM. Tractus de aure humano. Lugduna, Cap II. X, p 24, 1942.

49. Steinberg D, Neumann OG. Zur Genese der Otosklerose: eine Literatur Übersicht. HNO 1973;21:257–263.

50. Frazer GR. The causes of profound deafness in childhood. Baltimore: Johns Hopkins University Press, 1976.

51. Mengel MC, Konigsmark BW, McKusick VA. Two types of congenital recessive deafness. EENT Monthly 1969;48:301–305.

52. Konigsmark BW, Mengel MC, Haskins H. Familial congenital moderate neural hearing loss. J Laryngol 1970;84:495–505.

53. Konigsmark BW. Congenital nonprogressive moderate neural hearing loss. Birth Defects 1971;7(4):140.

54. Barr B, Wedenberg E. Prognosis of perceptive hearing loss in children with respect to genesis and use of hearing aid. Acta Otolaryngol (Stockh) 1964;59:462–474.

55. Mengel MC, Konigsmark BW, Berlin CI, McKusick VA. Recessive early onset neural deafness. Acta Otolaryngol (Stockh) 1967;64:313–326.

56. Dow GS, Poynter CI. The DAR family. Eng News 1930;15:128–130.

57. Frazer GR. Sex-linked recessive congenital deafness and the excess of males in profound childhood deafness. Ann Hum Genet 1965;29:171–196.

58. McRae KN, Uchida IA, Lewis M. Sex-linked congenital deafness. Am J Hum Genet 1969;21:415–422.

59. Mohr J, Mageroy K. Sex-linked deafness of a possible new type. Acta Genet (Basel) 1960;10:54–62.

60. Livan M. Contributo alla conoscenza delle sordita ereditarie. Arch Ital Otol 1961;72:331–339.

61. Pelletier LP, Tanguay RB. X-linked recessive inheritance of sensorineural hearing loss during adolescence. Am J Hum Genet 1975;27:609–613.

62. Nance WE, Setleff RC, McLeod A, Sweeney A, Cooper C, McConnel F. X-linked mixed deafness with congenital fixation of the stapedial footplate and perilymphatic gusher. Birth Defects 1971;7(4):64–69.

63. Glasscock ME. The stapes gusher. Arch Otolaryngol 1973;98:82–91.

64. Brown MR. The factor of heredity in labyrinthine deafness and paroxysmal vertigo. Ann Otol Rhinol Laryngol 1949;58:665–670.

65. Bernstein JM. Occurrence of episodic vertigo and hearing loss in families. Ann Otol Rhinol Laryngol 1965;74:1011–1021.

66. McKusick VA. Mendelian inheritance in man. 7th ed. Baltimore: Johns Hopkins University Press, 1971.

67. Lindsay JR. Inner ear pathology in congenital deafness. Otolaryngol Clin North Am 1971;4(2):249–290.

68. Paparella MM, Schachern PA. Sensorineural hearing loss non-genetic and genetic. In: Paparella MM, Shumrick DA, Gluckman JL, Meyerhoff WI, eds. Otolaryngology, Vol II: Otology and neuro otology. 3rd ed. Philadelphia: WB Saunders, Chaps 40–41, 1991; II:1561–1599.

69. Frazer GR. The genetics of congenital deafness. Otolaryngol Clin North Am 1971;4(2):227–247.

7/ Variations and Anomalies Involving the Facial Canal

All components of the temporal bone are subject to variations and anomalies. These aberrations involve the formation of the bony portions that together constitute the temporal bone, the extent of pneumatization, the size and configuration of the middle ear cavity, the differentiation of the middle ear structures, and the development of the otic and vestibular capsule. They also involve the location and anatomy of the facial canal, the architecture of the internal and external auditory meatus, the position of the endolymphatic sac, the localization of the major blood vessels, and the persistence of certain embryonic vascular structures.

The facial canal, as it traverses the temporal bone, may display congenital bony dehiscences and variations and anomalies of its usual course and, in a rare instance, include a large persisting embryonic artery or vein. Each of these features may have clinical and surgical significance. The otologic surgeon needs to be familiar with, suspect of, and identify these variations and anomalies preoperatively, in order to avoid an injury to the facial nerve.

CONGENITAL BONY DEHISCENCES IN THE FACIAL CANAL

It is not surprising that the facial canal may be defective, since it is composed of two separate embryologic structures, the primordial otic capsule and Reichert's cartilage from the second branchial arch (1). In the 10-week-old fetus, the facial "canal" is a deep sulcus in the canalicular portion of the primordial otic capsule. At that time the otic capsule is entirely cartilaginous. Reichert's cartilage becomes attached to the otic capsule and provides the remaining cartilaginous circumference to the labyrinthine and the tympanic segment of the facial canal. Its ossification begins just about at that time. This contribution from Reichert's cartilage persists as a readily identifiable histologic structure through the first postnatal year. By the end of the first year, ossification is generally completed. In some instances, closure of the facial canal is never fully accomplished, and in localized areas or dehiscences the canal remains open to the mucoperiosteum of the middle ear just as in fetal life the tissue of the facial sulcus is continuous with the mesenchyme beneath the epithelium of the expanding tympanic cavity (1).

A gap in the continuity of the osseous wall may be observed in any portion of the facial canal; most gaps, however, are observed along the tympanic segment (Fig. 7.1). Such dehiscences may involve the inferior, lateral, and medial walls. They are located most frequently above and posterior to the oval window and occasionally at the cochleariform process over the lateral aspect of the geniculate ganglion. The remaining gaps are found along the mastoid segment and, very rarely, over the superior aspect and medial to the geniculate ganglion. Their great-

est width varies from 0.5 to 3 mm. As a rule, they are less numerous and smaller in a well-pneumatized temporal bone, and they are regularly observed bilaterally, symmetrical in size and location. The presence of more than one dehiscence is not unusual.

The most accurate information concerning their incidence, size, and location has been derived from histological examination of serially sectioned temporal bones. Baxter (2) examined 535 temporal bones from 332 individuals from the collection of the Massachusetts Eye and Ear Infirmary. His observation revealed an incidence of 55%. Ninety-one percent of dehiscences were located in the tympanic segment, and 9% were located in the mastoid segment. Of all dehiscences in the tympanic segment, 83% were located adjacent to the oval window and involved the lateral, inferior, and medial portions of the canal, with the facial nerve protruding from its canal in 26%. Their greatest diameter ranged from 0.5 to 3.1 mm. In less than 1% (0.8%) did a dehiscence involve the entire length of the tympanic segment. Of all the dehiscences in the mastoid segment, 79% opened into the facial recess, and 21% opened into the tympanic sinus or into the retrofacial cells, with the nerve protruding from its canal in 12%. Their greatest diameter ranged from 0.4 to 2 mm. Baxter's findings are very similar to those of Dietzel's (3) who had examined 211 temporal bones and found an incident of 57%, identical predilective sites, and comparable dimensions. The frequency of dehiscences in the facial canal is, therefore, sufficient to regard them as a variation rather than as an anomaly.

Guild (4) emphasized the clinical and surgical significance of congenital bony dehiscences. Since Politzer (5) wrote about them in his textbook in 1894, numerous aural surgeons have reported observation of these dehiscences.

Dehiscences in the tympanic segment of the facial canal may lead to an inferior protrusion of the nerve from its canal (Figs. 7.1–7.4). This protrusion may vary from a slight bulge of the nerve through a small opening, to a situation in which the greater portion of the nerve has emerged from the facial canal and has come to lie on the superior aspect of the crural arch and on a portion of the footplate of the stapes (Figs. 7.3 and 7.4). Occasionally, the entire lateral and inferior circumference of the facial canal may be missing around the posterior crus of the stapes, leaving the facial nerve widely exposed (Fig. 7.5). That such an exposed nerve has a higher risk of becoming involved in an inflammatory process (Fig. 7.6) or any form of injury is readily understandable. Similarly, a facial nerve injury may result, for instance, from elevation of the middle cranial fossa dura during an approach to the trigeminal nerve in a patient with a bony dehiscence in the labyrinthine segment of the facial canal, above or just medial to the geniculate ganglion (Fig. 7.7). The observation that in a dehiscence the mucoperiosteum of the middle

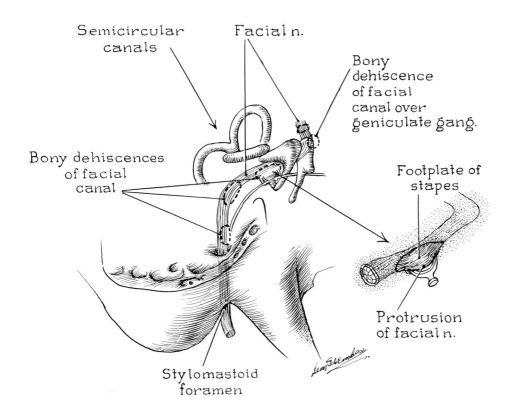

Figure 7.1. Locations of bony dehiscences in facial canal.

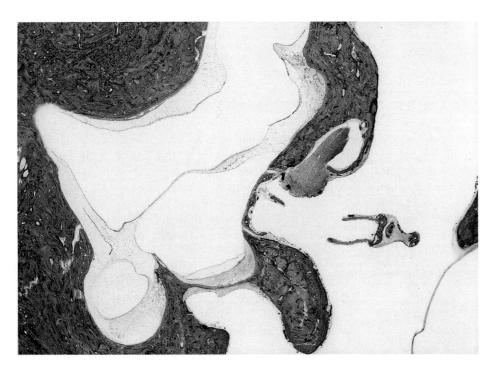

Figure 7.2. Vertical section through left temporal bone at level of vestibular and cochlear fenestrae in adult. Facial nerve partially protrudes through congenital dehiscence in the inferior wall of the tympanic segment of the facial canal. (Hematoxylin and eosin, ×16.)

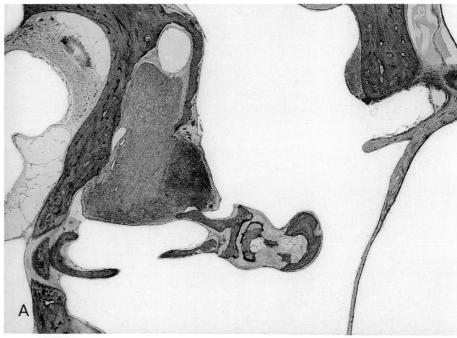

Figure 7.3. A. Vertical section through left temporal bone at posterior end of stapes footplate in an adult. Abnormal vein (persistent lateral capital vein) occupies one-third of facial canal. Major portion of facial nerve lies outside canal on posterior crus of stapes. Its lateral portion reveals early asymptomatic schwannoma. (Hematoxylin and eosin, ×12.)

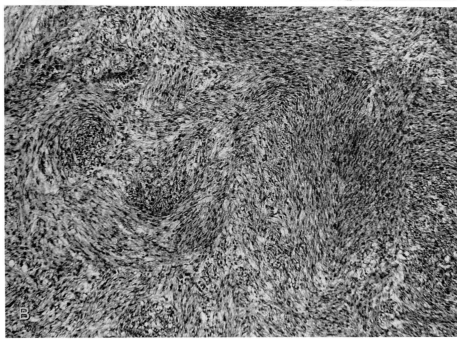

Figure 7.3. B. Tumor is composed of interwoven bundles of long biopolar spindle cells with ovoid or rod-shaped central nuclei containing variable amounts of chromatin and inconspicuous nucleoli (type A tissue of Antoni). (×250.)

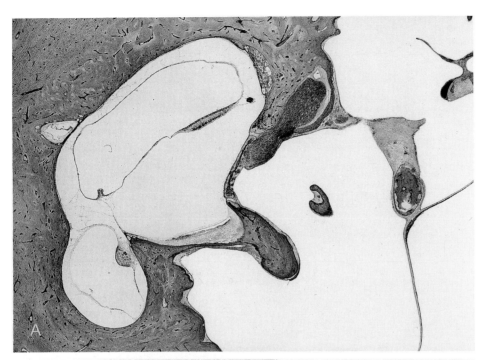

Figure 7.4. A. Vertical section through left temporal bone at center of stapes footplate in an adult. Almost half of the facial nerve protrudes into the oval window niche through a congenital dehiscence in the floor of the facial canal. (Hematoxylin and eosin, ×15.)

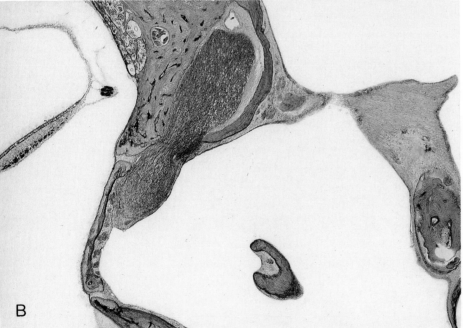

Figure 7.4. B. Extracanalicular portion of facial nerve covers cranial half of stapes footplate in its entire length. There is no separation between epineurium of nerve and mucoperiosteum of footplate. (×30.)

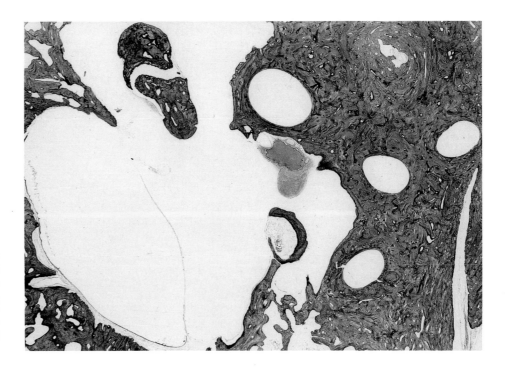

Figure 7.5. Vertical section through right temporal bone at junction of tympanic membrane with mastoid segment of facial canal in an adult. Congenital absence of the lateral, the inferior, and some of the medial portion of the bony canal wall resulted in almost total exposure of the facial nerve in that location. (Hematoxylin and eosin, ×12.)

ear is in direct apposition to the epineurium may explain the potential effect on the facial nerve of a local anesthetic in the middle ear. The inferior sagging of the seventh nerve through a bony defect above the oval window (Fig. 7.1) should not be confused with an aberrant course of the facial canal in that particular area (see Fig. 7.9G).

A dehiscence in the lateral wall of the facial canal at the geniculate ganglion exposes the nerve to the anterior epitympanic recess. Care, therefore, must be exercised when disease is eradicated from that area (6). Similarly, the aural surgeon must be aware of the frequent occurrence of dehiscences in the lateral, inferior, and medial walls of the facial canal above and posterior to the oval window (4, 7). A dehiscence over the vestibular fenestra may be so large as to permit the facial nerve to slide out of its bony canal and rest on the stapedial arch, where it may produce a conductive hearing loss (Fig. 7.3). Marked protrusions of an exposed facial nerve have been observed by many surgeons and reported in the literature (8). Their occasional presence in middle ear dysplasia is well recognized (9). Many years ago, the author discovered a small asymptomatic schwannoma in a herniated facial nerve in this location in the left temporal bone of a patient (Fig. 7.3). A subsequent report of a tumor-like herniation of the tympanic portion of the right facial nerve in a 17-year-old girl (10) raises the question of a possible causal relationship. Of interest in this respect are the observations by Babin et al. (11) of "traumatic" neurinomas of the facial nerve in such a herniation in two patients with a history of long-standing chronic otitis media.

ANATOMICAL VARIATIONS IN THE COURSE OF THE FACIAL CANAL

The labyrinthine segment of the facial canal extends from the fundus of the internal acoustic meatus to the geniculate ganglion across the long axis of the petrous pyramid. It varies in length between 2.5 and 6 mm (12). The tympanic segment runs from the geniculate ganglion posteriorly to the lateral semicircular canal in a more or less inclined plane parallel to the axis of the pyramid. As it courses along the medial wall of the tympanic cavity above the oval window, it follows an oblique direction from inside out. It varies in length from 7 to 11 mm (12). The mastoid segment generally runs straight downward from the posterior margin of the oval window to the stylomastoid foramen. Its length varies between 9 and 16 mm (13). It may form a slight anterior, posterior, or medial curve when viewed laterally (Fig. 7.8C–E). In most instances, its course is straight downward. In some patients, however, the stylomastoid foramen is located more laterally, when viewed from behind, and in such instances the mastoid segment of the facial canal follows an outward oblique direction instead of a vertical direction (Fig. 7.8F). Rarely does the mastoid segment follow an inward oblique course.

ANATOMICAL ANOMALIES OF THE COURSE OF THE FACIAL CANAL

In addition to the variations, there are a number of recognized anomalies involving the course of the facial canal. These anomalies are seldom encountered in the normally developed temporal bone but are frequently observed in its malformations.

Fowler (14) collected the most pertinent forms from the literature and depicted them in a diagrammatic manner. Whereas the observations involving the mastoid segment may be found in a normally developed temporal bone, the ones involving the tympanic segment are frequently associated with dysplasia of the stapes, lack of differentiation, or agenesis of the oval window. Severe dysplasia of the middle and the inner ear is, with few exceptions, regularly accompanied by an aberrant course of the facial canal. The anomalies of the course of the facial canal may be conveniently classified according to the level at which they involve the facial nerve or the segment of the facial canal in which they are encountered.

Canalicular Segment Anomalies

In an exceptional instance the facial nerve, instead of entering through the internal acoustic meatus, may enter the petrous pyramid across the subarcuate fossa and run through the center of the superior semicircular canal to the stylomastoid foramen, bypassing the middle ear cavity (Fig. 7.9A) (15). Rarely, a bifurcation of the nerve may be encountered within the internal auditory canal.

Labyrinthine Segment Anomalies

Rare cases of a bifurcation of the facial nerve within the labyrinthine segment of the facial canal were described by Altmann (16) and by Miehlke and Partsch (17).

Tympanic Segment Anomalies

Aberrations in the course of the facial nerve in the tympanic segment of the facial canal can be subdivided into the following categories:

1. Facial nerve coursing along the superior aspect of the lateral semicircular canal (Fig. 7.9B)
2. Bifurcation of the facial nerve anterior or proximal to the oval window (Fig. 7.9C–F)
3. Facial nerve coursing horizontally over the oval window (Fig. 7.9G)
4. Facial nerve coursing through the stapedial arch (Fig. 7.9H and I)
5. Facial nerve coursing posteriorly between the oval and the round window (Fig. 7.9J)
6. Facial nerve coursing posteriorly inferior to the round window (Fig. 7.9K)
7. Facial nerve coursing from the geniculate ganglion straight downward over the promontory (Fig. 7.9L)
8. Hypoplasia of the facial nerve (Fig. 7.9N, X, and Y)

H. P. House (personal communication) has seen the facial nerve coursing along the superior aspect of the lateral semicircular canal in two instances (Fig. 7.9B). One observation was in a cadaver; the other was in a patient scheduled for a fenestration operation.

Bifurcation of the facial nerve anterior to the oval window is commonly associated with developmental anomalies of the vestibular fenestra and stapes wherein the greater or lesser portion of the nerve may run above or below the totally or partially

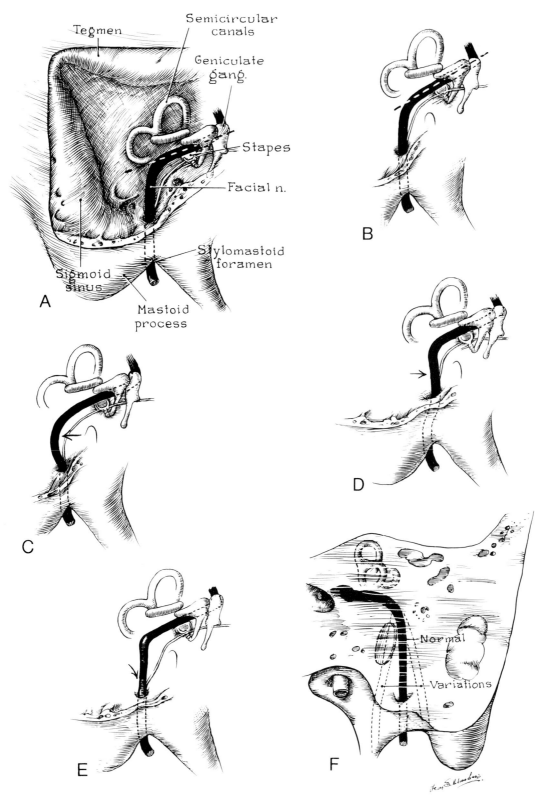

Figure 7.8.   Variations in course of facial nerve.

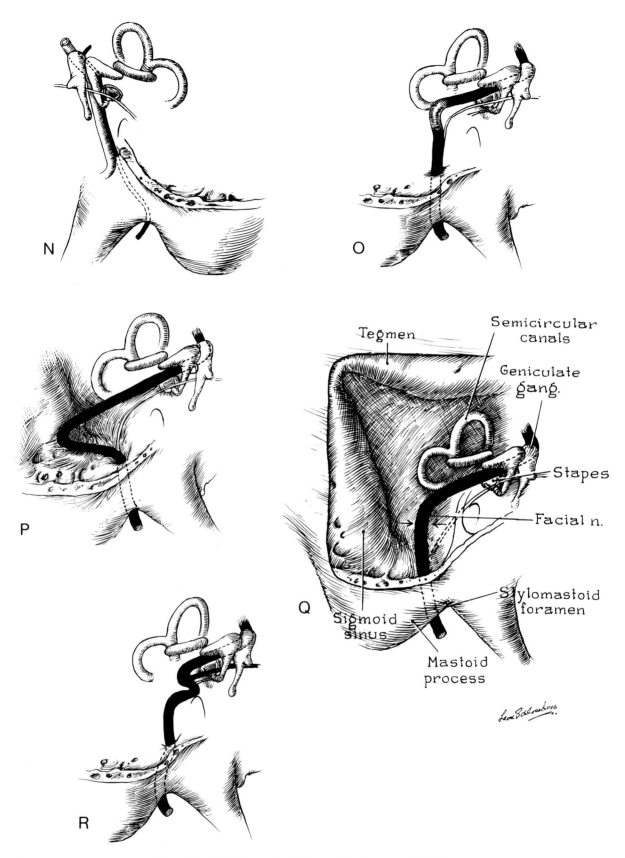

Figure 7.9.   N–Q. Anatomical abnormalities in course of facial nerve.

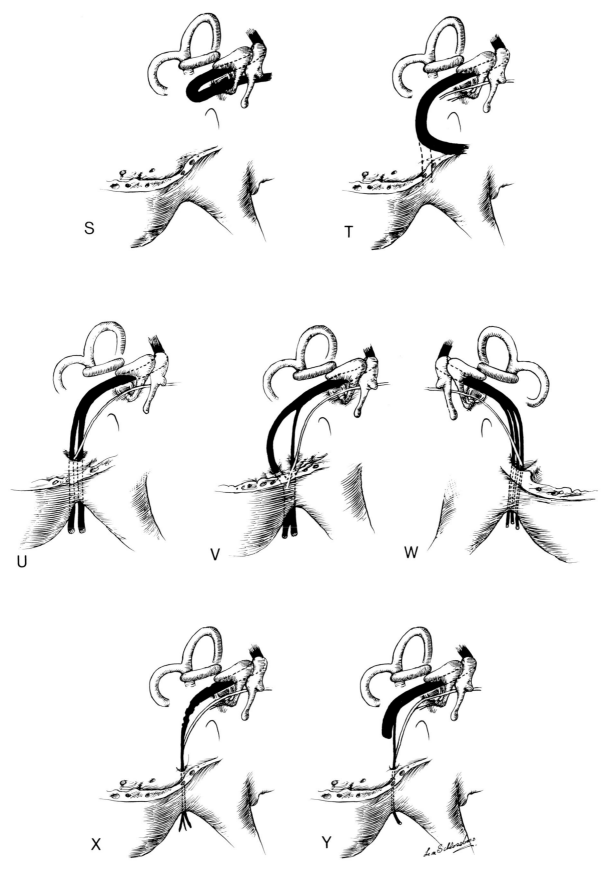

Figure 7.9.   R–Y. Anatomical abnormalities in course of facial nerve.

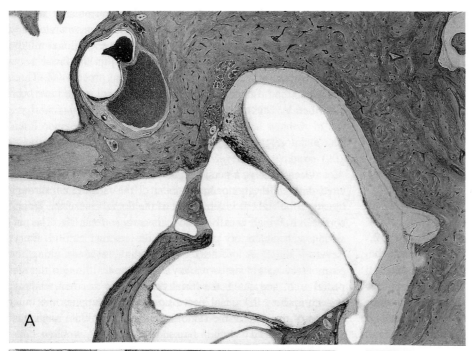

Figure 7.10. **A.** Vertical section through right temporal bone at level of cochleariform process in an adult. Abnormally large vein (persistent lateral capital vein) occupies half of lumen of tympanic segment of facial canal. (Hematoxylin and eosin, ×10.)

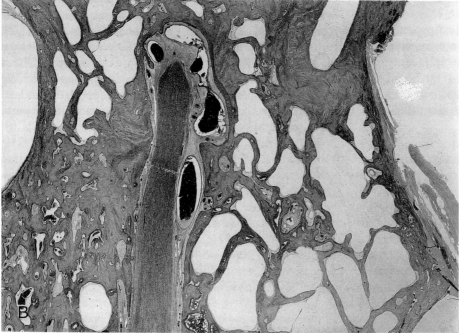

Figure 7.10. **B.** Same abnormal vein is seen accompanying right facial nerve in mastoid segment of facial canal. (×10.)

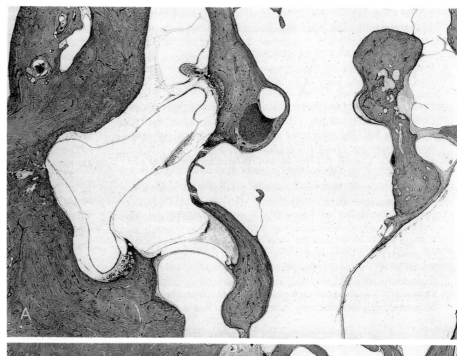

Figure 7.11.   A. Vertical section through left temporal bone of same patient as in Figure 7.10A at level of oval and round windows. Abnormal vein, accompanying facial nerve, is well recognized. (Hematoxylin and eosin, ×12.)

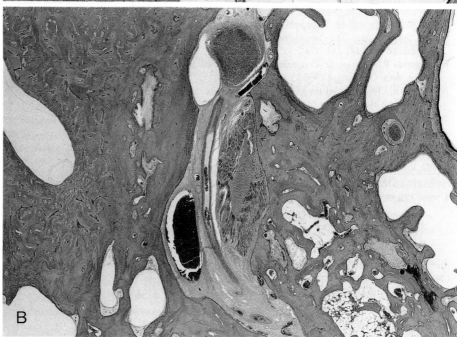

Figure 7.11.   B. Same abnormal vein accompanies left facial nerve and stylomastoid artery in mastoid segment of facial canal. (×16.)

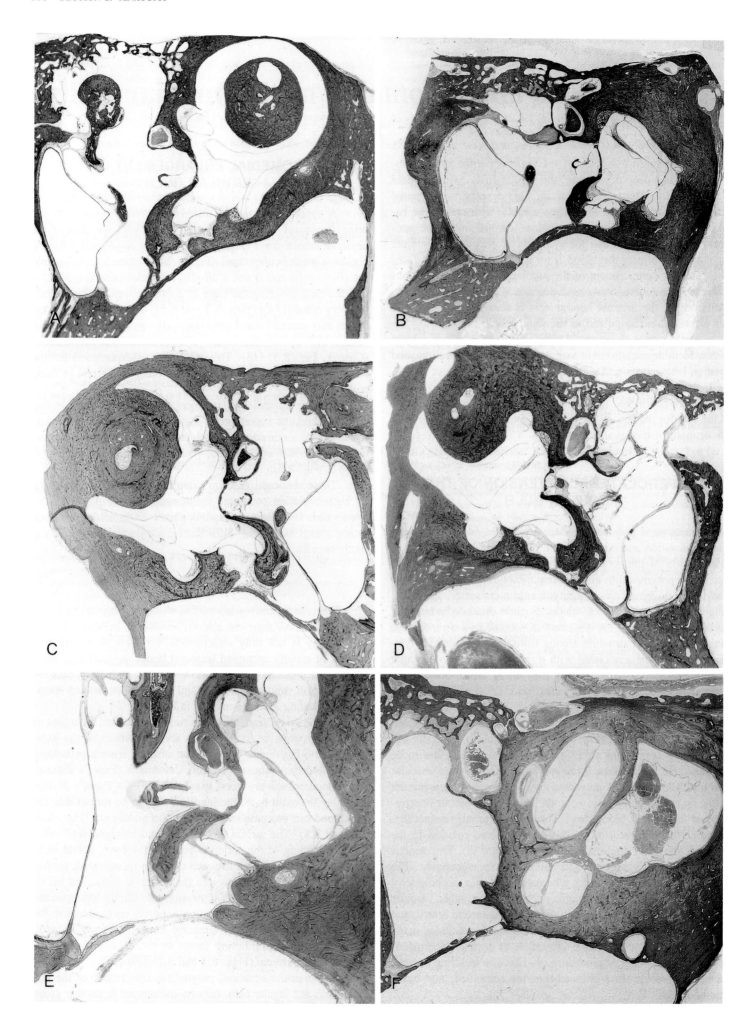

Figure 8.1 *(opposite page).* **A.** Vertical section through right temporal bone at level of superior semicircular canal in a 67-year-old man. A superomedial extension of the jugular bulb has eroded the posterior cortex of the pyramid and exposed the posterior fossa dura and endolymphatic sac. **B.** Vertical section through right temporal bone near center of oval window in a 48-year-old man. The superolateral extension of the jugular bulb caused a complete occlusion of the round window at this level. **C.** Vertical section through left temporal bone at level of oval and round windows in a 42-year-old man. A superolateral extension of the jugular bulb resulted in an elevation and obvious atrophy of the floor of the hypotympanum and an almost total obliteration of the round window niche. **D.** Vertical section through left temporal bone at level of superior semicircular canal in a 44-year-old woman. The severe superomedial and lateral distension of the jugular bulb caused a marked atrophy of the floor of the middle ear cavity and a subtotal occlusion of the round window. **E.** Vertical section of right temporal bone at level of oval and round windows in a 52-year-old man. The obvious elevation of the floor with its near-total bony destruction resulted from a marked superior extension of the jugular bulb. **F.** Vertical section through right temporal bone in a 48-year-old man. The partial destruction of the elevated floor of the hypotympanum and erosion of the posterior cortex of the petrous pyramid have been caused by an obvious superior, medial, and lateral extension of the jugular bulb. (Hematoxylin and eosin, ×7.5, ×7.5, ×7.5, ×7.5, ×7.5, and ×8, respectively.)

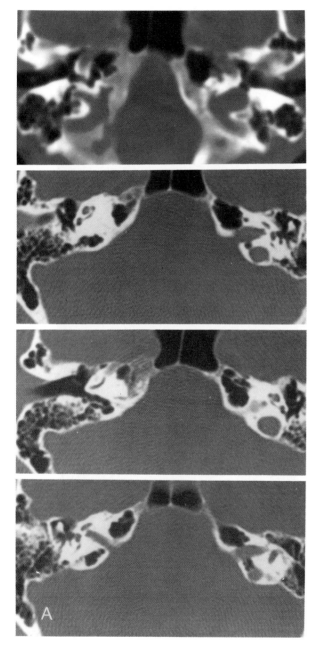

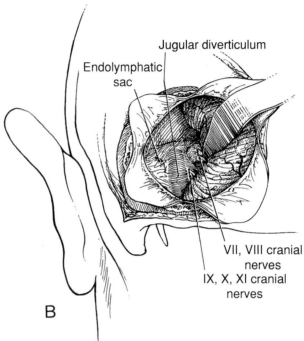

Endolymphatic sac

Jugular diverticulum

VII, VIII cranial nerves

IX, X, XI cranial nerves

B

Figure 8.5. **A.** Axial CT scans of the petrous pyramids reveal funnel-shaped medial enlargement of the left IAC. Just posterior to the IAC, one recognizes the medial extension of the jugular bulb *(arrows).* **B.** Drawing of observations during exploration of left cerebellopontine angle. The superior and medial enlargement of the jugular bulb extends behind the IAC up to the level of the roof of the acoustic meatus. It has exposed the meatal dura and is protruding slightly into the canal lumen. The vestibular schwannoma is just pouting out from the porus acusticus. (Courtesy of Dr. D. W. Kennedy.)

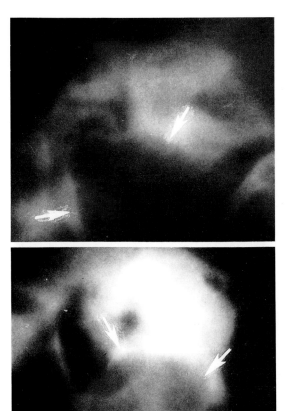

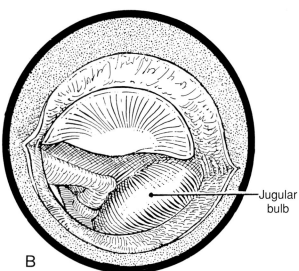

Jugular
bulb

Figure 8.6.   A. The anteroposterior *(upper left)* and lateral *(lower left)* multiplanar tomograms of the right temporal bone demonstrate the marked superior, medial, and lateral distension of the jugular bulb and its close relationship to the vertical segment of the Fallopian canal *(upper left)* and to the posterior fossa dura *(lower left)*. **B.** Drawing of findings encountered at right exploratory tympanotomy. The jugular bulb displays a remarkable superior and lateral extension into the middle ear cavity to the level of the inferior oval window margin. It completely obliterates the round window niche and is totally covered by bone. (Courtesy of Dr. D. W. Kennedy.)

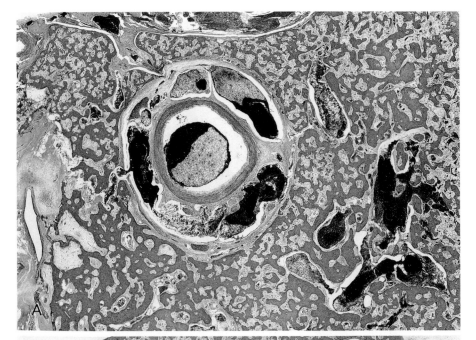

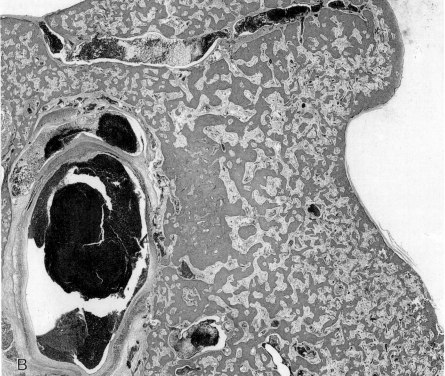

Figure 8.9.   A and **B.** Vertical sections through right petrous apex near anterior wall of IAC in a 74-year-old woman with widespread active Paget's disease. Several large venous lakes and channels representing extensive arteriovenous shunting collect blood from many areas and empty into a markedly distended pericarotid venous plexus that, in turn, drains into the enormously enlarged internal jugular vein, bilaterally (see Fig. 8.8*B*). (Hematoxylin and eosin, ×8.)

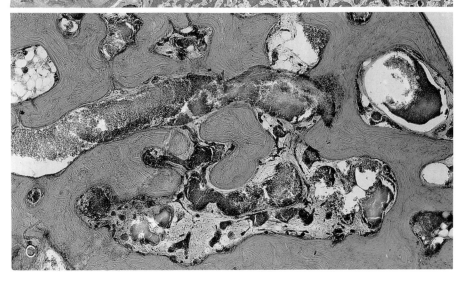

Figure 8.9.   C. Numerous arteries within the bone ramify and shunt arterial blood across venous lakes of varying size into the pericarotid venous plexus (×40.)

of abnormal bone remodeling processes including certain craniotubular scleroses, sclerosteosis (Van Buchem's disease), and osteopetroses (16, 17). In these instances, increased deposition of lamellar bone and lack of bone resorption lead to progressive narrowing of the vascular and neural foramina in the base of the skull (Fig. 8.10). This eventually leads to impairment of cranial nerve function, reduction of venous drainage from the brain, and, finally, a steady increase of intracranial pressure (16). Certain disorders of bone remodeling may, therefore, produce either an acquired enlargement, deformity, and herniation of the jugular bulb into the middle ear or IAC or a progressive narrowing of the IAC, other neural foramina, the sigmoid sinus, and the jugular foramen (16, 17).

Case Reports

The following two cases demonstrate the surgical consequences of an abnormal extension of the jugular bulb.

Case 1. *Left intracanalicular vestibular schwannoma with funnel-shaped enlargement of internal auditory canal (IAC). Medial and superior extension of enlarged jugular bulb behind IAC to level of roof of meatus with protrusion into canal lumen. Removal of tumor through a suboccipital approach with preservation of near-normal hearing and discrimination.*

A 51-year-old woman with persistent unsteadiness was seen. Cochlear function studies of the left ear revealed a minimal high-frequency sensorineural loss, a normal discrimination score, a Short Increment Sensitivity Index (SISI) score, acoustic reflexes, and absence of tone decay. The auditory brain stem responses, however, disclosed a wave V latency delayed more than for standard deviations. Electronystagmography disclosed a mild spontaneous left-beating nystagmus but bilateral normal semicircular canal reflexes to caloric stimulation.

The enhanced CT scan showed enlargement of the left IAC (Fig. 8.5A). The jugular bulb was larger on the left side and extended to the level above the floor of the IAC. A contrast cisternogram disclosed a filling defect of the IAC extending slightly outside the porus acusticus (Fig. 8.5B).

The suboccipital approach to the IAC was chosen. The intracanalicular tumor extended to the porus acusticus. Elevation of the posterior fossa dura uncovered a bluish superior and medial extension of the jugular bulb, posterior to the midportion of the IAC, to the

level of the roof of the meatus. The tumor was totally removed. During displacement of the jugular bulb, a small laceration of the sinus wall occurred. Bleeding was easily controlled.

Postoperatively, the audiogram revealed a slight increase of the preexisting high-frequency loss in the left ear. The speech reception threshold (SRT) was 25 dB, and the discrimination score was 88%. The histologic diagnosis was schwannoma (Fig. 8.5A and B).

Case 2. *Unusually marked enlargement of right jugular bulb superiorly, medially, and laterally, covered by a thin shell of bone extending into the middle ear cavity to inferior oval window margin. Complete obliteration of round window niche. No impingement on ossicular chain. Conductive hearing loss in right ear. Findings compatible with a congenital anomaly of the right jugular bulb.*

A 24-year-old woman with a history of decreased hearing in the right ear, first noticed in childhood when she also had multiple episodes of acute otitis media, was seen. A right exploratory tympanotomy done elsewhere at the age of 12 showed apparently no evidence of a middle ear anomaly and an intact and mobile ossicular chain. A right traumatic tympanic membrane perforation in her adolescence healed spontaneously.

Otoscopic examination disclosed a right tympanic membrane with a localized retraction of a flaccid posterior pars tensa, adherent to the long crus of the incus. No abnormalities of the middle ear structures were identified. Cochlear function studies showed a flat mixed hearing loss in the right ear with an SRT of 35 dB and a discrimination score of 100%. Hearing was normal on the left. The tuning fork referred from the vertex to the right, where bone conduction was greater than air conduction. The acoustic reflex was absent when measured from the right ear with the left ear stimulated.

Conventional x-rays of the right temporal bone showed decreased pneumatization and secondary sclerosis of the air cells system. Multiplanar tomograms disclosed an unusually large right jugular bulb but no other abnormalities (Fig. 8.6A).

At *operation*, reexploration of the right ear was elected with the anticipation of finding a fibrous or bony fixation of the ossicular chain or a blockage in the attic. Reflection of the tympanic membrane disclosed a normally mobile ossicular chain but an abnormally enlarged jugular bulb covered by a thin shell of bone. The bulb extended superiorly to the inferior oval window margin. It completely obliterated the round window niche (Fig. 8.6B). No attempt was made to displace the jugular bulb inferiorly. The procedure was terminated after the small retraction pocket had been medially reinforced with a fascial graft.

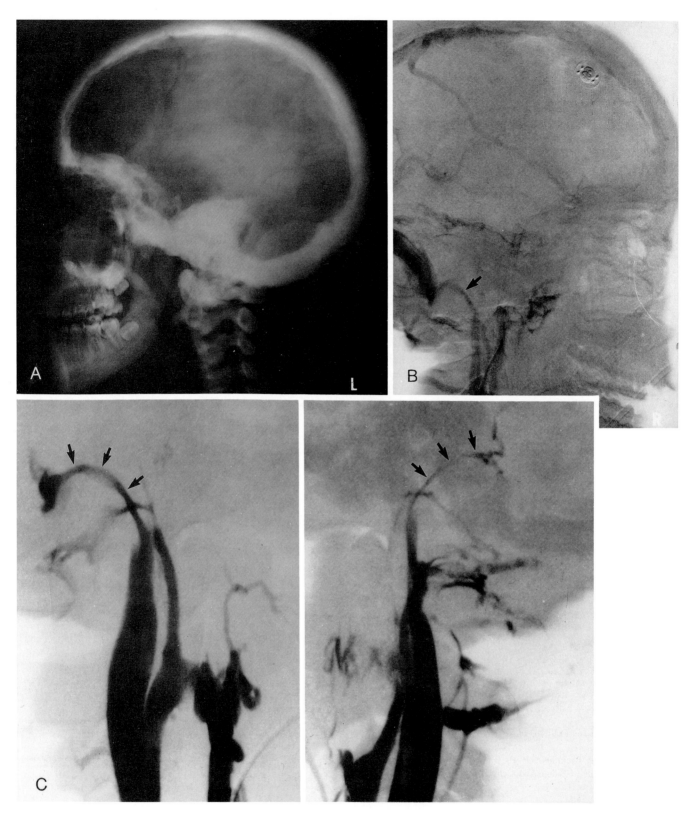

Figure 8.10. **A.** Lateral radiograph of the skull of a girl 10 years 9 months old with sclerosteosis and a family history of three distant relatives reported to have the same disease. The striking increase in thickness and density of most bones is most prominent in the base of the neurocranium, especially in the temporal bones. No mastoid air cells are visible. The hyperostenosis and sclerosis of the inner and outer table of the calvaria apparently obliterated the diploë. **B.** Venous phase of carotid angiogram, right lateral subtraction study. The almost-total occlusion of the right sigmoid sinus and jugular bulb is clearly evident *(arrows).* It resulted from concentric narrowing of the osseous vascular channel by the progressive apposition of periosteal bone. **C.** The right and left retrograde jugular venograms confirm the thread-like lumen of the left jugular bulb and sigmoid sinus *(arrows)* and the extreme narrowing of the right jugular bulb *(arrows).*

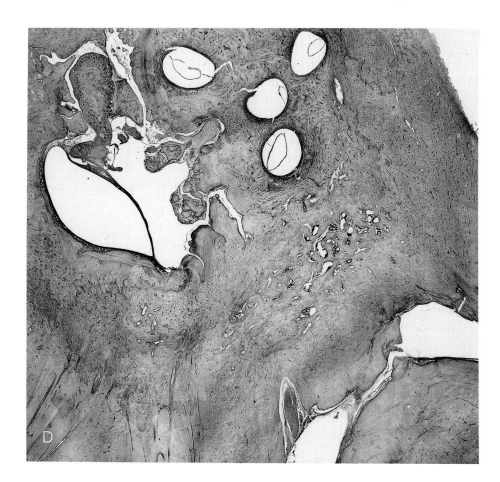

Figure 8.10. D. Vertical section through right temporal bone at level of jugular bulb of a 31-year-old Afrikaner who died suddenly, presumably from acute compression of the medulla oblongata associated with progressive increase of intracranial pressure. A broad-based hemispherical proliferation of periosteal bone almost completely obliterated the already severely reduced vascular lumen *(arrow)*. (Hematoxylin and eosin, ×4.8.)

References

1. Beck C. Antomie und Histologie des Ohres. In: Berendes J, Link R, Zöllner F, eds. Hals-Nasen-Ohrenheilkunde in Praxis und Klinik. Ohr I. Stuttgart: Georg Thieme, Chap 2, 1979;5:1–60.

2. Gejrot T. Retrograde jugulography in the diagnosis of abnormality of the superior bulb of the internal jugular vein. Acta Oto-laryngol (Stockh) 1964;57:177–80.

3. Abul-Naga G. Transbasale Venenabflüsse im und am Foramen jugulare. Anat Anz 1964;113:369.

4. Overton A, Ritter F. A high placed jugular bulb in the middle ear: a clinical and temporal bone study. Laryngoscope 1973;83:1986–1991.

5. Zorzetto NL, Tamega OJ. The anatomical relationship of the middle ear and the jugular bulb. Anat Anz 1979;146:470–482.

6. Hentzer E. Objective tinnitus of the vascular type. Acta Otolaryngol (Stockh) 1968;66:273–281.

7. Chandler J. Diagnosis and cure of venous hum tinnitus. Laryngoscope 1983;199:892–895.

8. Much O. Über die Beeinflussung der Blutzirkulation im Schädelinnern durch die sogenannte Sternocleidostellung des Kopfes. Münch Med Wochenschr 1912;1:151.

9. Page JR. A case of probable injury to the jugular bulb following myringotomy in an infant ten months old. Ann Otol Rhinol Laryngol 1941;23:61–63.

10. Robin PE. A case of upwardly situated jugular bulb in the left middle ear. J Laryngol 1972;186:1241–1246.

11. Hough JVD. Congenital malformations of the middle ear. Arch Otolaryngol 1963;78:335–343.

12. Smyth GD, Black JHA. A case report of protruding jugular bulb. Laryngoscope 1965;75:669–672.

13. Stern J, Goldberg M. Jugular bulb diverticula in medial petrous bone. AJR 1980;134:959–961.

14. Kennedy DW, El-Sirsi HH, Nager GT. The jugular bulb in otologic surgery: anatomic, clinical and surgical considerations. Otolaryngol Head Neck Surg 1986;94(1):6–15.

15. Nager GT. Paget's disease of the temporal bone. Ann Otol Rhinol Laryngol Suppl 22 1975;84(4):1–32.

16. Nager GT, et al. Sclerosteosis involving the temporal bone. Clinical and radiologic aspects. Ann J Otolaryngol 1983;4(1):1–17.

17. Nager GT. Sclerosteosis involving the temporal bone: histopathologic aspects. Ann J Otolaryngol 1986;7(1):1–16.

9/ Variations, Anomalies, and Pathology of the Intratemporal Carotid Artery

ANEURYSM

Aneurysms involving the intratemporal segment of the internal carotid artery have been reported in increasing numbers in recent years. Most of these aneurysms are congenital. They may be associated with a congenital defect in the walls of the carotid artery or with a preceding injury of the temporal bone (1). One predilective site is at the base of the skull just below the carotid foramen. They may be observed at any age, as early as during the second decade. They usually manifest themselves with transient ischemic episodes and Eustachian tubal obstruction. Extension of the aneurysm medially may eventually involve the optic chiasm. As the aneurysm extends laterally, it may block the Eustachian tube, involve the middle ear, and appear as a bright-red pulsating mass behind the lower tympanic membrane, occasionally impinging on the drum. It can therefore be mistaken for a paraganglioma. An aneurysm can suddenly thrombose or rupture and cause a massive hemorrhage through the Eustachian tube. Carotid angiography is indispensable in establishing the diagnosis and evaluating the situation. The management involves resection of that vascular segment and replacement by a graft from the saphenous vein inserted over a temporary polyethylene bypass (2).

ABERRANT LOCATION

An aberrant location of the internal carotid artery in the hypotympanum and lower mesotympanum may occasionally be encountered (see Fig. 9.10) (3–6). This situation may represent the sole abnormality. In other instances, it may result from a dysgenesis of the internal carotid artery, associated with a compensatory hypertrophy of the ascending pharyngeal, inferior tympanic, and caroticotympanic arteries (2). In the absence of the usual vascular connection between the internal maxillary artery and the middle meningeal artery, the latter receives blood from the petrosal artery via a persisting hypertrophic stapedial artery. No treatment is indicated in such situations. Ligation of

the stapedial artery is to be avoided, as this vessel may contribute significantly to the blood supply of the ipsilateral cerebral hemisphere. The carotid angiogram again clarifies the situation. The differential diagnosis includes a paraganglioma, other vascular neoplasms, and a high, exposed jugular bulb.

ABSCESS AND INFLAMMATORY NECROSIS

Rarely, coalescent osteitis in the petrous pyramid, more common in the apex region, can lead to an inflammation of the vessel wall with one or several abscesses and necrosis. Another source for a vasculitis can be an empyema in an adjacent pericarotid air cell or a thrombophlebitis of the pericarotid venous plexus as a complication of a chronic mastoiditis, a meningitis, and/or a thrombophlebitis of the superior longitudinal or lateral sinus (Fig. 9.1). Necrosis of the arterial wall may give rise to repeated hemorrhages (3–10).

TRAUMATIC LACERATIONS

Traumatic injuries are rare and may result from an extensive comminuted fracture or evulsion of the petrous pyramid or from a ballistic injury of the temporal bone. Such injuries are generally accompanied by massive arterial bleeding through the Eustachian tube.

ATHEROSCLEROSIS, MORPHOLOGIC CHANGES, AND ADHESIONS INVOLVING THE ARTERIAL WALL

The intratemporal segment of the carotid artery, as with other segments of this vessel, is often the site of arteriosclerotic changes that may lead to thickening, ulceration, calcification, and metaplastic ossification of the arterial wall. These changes, in turn, may give rise to thrombosis and partial or total occlusion of the vascular lumen (Figs. 9.2–9.4).

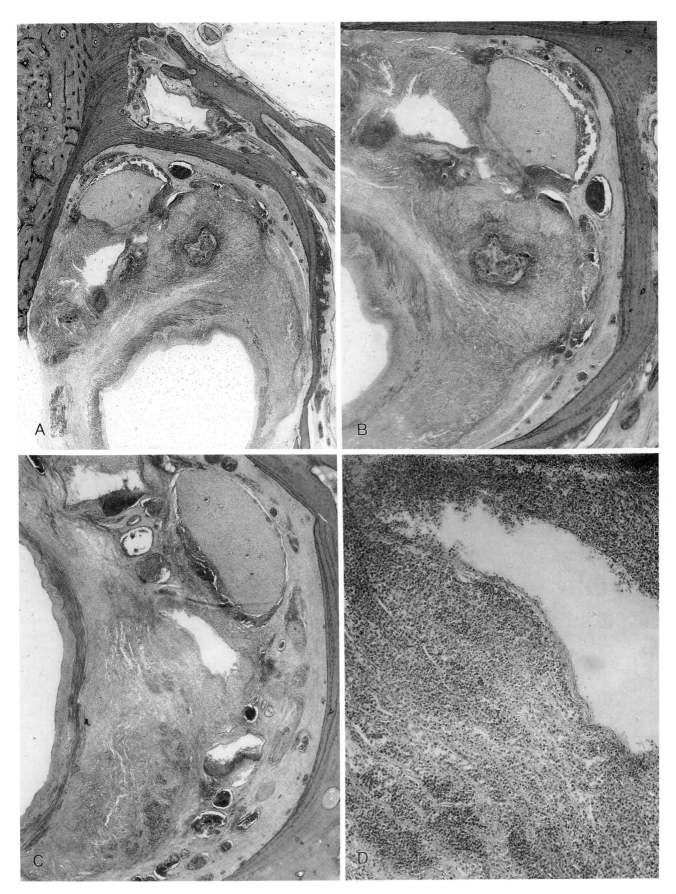

Figure 9.1. **A.** Vertical section through left petrous pyramid with cross-section through horizontal segment of internal carotid artery in a 30-year-old woman who died from purulent pachymeningitis and leptomeningitis. The meningitis was a complication of pansinusitis extending to both orbits and the superior longitudinal sinus. It shows a diffuse cellulitis involving the wall of the carotid and its pericarotid connective tissue sheath. **B.** A central abscess developed in the diffuse cellulitis involving the tunica ad-ventitia of the artery and its pericarotid sheath. **C.** Several of the veins that constitute the pericarotid venous plexus show evidence of acute throm-bophlebitis. **D.** Cross-section through a vein of the pericarotid venous plexus with evidence of acute thrombophlebitis. Necrosis and destruction of the venous wall have given rise to the pericarotid cellulitis and its central abscess. (Hematoxylin and eosin, ×25, ×27, ×50, and ×115, respectively.)

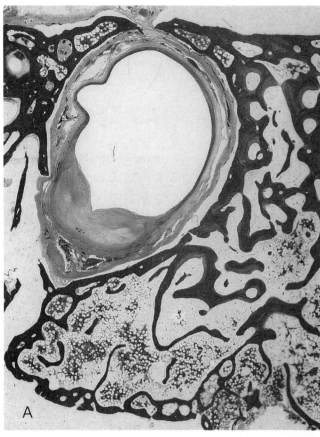

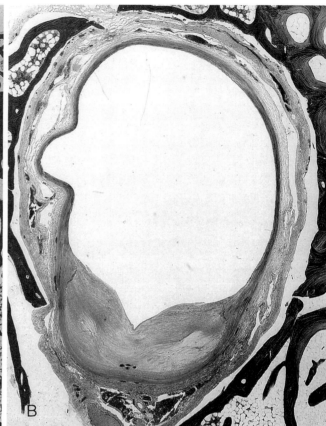

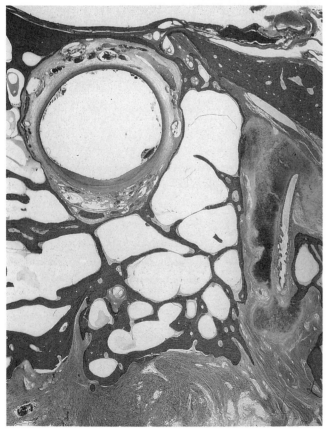

Figure 9.2. **A.** Vertical section through right petrous apex of a 24-year-old man who died from pulmonary tuberculosis. The intratemporal internal carotid artery reveals a circumscribed semilunar area of medial hypertrophy and intimal thickening with fibrosis, hyalinization, and beginning calcification. **B.** The tunica intima and the media are primarily affected. (Hematoxylin and eosin, ×7 and ×23, respectively.)

Figure 9.3. Vertical section through left petrous pyramid of a 43-year-old man who died from bilateral pulmonary tuberculosis. The intratemporal internal carotid artery exhibits a localized hypertrophy of the intima and the media. (Hematoxylin and eosin, ×6.5.)

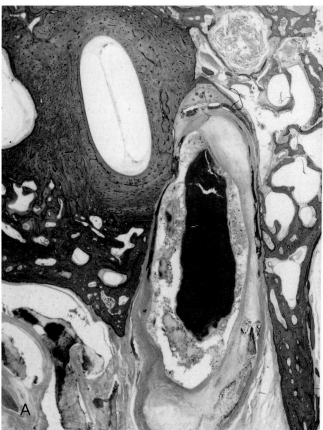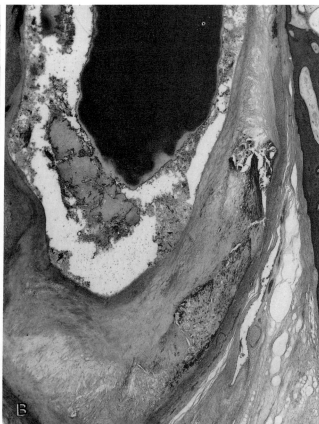

Figure 9.4. **A.** Vertical section through left temporal bone at level of bend of intratemporal internal carotid artery in a 78-year-old man who died from cerebral and bilateral frontal subdural hemorrhage with arteriosclerosis. The artery demonstrates extensive atheromatous changes with marked fibrosis, hyaline degeneration, and metaplastic calcification. **B.** Ulcerations of the intima and necrosis of the media resulted in obliterating thrombosis. (Hematoxylin and eosin, ×7 and ×27, respectively.)

Localized adhesions and atrophies of the vessel to the medial wall of the carotid canal are also of special interest to the neuro-otologic surgeon as he or she exposes and plans to displace that artery during procedures involving the petrous pyramid. Several examples in our collection portray this anomaly (Figs. 9.5–9.8). They may occur bilaterally, and their location near the junction of the ascending and the horizontal vascular segment is quite constant. In that region the medial wall of the artery can be extremely thin, represented only by the intima or a remaining portion of it or by a calcified plaque replacing it, firmly adherent to the underlying irregular bony surface (Figs. 9.5–9.8). The artery in that location also lacks its usual broad surrounding protective sheath of connective tissue containing the pericarotid venous and sympathetic nerve plexus (Figs. 9.5–9.8). The underlying bone of the cochlear capsule frequently displays a somewhat irregular protrusion into the lumen of the carotid canal (Figs. 9.6–9.8). It is presently unclear whether these bony irregularities play a role in the etiology of these localized vascular changes or whether they are a secondary phenomenon. These changes have been elegantly described by Guild (11, 12). Whereas circumscribed atrophy of the arterial wall, calcified plaques, or

both, without adhesions, has been observed in many instances, firm adhesions of the vessel to the underlying bone are not so rare, and the actual incidence has yet to be determined. They have been observed at all adult ages (personal observation). The surgeon, aware of such a situation, will remove the bone between the lateral cochlear capsule and the medial wall of the carotid canal with appropriate care. In some of our examples where the bony adhesion was associated with a subtotal or complete defect of the arterial wall, it would not have been possible to free the carotid artery successfully from the osseous canal wall. Even in situations where the carotid artery tends to resist forward displacement, the surgeon aware of the underlying factors will proceed with extreme caution, prepared to handle a vascular laceration and segmental resection by a saphenous vein graft over a temporary polyethylene bypass.

In rare instances, the wall of the internal carotid artery may exhibit a transverse ridge and/or longitudinal ridge that can protrude markedly into the vascular lumen. These ridges represent a duplication of the vessel wall and theoretically could have an influence on the hemodynamics (Fig. 9.9)

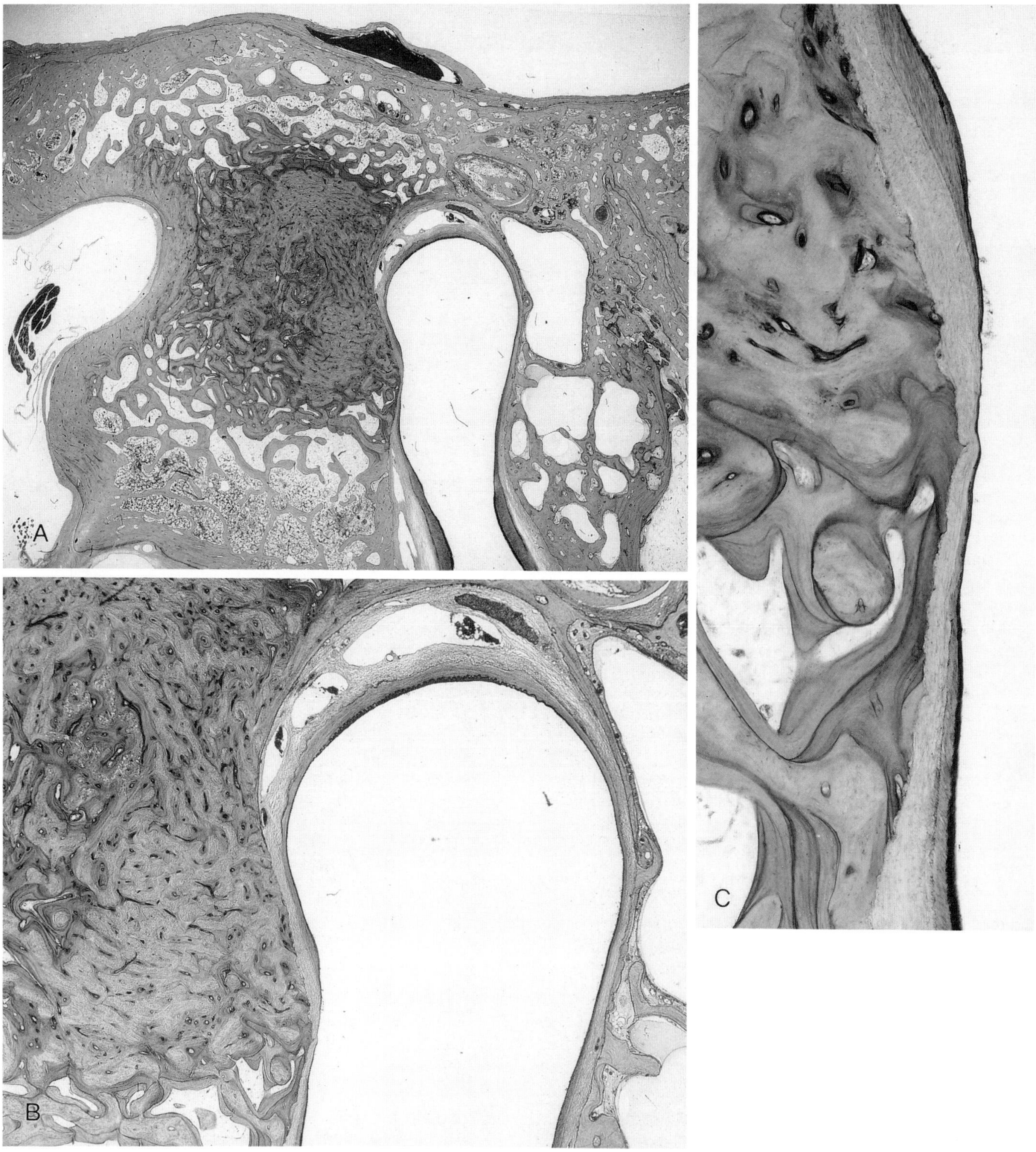

Figure 9.5. **A.** Vertical section through left temporal bone at level of ascending internal carotid artery in an 8-year-old girl. At the junction of the vertical and horizontal vascular segments, the arterial wall exhibits an obvious thinning, medially and laterally. **B.** The medial wall of the carotid reveals a more extensive atrophy. Its location is over a protrusion of the cochlear capsule. The pericarotid sheath of connective tissue, which contains the pericarotid venous and sympathetic plexus, is missing in both places where the vascular wall is atrophic. **C.** Atrophy of the carotid wall involves the tunica media and tunica intima most severely. (Verhoff stain, ×6, ×15, and ×55, respectively.)

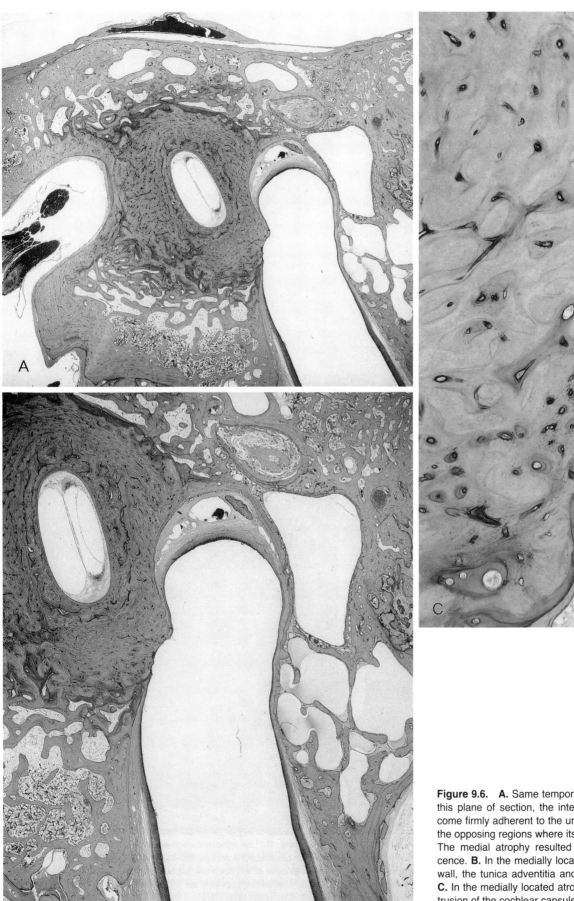

Figure 9.6.   A. Same temporal bone as in Figure 9.5. In this plane of section, the internal carotid artery has become firmly adherent to the underlying bony canal wall in the opposing regions where its wall has become atrophic. The medial atrophy resulted in a circumscribed dehiscence. **B.** In the medially located atrophy of the vascular wall, the tunica adventitia and tunica media are lacking. **C.** In the medially located atrophy overlying a lateral protrusion of the cochlear capsule, the irregular bony surface is covered solely and incompletely by an atrophic tunica intima. (Verhoff stain, ×6, ×15, and ×55, respectively.)

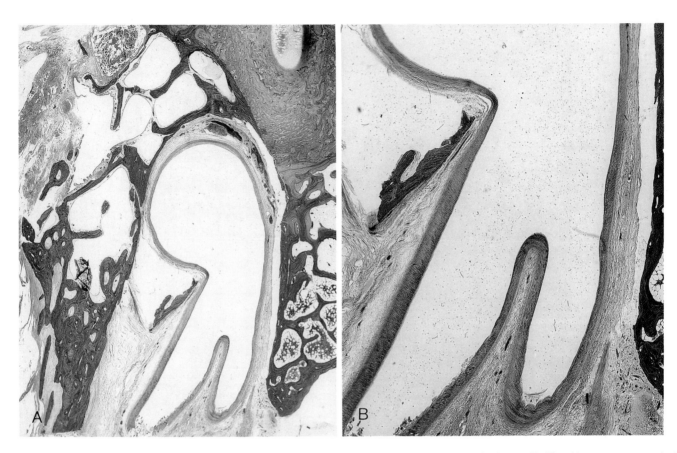

Figure 9.9. **A.** Vertical section through right temporal bone at level of anterior tangent of lower basal turn of cochlea in a 43-year-old man. The internal carotid artery displays two longitudinal ridges of the vessel wall that protrude into the vascular lumen. **B.** The ridges represent a duplication of the arterial wall, each with a three-layered structure. (Hematoxylin and eosin, ×7 and ×27, respectively.)

Case Report

Case 1. *Abnormal course of right intratemporal internal carotid artery presenting as a spherical, pulsating, pinkish-red mass in the mesotympanum. Abnormal origin of right occipital artery and middle meningeal artery from internal carotid artery. Conductive hearing loss in right ear. Preauricular appendices and bifid tragal cartilage deformity. Congenital ptosis.*

An 8-year-old girl born with congenital ptosis, bilateral preauricular appendices, and bifid tragal cartilage deformity was referred for evaluation of right congenital conductive hearing loss.

Otologic examination showed bilateral preauricular appendices and bifid tragal cartilage deformity. Otoscopy disclosed a pinkish-red, spherical, pulsating mass arising from the right hypotympanum be-hind an intact tympanic membrane. It was impinging on the umbo. Cochlear function studies disclosed a 35-dB conductive hearing loss in the right ear but normal hearing in the left ear.

Axial computed tomography (CT) scanning of the petrous pyramids demonstrated a bony dehiscence between the ascending right carotid canal and the middle ear, with a posterior location of the internal carotid artery in the mesotympanum overlying the inferior promontory (Fig. 9.10). Otherwise, there was no vascular abnormality to suggest a vascular tumor. Both internal carotid arteries displayed a symmetrical bulbous enlargement, considered to be an anatomical variation.

A *four-vessel carotid angiogram* demonstrated the abnormal course of the right internal carotid artery through the middle ear and the right occipital and middle meningeal artery proceeding from the internal carotid artery.

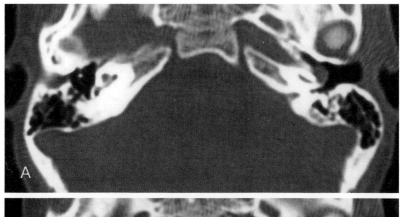

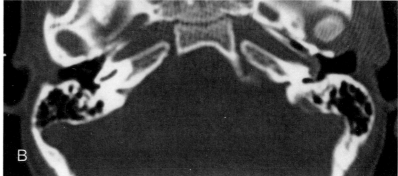

Figure 9.10. Axial CT scan of petrous pyramids. The abnormal position of the right intratemporal internal carotid artery is readily seen as the artery ascends through the mesotympanum over the promontory and bends forward to continue its horizontal course through the petrous apex.

References

1. Roland PS, Glasscock ME III. Surgery of the cranial base. In: Paparella MM, Shumrick DA, Gluckman JL, Meyerhoff WL, eds. Otolaryngology, Vol II: Otology and neuro-otology. 3rd ed. Philadelphia: WB Saunders, Chap 55, 1991:1789–1807.
2. Fisch U, Mattox D. Microsurgery of the skull base. Stuttgart: Georg Thieme, 1988.
3. Marx H. Monatsschr Ohrenheilkd 1899:251, cited in Kecht B. Die Bedeutung der Arteria carotis interna in der Hals-, Nasen-, Ohrenheilkd. Arch Ohren- Heilkd 1937;143:3.
4. Rozier. Thesis, Paris 1902, cited in Kecht B. Die Bedeutung der Arteria carotis interna in der Hals-, Nasen-, Ohrenheilkd. Arch Ohren- Heilkd 1937;143:3.
5. Hansen. Münch Med Wochenschr 1903;1:949, cited in Kecht B. Die Bedeutung der Arteria carotis interna in der Hals-, Nasen-, Ohrenheilkd. Arch Ohren- Heilkd 1937;143:3.
6. Kecht B. Die Bedeutung der Arteria carotis interna in der Hals-, Nasen-, Ohrenheilkd. Arch Ohren- Heilkd 1937;143:3.
7. Ramadier J, Leroux R, Bousquet M. Particuliarités structurales des parois de la carotide interne intrapétreuse. Soc Anat Paris February 2nd, 1933.
8. Tato E, Soubiron V. Monatsschr Ohrenheilkd 1935:1454, cited in Kecht B. Die Bedeutung der Arteria carotis interna in der Hals-, Nasen-, Ohrenheilkd. Arch Ohren- Heilkd 1937;143:3.
9. Podesta R, Tato JM. Histopathologischer Bericht über einen Fall von Petrositis (Operation nach Ramadier). Riss und Blutung der Carotis interna. Eiterige Hirnhautentzündung. Acta Otolaryngol (Stockh) 1937;25:254.
10. Mayer O. Die Pyramidenzellen Eiterungen. Z Hals-, Nasen-, Ohrenheilkd Kongressbericht 1937;42(1):1–93.
11. Guild SR. The anatomy of the petrous pyramid. Ann Otol Rhinol Laryngol 1935;44:1011.
12. Guild SR. A hitherto unrecognized danger in the operation of Ramadier for suppuration of the petrous pyramid. Acta Otolaryngol 1937;25:561–567.

SECTION II

INFLAMMATORY DISEASES

an exudative crust. The mycelia extend below the necrotic surface but do not invade the deeper layers of the tissue. The meatal lining is edematous and infiltrated with mononuclear cells. The skin appendages are generally not involved.

SEBORRHEIC DERMATITIS

The association of a desquamative inflammatory dermatitis that involves the cavum conchae, the entrance to the external meatus, the adjacent portion of the external canal, and the retroauricular crease with an itchy dandruffy scalp readily establishes the diagnosis. In the form that is free from moisture, the scales are dry and greasy. In the moist and more sebaceous form, the scales are more yellow in color and may have a strong odor. The greater inflammatory reaction in the underlying skin gives rise to vesiculation, fissures, focal cellulitis, and regional lymphadenitis. The etiology remains unknown.

Microscopically, the epidermis appears thickened and exhibits various stages of intracellular and intercellular edema and, occasionally, vesicles and parakeratosis. The dermis shows some distension of the most superficial papillary vessels surrounded by mononuclear exudate. The sebaceous glands show no pathologic changes (2).

BACTERIAL ECZEMA

Bacterial eczema is the most frequent of the dermatoses involving the external ear. It is more often encountered in warm and humid climates. *Pseudomonas aeruginosa* is the prevalent causative organism (2). The predisposing factor that facilitates the growth of this organism is considered to be the change in the pH of the surface of the external ear (2). This change results from the decrease in serum production and consequent loss of acidity caused by an atrophy of the skin appendages, especially of the ceruminous glands, observed repeatedly in skin biopsy material. The clinical characteristics are vesication and varying stages of exudation. At times, it may accompany or be the sequela of an exudative otitis media.

Microscopically, the vesicles assume a superficial location in the epidermis. They result from an accumulation of intercellular fluid and include a certain amount of exudate. By contrast, the vesicles in virus diseases result from changes within the epithelial cells themselves from an intracellular accumulation of fluid, and they are usually loculated. In pemphigus, the vesicles are due to accumulation of fluid, either in the basal layer or between the basal layer and the dermis, elevating the entire epidermis into a large, nonloculated bulla. The epithelium displays some parakeratosis and an increase in surface keratin. The dermis shows some distension of the papillary vessels and a perivascular edema that, in the presence of an underlying allergy, may include eosinophils (2).

References

1. Friedmann I. Otomycosis. In: Pathology of the ear. Oxford: Blackwell Scientific Publications, 1974.
2. Ash JE. Pathology of the ear. In: English GM, ed. Otolaryngology. Philadelphia: Harper & Row, Chap 4, 1986;1:1–69.

Part 3
Necrotizing ("Malignant") Granulomatous External Otitis and Osteomyelitis

DEFINITION

The necrotizing malignant granulomatous external otitis (NEO) is a particularly virulent, potentially lethal form of external otitis. It begins as a superficial infection, often following a minor epithelial laceration, and progresses to a deep-seated diffuse cellulitis involving the outer ear canal. Without early and proper treatment, it progressively involves adjacent soft tissues and bone. It extends to the soft tissues in the neck across the junction of the cartilaginous and osseous portions of the external auditory canal wall and through the fissures of Santorini of the conchal cartilage. It frequently involves the facial nerve, parotid gland, internal carotid artery, jugular vein, and nasopharynx. It often extends to the temporomandibular joint, the petrous and mastoid portions of the temporal bone, and can affect other cranial nerves, i.e., V, VI, and IX–XII. It can spread to adjacent bony structures of the skull base and cervical spine and eventually leads to thrombophlebitis of the lateral and cavernous sinus, giving rise to septicemia and to meningitis, brain abscess, and death. It is caused uniformly by the Gram-negative organism, *Pseudomonas aeruginosa*. Although observed in any age group, it affects primarily elderly diabetics or patients whose immune system has become otherwise compromised.

The present management includes long-term treatment with two intravenous antibiotics and periodic meticulous debridement of the outer ear canal over a period of at least 2 months, determined by clinical signs and laboratory tests, until the indium-III-labeled white blood cell (WBC) scan has become normal. The underlying diabetes requires careful adjustment.

If NEO is not properly treated, it is likely to recur, either in the external auditory canal or in the bone of the base of the skull. Early recognition and appropriate management, in the past two decades, resulted in a conversion of a disease process that was once regarded with fear because of its high morbidity and mortality to one that has become routinely curable.

PATHOGENESIS

The organism almost exclusively responsible is the *P. aeruginosa*. It is often cultured in the presence of an external otitis after swimming or minor injury of the canal skin. In certain elderly, debilitated diabetic patients it may lead to a progressive cellulitis involving soft tissues, cartilage, and bone, a disease that only three decades ago had a mortality rate approaching 60%. Two factors have so far been identified as being essential for the development of NEO: (a) a laceration of the skin covering the external meatus, i.e., a tear with a hairpin, match, or Q-tip (during an attempt to remove cerumen or relieve itching) or a scratch from an ear mold; and (b) an impairment of the host's defense mechanism caused by an underlying defect of the body's immune system.

P. aeruginosa is not regularly cultured from an intact external auditory canal. However, in chronic external otitis, frequently encountered in a warm and humid climate, maceration or laceration of the meatal skin predisposes to bacterial superinfection and colonization with *Pseudomonas*. *Pseudomonas* is a virulent organism and difficult to eradicate on account of its protective polysaccharide layer, which inhibits phagocytosis and the effect of antibiotics (1). Potent endotoxins and exotoxins and elastolytic and collagenolytic enzymes released by the *Pseudomonas* organism produce a rapid degradation of tissues and a necrotizing vasculitis. The neurotoxin secreted by the organism may contribute to the neuropathy involving the cranial nerves (2).

Diabetes mellitus is a systemic disease that causes an obliterative endarteritis of the small vessels throughout the body. The resulting interference with phagocytosis and chemotaxis of the leukocytes leads to an impairment of the inflammatory response. The functional defect of the neutrophilic polymorphonuclear leukocytes has been identified as an impairment in their migration capability (3). The combination of the diabetic microangiopathy, necrotizing vasculitis, and functional defect of the neutrophilic polymorphonuclear leukocytes sets the stage for the development of the NEO. Once the cellulitis is established, it spreads to the adjacent cartilage and along its dehiscences, the fissures of Santorini, to the soft tissues in the neck and to the bony structures of the temporal bone, skull base, and cervical spine. The soft tissue structures affected in the neck include the facial nerve, at and below the stylomastoid foramen (Fig. 10.3.1), the parotid gland, the cervical lymph nodes, the muscles, the great vessels (Fig. 10.3.2), and the temporomandibular articulation (see Figs. 10.3.3 and 10.3.5).

In a very rare instance, NEO can affect a nondiabetic patient whose immune system may be otherwise compromised by severe peripheral arteriosclerosis, chronic lymphoblastic leukemia, granulocytopenia, chronic steroid dependence, anemia and malnutrition, etc. In a rare instance, organisms other than *Pseudomonas*, e.g., *Serratia, Proteus, Staphylococcus aureus*, and *Aspergillus*, have been identified. Although NEO is primarily a disease of the elderly, it has been reported in a few children either with or without juvenile diabetes or in association with severe systemic illness (4–10). In some of these nondiabetic children, a decreased immunocompetence is considered primarily responsible for the susceptibility, regional behavior, and distal complication of the infection.

MACROSCOPIC APPEARANCE

The salient macroscopic features are the inflammatory edema involving the auricle and periauricular area, the swelling and induration of the meatal skin, and the presence of exophytic granulation tissue over exposed, osteitic and necrotic bone along the floor and anterior external auditory canal wall (see Figs. 10.3.3, 10.3.5, and 10.3.6).

MICROSCOPIC APPEARANCE

In comparison to the benign external otitis, which involves primarily the cartilaginous portion of the external meatus, the NEO begins more often in the osseous portion, spreading thereafter quickly to the cartilaginous portion (11). Histologic examination of the meatal skin reveals a thickened, hyperplastic epidermis with acanthotic changes and pseudoepitheliomatous hyperplasia (11). The subcutis displays a diffuse acute and chronic inflammation with massive infiltration of polymorphonuclear neutrophils, lymphocytes, and plasma cells. As the disease progresses, the skin becomes ulcerated, cartilage and bone undergo rapid massive necrosis, and there is development of an exophytic inflammatory granulation tissue overlying osteitic bone (see Figs. 10.3.3 and 10.3.5). Necrotizing vasculitis is a frequent observation, and sequestra of devitalized cartilage and bone may be encountered (see Fig. 10.3.10). In the early stage of the disease, the clinician may observe a layer of poorly vascularized or avascular, degenerated fibrous connective tissue covering cartilage and bone. This has led to the assumption that in NEO the basic mechanism is an invasion by an opportunistic Gram-negative organism of a tissue that previously became devitalized as a result of the microangiopathy encountered, i.e., in diabetes mellitus (12, 13).

CLINICAL MANIFESTATIONS

NEO is a disease primarily of the elderly, almost exclusively diabetic person with an average age of 70 years. Males are more frequently affected, with the ratio being about 4:1 to 5:1. Onset is insidious and often follows a minor trauma that causes a laceration of the meatal skin. There is progressive pain and purulent, occasionally serosanguinous discharge from the affected ear. *P. aeruginosa* is cultured almost uniformly and identified as the causative organism. Beginning in the external canal, the cellulitis destroys cartilage and bone. Extension beyond the outer ear canal leads to cellulitis of adjacent soft tissues involving the parotid gland, lymph nodes, muscles, nerves, and major blood vessels in the neck. Excursions in the temporomandibular joint become increasingly painful and may be accompanied by trismus. There is marked tenderness on deep palpation of the infra-auricular and retromandibular area. If not controlled, progressive osteitis of the temporal bone and base of the skull may lead to multiple unilateral and bilateral cranial nerve involvement (Figs. 10.3.1 and 10.3.2), thrombosis of the major vessels, meningitis, brain abscess, and death. Death results almost exclusively from involvement of the central nervous system, only occasionally from septicemia. In the advanced stage, an inflammatory edema often involves the soft tissue of the nasopharynx and parapharyngeal space. Occasionally, the nasopharyngeal orifice of the Eustachian tube is surrounded by an ulcerating granulation tissue (Fig. 10.3.6), and *Pseudomonas* can be cultured from that area and from the nasal secretions. The hallmark is the presence of recurrent inflammatory granulation tissue over exposed devitalized and osteitic bone, along the floor and anterior wall of the external auditory canal at the osseous-cartilaginous junction. Paralysis of the facial nerve is a characteristic feature whereby the neural involvement is at the level of the stylomastoid foramen or below (Fig. 10.3.1). It was once considered an ominous prognostic sign. Whereas the extension of the osteitic process to the petrous apex may lead to involvement of cranial nerves II, III, V, and VI, spread to the neural compartment of the jugular foramen and soft tissues at the base of the skull may give rise to paralysis of cranial nerves IX–XII (Fig. 10.3.2).

The diagnosis is established on the following bases: *(a)* a refractory purulent external otitis in an elderly patient with a history of diabetes or an abnormal glucose tolerance test or an

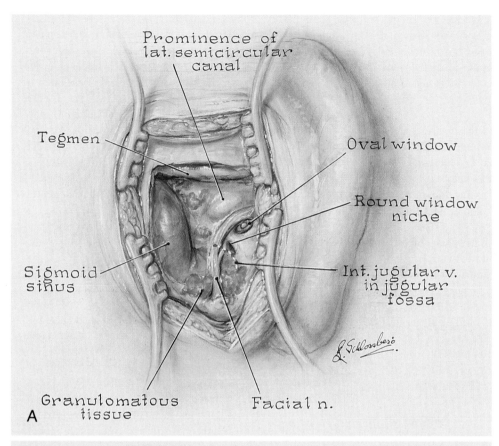

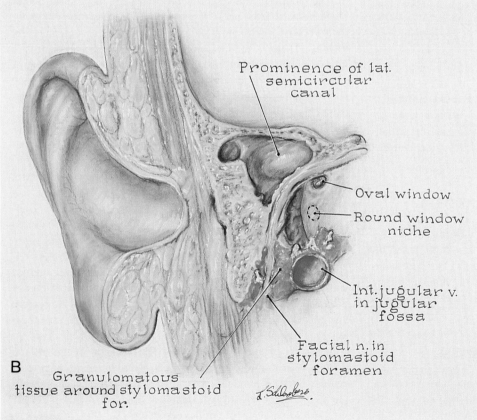

Figure 10.3.1. Illustration of location of facial nerve involvement in NEO immediately above, at, or below stylomastoid foramen.

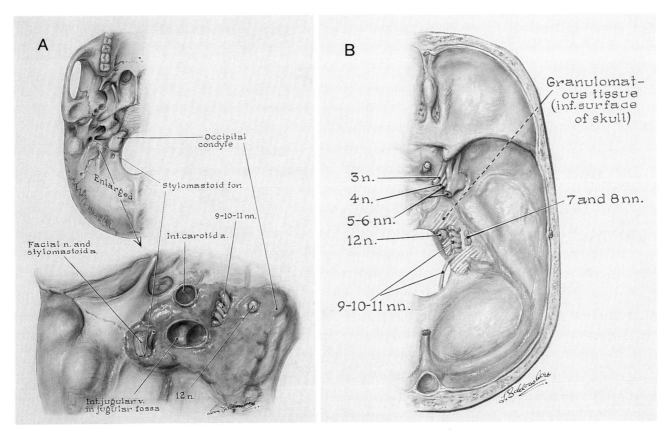

Figure 10.3.2. Illustration of site of involvement of cranial nerves IX–XII in NEO caused by osteitis of surrounding bone or inflammatory granulation tissue at base of skull.

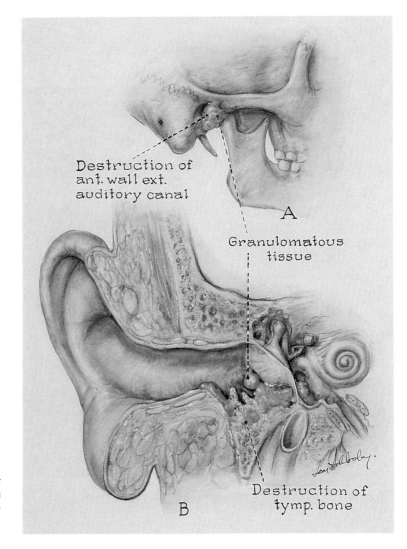

Figure 10.3.3. Illustration of the osteitic process involving the floor and anterior external auditory canal wall, covered by granulation tissue, and anterior dislocation of the mandibular condyle associated with adjacent cellulitis.

individual with some other immune deficiency, *(b)* a deep-seated otalgia characteristically aggravated during the night, *(c)* marked tenderness in the infra-auricular area and retromandibular fossa, *(d)* the presence of an acute inflammatory granulation tissue overlying a bony defect along the floor and anterior external canal wall, frequently leading into the temporomandibular joint and continuous with a cellulitis of soft tissue at the base of the skull, and *(e)* identification of the bacillus *P. aeruginosa.*

OTOLOGIC EXAMINATION

The otologic examination reveals an inflammatory swelling of the periauricular region and meatal skin. The meatal skin initially has an indurated granular appearance. Thereafter, it is being replaced in some areas by an exophytic bluish-gray granulation tissue that covers diseased, superficially necrotic bone at the cartilaginous-osseous junction (see Figs. 10.3.3 and 10.3.5). The tympanic membrane is generally intact though thickened, edematous, and restricted in mobility. The middle ear often displays a serous exudate and an inflammatory edema of the mucoperiosteum commonly associated with a conductive hearing loss. Trismus and tenderness over the temporomandibular joint reflect involvement of that articulation. Nasopharyngoscopy may disclose a localized or diffuse inflammatory thickening of the mucosa and granulation tissue that resembles a vascular neoplasm, surrounding the Eustachian tubal orifice (see Fig. 10.3.6C). The WBC generally reveals a mild leukocytosis with a shift to the left. The sedimentation rate is routinely markedly elevated. The facial palsy is a reflection of neural involvement at or below the stylomastoid foramen (Fig. 10.3.1).

RADIOGRAPHIC ASPECTS

Radiographic evaluation is essential in identification and management of this grave and potentially lethal disease. Serial axial and coronal tomograms provide satisfactory visualization of the mastoid cells, middle ear cavity, temporomandibular articulation, external ear canal, nasopharynx, and parapharyngeal space. They may demonstrate bone destruction in the various regions of the temporal bone (Figs. 10.3.4 and 10.3.8), adjacent bones (Fig. 10.3.8), center of the skull base, opposite temporal bone, and cervical spine. Their value in diagnosing osteomyelitis is limited, however, since osteolysis can only be detected after about half of the trabecular bone has been resorbed (1). They generally demonstrate a moderately enhancing soft tissue mass within and around the outer ear canal and stylomastoid foramen that may extend posteriorly, over the mastoid cortex, and displace the mandibular condyle anteriorly (Figs. 10.3.4 and 10.3.8). Besides clouding of the mastoid process (Fig. 10.3.7), they may show an enhancing soft tissue swelling in the epipharynx and parapharyngeal compartments that is continuous with the soft tissue mass around the external auditory canal. The structural changes observed in the computed tomography (CT) scans are in decreasing frequency: *(a)* changes in the external auditory canal, *(b)* inflammatory edema of the middle ear and mastoid mucoperiosteum, *(c)* anterior displacement of the condyloid ramus, *(d)* involvement of the petrous apex, *(e)* soft tissue swelling in the nasopharynx and parapharyngeal space, *(f)* erosion of the central skull base, and *(g)* erosion of the jugular foramen and carotid canal. Whereas the CT scan can certainly demonstrate resolution of the central soft tissue swelling in the neck area during con-

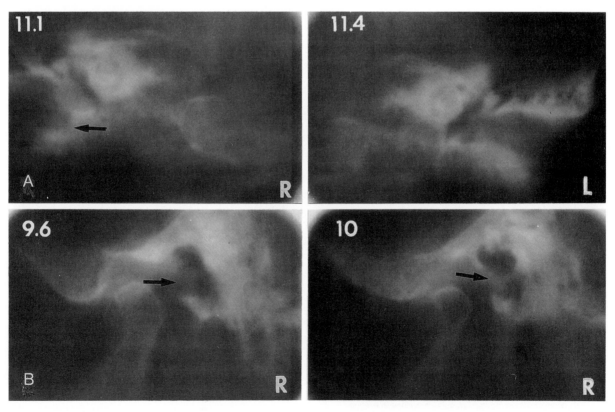

Figure 10.3.4. Anteroposterior (AP) and lateral multidirection tomograms of right and left temporal bones. They demonstrate the bony erosion of the floor and anterior canal wall (**A**, *11.1;* **B**, *9.6*), the soft tissue mass in the right external meatus and middle ear (**A**, *11.1*), and the anterior displacement of the mandibular condyle.

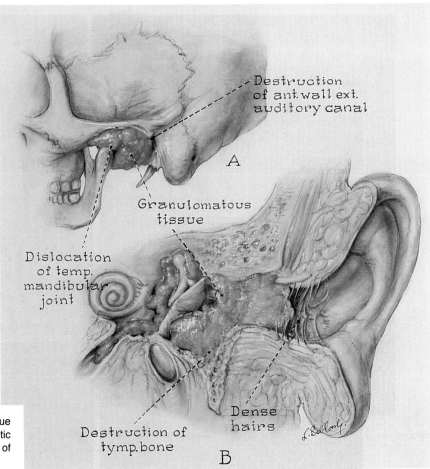

Figure 10.3.5. Illustration of exophytic granulation tissue in the outer ear canal and middle ear, overlying the osteitic tympanic bone **(B),** and anterior subluxation of the head of the condyloid ramus **(A).**

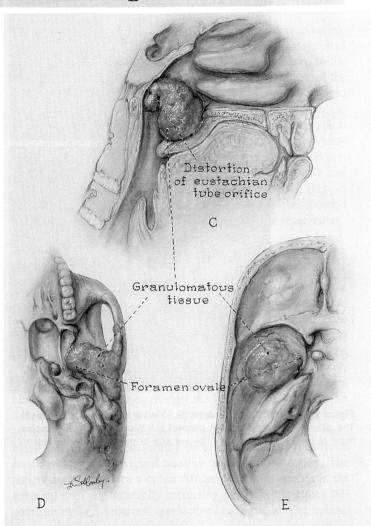

Figure 10.3.6. Illustration of inflammatory granulation tissue in left fossa of Rosenmüller, surrounding the tubal orifice **(C),** and the osteitic process involving the skull base and root of zygoma, covered by granulation tissue **(D and E).**

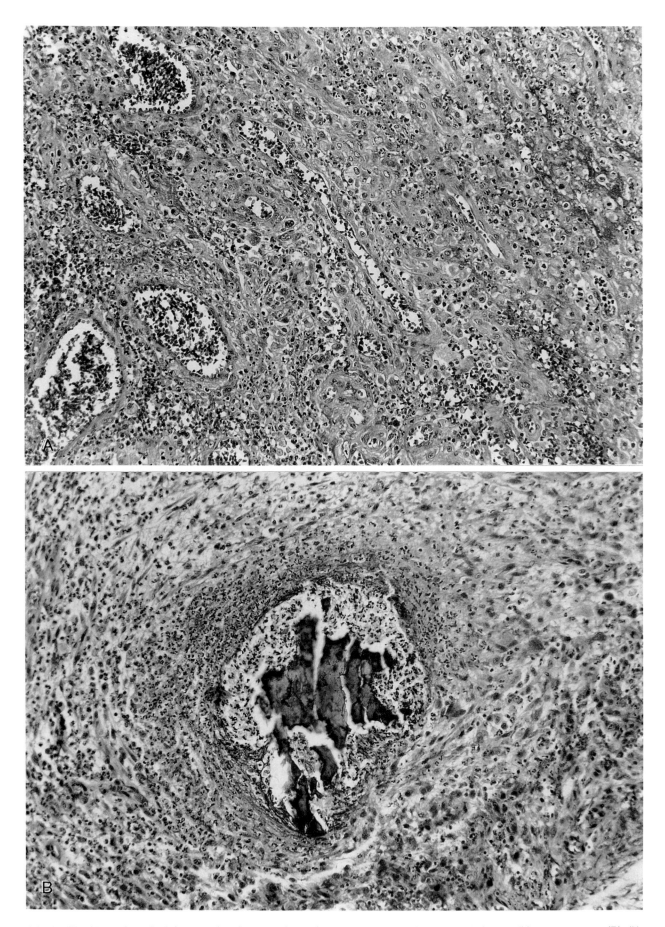

Figure 10.3.10. The biopsy from the left external auditory canal reveals a vascular granulation tissue with acute inflammation and occasional areas of vasculitis **(A)**. It also includes small bony sequestrae **(B)**. (Hematoxylin and eosin, ×250 for both.)

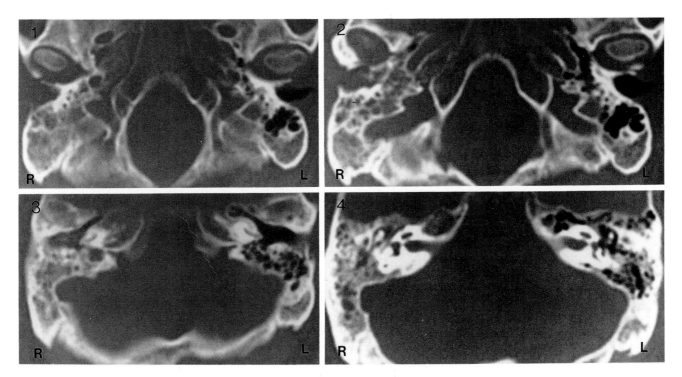

Figure 10.3.11. Serial axial CT scans of the temporal bones, showing the left external auditory canal, middle ear cleft, and mastoid air cells dif- fusely opacified. There is marked erosion involving the right anterior, in- ferior, and posterior bony canal wall. (Courtesy of Dr. D. Mattox.)

chemic ulcerations involving the plantar surface of both feet and the loss of several toes were noted. The patient had no ear problems until 4 weeks prior to admission when he developed symptoms of right external otitis with itching, swelling, pain, discharge, loss of hearing, and a diffuse periaural edema, redness, and tenderness. While being treated with local and systemic antibiotics for 2 weeks, he developed progressively severe pain on chewing and palpation of right retromandibular, infra-auricular, and retroauricular areas that became unbearable at night when lying on that ear.

Otologic examination showed an inflammatory edema involving the right cavum conchae and periauricular region. There was tender- ness over the temporomandibular articulation and preauricular and postauricular areas. The entire external auditory canal was occupied by a characteristic bluish-gray, friable, easy-bleeding granulation tis- sue surrounded by a malodorous exudate. It totally obstructed the view of the tympanic membrane. Cochlear function studies revealed a combined hearing loss in the right ear with a speech reception threshold (SRT) of 35 dB and a discrimination score of 98%. The left ear showed a mild combined hearing loss. There was no spon- taneous nystagmus, and cranial nerves III–XII were intact. Results of laboratory studies were: WBC, 7,100–10,200; serum glucose, 89– 273 mg/dl; creatinine, 2.5–3.4 mg/dl.

Radiologic examination. The CT scan of the temporal bones dis- closed a diffuse opacification of the right external auditory canal, middle ear cleft, and mastoid air cells. There was evidence of bone destruction involving the anterior and inferior canal wall with a soft tissue mass involving the right preauricular area (Fig. 10.3.11).

A three-phase bone imaging with 20.0 mCi technetium-99m methylene diphosphate displayed an increased activity in the area of the right tympanic and mastoid bone on the flow, blood pool, and static images characteristic of osteomyelitis (Fig. 10.3.12).

Gallium imaging with 4.6 mCi gallium-67 citrate 24 hours after intravenous administration showed an abnormal focal area of in- creased radiotracer uptake in the area of the right temporal bone. It corresponded with the area of increased radiotracer uptake on the bone scan and confirmed the diagnosis of osteomyelitis (Fig. 10.3.12).

Operation. A right modified radical mastoidectomy was per- formed. The external auditory canal was occupied by a densely packed granulation tissue surrounded by purulent exudate and outlined by mostly devitalized squamous epithelium. There was widespread de- struction of cartilage and bone involving the anteroinferior and pos- terior canal wall. The granulation tissue extended anteriorly into the parotid gland and posteriorly into the mastoid and from there into the antrum and forward along the aditus to the attic. The tympanic membrane revealed a central necrosis. The tegmen antri disclosed a localized destruction with an underlying extradural collection of in- flammatory granulation tissue (abscess) and destruction of the dura. All osteitic bone was removed.

Histologic examination of the different intraoperative specimens reveals: *(a)* meatal squamous epithelium with extensive acute and chronic inflammation, *(b)* mastoid granulation tissue with acute and chronic inflammation, and *(c)* mastoid and tympanic bone with evi- dence of osteomyelitis and bone remodeling. There is no evidence of vasculitis (Fig. 10.3.13).

References

1. Kraus DH, Rehm SJ, Kinney SE. The evolving treatment of necrotizing external otitis. Laryngoscope 1988;98:934–939.
2. Damiani JM, Damiani KK, Kinney SE. Malignant external otitis with multiple cranial nerve involvement. Am J Otol 1979;1(2):115–120.
3. Corberand J, Nguyen F, Fraysse B, Enjalbert L. Malignant external otitis and polymorphonuclear leukocyte migration impairment. Arch Otolaryngol 1982;108:122–124.
4. Joachims H. Malignant external otitis in children. Arch Otolaryngol 1976;102:236–237.
5. Rubin J, Yu VL, Stool SE. Malignant external otitis in children. J Pediatr 1988;113(6):965–970.
6. Ganz H. Malignant external otitis in a young diabetic. Successful azlocillin treatment. HNO 1984;32:431–432.
7. Horn KL, Gherini S. Malignant external otitis of childhood. Am J Otol 1981;2(4):402–404.
8. Sherman P, Black S, Grossman M. Malignant external otitis due to *Pseudomonas aeruginosa* in childhood. Pediatrics 1980;66(5):782–783.
9. Coser PL, Stamm AE, Lobo RC, Pinto JA. Malignant external otitis in infants. Laryngoscope 1980;90(2):312–316.
10. Gignore P, Rouillard G. Malignant bilateral external otitis in a 10 year old girl. J Otolaryngol 1976;5(2):159–166.
11. Bernheim J, Sadé J. Histopathology of the soft parts in 50 patients with malignant external otitis. J Laryngol Otol 1989;103:366–368.
12. Kohut RI, Lindsay JR. Necrotizing malignant external otitis. Histopathologic processes. Ann Otol Rhinol Laryngol 1979;8:714–720.
13. Ostfeld E, Segal M, Czernobilsky B. Malignant external otitis: early histopathologic changes and pathogenic mechanism. Laryngoscope 1981;91:965–970.
14. Gold S, Som PM, Lucente FE, Lawson W, Mendelson M, Parisier SC. Radiographic findings in progressive necrotizing "malignant" external otitis. Laryngoscope 1984;94(3):363–366.
15. Gherini SG, Brackmaun DE, Bradley WG. Magnetic resonance imaging and computerized tomography in malignant external otitis. Laryngoscopy 1986;96:542–548.
16. Meltzer PE, Kelemen G. Pyocyaneus osteomyelitis of the temporal bone, mandible and zygoma. Laryngoscope 1959;69:1300–1316.
17. Schilling R. Über Osteomyelitis der flachen Schädelknochen im Anschluss an Entzündungen der Stirnhöhle und des Mittelohres. Z Ohrenheilkd Krankh Luftwege 1904;48:52–100.
18. Schilling R. Die septische Osteomyelitis des Felsenbeins. Die Erkrankungen des Gehörorgans. In: Denker A, Kahler O, eds. Handbuch der Hals-Nasen-Ohren-Heilkunde. Berlin: Julius Springer, 1926;7(2):179–203.
19. Neff N. Beitrag zur Lehre von der otogenen, akuten, progressiven Osteomyelitis des Schläfenbeines beim Kinde und beim Erwachsenen. Z Ohrenheilkd Krankh Luftwege 1920;80:14–55.
20. Chandler JR. Malignant external otitis. Laryngoscopy 1968;78:1257–1294.
21. Chandler JR. Pathogenesis and treatment of facial paralysis due to malignant external otitis. Ann Otol Rhinol Laryngol 1972;81:1–11.
22. Chandler JR. Malignant external otitis: further considerations. Ann Otol Rhinol Laryngol 1986;84:417–428.
23. Chandler JR. Malignant external otitis and osteomyelitis of the base of the skull. Am J Otol 1989;10:108–10.
24. Rehm SJ, Weinstein AJ. Home intravenous antibiotic therapy: a team approach. Ann Intern Med 1983;99:388–392.

Part 4

Keratitis Obturans (Cholesteatoma of the External Ear Canal)

In keratosis obturans the lesion consists of a concentric accumulation of desquamated epithelial debris arranged in a lamellar onion-skin-like fashion. The condition is rare, mainly accounted in the older age group, and develops in the bony portion of the external ear canal. As it gradually increases in size by continuous peripheral apposition of keratinous material, it begins to erode and enlarge the osseous canal. The expansion lends to ulceration and destruction of the meatal epithelium, formation of an inflammatory granulation tissue, and superficial bone necrosis. When the bone erosion is irregular and scalloped, the keratinous plug becomes firmly affixed and adherent, difficult and painful to remove. The clinical features usually include pain, conductive hearing loss, and malodorous otorrhea. The concentric lamellar structures of keratin lend the lesion a glistening, pearly-white appearance identical with the one of the middle ear cholesteatoma and the epidermoid. Since the lesion shares the identical etiology, pathogenesis, and regional behavior with the papillary cholesteatoma of the middle ear, the term, primary cholesteatoma of the external auditory, which it was first given in 1887 (1, 2), in the presence of an intact tympanic membrane, appears correct. External cholesteatomas may be encountered in congenital or acquired atresia of the ear canal and in the association with certain bone dysplasias involving the tympanic bone. Osteitis deformans and fibrous dysplasia are such examples (3, 4). The rare simultaneous occurrence of an external cholesteatoma and a papillary cholesteatoma of the middle ear should not be surprising, since both can arise from the squamous epithelium adjacent to the tympanic membrane, which is recognized for its persisting and usual growth potential (5).

References

1. Kall M. Mitteilungen über die Tätigkeit der Univ Poliklinik für Ohrenkranke zu Bonn im Etatsjahre 1866/67. Arch Ohrenheilkd 1887;25:73.
2. Oltersdorf U. Das Gehörgangscholesteatom und seine Deutung. Arch Ohren-Nasen- Kehlkopfheilkd 1956;169:420.
3. Nager GT, Kennedy DW, Kopstein E. Fibrous dysplasia. A review of the disease and its manifestations in the temporal bone. Ann Otol Rhinol Laryngol (Suppl 92) 1982;91(3):5–52.
4. Nager GT. Paget's disease of the temporal bone. Ann Otol Rhinol Laryngol 1975;84(Suppl 22)(4):1–32.
5. Schätzle W, Haubrich J. Pathologie des Ohres. In: Doerr W, Seifert G, Uehlinger E, eds. Spezielle pathologische Anatomie. Berlin: Springer Verlag, 1975.

Part 5

Myringitis (Diseases of the Tympanic Membrane)

Depending on the etiology, diseases of the tympanic membrane may be divided into myringitis of viral, bacterial, fungal, and other possible origin.

VIRAL MYRINGITIS

Viral myringitis may be a manifestation of an infection with an influenza, chickenpox, herpes zoster, herpes simplex, and possibly other viruses.

Influenza Myringitis

The influenza myringitis is characterized by a hemorrhagic bullous inflammation of the tympanic membrane. It is usually a manifestation of an underlying hemorrhagic otitis media, a frequent complication of an influenza upper respiratory infection. The condition is regularly observed during influenza epidemics and pandemics. Children and adults can be affected. The causative virus is transmitted by the respiratory route by transfer of virus-containing respiratory secretions. Influenza virus types A, B, and C belong to the Orthomyxoviridae. Influenza virus type A is the most frequent single virus involved in clinical influenza. Influenza virus type B, paramyxoviruses, rhinoviruses, or echoviruses are less frequently responsible.

In hemorrhagic bullous myringitis, more than one blister is usually encountered. As blisters involve the tympanic membrane, they may extend to the adjacent meatal skin and give rise to a hemorrhagic external otitis (1). They have a characteristic dark-red or black-blue color and can lead to partial occlusion of the bony external auditory canal. Their spontaneous rupture produces a serosanguineous discharge.

The appearance of blisters is accompanied by pain, aural fullness, and, sometimes, partial loss of hearing. The pain is typically continuous and can be extraordinarily severe. It may be associated with constitutional symptoms of the virus infection, but in general it is not accompanied by fever. The characteristic histopathologic features are marked vascular hyperemia and extravasation of blood in the subcutis, submucosa, and adjacent tissues. Accumulation of blood within the tympanic membrane leads to dissection and elevation of the epidermal layer in circumscribed areas and to the formation of hemorrhagic blisters on the pars tensa and adjacent meatal skin.

A hemorrhagic bullous myringitis and external otitis may also develop independently in the absence of an underlying acute otitis media. This, however, occurs less frequently.

Chickenpox (Varicella) and Herpes Zoster Myringitis

Varicella and herpetic lesions in herpes zoster otitis may occasionally be encountered in the external auditory canal and on the tympanic membrane (2). Otic and ophthalmic zoster are variations of cephalic herpes zoster. Varicella and herpes zoster are caused by the varicella-zoster virus, where "varicella" represents the acute invasive phase, and "herpes zoster," a reactivation of the latent phase. In each instance the initial rash, a macular eruption, develops within a few hours to papules and monolocular "teardrop" vesicles that contain a clear fluid and stand out on an erythematous base. They begin to dry and form a scab about the fifth day after their appearance and leave an adherent crust that persists for 7–10 days.

The otic zoster manifests itself by the appearance of clusters of vesicles involving the concavity of the auricle, the entrance to the external meatus, and the external auditory canal. The ear lobe, the skin over the mastoid process, and the postauricular crease are less often affected. Isolated blisters may be encountered on the tympanic membrane. The rash is nearly always unilateral and limited to the distribution of the sensory branch of the facial nerve. In addition to the geniculate ganglion, the Gasserian ganglion of cranial nerve V and the spiral and vestibular ganglia of cranial nerve VIII and, occasionally, cranial nerves I, VI, IX, X, and XI may become involved. Consequently, the otic zoster may be associated with severe ear pain, paralysis of the facial nerve, loss of hearing, and disturbance of vestibular function. The hearing loss may be permanent or partial, or there may be total recovery. The vertigo may last for days to several weeks, and facial paralysis may be transient or permanent. Some degree of meningeal involvement is common,

and the cerebrospinal fluid may contain lymphocytes and show an elevated protein content. Some patients may exhibit evidence of mild generalized encephalitis. Prodromal symptoms of fever, malaise, sometimes gastrointestinal disturbances, and severe ear pain in the region of the future eruption may be present for 3–4 days before the distinctive features of the disease become manifest. Otic zoster of the geniculate ganglion has to be differentiated from herpes simplex.

Herpes Simplex Myringitis

Herpes simplex occurs most commonly about the mouth and on the lips as a so-called "cold sore," but occasionally it may affect the skin of the auricle and external auditory canal. The affecting agent is the relatively large herpes simplex virus (HSV-1). After a short period of tingling discomfort, itching, or burning, single or multiple clusters of small vesicles filled with a clear fluid appear on a slightly elevated, hemorrhagic base. After a few days they begin to dry up and leave a thin yellowish crust. The diagnosis is confirmed by the determination of a progressive increase in serum antibodies and by biopsy findings. Herpes simplex affects children and adults and tends to recur, whereas herpes zoster is most common in adults after the age of 50 years and rarely recurs. Herpetic eruptions can be precipitated by a variety of factors.

BULLOUS MYRINGITIS

Bullous myringitis is a complication of an upper respiratory infection of viral or bacterial origin including influenza and β-hemolytic streptococci and *Streptococcus pneumoniae*. The condition is frequently observed during epidemics, and children are particularly affected. The inflammation involves the drum and the adjacent canal skin. Epidermal layers of the tympanic membrane are dissected loose and elevated, and the accumulation of serum produces the characteristic blisters. As the middle ear is not involved, the hearing loss is minor. The condition is self-limiting and resolves in a matter of a few days (Figs. 10.5.1 and 10.5.2).

BACTERIAL MYRINGITIS

Acute bacterial myringitis may represent either a primary or a secondary inflammation of the eardrum. In the primary form, the inflammatory process is limited to the eardrum, and the tympanic cavity is not involved. In the secondary form, the infectious process develops initially in the middle ear cavity, and the tympanic membrane becomes secondarily involved. In either form, the eardrum may become affected in a diffuse or more localized fashion. In most instances, the posterior superior quadrant of the eardrum is involved. The milder form of myringitis is characterized by the development of several ecchymoses or blisters containing a serous exudate. Some streptococci produce a dark-red hemorrhagic exudate. The more severe form of myringitis can lead to the formation of larger blisters or to one or several interstitial abscesses. The blisters and abscess may rupture into the outer ear canal, or their content may be resorbed. Very rarely does an abscess perforate into the middle ear cavity.

Otoscopic examination reveals an inflammatory swelling of the posterior superior portion of the drum, which, depending

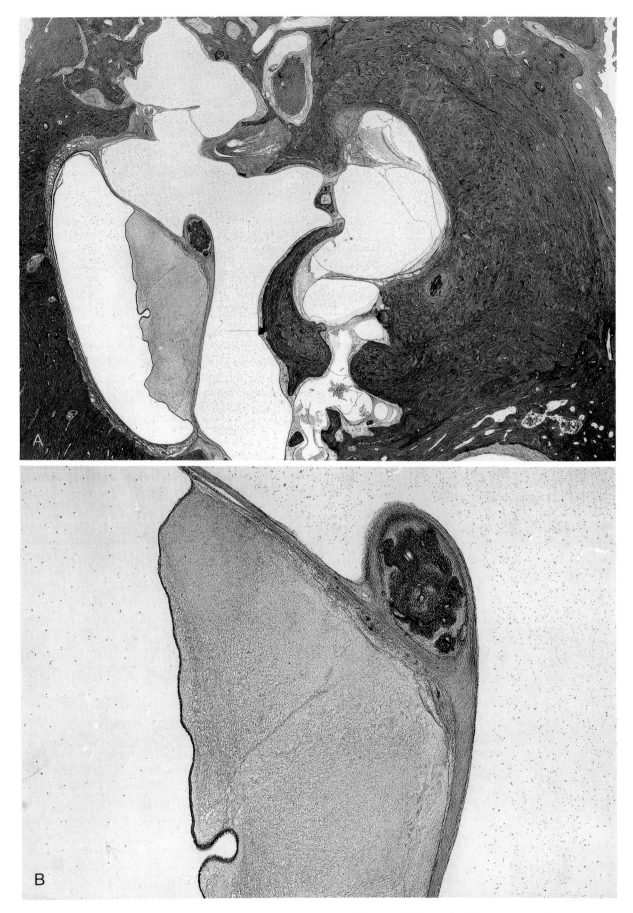

Figure 10.5.1.   A. Vertical section through right temporal bone at anterior margin of oval window of a 52-year-old man who died 2 days after removal of a deep-seated glioma from the right temporal lobe. The tympanic membrane reveals a large single vesicle in the outer epidermal layer. There is no evidence of otitis media. **B.** The vesicle developed by separation or cleavage of the epidermis. It contains a translucent fibrinous fluid. (Hematoxylin and eosin, ×10 and ×35, respectively.)

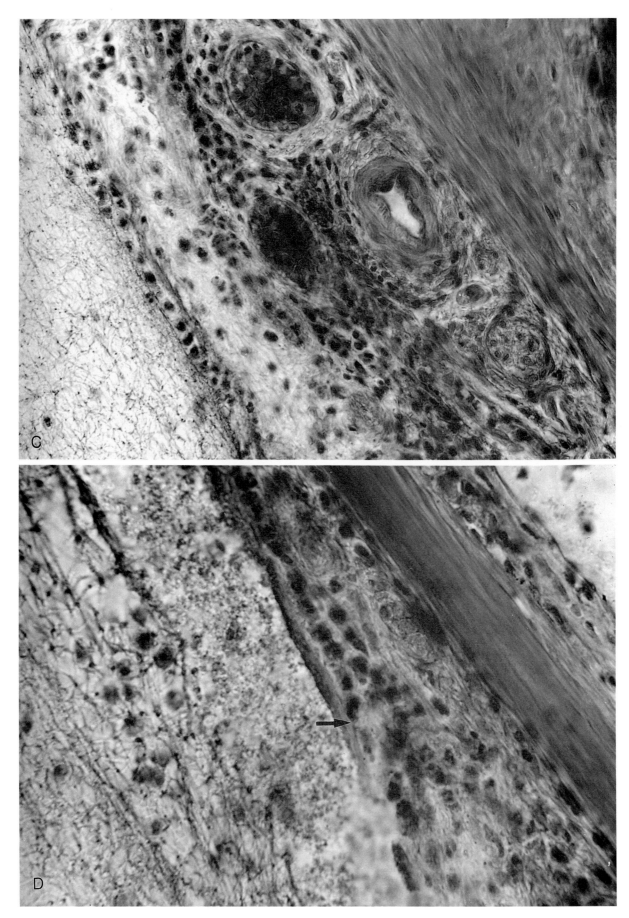

Figure 10.5.1. C. The outer vascular network of the eardrum in the dermal base of the vesicle is quite hyperemic. The arterioles and venules are distended and surrounded by perivascular accumulations of lymphocytes, plasma cells, and polymorphonuclear cells. Rupture of capillaries led to hemorrhages into the edematous tissues. **D.** Rupture of a capillary *(arrow)* resulted in extravasation of blood into the adjacent tissue and vesicle. (×500 and ×750, respectively.)

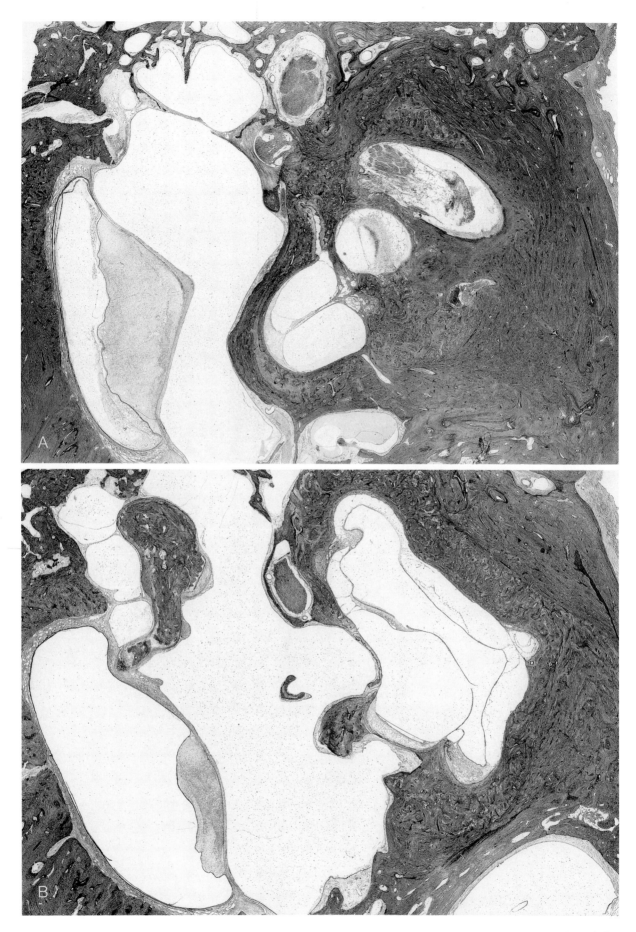

Figure 10.5.2. **A.** Vertical section through right temporal bone at level of fissula ante fenestram. The vesicle, which contains a translucent fibrinous exudate, involves the entire pars tensa of the tympanic membrane. **B.** Vertical section through right temporal bone near center of oval window. The single vesicle is a manifestation of an acute primary bullous myringitis of viral origin, not associated with an underlying otitis media. (Hematoxylin and eosin, ×10 and ×10, respectively.)

on the serous or purulent nature of the underlying exudate, may lend the blister a yellowish translucent or a more greenish-red color. In the presence of an abscess, which generally develops in the deeper layers of the eardrum and extends over a wider area, the epidermis of the pars tensa displays a generalized inflammatory edema and a dark-red color.

The primary myringitis is associated with severe lancinating pains that may radiate to the vertex and neck, with a sensation of aural fullness and pressure, with tinnitus, with some impairment of hearing, and, in children, often with a mild fever. Characteristically, the degree of hearing loss is disproportionally mild, compared with the extent of the inflammatory changes involving the eardrum. Its course differs more from that of a secondary myringitis in the rapid decrease of the inflammatory symptoms and the complete healing within 3–4 days. The diagnosis of primary acute myringitis can only be made with certainty within the first 2 days of the infection and if major inflammatory changes are associated with a disproportionally mild hearing loss. In the acute otitis media and secondary myringitis in which the inflammatory process begins in the middle ear, the copious exudate produces a significant conductive hearing loss from the beginning (Fig. 10.5.3).

Chronic bacterial myringitis is infrequently observed. It may develop after an acute primary myringitis. More often, it is the residue of a chronic external otitis. At times, however, it develops in the presence of a severe underlying or a terminal illness. Occasionally, it may be limited to a certain area of the tympanic membrane and then tends to involve the adjacent meatal skin. The deepithelialized surface of the eardrum has a moist glistening appearance with a pinkish-red color and is covered by a serous exudate. The chronic myringitis occasionally assumes a special form distinguished by its clinical appearance and morphologic changes, recognized as the granular myringitis.

Chronic Granulomatous Myringitis

The chronic granular myringitis was first recognized in the late 19th century (3, 4) and has since been discussed on several occasions (5–7). It is seen infrequently, runs a chronic course over weeks and months, and is usually associated with a sensation of itching, slight discomfort, aural fullness, mild loss of hearing, and intermittent serous discharge. The epidermal layer of the eardrum is replaced by a sheath of proliferating, nodular, papular inflammatory granulation tissue. In later stages, the middle fibrous layer and the inner mucosal layer of the tympanic membrane may become involved. Occasionally, the granulomatosis process involves primarily the inner, mucosal layer. Characteristically, the granular myringitis extends to and involves the adjacent external canal skin and is regularly accompanied by a chronic external otitis. The tympanic membrane maintains its

mobility. The hearing loss is mild, and the middle ear is not involved except for an occasional underlying localized inflammatory reaction. If it is not treated or if the underlying cause is not recognized and eliminated, progressive reactive hyperplasia of fibrous tissue over a period of time can lead to stenosis of the medial end of the ear canal. Long-term application of topical and systemic antibiotic and anti-inflammatory medication and, where indicated, surgical removal of the granulation tissue with subsequent skin grafting will control the disease. The etiology is not always clearly understood.

Three examples of a situation in which a granular myringitis was the initial manifestation of a serious underlying disease are worth mentioning here briefly. In one instance, a granular myringitis developed as a manifestation of an invasion of the hypotympanum, adjacent tympanic membrane, and meatal skin by an endotheliomatous meningioma. This meningioma had originated from the opposite (right) sphenoid ridge. The tumor had compressed the right frontal and temporal lobe, infiltrated the meninges and right cavernous sinus, and invaded the underlying bones of the skull, including the floor of the right anterior and middle cranial fossa and the entire right temporal bone. It had invaded the right parietal bone, sella turcica, and right sphenoid sinus and had extended across the midline to the hypotympanic region of the opposite (left) temporal bone (Fig. 10.5.4). In another instance, the granular myringitis had developed as a manifestation of an adjacent metastasis in the fibrous annulus and nearby meatal skin from a squamous cell carcinoma originating in the left vocal cord. The tumor had massively infiltrated the left larynx, destroyed the left thyroid cartilage, and metastasized to the regional lymph nodes of the neck to the skin at the annulus of the left external ear canal. The tympanic membrane was mobile, hearing was not significantly affected, and the underlying bone and the middle ear cavity were not involved. The initial two biopsies from the meatal skin at the annulus were negative, but the third specimen disclosed a squamous cell carcinoma morphologically identical with the primary lesion. In the third instance, the granular myringitis heralded an underlying cholesterol granuloma involving the entire middle ear cleft and destroyed a vast area of the mastoid process and cortex and of the bony wall of the lateral sinus and tegmental region. It had involved the mucosal and fibrous layer and given the outer, partially deepithelialized surface of the tympanic membrane a granular, nodular appearance. In a few other instances, the granular myringitis involved primarily the mucosal layer of the eardrum, and bacteriologic studies and biopsies failed to identify an underlying specific granulomatous or neoplastic disease. The conditions were controlled with local and systemic antimicrobial medications. Granulomatous myringitis may, therefore, be a form of chronic bacterial inflammation or a manifestation of an underlying neoplastic or granulomatous process whereby the etiology is not always clearly understood.

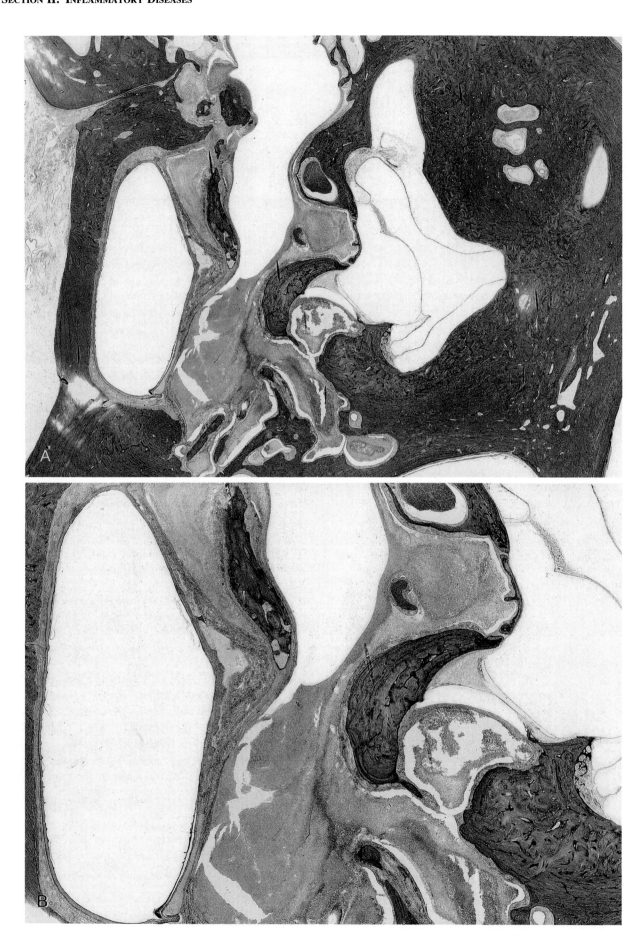

Figure 10.5.3. A. Vertical section through right temporal bone at level of oval and round windows in a 35-year-old man with acute purulent otitis media and secondary acute myringitis. The niches of the vestibular and cochlear fenestrae and the hypotympanum are filled with purulent exudate. A diffuse abscess is recognized within the tympanic membrane. **B.** The abscess developed between the epidermis and dermis of the epidermal layer of the eardrum. It has partially destroyed the overlying epidermis and the underlying fibrous or middle layer of the tympanic membrane and is about to perforate into the external auditory canal. (Hematoxylin and eosin, ×8, and ×15, respectively.)

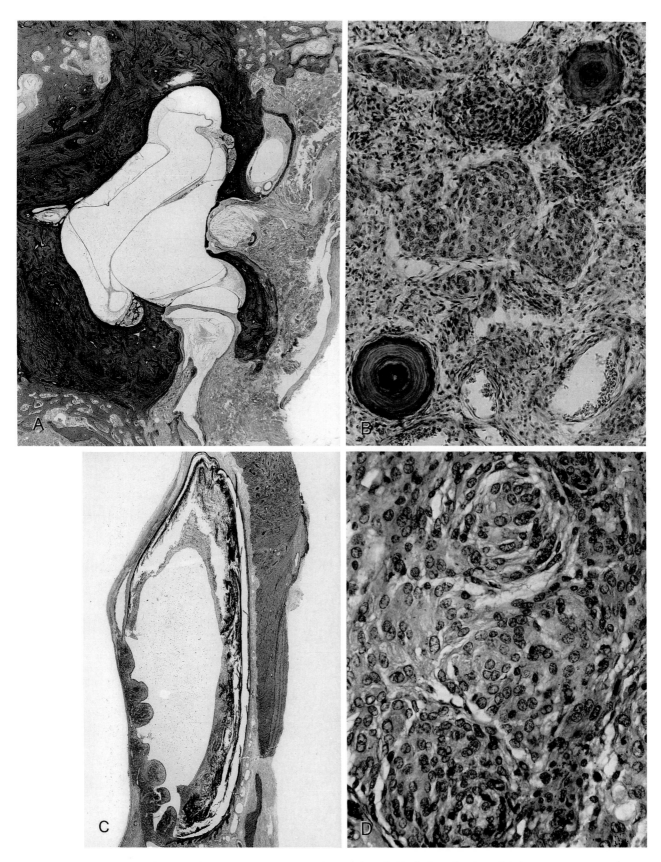

Figure 10.5.4. **A.** Vertical section through left temporal bone at level of oval and round windows in a 41-year-old man with a meningioma that had originated from the right sphenoid ridge. It had invaded the entire underlying right temporal bone and, extending across the midline, had partially invaded the opposite (left) temporal bone. Destruction of the tegmental bone allowed the meningioma to occupy the entire right middle ear cavity. **B.** Same section as in **A.** The meningioma is of the endotheliomatous variety. **C.** Vertical section through left tympanic membrane and external auditory canal. The endotheliomatous meningioma that had invaded the left hypotympanum, adjacent tympanic membrane, and external meatus has given rise to a chronic granular myringitis and external otitis. **D.** Same section as in **C.** The tumor invading the left tympanic annulus displays the same endoetheliomatous pattern. (Hematoxylin and eosin, ×10, ×100, × 20, and ×400, respectively.)

References

1. Burian K. Otitis haemorrhagica externa. Monatsschr Ohrenheilkd 1952;32:226.
2. Becker A. Die virusbedingten Erkrankungen im Hals-Nasen-Ohrenbereich. Arch Ohren-Nasen-Kehlkopfheilkd 1955;167:106.
3. Politzer A. Die Entzündungen des Trommelfells. In: Politzer A, ed. Lehrbuch der Ohrenheilkunde für Praktische Ärzte und Studierende. 5th ed. Stuttgart: Ferdinand Enke, 1908:234–241.
4. Bezold F. Erkrankungen des Trommelfells. In: Bezold F, Lehrbuch der Ohrenheilkunde für Ärzte und Studierende. Wiesbaden: JF Bergmann, 14 Vortrag. 1906:135–142.
5. Moffett AJ. Granulating myringitis—an unusual affection of the ear drum. J Laryngol 1943;58:453–456.
6. Senturia BH. Diseases of the external ear. Springfield, Illinois: Charles C Thomas, 1957.
7. Brown OE, Meyeroff WL. Diseases of the tympanic membrane. In: Paparella MMP, Shumrick DA, Gluckman JL, Meyeroff WL, eds. Otolaryngology, Vol II: Otology and neuro-otology. 3rd ed. Philadelphia: WB Saunders, Chap 25, 1991:1271–1288.

11/ Otitis Media with Effusion (Serous Otitis)

DEFINITION

Otitis media with effusion, also known as serous otitis (1), is a disease that involves both the Eustachian tube and middle ear. It results from a dysfunction of the Eustachian tube, where the causes are manifold and often suggest a complex interaction of several contributing factors. Depending on the nature of the exudate or transudate in the middle ear space, it may manifest itself under different forms. It often follows an episode of acute otitis media in children 2 years old or younger (2, 3), but it is to be differentiated from the purulent otitis media.

AGE INCIDENCE AND SEX DISTRIBUTION

Otitis media affects primarily infants and young children with the highest incidence between 6 and 24 months. Over 60% have had otitis media before the age of 2 years. Boys are affected more frequently than girls (4).

ETIOLOGY AND PATHOGENESIS

Serous otitis media is, in most instances, associated with a malfunction or partial or total occlusion of the Eustachian tube. The etiology of tubal obstruction varies considerably and includes inflammatory diseases and anatomical, mechanical, and a variety of other contributing factors. An abnormal development or underdevelopment of the temporal bone, an intrinsic or extrinsic compression of the Eustachian tube by a bone dysplasia or a neoplastic process, and a fracture of the petrous apex can cause an obstruction of the tubal lumen. Hyperplasia of the adenoids or lymphoid tissue involving the nasopharyngeal ostium or lumen of the Eustachian tube, a neoplastic process arising in those locations, or postadenoidectomy scars and adhesions can block the Eustachian passage. Similarly, a sinusitis, rhinopharyngitis, or allergy, by producing a mucosal edema, may interfere with the tubal patency. Other contributing elements include seasonal, socioeconomic, immunologic, microbiologic, and genetic factors, lack of transmission of specific immunoglobulins during breast feeding, and dysfunction of the tensor and levator veli palatini muscles associated with a cleft palate. In children, adenoid hyperplasia is the most prominent predisposing factor, and rhinopharyngitis is the most frequent cause.

The occlusion of the Eustachian tube produces a decrease in intratympanic pressure and air exchange in and to the middle ear. The negative intratympanic pressure results from resorption of oxygen by the mucoperiosteum of the middle ear. The decrease in intratympanic pressure produces an occlusion of the tubal isthmus by suction and collapse of its mucosal walls. Under normal circumstances, a slight increase in the nasopharyngeal pressure readily overcomes a suction-locking effect up to about −25 mm Hg. In the presence of an edema of the tubal mucosa, caused by an inflammatory, allergic, or some other condition, the identical increase in nasopharyngeal pressure is no longer able to overcome an even lower negative intratympanic pressure of only −5 mm Hg (3, 5).

A persisting negative middle ear pressure may give rise to extravasation of fluid from the vascular bed into the surrounding mucoperiosteal tissue, intercellular spaces, and air spaces of the middle ear. The pressure differential between external and middle ear results in a retraction of the tympanic membrane, in abolition of the triangular light reflex, and in a vascular hyperemia of the vessels of the drum, all characteristic features of serous otitis media. The resulting stiffness of the ossicular chain may be reflected by the presence of a conductive hearing loss.

MICROSCOPIC APPEARANCE

The serous otitis media is characterized histologically by vascular hyperemia and edema of the mucoperiosteum, by epithelial desquamation, by round cell infiltrations, and by accumulation of an exudate in the middle ear cleft (Figs. 11.1 and 11.2). As the inflammatory process persists, the originally flat cuboidal epithelium undergoes a progressive metaplasia and transition to a columnar ciliated epithelium with goblet cells that under normal circumstances are only present around the tympanic orifice of the Eustachian tube and in the adjacent hypotympanum. The ciliated and cuboidal cells have a dark cytoplasm because of their higher concentration of intracellular organelles. The nonciliated cells are cylindrical or cuboidal. Microvilli instead of cilia project from their surface into the middle ear cavity (3). Below these cells and the basement membrane are the basal cells that are the precursors of the epithelial cells. Between the basement membrane and the periosteum lies the subepithelial layer that contains the blood vessels, the capillary network, the nerve fibers of the tympanic plexus, and the connective tissue elements.

In serous otitis media, the spaces between epithelial cells are distended and occupied by fluid that communicates with the middle ear exudate. The increase in thickness of the subepithelial layer results from an interstitial edema and a distension and hyperemia of the vascular network (Figs. 11.1C and 11.2C). Few inflammatory cells are generally encountered (3). In the mucoid form of chronic serous otitis media, the ciliated columnar epithelium predominates, and goblets cells are frequently encountered.

MICROORGANISMS

The bacterial pathogenes most frequently identified in serous otitis media include: *Streptococcus pneumoniae, Haemophilus influenzae,* group A streptococcus, *Staphylococcus aureus, Staphylococcus epidermidis, Branhamella catarrhalis,* and Gram-negative enteric bacilli. Viruses are also involved (3).

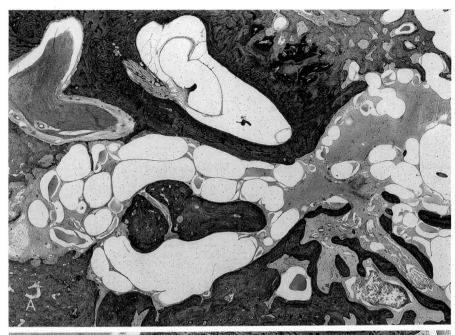

Figure 11.3.   A. Horizontal section of left temporal bone of a 63-year-old man with chronic serous otitis. The middle ear exudate has undergone progressive resorption and replacement by ingrowth of a fibrous connective tissue. (Hematoxylin and eosin, ×10.)

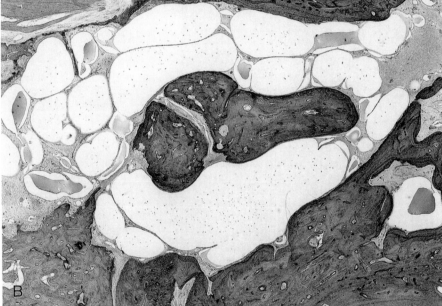

Figure 11.3.   B. In the epitympanic recess the malleus and incus are involved in a network of fibrous strands and adhesions, with some of the compartments still containing remnants of the exudate. (×25.)

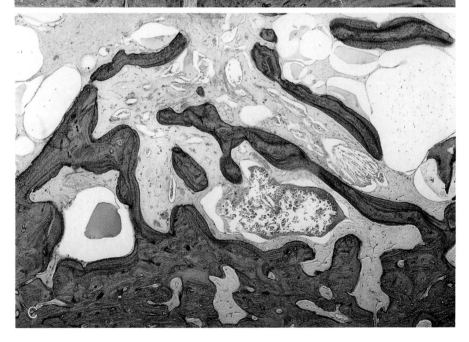

Figure 11.3.   C. The mastoid antrum includes large sheets of fibrous scar tissue, areas where the exudate is undergoing decomposition and resorption, and a region where the disintegration of the exudate has given rise to the formation of cholesterol crystals. (×25.)

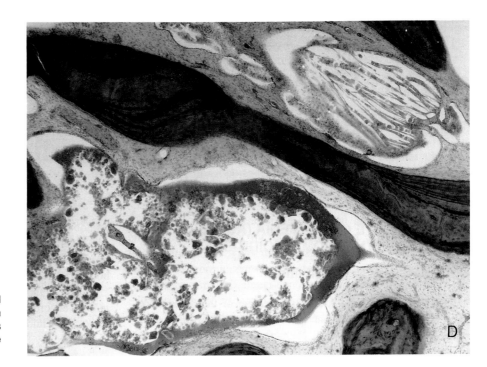

Figure 11.3. **D.** The area of multiple longitudinal clefts within a cystic space of the mucoperiosteum represents an accumulation of cholesterol crystals that were dissolved during the preparation of the sections. (×65.)

CHRONIC SEROUS OTITIS

At times, it may be difficult to differentiate between recurrent attacks of acute serous otitis and a single episode that continues over several months. In the latter case, the tympanic membrane tends to become increasingly retracted. The originally serous exudate, which derived primarily from blood serum, becomes steadily more viscous. Subsequently, organization of this gelatinous exudate by ingrowth of a vascular connective tissue leads to adhesions and scar formations between the middle ear ossicles and walls of the tympanic cavity, a condition recognized as a middle ear adhesive process (Fig. 11.3) (6–9). In many instances, this is associated with a partial or complete obstruction of the Eustachian tube.

The introduction of antimicrobial agents after some time brought about a certain change in the behavior and course of some forms of acute otitis media. In instances where an acute infection could not be readily controlled, transitions into a serous otitis could be observed in increasing numbers.

Except for the development of a retraction pocket of the drum, which in turn can lead to a cholesteatoma, the formation of a cholesterol granuloma, and a conductive hearing loss, the serous otitis does not predispose to serious complications (6).

The "idiopathic hematotympanum" may be considered a sequel of chronic serous otitis media, as it frequently develops on that basis. The condition is characterized by a dark reddish-blue discoloration of the tympanic cavity, usually accompanied by a conductive hearing loss and a chronic course. The appearance of the drum is due to the presence of an inflammatory exudate in the middle ear that contains fresh and partially metabolized blood. It reflects the existence of an underlying cholesterol granuloma. The granuloma is a reaction to the presence of cholesterol crystals. Cholesterol crystals may develop from the middle ear exudate that derives from the blood serum or from the dis-integration of macrophages and other cell material. They also develop from extravasation of blood and breakdown of erythrocytes. Bleeding into the middle ear results from desquamation of the epithelium with exposure and damage of the underlying vessels (5, 10). Cholesterol crystals are irritative foreign bodies that become engulfed by histiocytes and lead to the formation of cholesterol foreign body granulomas. As the cholesterol granulomas include numerous abnormally friable blood vessels, they in turn become the source of recurrent hemorrhages and formation of more cholesterol crystals and granulomas and thus promote a vicious circle.

References

1. Zöllner F. Anatomie, Physiologie, Pathologie und Klinik der Ohrtrompete und ihrer diagnostisch-therapeutischen Beziehungen zu allen Nachbarschaftserkrankungen. Berlin: Springer, 1942.
2. Pelton SI, Shurin PA, Klein JO. Persistence of middle ear effusion after otitis media. Pediatr Res 1977;11:504.
3. Paparella MM, Jung TTK, Goycoolea MV. Otitis media with effusion. In: Paparella MM, Shumrick DA, Gluckman JL, Meyerhoff WL, eds. Otolaryngology, Vol II: Otology and neuro-otology. 3rd ed. Philadelphia: WB Saunders, Chap 27, 1991;1317–1342.
4. Stewart I, Kirkland, C, Simpson A, Silva P, Williams S. Some factors of possible etiologic significance related to otitis media with effusion. In: Lim DJ, Bluestone CD, Klein JO, Nelson JD, eds. Recent advances in otitis media with effusion. Philadelphia: BC Decker, 1984;25–27.
5. Ingelsted S. Chronic adhesive otitis. Acta Otolaryngol (Stockh) 1963;188(Suppl):19.
6. Schätzle W, Haubrich J. Tubenmittelohrkatarrh. In: Doerr W, Seifert G, Uehlinger E, eds. Spezielle pathologische Anatomie, Pathologie des Ohres. Berlin: Springer, 1975;68–72.
7. Sirala U. Adhesive otitis. Acta Otolaryngol (Stockh) Suppl 1960;158:301.
8. Sirala U. Restoration of air-filled tympanum. Ann Otol Rhinol Laryngol 1963;72:97.
9. Sirala U. Otitis media adhesiva. Arch Otolaryngol 1964;80:287.
10. Matzker J. Das "idiopathische Hematotympanum." Z Laryngol Rhinol 1964;40:532.

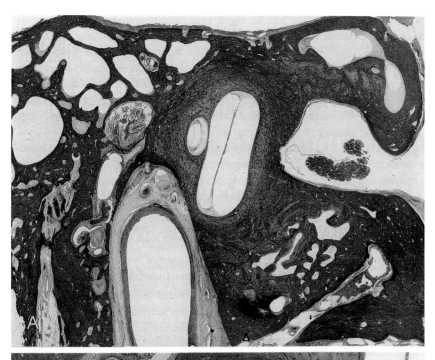

Figure 12.1. A. Vertical, anterior paramodiolar section through right temporal bone of a 35-year-old man with an early stage of acute otitis media and Eustachian salpingitis. (Hematoxylin and eosin, ×6.)

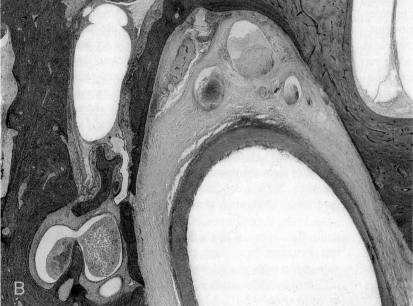

Figure 12.1. B. Purulent exudate lines the floor of the Eustachian tube and occupies two infratubular cells. (×10.)

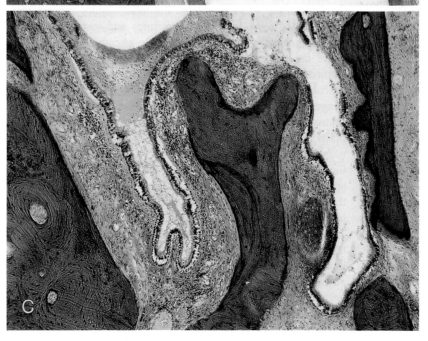

Figure 12.1. C. The submucosa of the mucoperiosteum lining the floor of the Eustachian tube is greatly thickened by an inflammatory edema. (×80.)

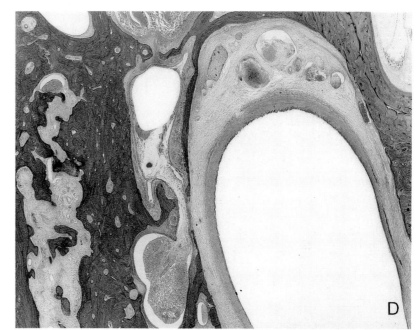

Figure 12.1.   D. Vertical section of same specimen as in *A–C* through Eustachian tube and adjacent carotid artery. A dehiscence in the osseous carotid canal, as shown here, can lead to the spread of an infection in the peritubal cells to the pericarotid venous plexus and cavernous sinus. (×10.)

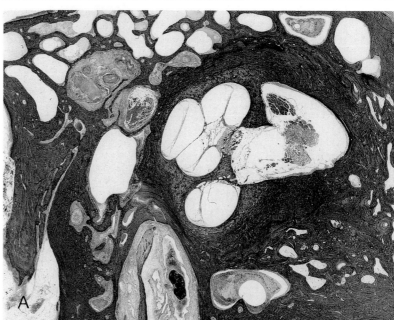

Figure 12.2.   A. Vertical, anterior paramodiolar section of same specimen as in Figure 12.1. Most peritubal and some perilabyrinthine air cells contain an inflammatory exudate. (Hematoxylin and eosin, ×6.)

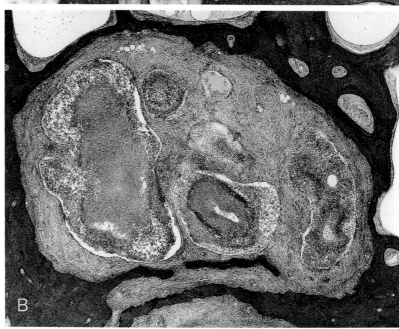

Figure 12.2.   B. A large air cell lateral to the tensor tympani muscle includes an encapsulated empyema. (×30.)

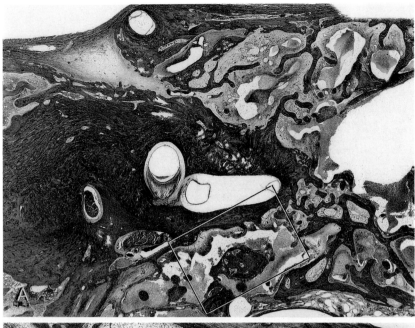

Figure 12.6. A. Horizontal section through right temporal bone at level of superior margin of vestibular fenestra in a 7-month-old infant with acute purulent otitis media. The tympanic cavity, mastoid antrum, and periantral cells are filled with purulent exudate. (Hematoxylin and eosin, ×5.)

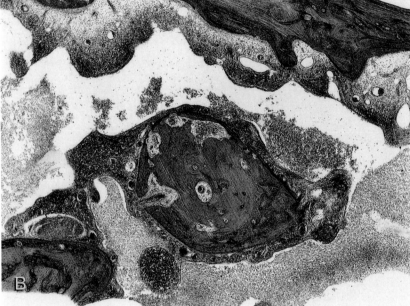

Figure 12.6. B. Note the polypoid thickening of the mucoperiosteum covering the promontory and middle ear ossicles. The inflammatory process extends from the mucoperiosteum to a marrow space in the long process of the incus along a vascular channel. (×35.)

become involved in the ossification process. Whether or not new bone is laid down depends on the reaction of the connective tissue. Thus, a defect following osteoclastic bone resorption may be filled in with connective tissue only or with new bone.

In the uncomplicated chronic mucoperiosteitis, the middle ear ossicles are, in general, less frequently involved. In the persistent mucoperiosteitis associated, for instance, with a cholesteatoma, osteitis is always present, the blood supply of the ossicles is often affected, and sooner or later the ossicles are eroded or destroyed (Fig. 12.7). The long process of the incus is particularly prone to destruction. Firm scar tissue, at times, may splint the bony defect and restore some of the initially lost stability of the ossicular chain (Figs. 12.8 and 12.9). An osteitic process in the wall of the epitympanic recess may lead to a secondary bony union between the head of the malleus and the tegmen and to the lateral or the medial wall of the attic (Fig. 12.10). In general, the incidence of involvement of the auditory ossicles steadily increases from the simple, nonperforative otitis media to the chronic otitis media associated with osteitis.

In the mastoid cells, the inflammatory process may heal without complications. In the presence of persisting infection, inadequate drainage, and retention of the inflammatory exudate, the mucoperiosteum may be destroyed and replaced by an osteoclastic granulation tissue. Consequently, bone is being destroyed by lacunar resorption along vascular channels and along the surface of the trabeculae and walls of the mastoid cells (Fig. 12.11). This leads to destruction of cell partitions and coalescence. Subsequently, osteoid bone is deposited within this granulation tissue and on the walls of the remaining bone, and gradually smaller or larger areas undergo secondary sclerosis (Fig. 12.12). The characteristic histologic findings in chronic otitis are, therefore, (a) the simultaneous occurrence of every stage of the inflammatory process and of bone destruction and (b) the repair by new bone formation.

The surgical observations coincide entirely with the histologic findings. Areas of coalescence may be encountered next to mastoid cells containing purulent exudate or fibrous or polypoid granulation tissue or simply showing an inflammatory edema.

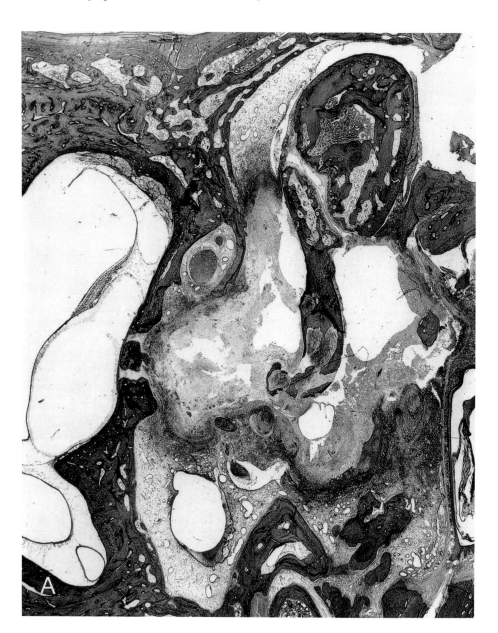

Figure 12.7 A. Vertical section through left petrous pyramid at level of incudomalleolar articulation of a 20-month-old girl with chronic purulent otitis media. The severe polypoid thickening of the mucoperiosteum, the localized necrosis of the epithelium, the dense infiltration with inflammatory cells, and the cyst formation are characteristic features of the chronic form of otitis media. (Hematoxylin and eosin, ×8.5.)

Bone undergoing destruction has a decayed, crumbly texture, whereas newly formed osteoid bone possesses a soft pumice-stone-like consistency. The experienced surgeon recognizes the significance of the differences between these bony textures.

Factors that also influence the development of chronic otitis media include a remaining defect of the drum and a usually severe form of the initial acute otitis media. A persistent tympanic membrane perforation predisposes to external reinfections and introduction of foreign material from the nasopharynx (5). Certain necrotizing forms of acute otitis media as observed many decades ago with scarlet fever, diphtheria, and tuberculosis, in which the tympanic membrane and middle ear mucoperiosteum underwent rapid and often total destruction, have frequently led to a very severe form of chronic middle ear disease.

Two forms of chronic otitis media may be distinguished, depending on whether the inflammation is limited to the mucoperiosteum or involves bone. The former affects primarily the mesotympanum and is associated with a central, usually inferior, occasionally anterior pars tensa perforation and a mucopurulent, generally odorless discharge. It may continue for months but eventually subsides and does not lead to serious complications. The latter form of chronic otitis media affects primarily the epitympanum. It is associated with a marginal perforation of the pars tensa or Shrapnell's membrane and regularly by an osteitic destruction of the posterior superior bony canal wall or lateral wall of the attic. In most instances, it is accompanied by a cholesteatoma and, therefore, predisposes to a variety of serious complications (5).

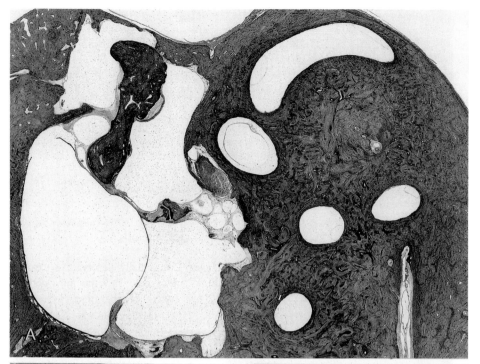

Figure 12.10. **A.** Vertical section through right temporal bone at level of malleus of a 45-year-old woman with a history of recurrent otitis media in childhood. The otologic examination of the right ear had revealed *(a)* a partially fixed malleus, *(b)* a central atrophic scar in the inferior pars tensa, and *(c)* a moderate conductive hearing loss. The localized, postinflammatory synostosis between the head of the malleus and tegmen tympani and the atrophic scar in the tympanic membrane are clearly recognized. (Hematoxylin and eosin, ×4.5.)

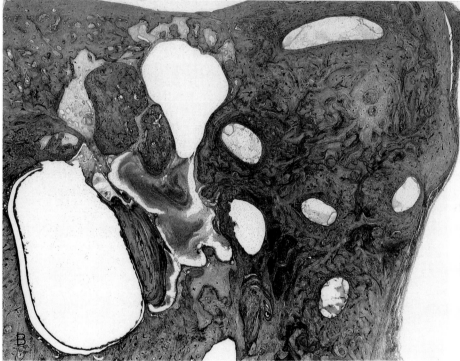

Figure 12.10. **B.** Vertical section through right temporal bone at level of incudomalleolar articulation in a 25-year-old man with chronic otitis media. The beginning postinflammatory synostosis between the head of the malleus and the tegmen tympani is clearly visible. (×8.5.)

Chronic Otitis Media with Predominant Involvement of the Mucoperiosteum

Chronic otitis media with predominant involvement of the mucoperiosteum is a disease characteristically associated with a persistent pars tensa peforation, the margins of which have become covered by squamous epithelium, therefore preventing healing by a spontaneous closure. The subepithelial layer of the mucoperiosteum is greatly thickened by an inflammatory edema (Fig. 12.13). The vessels are markedly distended and overflowing with blood. It contains dense localized and diffuse lymphocytic infiltrations (Fig. 12.13C). The epithelial lining consists of cuboidal or high columnar ciliated cells with goblet cells. The exudate is purulent with abundant polymorphonuclear leukocytes, lymphocytes, plasma cells, and macrophages. The mucoperiosteum often takes on a polypoid appearance (Fig. 12.13B, E, and F). The multiple cysts encountered throughout the submucosal layer result from invaginations and depressions of the epithelium that become separated and embedded in the deeper layers of the submucosa (Fig. 12.13B and D). They are lined with the same cuboidal secretory epithelial cells and contain a homogeneous eosinophilic fluid (Fig. 12.14A–F). In some places the gradual organization of the middle ear exudate with resorption and ingrowth of a vascular connective tissue from the adjacent epithelium can be followed. This newly formed connective tissue may lead to a constriction of the tympanic cavity, investment of the middle ear ossicles, and obliteration of the window niches. The loss of ossicular mobility and cover of the window regions will interfere with sound conduction. Also, localized necrosis of the long process of the incus, by leading to an interruption in the ossicular chain, will manifest itself with a conductive hearing loss. Regressive changes in the subepithelial layer of the mucoperiosteum can give rise to metaplastic calcification and ossifications (5).

In this form of chronic otitis media the hyperplastic polypoid mucosa may occasionally protrude through the central perforation into the outer ear canal and give the appearance of a pedunculated polyp lined by a ciliated epithelium with goblet cells or covered by squamous epithelium. It can also be associated with a highly vascular inflammatory granulation tissue that typically lacks an epithelial cover and whose capillaries are exposed to the surface. This tissue, therefore, bleeds readily on the slightest touch with a suction tip (5). Cholesterol granulomas are also frequently part of this disease. They represent a foreign body tissue reaction to the presence of cholesterol crystals. They are characterized histologically by giant cells, fibroblasts histiocytes, and, occasionally, hemosiderin deposits.

Tympanosclerosis

A significant consequence occasionally observed in chronic otitis media with predominant involvement of the mucoperiosteum is the localized or diffuse hyalin degeneration of the mucoperiosteum with subsequent calcification and ossification, a process generally recognized as tympanosclerosis (Fig. 12.15). It was first described in 1873 (6) and has since been the topic of frequent discussions (5, 7–10). It is characterized histologically by ossification and calcification of a previously fibrosed and hyalinized mucoperiosteum in an onion-skin-like lamellar arrangement. This peculiar connective tissue reaction might reflect an allergic phenomenon. It is generally most prominent in the epitympanic recess (Fig. 12.15B), around the middle ear ossicles (Fig. 12.15E, G, and H), over the promontory (Fig. 12.15B, C, J, and K), in the oval window region (Fig. 12.15B, C, and L), and in the tympanic membrane (Fig. 12.15D–I). It may greatly increase the mass of the eardrum and totally immobilize it. By involving the oval window it may firmly fix the stapes (Fig. 12.15C and L). It can lead to solid encasement of the entire ossicular chain and totally obliterate the tympanic cavity (5, 10).

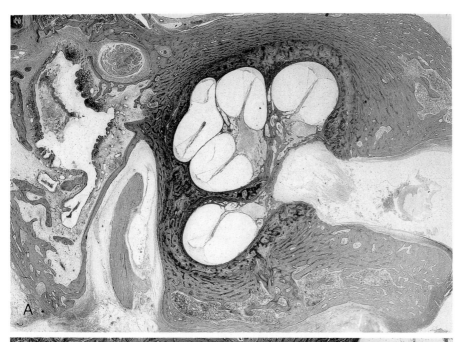

Figure 12.13. A. Vertical midmodiolar section through right petrous pyramid of a 3-month-old boy with bilateral chronic purulent otitis media, labyrinthitis, and meningitis. (Hematoxylin and eosin, ×9.)

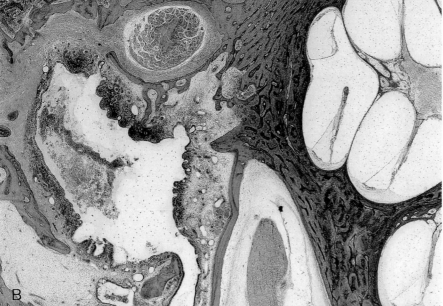

Figure 12.13. B. The mucoperiosteum outlining the tympanic orifice of the Eustachian tube and the anterior mesotympanum reveals a marked inflammatory edema. Purulent exudate occupies the middle ear space. (×14.)

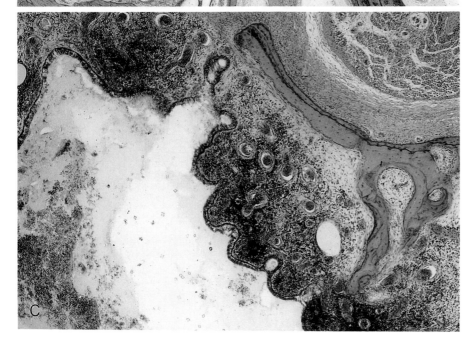

Figure 12.13. C. The mucoperiosteum displays a large number of greatly dilated, hyperemic blood vessels and localized and diffuse lymphocytic infiltrations. (×65.)

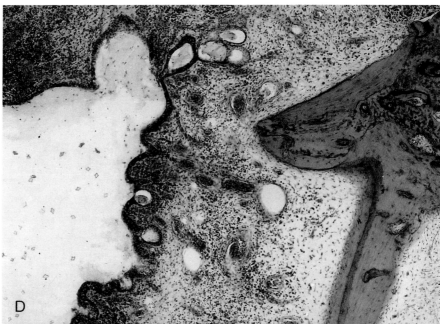

Figure 12.13. D. Invagination and protrusions of the epithelium into the underlying submucosal layer and subsequent separation lead to the formation of multiple cysts scattered throughout the submucosa. (×65.)

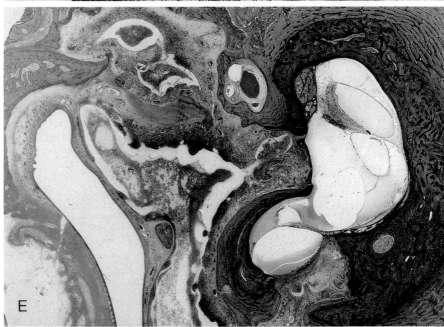

Figure 12.13. E. Vertical section at level of vestibular and cochlear fenestrae. The middle ear cavity is lined by a polypoid, greatly thickened, inflammatory mucoperiosteum that completely obliterates the oval and round window niches. (×10.)

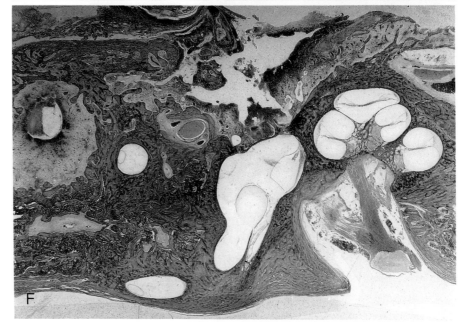

Figure 12.13. F. Horizontal, superior paramodiolar section through left temporal bone of the same patient. The chronic inflammatory changes are identical throughout the middle ear cleft. The meningitis is characterized by the presence of an inflammatory exudate in the subarachnoid space of the internal auditory canal. (×6.)

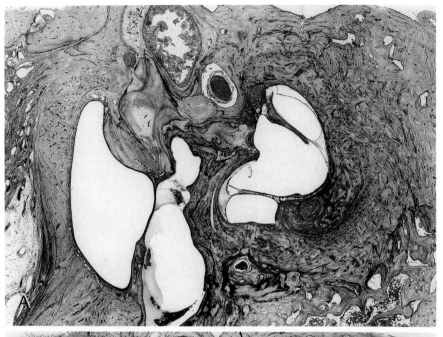

Figure 12.15. A. Vertical section through right temporal bone near anterior border of vestibular fenestra of a 34-year-old woman with a history of acute perforative otitis media at the age of 12, extensive tympanosclerosis, and a maximal conductive hearing loss. (Hematoxylin and eosin, ×10.)

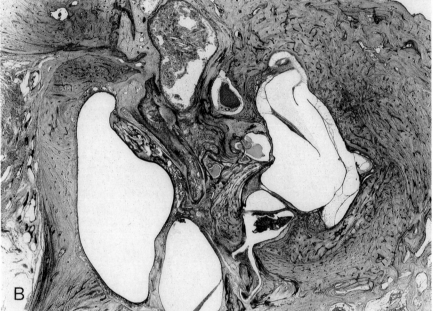

Figure 12.15. B. Vertical section near center of vestibular and cochlear fenestrae. The pars tensa of the tympanic membrane and the mucoperiosteum of the middle ear had been replaced by a solid mass of fibrous connective tissue revealing extensive hyaline degeneration and calcification. (×10.)

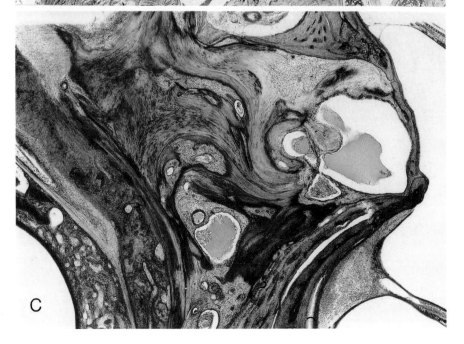

Figure 12.15. C. The middle ear cavity and the niche of the oval window are completely obliterated by masses of tympanosclerosis displaying a characteristic lamellar arrangement. This resulted in total immobilization of the stapes. (×35.)

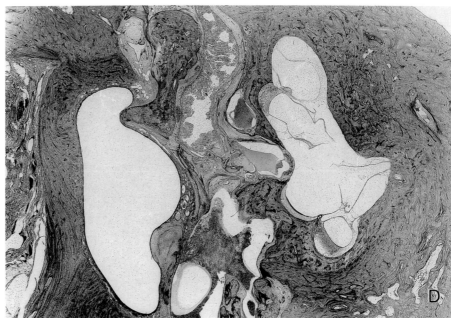

Figure 12.15. **D.** Vertical section near posterior border of oval window. A recent hemorrhage has occurred into the medial compartment of the epitympanum. The hypotympanum is occupied by purulent exudate. (×10.)

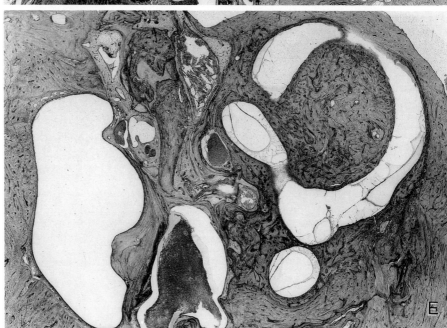

Figure 12.15. **E.** Vertical section at level of incudomalleolar articulation. Malleus and incus are solidly embedded in tympanosclerotic masses. An exophytic tympanosclerotic process involves the lower half of the tympanic membrane. (×10.)

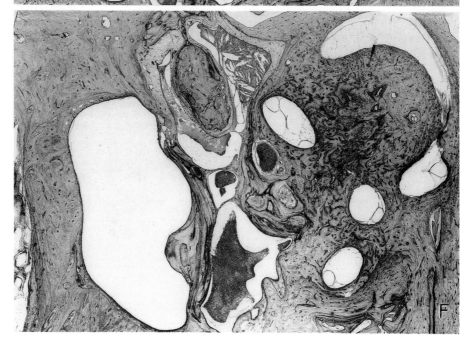

Figure 12.15. **F.** Vertical section at level of superior canal. In the medial compartment of the attic between the body of the incus and the lateral semicircular canal, a cholesterol granuloma has developed within the enclosed space of an old hemorrhage. (×10.)

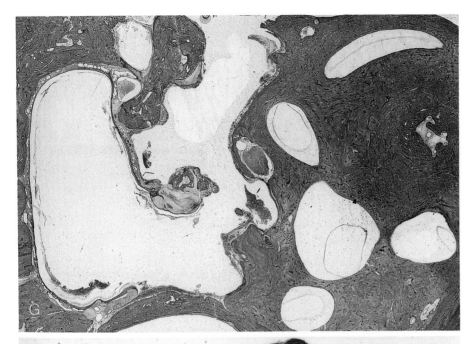

Figures 12.15. G. Vertical section through right temporal bone of a 37-year-old man with chronic otitis media, subtotal marginal tympanic membrane perforation, and extensive tympanosclerosis. (Hematoxylin and eosin, ×7.5.)

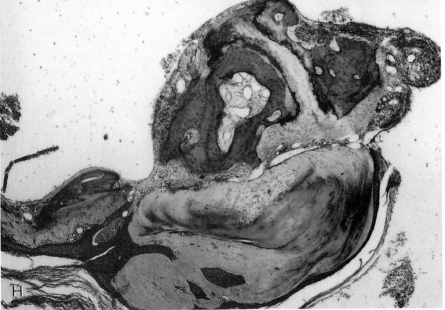

Figure 12.15. H. Several tympanosclerotic lesions involve the mucoperiosteum lining the auditory ossicles, their articulations, and the walls of the middle ear cavity. (×45.)

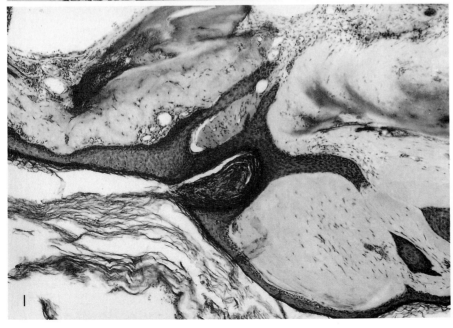

Figure 12.15. I. The tympanosclerotic lesion involving the superior margin of the tympanic membrane perforation and adjacent incudostapedial articulation has been invaded by an epidermal papilla from the outer layer of the drum. This papilla in turn has given rise to a small epidermoid cyst or beginning cholesteatoma *(arrow).* (×95.)

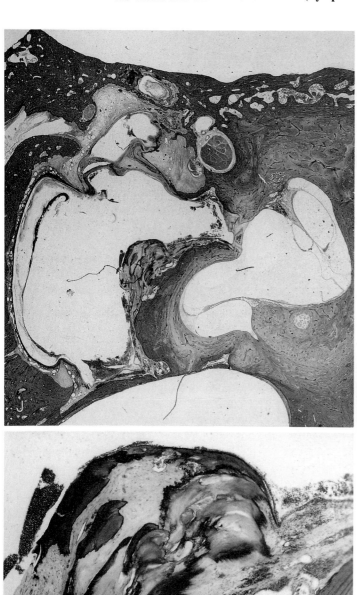

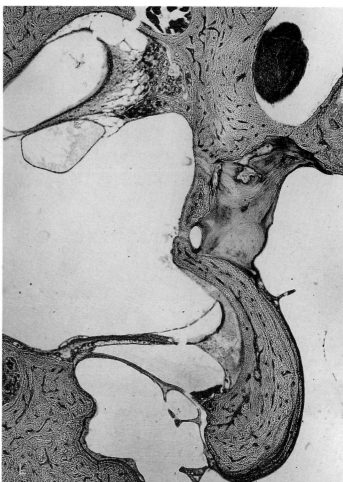

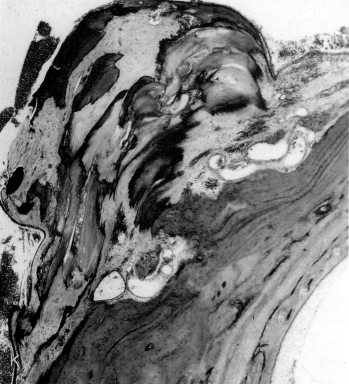

Figure 12.15.   J. An extensive tympanosclerotic mass is covering the promontory. **K.** Typical layered structure of hyalinized and partially calcified connective tissue and its propensity to erode underlying cochlear capsule. **L.** Vertical section through left temporal bone of a 28-year-old woman with chronic otitis media and massive tympanosclerotic lesion totally obliterating the oval window and solidly embedding the stapes, causing a maximal conductive hearing loss. (Hematoxylin and eosin, ×8, ×50, and ×25, respectively.)

Chronic Otitis Media with Involvement of the Mucoperiosteum and Bone

Chronic otitis media with involvement of the mucoperiosteum and underlying bone is a disease characteristically associated with *(a)* marginal perforation of Shrapnell's membrane or the posterior superior portion of the pars tensa and *(b)* the presence of a cholesteatoma. The perforation in Shrapnell's membrane is regularly accompanied by an osteitic destruction of the lateral wall of the attic. The posterior superior pars tensa perforation is routinely accompanied by osteolytic destruction of the posterosuperior bony canal wall. The portions of the underlying ossicular chain that secondarily become involved are, in order of decreasing frequency: *(a)* the lenticular and long process of the incus, *(b)* the stapedial superstructure, and *(c)* the body of the incus and the head of the malleus. The osteitic defects are frequently covered by an inflammatory vascular granulation tissue (Figs. 12.7 and 12.10). The secretions are purulent, creamy, and malodorous. As the disease progresses within the temporal bone, the osteolytic process can involve the tegmen tympani and tegmen antri, the cortical bone of the mastoid process and petrous pyramid, the region of the sinodural angle, and the Fallopian canal. It can involve the vestibular capsule, most frequently the lateral semicircular canal, the regions of the oval and round windows, and the cochlear capsule, especially the lower basal turn. Depending on the location, an osteitic process may give rise to regional, endocranial, and, via the bloodstream, systemic complications. The factors involved in bone resorption include: *(a)* the osteoclastic effect of the inflammatory process, particularly near the matrix of a cholesteatoma with its irritative influence of the cholesterol esters and fatty acids it contains, and *(b)* the pressure resulting from the increasing accumulation of keratinous material (4). This form of chronic otitis, because of its predisposition to complications is, therefore, more serious. A far less frequent variant of chronic otitis with involvement of mucoperiosteum and bone but not associated with a cholesteatoma leads to fewer and less severe complications and occasionally may heal spontaneously (5).

Sequelae of Chronic Otitis Media

The sequelae from chronic otitis media may involve the tympanic membrane, the mucoperiosteum of the middle ear cleft, and the ossicular chain. It may affect the regions of the vestibular and cochlear fenestrae and the osseous structure of the temporal bone. The tympanic membrane can heal with an atrophic or hypertrophic tympanosclerotic scar or with a partial or total perforation (Fig. 12.16). In the healing process it may become adherent to the ossicular chain or to the promontory (Figs. 12.17 and 12.18). Regressive changes within the mucoperiosteum may lead to localized calcifications and metaplastic ossification. Obliteration of the attic by connective scar tissue will separate the epitympanic space from the retrotympanic space, will cause retention of inflammatory secretions, and thereby can give rise to the formation of cholesterol granulomas (Figs. 12.19 and 12.20). The middle ear ossicles may be partially or totally destroyed or may become embedded and immobilized by scar tissue. The oval and round window niches frequently become obliterated by fibrous connective tissue (Figs. 12.21 and 12.22). In the presence of a larger pars tensa perforation the middle ear cavity often becomes relined by the ingrowth of squamous epithelium from the outer ear canal (Figs. 12.21*B* and *C* and 12.22). Accumulation of keratinous debris can, in turn, give rise to formation of a cholesteatoma (Fig. 12.20). The new bone that has replaced a previous osteolytic defect displays a very different trabecular pattern from the surrounding original bone. This is clearly noticeable in the epitympanic, hypotympanic, and mastoid regions but may also be observed in other areas of the temporal bone (Figs. 12.21*A* and *D* and 12.22).

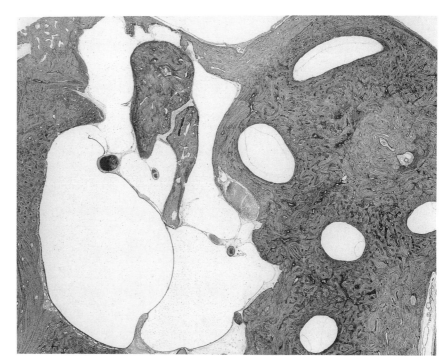

Figure 12.16. Vertical section through right temporal bone at level of incudomalleolar articulation of a 33-year-old man with a distant history of perforative otitis media that resulted in destruction of the greater portion of the pars tensa of the tympanic membrane. A monomeric scar has become adherent to the long crus of the incus, which shows some postinflammatory fibrous replacement of bone. (Hematoxylin and eosin, ×8½.)

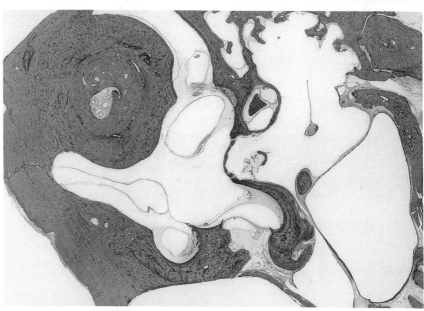

Figure 12.17. Vertical section through left temporal bone at level of oval and round windows of a 17-year-old woman with a distant history of otitis media. It resulted in retraction and fixation of the handle of the malleus and tympanic membrane to the promontory and in partial fibrous occlusion of the round window niche. (Hematoxylin and eosin, ×8½.)

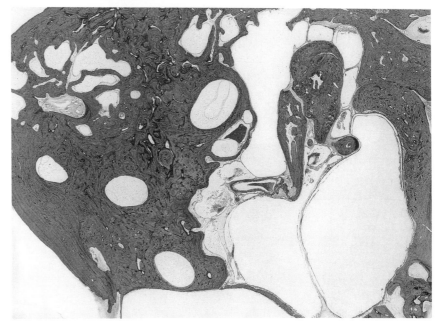

Figure 12.18. Vertical section through left temporal bone at level of ossicular chain in an adult man with a distant history of otitis media. It shows the investment of the stapedial arch in fibrous scar tissue. (Hematoxylin and eosin, ×8½.)

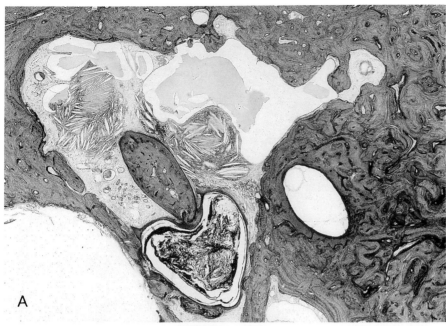

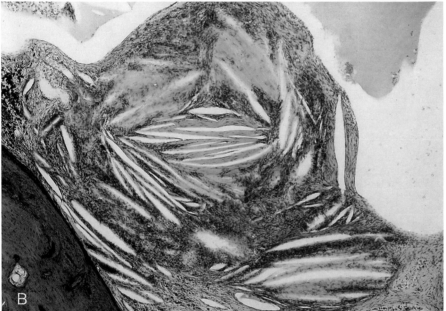

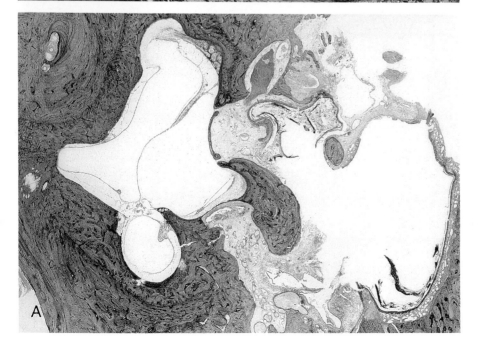

Figure 12.19. A. Vertical section through right temporal bone at level of aditus ad antrum of a 45-year-old man with bilateral chronic otitis media associated with an attic cholesteatoma. This cholesteatoma, by extending toward the antrum, created an attic block that in turn gave rise to the development of a cholesterol granuloma. (Hematoxylin and eosin, ×12.)

Figure 12.19. B. The cholesterol granuloma is a reaction to the presence of cholesterol crystals that develop during breakdown of erythrocytes and during disintegration of other cell material. (×50.)

Figure 12.20. A. Vertical section through left temporal bone at level of vestibular and cochlear fenestrae in the same patient as in Figure 12.19, with chronic otitis media associated with a marginal pars tensa perforation and a middle ear cholesteatoma. (Hematoxylin and eosin, ×8½.)

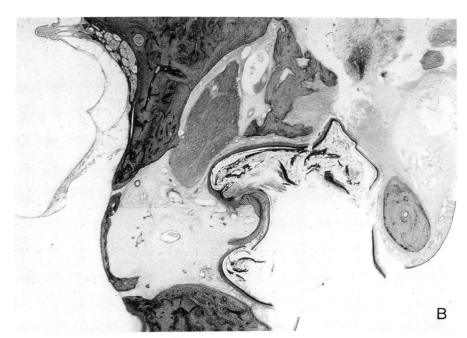

Figure 12.20. B. Both window niches are obliterated by fibrous connective tissue. The stapedial arch is covered by the matrix of the cholesteatoma. (×17.)

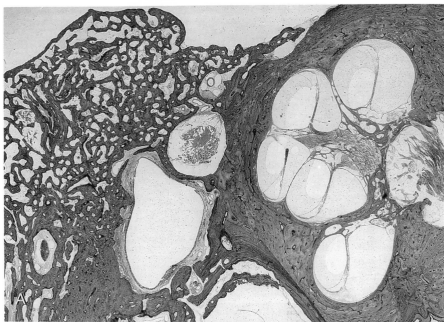

Figure 12.21. A. Vertical midmodiolar section through right petrous pyramid in a 43-year-old man with a distant history of chronic bilateral otitis media and evidence of bone remodeling following osteitis involving the floor of the middle cranial fossa. The trabeculae display a characteristic irregular dense mesh work. (Hematoxylin and eosin, ×6½.)

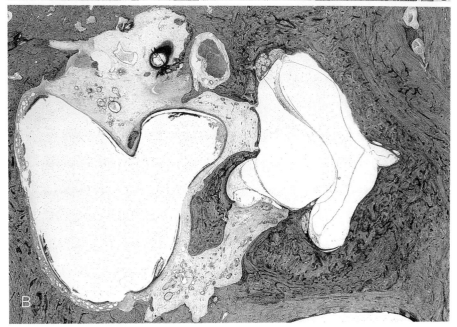

Figure 12.21. B. Vertical section at level of right oval and round windows. The persistent subtotal pars tensa perforation resulted in lining of the middle ear cavity with squamous epithelium from the outer ear canal. (×6½.)

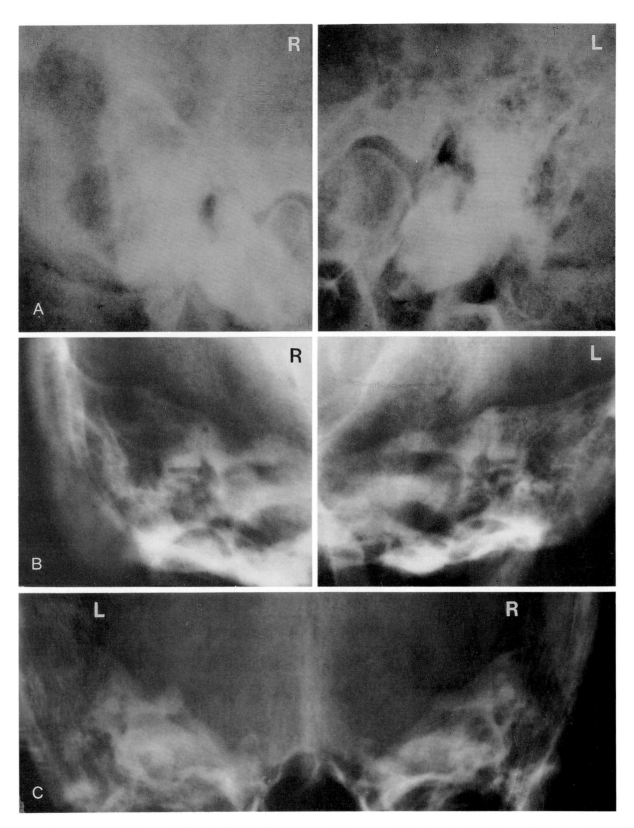

Figure 12.24.   Same patient as in Figure 12.23. In the Schüller, Stenvers, and anteroposterior (AP) projections of the temporal bone, the widespread inflammatory destruction involving the mastoid and posterior portion of the petrous bone and their cortices are well recognized.

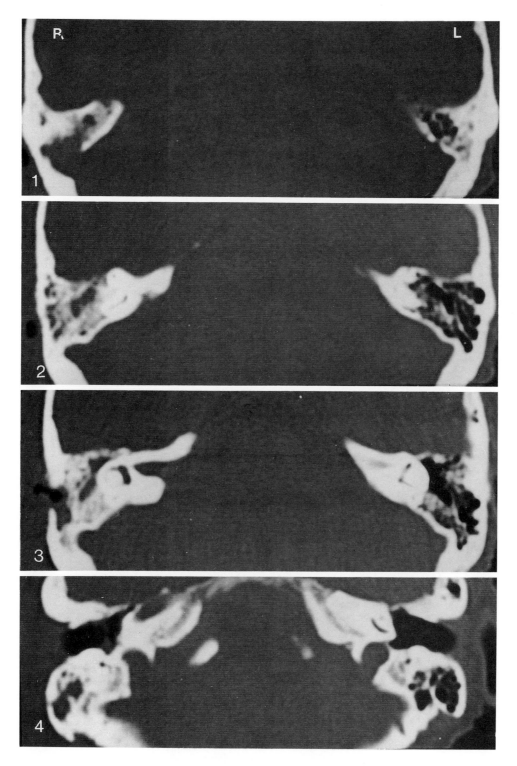

Figure 12.25. Same patient as in Figure 12.23. In the axial computed tomography (CT) scan of the temporal bone, the coalescent osteitic process with destruction of the lateral and the medial cortex is clearly visible.

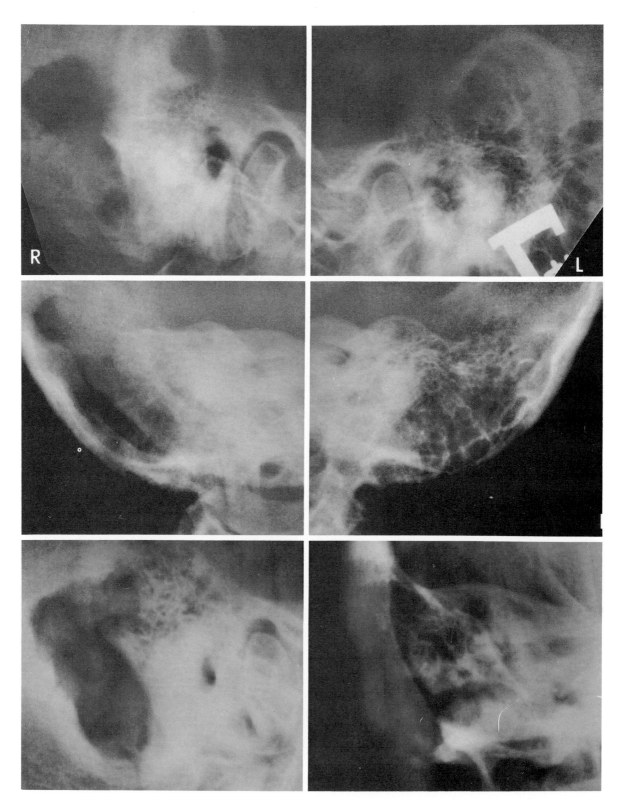

Figure 12.26. This 45-year-old woman presented with a long history of chronic, purulent, right tympanomastoiditis. At operation, an extensive osteitis and osteomyelitis with widespread coalescence involving the mastoid bone and a large abscess overlying the dura of the middle cranial fossa were encountered. The extent of the inflammatory osteolytic process is well demonstrated in the Schüller and Stenvers projections of the right temporal bone.

Osteitis of the Temporal Bone in Other Locations

Osteitis involving the root of the zygoma and the squamous portion of the temporal bone simply represents an osteitic process in another location. Its occurrence is rare, but the clinical manifestations are characteristic.

LABYRINTHITIS

Involvement of the labyrinth is the next most frequent complication of otitis media. It arises more often from a chronic than an acute otitis media, and in the majority of instances it is associated with a cholesteatomatous or necrotizing form of chronic otitis media (Figs. 12.27 and 12.28). The inflammatory process may reach the vestibule and cochlea through the vestibular and cochlear fenestrae, where the oval window represents the more common avenue (Fig. 12.28). The pathway through a fenestra has been documented on many occasions during acute otitis media or an acute exacerbation of uncomplicated chronic otitis media. In the chronic, cholesteatomatous otitis media, perforations usually occur through the labyrinthine capsule, primarily through one of the semicircular canals. Transgression of microorganisms or the mere diffusion of bacterial toxins through the annular ligament or round window membrane suffices to induce labyrinthitis, although sooner or later necrosis and destruction of these structures may follow (Figs. 12.27 and 12.28). Invasion of a semicircular canal usually results from a localized, destructive osteitis, whereas extension of the inflammatory process to the cochlea generally occurs along preformed vascular channels. At times, several perforations into the inner ear capsule develop simultaneously. Within the labyrinth and cochlea the inflammatory process may remain localized or may spread in a diffuse manner. Depending on the nature of the inflammation, the exudate may be serous, hemorrhagic, fibrinous, or purulent, and the character of the inflammatory process may be productive or necrotizing and destructive.

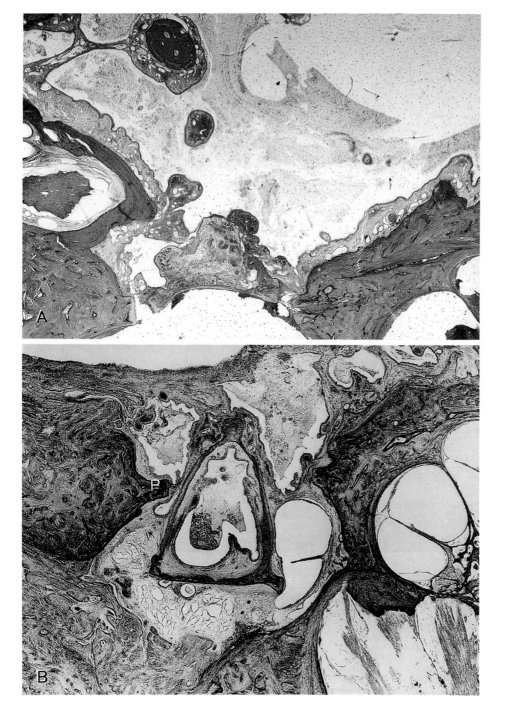

Figure 12.28. A. Horizontal section through left temporal bone at level of oval window of a 9-year-old boy with a history of chronic otitis media followed by otogenic labyrinthitis and lethal meningitis. The destruction of the annular ligament by the inflammatory process opened the pathway for the spread of the infection to the membranous labyrinth and subarachnoid space. (Hematoxylin and eosin, ×17.)

Figure 12.28. B. Horizontal section through left temporal bone at level of oval window of a 20-year-old woman with a history of chronic cholesteatomatous tympanomastoiditis. After a left radical mastoidectomy during which the stapes was accidentally dislocated medially, the patient developed a labyrinthitis and subsequently died from an otogenic meningitis. The displaced stapes is recognized in the vestibule, surrounded by inflammatory granulation tissue. (×20.)

The purulent labyrinthitis invariably leads to total loss of cochlear and vestibular function and occasionally to partial or complete obliteration of the perilymphatic and endolymphatic compartments with connective and osseous tissue (Figs. 12.29 and 12.30). The hearing loss in chronic otitis media, on the other hand, is usually due to impairment of both sound conduction and perception. A perceptive component is identified in about 75% of patients (3, 4). Its incidence is highest in chronic otitis media with cholesteatoma. The recurrence of infections, the bacterial infiltration of the round window membrane, and the persisting effect of toxic substances are thought to be responsible. The secondary tympanic membrane has long been considered a semi-permeable membrane for bacterial and other toxins (4). There is ample clinical and experimental evidence that diffusion of toxins across the round window membrane can affect cochlear and vestibular functions. It has also been shown that an inflammatory process of the mucoperiosteum or of granulation tissue in close proximity to the lateral semicircular canal and mastoid antrum can affect cochlear function and that the resulting sensorineural loss decreases after the surgical eradication of the inflammatory process (4). The effects of bacterial toxins and other toxic substances are reversible in some instances but in the long run may lead to degeneration of the sensorineural cells and their afferent nerve fibers.

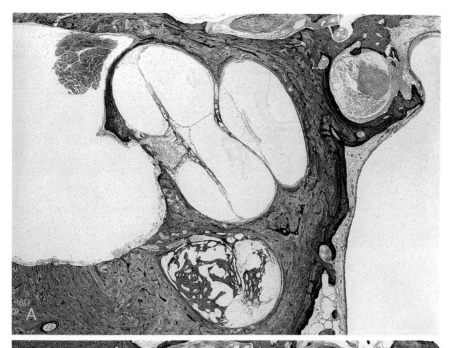

Figure 12.30.   A. Vertical, posterior paramodiolar section through left temporal bone of a 28-year-old man with a distant history of left tympanomastoiditis in early childhood, resulting in total loss of hearing and requiring a transcortical mastoidectomy. (Hematoxylin and eosin, ×16.)

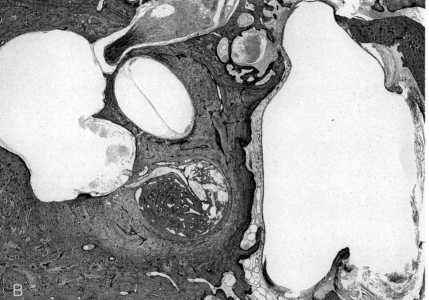

Figure 12.30.   B. The lower basal turn of the cochlea reveals a very circumscribed fibrous and osseous obliteration that resulted from a regional inflammatory process. (×16.)

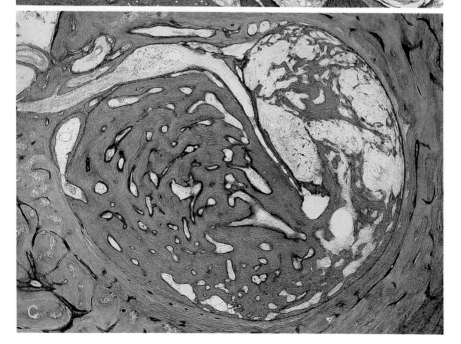

Figure 12.30.   C. The scala vestibuli, scala media, and scala tympani are almost totally obliterated by fibrous tissue and membranous, metaplastic bone. (×45.)

PARALYSIS OF THE FACIAL NERVE

Paralysis of the facial nerve may be a complication of acute or chronic otitis media. It if develops within the first few days of acute otitis media, it is generally caused by an inflammatory edema of the nerve within an intact bony canal. The edema interferes with the blood supply to the nerve and leads to paresis and, ultimately, to paralysis. The acute inflammation in the middle ear may extend to the nerve through one of the usually existent dehiscences in the tympanic or mastoid segment of the Fallopian canal (Fig. 12.31) (11). If the facial nerve palsy develops later during the course of an acute middle ear infection, it is generally caused by an erosion of the Fallopian canal with subsequent involvement of the nerve by the suppurative process.

Paralysis of the facial nerve as a complication of chronic otitis media results from erosion of the Fallopian canal by either a middle ear cholesteatoma, osteitis, or osteomyelitis of the mastoid process or petrous pyramid with an ensuing extension of the infection to the nerve. The perineurium and epineurium generally disclose a cellular infiltration, and the nerve may ultimately undergo partial or total destruction. In the past, tuberculous osteitis and luetic osteitis and, more recently, *Pseudomonas* osteitis in the elderly, severe diabetic patient are other typical examples (Fig. 12.32). On the other hand, there are many known instances in which the Fallopian canal has been widely eroded and the nerve has become completely surrounded by a cholesteatoma and the inflammatory process, without the slightest loss of its function. Paralysis of the facial nerve, which is more often a complication of chronic than acute otitis media, has become a very rare observation.

Endocranial Complications

The source of many endocranial complications is an inflammatory process in the middle ear, mastoid process, petrous pyramid, labyrinth, or sigmoid sinus and its contributing petrosal sinuses. The nature of the complication is determined to a great extent by the character and pathway of the inflammatory process. The three endocranial complications to be considered, in order of decreasing frequency, are: (a) meningitis, (b) sinus thrombophlebitis, and (c) brain abscess.

OTOGENIC MENINGITIS

The origin of an otogenic meningitis may be an acute or a chronic inflammatory process in the middle ear, where both are involved with about equal frequency and neither has a more detrimental influence on the course and severity of a meningeal complication. The following pathways for the spread of infection from the middle ear to the meninges should be considered.

An osteitic process can involve the adjacent dura and from there extend to neighboring structures. These localized osteitic lesions have certain predilective sites. They occur in mastoid cells around the sigmoid sinus and in the roof of the middle ear and antrum. The infection can thus spread through the sinus plate or tegmen to the meninges of the posterior or middle cranial fossa. Osteitic lesions may occasionally develop in the walls of perilabyrinthine and peritubal cells and in the petrous apex and involve the dura in those areas. These particular pathways are hidden and often recognizable only under the microscope, but they play an important role. Natural dehiscences in the osseous structure of the temporal bone are considered to be of lesser importance. Such dehiscences occur in the tegmen, in the petrosquamous fissure, and wherever middle ear mucosa covers the outer surface of the dura.

An important pathway for the propagation of infection begins in the labyrinth. In labyrinthitis after otitis media, the inflammatory process reaches the meninges, in most instances, along the perineural spaces and the internal acoustic meatus and, less frequently, across the endolymphatic and perilymphatic ducts (Figs. 12.33–12.37). In this manner the infection invades the lateral and pontine cisterns directly. An osteitic process originating from labyrinthitis can develop in different regions of the labyrinthine capsule and, like an empyema of the endolymphatic sac, can produce an epidural, intradural, and subdural or subarachnoidal inflammation. Many decades ago, labyrinthitis was responsible for about 60% of all otogenic meningeal complications. Today, it accounts for about 15% or less.

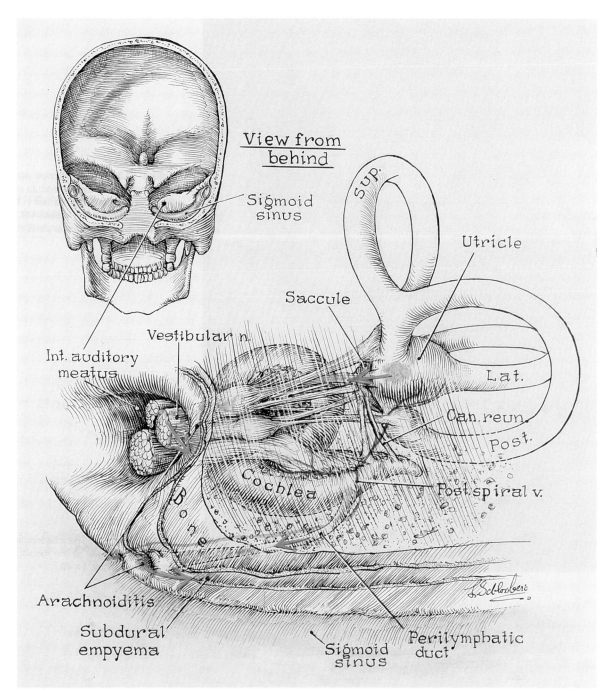

Figure 12.33.   Illustration of right membranous labyrinth, cochlea, and perilymphatic duct (cochlear aqueduct) and their relation to posterior cranial fossa. A labyrinthitis involving the saccule and utricle may extend along the perineural spaces to the internal acoustic meatus. A suppuration within the cochlea may spread via the perilymphatic duct to the meninges.

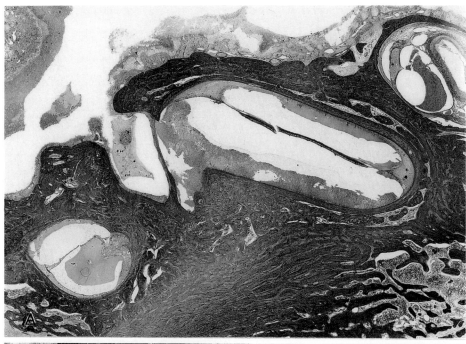

Figure 12.35.   A. Horizontal section through left pyramid of a patient with meningitis occurring after labyrinthitis. Note the inflammatory exudate in the middle ear and in the scala vestibuli and scala tympani of the lower basal turn. (Hematoxylin and eosin, ×14.)

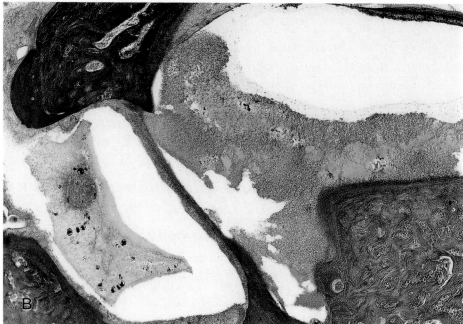

Figure 12.35.   B. The inflammatory exudate in the scala tympani continues into the cochlear orifice of the cochlear aqueduct. The blood vessel near the right lower corner is the vein accompanying the cochlear aqueduct. It opens into the inferior petrosal sinus. (×40.)

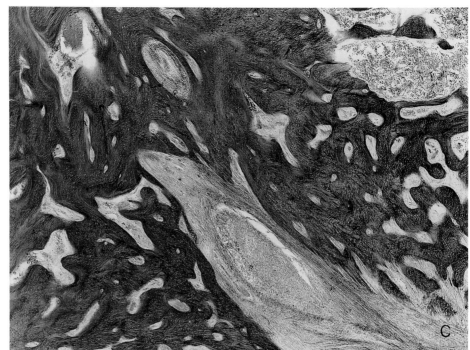

Figure 12.35. C. Horizontal section through left cochlear aqueduct midway between the cochlear and cranial aperture. Its lumen is filled with pus. (×40).

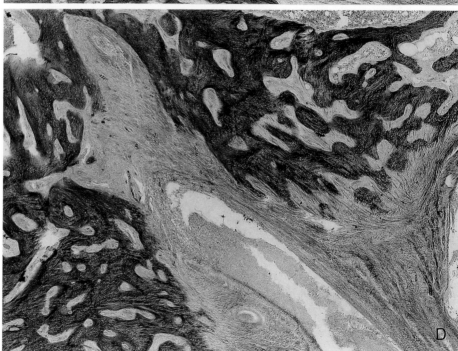

Figure 12.35. D. Horizontal section through left cochlear aqueduct in the region of emergence of glossopharyngeal nerve. Note the purulent exudate pouring into the subarachnoid space of the basilar cistern. (×40.)

The spread of infection along vascular channels occurs more frequently than generally recognized, and therefore deserves greater consideration. Blood vessels connect the vascular network of the temporal bone with the vascular bed of the dura and with the system of venous sinuses. In some instances, direct vascular connections exist between the mucoperiosteum of the middle ear and dura. These veins drain mainly into the pericarotid venous plexus and the jugular bulb. The vascular pathway is of considerable importance in the etiology of meningitis. It plays a significant role in the development of a hematogenous subdural inflammation and a localized meningitis, especially when the circumscribed meningitis is removed from the original source of infection (Fig. 12.38).

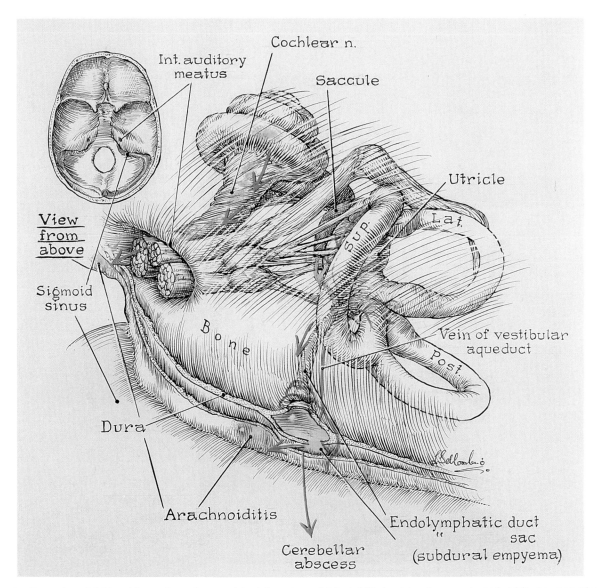

Figure 12.36. Illustration of right cochlea and membranous labyrinth and their relation to posterior cranial fossa. A suppuration within the cochlea may extend along the perineural spaces to the internal acoustic meatus. A labyrinthitis involving the saccule and utricle may spread via the endolymphatic duct system to the meninges, which give rise to a number of endocranial complications.

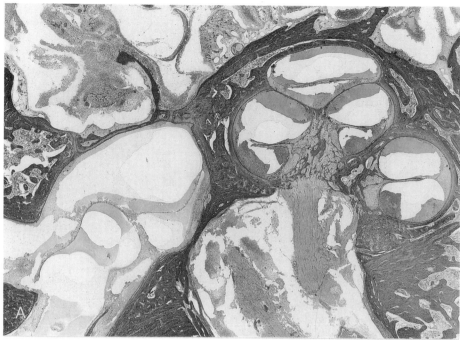

Figure 12.37. A. Horizontal section through left membranous labyrinth at level of origin of endolymphatic duct in a patient with meningitis occurring after labyrinthitis. (Hematoxylin and eosin, ×14.)

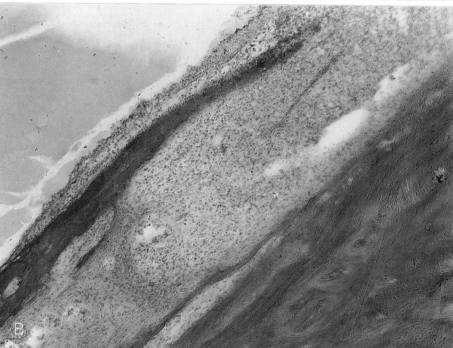

Figure 12.37. B. The purulent exudate within the saccule can be traced into the vestibular opening of the endolymphatic duct. (×100.)

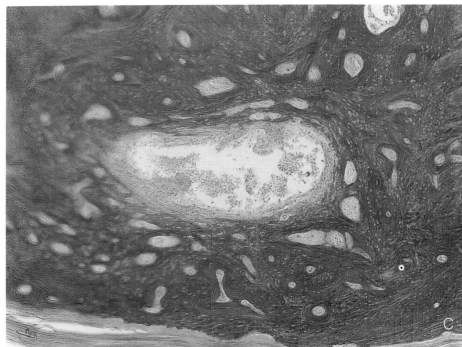

Figure 12.37.   C. Horizontal section through left endolymphatic duct that contains a mass of polymorphonuclear cells. The blood vessel in the right upper corner is the vein of the vestibular aqueduct. (×100.)

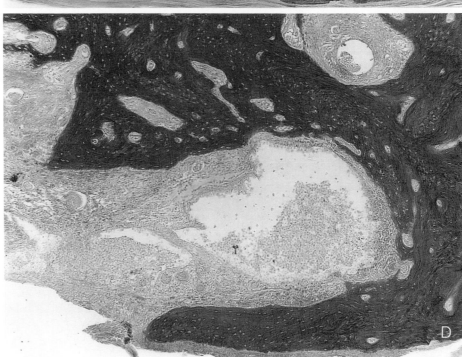

Figure 12.37.   D. Horizontal section through left endolymphatic sac with empyema. This empyema is an intradural abscess that can be the source of a number of endocranial complications. (×100.)

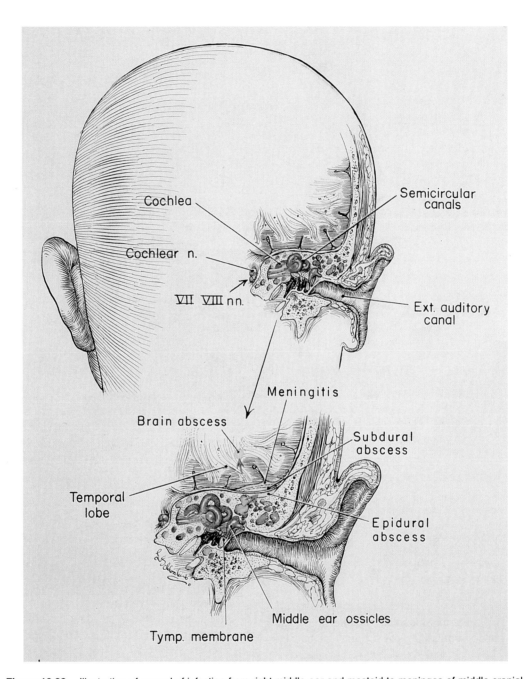

Figure 12.38. Illustration of spread of infection from right middle ear and mastoid to meninges of middle cranial fossa, temporal lobe, petrous apex, and jugular bulb.

Pachymeningitis

Three forms of pachymeningitis may be distinguished: *(a)* epidural, *(b)* intradural, and *(c)* subdural (see Figs. 12.38, 12.43, and 12.48). Epidural inflammation, by far the most frequent, occurs as a proliferative process with formation of granulation tissue on the outer surface of the dura or as an exudative process with an epidural abscess (see Figs. 12.43 and 12.48). At times, the extradural abscess can develop even after the original middle ear infection has subsided.

Thrombophlebitis of the lateral and petrosal sinuses and empyema of the endolymphatic sac are typical examples of an intradural inflammation (see Figs. 12.36 and 12.59). Other etiologic factors are thrombophlebitis in smaller vessels and osteitic lesions. These processes may involve cranial nerves at their point of penetration through the dura.

The internal pachymeningitis, either a proliferative or an exudative inflammation on the inner surface of the dura, is often associated with an extradural and meningeal infection and thus can hardly be considered an independent entity. The exudative inflammation occurs less frequently. In the localized form of pachymeningitis, it can, by colliquation necrosis, lead to a cortical brain abscess. In its diffuse form, a subdural empyema can extend over an entire hemisphere. In the middle cranial fossa, the origin of a subdural empyema frequently is a cholesteatomatous middle ear disease, whereas in the posterior fossa, chronic labyrinthitis or petrous apicitis is the usual source of infection.

Leptomeningitis

Any form of middle ear infection, acute or chronic, may give rise to either a localized or a diffuse leptomeningitis (see Figs. 12.33, 12.36, 12.38, 12.41, and 12.43). The inflammatory process often begins as a basal meningitis, which subsequently may become diffuse and expand over an entire hemisphere. Diffuse meningitis occurs more frequently and often develops as a hematogenous complication, whereas localized meningitis usually originates from a subdural abscess. The subarachnoidal cisterns at the base of the brain and the subarachnoidal spaces of the Sylvian fossa and central sulcus of Rolando are preferential sites for otogenic meningitis (Figs. 12.33 and 12.36).

The responsible bacterial organisms, in order of decreasing frequency, are: streptococci (particularly the hemolytic group A), pneumococci, staphylococci, and a few others, e.g., *Escherichia coli* and anaerobic organisms.

Viral infections are playing an increasingly important part. A virus may affect middle ear and meninges simultaneously, in which case the two sites simply represent different hematogenous localizations of the same malady. Alternatively, the virus may first affect the middle ear, and the otitis media in turn may later lead to a viral endocranial complication. On the other hand, a virus-induced otitis media may become superinfected and lead to a bacterial endocranial complication. Thus it may be difficult to differentiate between primary and secondary viral complications of otogenic origin. Case 1 is a classic example of a chronic, nonperforative otitis media that has progressed to a labyrinthitis and petrositis, which in turn has led to a lethal meningitis.

OTOGENIC SINUS THROMBOPHLEBITIS

Thrombophlebitis of the lateral sinus ranks second among the otogenic intracranial complications. It is more often encountered in the younger age group and affects men more frequently than women (2:1). No one sinus has predominance over the localization of the disease.

Thrombophlebitis generally arises as a complication of a chronic rather than an acute tympanomastoiditis. The inflammation can reach the sinus in one of the following ways (Fig. 12.39). In most instances, the phlebitis arises in the posterior wall of the petrous pyramid or from a small fistula of the otic capsule. Another avenue is the metastatic route via vascular channels. It can reach the lateral sinus directly or via the superior petrosal sinus that receives veins from the petrous pyramid and mastoid process. Occasionally, the superior petrosal sinus alone becomes involved. Vascular anastomoses and bony dehiscences in the floor of the middle ear can give rise to thrombophlebitis of the jugular bulb. The caroticotympanic canaliculi, in a few instances, can provide a pathway to the pericarotid venous plexus and cavernous sinus. An osteitic process in the labyrinthine capsule or an empyema of the endolymphatic sac can cause thrombophlebitis. Finally, sinus thrombophlebitis, in a rare instance, may develop in a retrograde direction via a cavernous sinus thrombophlebitis of facial origin.

Depending on the character of the middle ear infection, the wall of the sinus can be involved in a granulomatous or necrotizing process, which in turn induces formation of a thrombus. As the infection spreads both within the wall and within the lumen of the sinus, the phlebitis extends into, with, or against the bloodstream. With the bloodstream, it may reach the jugular bulb, the superior vena cava, and the veins in the neck. Against the bloodstream, it can extend to the torcular herophili, the sagittal sinus, and even the opposite lateral sinus. Anteriorly, it may involve the cavernous sinus via the superior petrosal sinus (Fig. 12.39). As the cerebellar veins drain into the lateral sinus, a cerebellar thrombophlebitis or a cerebellar abscess can develop by retrograde extension. Similarly, a thrombophlebitis of the superior petrosal sinus can be the forerunner of a cerebral thrombophlebitis or brain abscess. If cortical thrombophlebitis spreads farther, one or several brain abscesses can develop in areas far removed from the original source of infection and the point of vascular invasion. Such extensive thrombophlebitis is usually associated with chronic otitis media, whereas in an acute otitis media the phlebitis is generally limited to the lateral sinus.

Sinus thrombophlebitis is almost always accompanied by septicemia, which may produce embolic abscesses in visceral organs, pleuroperitoneal cavities, joint cavities, and subcutaneous tissue. Any of the pyogenic organisms encountered in acute or chronic ear infections can cause sinus thrombophlebitis. Only the organism cultured from the bloodstream or from the thrombus can be regarded as the true bacterial agent.

In about 40% of cases, sinus thrombophlebitis is associated with an inflammatory process in other areas, such as the meninges, subarachnoid space, cerebrum, and cerebellum. Leptomeningitis occurs in about 31% of the cases. The association with brain abscess is very rare (12).

OTOGENIC BRAIN ABSCESS

Brain abscess, although the least frequent of the otogenic endocranial complications, deserves special consideration, as it continues to be associated with a significant morbidity and mortality. The introduction of antibiotics resulted in a substantial decrease of brain abscesses, in all likelihood because of earlier

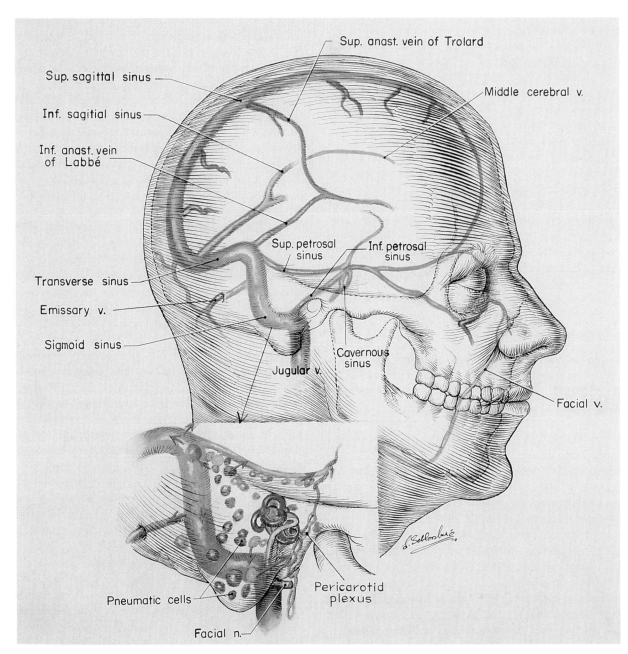

Figure 12.39. Illustration of locations in which an inflammatory process within the mastoid process or petrous pyramid may invade the sigmoid, superior, and inferior petrosal sinuses, the pericarotid venous plexus, or the jugular bulb. Thrombophlebitis may extend with or against the bloodstream and involve adjacent venous sinuses or cerebral or cerebellar veins.

and more accurate control of the primary infections in the middle ear cleft and paranasal sinuses. However, with the steadily increasing number of patients receiving immunosuppressive and cytotoxic therapy, patients that have undergone organ transplantation and patients with the acquired immune deficiency syndrome, a constant rise in brain abscesses by opportunistic pathogenes has been observed in recent years (13, 16).

Incidence, Age, and Sex Distribution

Brain abscess is observed about one-sixth as frequently as bacterial meningitis. In 1955, it was found to be a complication in 3% of patients with chronic otitis media compared with 0.5% of patients with acute middle ear disease (17). Infection of the middle ear, even in the present era of antibiotics, remains the most common single causative disease. Brain abscesses may occur at any age, but they are more common during the third and fourth decades of life. About one-fourth of all cases are observed in children under 15 years of age. They are infrequent in the first year of life and in old age (18). For reasons not fully understood, males are affected more frequently than females, with the ratio varying from 3:2 to 2:1, depending on the various statistics.

Pathogenesis

Four mechanisms are involved in the development of a brain abscess: *(a)* direct extension from a contiguous primary focus of infection in the skull, *(b)* hematogenous dissemination from a remote focus of infection, *(c)* complication of a cranial injury with laceration of the dura, and *(d)* no identifiable primary focus of infection (cryptogenic) (16).

Most brain abscesses arise from direct extension of an inflammatory process involving the cortical bone or the mucoperiosteum of the temporal bone or a paranasal sinus (19, 20). Recent statistics indicate that between 34% and 66% of all brain abscesses continue to be otogenic in origin (21, 22) and that infections of the paranasal sinuses account for 10–15% of brain abscesses. Most of the otogenic abscesses are associated with a chronic rather than an acute middle ear infection (23). Sixty-four percent of these abscesses are located in the temporal lobe, while 35% are located in the cerebellum (21). In 1% of cases an abscess may develop simultaneously in both locations.

Whereas an osteitic process of the tegmen usually leads to an inferior posterior temporal lobe abscess, the perisinus abscess tends to give rise to a posterior superficially located cerebellar abscess. A frontal sinusitis may lead to an anteriorly and inferiorly located frontal abscess, and an ethmoid sinusitis can cause a frontal or deep temporal lobe abscess. The sphenoid sinusitis usually leads to an abscess in the frontal or temporal lobe or in the pituitary gland. The maxillary sinus very rarely is the source of an abscess, and if it is, it is located in the frontal lobe.

Metastatic abscesses generally originate from the lungs, pleura, or heart but less often originate from septic foci in the skin, teeth, abdomen, or surgical wound. The most important cause is a chronic infection in the lungs and pleura, such as a lung abscess, bronchiectasis, or an empyema. Pleuropulmonary infections are the most common causes in adults, whereas congenital heart diseases, especially tetralogy of Fallot and transposition of the great vessels, are the most predisposing conditions in children (24).

Penetrating craniocerebral trauma and a craniotomy may occasionally be complicated by the development of a brain abscess.

In about 15–25% of cases, no primary source of infection can be identified (25), and the pathogenesis remains obscure. In many instances a nonidentifiable adjacent focus or a hematogenous seeding is suspected.

The temporal lobe abscess usually arises from an osteitis of the tegmen antri or tegmen tympani. At times, the vascular pathway plays a part (Figs. 12.14–12.27). The cerebellar abscess frequently originates from a labyrinthitis. The infection may spread through the endolymphatic sac or through a fistula in the otic capsule. It may also arise from a localized osteitis or meningitis at the petrous apex. These foci of infection usually give rise to the medially located, deep-seated cerebellar abscess. The laterally and superficially located cerebellar abscess is often the consequence of an osteitis in the sinodural angle. A lateral sinus thrombophlebitis and empyema of the cochlear aqueduct are other possible sources (Figs. 12.14–12.26).

Although the evolution of a brain abscess is a continuous process, four stages may be distinguished histologically: an early and a late stage of cerebritis, and an early and a late stage of capsular development.

The pathogenesis of a brain abscess, in brief, follows. The dura, which initially forms a barrier against an expanding extradural inflammation, eventually undergoes necrosis. This leads to a localized subdural empyema or to a meningitis from which the abscess originates. The abscess develops in the subcortical area of the brain, where the organisms penetrate the brain along the perivascular lymph spaces and cause a purulent encephalitis. Further development of the abscess depends to some extent on the reaction of the glial tissue and the vascular apparatus. The abscess may be characterized by diffuse purulent encephalitis, with formation of a so-called free abscess, or by formation of an abscess membrane, with development of a chronic encapsulated abscess. Encapsulated abscesses are usually associated with chronic otitis media, and diffuse abscesses, with acute otitis media. The most frequently cultured organisms are hemolytic streptococci, followed by staphylococci and pneumococci. However, mixed infections with Gram-negative and anaerobic bacilli may also be observed. In general, the abscess is adjacent to the source of infection, in the ipsilateral temporal lobe or in the ipsilateral cerebellar hemisphere. The temporal lobe abscess has a tendency to extend toward the lower horn of the lateral ventricle. Not infrequently, it breaks into the ventricle, thus causing a lethal ventricular meningitis. In 4–15% of instances, multiple abscesses are encountered (26); their development can be primary or secondary.

With the introduction of the antimicrobial agents, intratemporal and endocranial complications resulting from acute and chronic middle ear infections have been greatly reduced, and when they do occur, they generally no longer have the guarded prognosis of the past. Nevertheless, a certain number of these complications remain uncontrolled.

Inasmuch as successful therapy is based on understanding of the pathogenesis of a disease process, this chapter exclusively deals with the mechanisms and pathology of infectious processes in the middle ear, mastoid, and petrous pyramid. With this knowledge, the otolaryngologist is in an excellent position to contribute toward the eventual elimination of intratemporal and endocranial complications. Further improvement in otologic and neurosurgical techniques may provide an even larger number of operative cures. Cases 2 and 3 are classic examples and explain the pathogenesis of otogenic temporal lobe and cerebellar abscesses.

PROGNOSIS

Since the introduction of antimicrobial agents, intratemporal and endocranial complications have dramatically decreased, and when they do develop, they no longer elicit the guarded prognosis of the past. Nevertheless, some complications still escape control.

The otolaryngologist who comprehends the pathogenesis of these disease processes is in an excellent position to contribute significantly toward the eventual elimination of intratemporal and endocranial complications. The continuous refinement of otologic and neurosurgical techniques will, in turn, increase the number of operative cures.

Case Reports

Case 1. *Otogenic pneumococcal meningitis. Chronic purulent, nonperforative tympanomastoiditis of left ear. Necrosis of annular ligament and round window membrane. Purulent labyrinthitis and osteitis. Multiple fistulae into all semicircular canals and internal auditory meatus. Extension of inflammatory process to subarachnoid space of internal acoustic meatus along a bony fistula and perineural spaces of cochlear and vestibular nerves.*

A 58-year-old man 3 months prior to admission developed tinnitus and 2 weeks prior to hospitalization noticed a decrease of auditory acuity in the left ear and dizziness. On the morning of admission he woke up with a left-sided temporoparietal headache that progressed rapidly to nausea, vomiting, and severe ataxia.

On admission, *otologic examination* revealed an opaque left tympanic membrane and total loss of hearing on the left; the Weber test disclosed lateralization to the right ear. There was a spontaneous right-beating horizontal nystagmus. His stance and gait were broad-based with a tendency to fall to either side. He had some difficulties with rapid fine movements with his right hand. A brain scan revealed an abnormal uptake in the left posterior fossa of questionable significance. Electroencephalograms and echoencephalograms disclosed no abnormalities. Multidirectional polytomograms of the temporal bones were suggestive of left-sided chronic middle ear disease. A lumbar puncture produced a clear fluid with a protein of 45 mg/100 ml, a glucose of less than 25 mg/100 ml, a blood sugar of 105 mg/100 ml, and 3 polymorphonuclear leukocyte cells. A left cerebellopontine tumor was suspected. His past medical history included a right pneumonectomy and thoracoplasty for pulmonary tuberculosis, left lower lobe pneumonia, hematemesis associated with an endoscopically confirmed lesser curvature ulcer, a positive serum but a negative cerebrospinal fluid (CSF) serologic test for syphilis (STS), and high-output heart failure secondary to sideroblastic anemia. On the evening of the 17th hospital day, the patient complained of sudden onset of headache and chills. His temperature rose to 103°C, and he became obtundent and developed marked nuchal rigidity. A lumbar puncture showed a CSF pressure of 4 cm of water and "poor dynamics." The fluid was cloudy and formed a gelatinous precipitate, but no cells or organisms were seen on microscopic examination. The presumptive diagnosis of meningitis was made. Later in the evening the patient developed generalized seizures, became hypotensive, and died from cardiorespiratory arrest.

Postmortem examination of the cranial cavity disclosed a large amount of greenish creamy purulent exudate over the entire cortical and basal surfaces of the brain with a large pocket of pus in the left cerebellopontine angle (Fig. 12.40). There was increased vascular congestion of the dura about the entrance to the left internal auditory canal, which contained purulent exudate. A Gram stain revealed numerous neutrophils and scattered Gram-positive diplococci. Blood and CSF cultures taken postmortem grew diplococci. The extensive involvement about the brain stem (Fig. 12.40*B*) with obstruction of the foramen magnum was thought to explain the low CSF pressure and the "poor dynamics" at the time of the second lumbar puncture. Cut sections of the brain and cerebellum showed an overlying layer of thick purulent exudate (Fig. 12.40*C* and *D*) with thickening of the meninges and localized vasculitis but no thrombosis and no evidence of brain abscess, infarction, hemorrhage, or petechiae. There was no sign of bone destruction involving the left temporal bone. Microscopic examination of the meninges suggested that the meningitis had been present for several weeks before death.

Histologic examination of the left temporal bone reveals a chronic purulent tympanomastoiditis associated with labyrinthitis and chronic osteitis in the presence of a tympanic membrane *without a perforation* but with evidence of chronic inflammatory changes. The middle ear cleft and most of the formerly air-containing cells and marrow spaces contain a purulent exudate. The ensuing osteomyelitis and osteitis had resulted in the formation of several abscesses throughout the bone of the petrous pyramid and mastoid (Fig. 12.41). One of these abscesses is situated anterior and inferior to the cochlea. It had destroyed the medial bony wall of the canal for the internal carotid artery. The abscess extends into the perivascular space and to the pericarotid venous plexus (Fig. 12.41). The potential spread of the infection to the cavernous sinus and internal jugular vein is obvious. Another abscess, located in the roof of the internal auditory canal, communicates through a fistula tract with the internal meatus, where it has given rise to a meningitis and an abscess (Fig. 12.42). The pathway of the inflammation is along the lumen of a vein, a thrombophlebitis, and the perivascular space (Fig. 12.42*B*). The abscess within the internal acoustic meatus, in turn, had become the source for the diffuse lethal meningitis. The same abscess in the roof of the inner ear canal had also led, at a more posterior level, to the formation of an epidural abscess over the middle cranial fossa (Fig. 12.43*A*). The overlying dura, however, remained intact (Fig. 12.43*B*).

The chronic middle ear infection had caused a necrosis of the annular ligament and round window membrane and had enabled the infection to extend to the perilymphatic and endolymphatic spaces of the labyrinth and cochlea (Fig. 12.44). From the vestibule and cochlea, the inflammation spread along the perineural spaces of the vestibular and cochlear nerves into the subarachnoid compartment of the internal auditory canal (Fig. 12.43*C* and *D*).

An abscess near the subarcuate fossa had destroyed the osseous wall of the superior semicircular canal and permitted the spread of the infection into the perilymphatic space of that canal (Fig. 12.45*A*). In the bony wall of that abscess, the simultaneous occurrence of bone destruction and repair, side by side, can be observed (Fig. 12.45*B*–*D*). While superiorly the bone near the arcuate eminence is being resorbed by the activity of numerous multinucleated osteoclastic giant cells (Fig. 12.45*C*), new bone is being deposited along the inferior wall by osteoblasts rimming an irregular jagged surface (Fig. 12.45*D*). The lateral semicircular canal displays the largest fistula near its ampullated end (Fig. 12.46*A*–*C*), where the extension of the middle ear infection into the perilymphatic and endolymphatic compartments of that canal can readily be followed (Fig. 12.47*A*–*B*). A number of smaller fistulae and erosions can be seen along the superior and lateral as well as the posterior semicircular canals (Fig. 12.46*A*, *B*, and *D*).

An abscess in the mastoid antrum had destroyed the tegmental bone and exposed the overlying dura but had left it intact (Fig. 12.48).

The right, opposite temporal bone also displays evidence of a purulent meningitis. The subarachnoid space that surrounds the cochlear, vestibular, and facial nerve within the internal auditory canal contains an inflammatory exudate (Fig. 12.49). This exudate envelops the seventh nerve to the geniculate ganglion (Fig. 12.50). The same purulent exudate extends from the right basal cistern along the cochlear aqueduct into the scala tympani of the lower basal turn of the cochlea, where it has produced a beginning meningogenic inflammation of the cochlea and labyrinth (Fig. 12.51). No inflammatory cells are encountered in the perineural spaces of the eighth cranial nerve. The remarkable feature of this form of tympanomastoiditis is that it led to these serious local complications and, finally, to the lethal endocranial complications without ever producing a perforation of the tympanic membrane and purulent otorrhea.

Case 2. Otogenic abscess of right temporal lobe (B. proteus) resulting from destructive osteitis of the tegmen antri. Epidural and subdural abscess and circumscribed meningitis over right temporal lobe secondary to a middle ear cholesteatoma arising from a marginal pars tensa perforation extending to the mastoid antrum. Death from ventricular meningitis and cerebral edema 5 days after right temporal and occipital trephine.

A 16-year-old boy who at the age of 9 years had in succession measles and scarlet fever complicated by a right necrotizing otitis media, with a marginal pars tensa perforation and persistent purulent otorrhea, was seen. Three weeks prior to admission he developed increasingly severe frontal headaches, followed by malaise, nausea, vomiting, vertigo, diplopia, and nuchal rigidity, and eventually became delirious. Drainage from the right ear had ceased during the period of increasing symptoms. He then, for the first time, was seen by a physician who sent him to the hospital without delay.

On *admission,* his temperature was 99°F; pulse, 60; and respiration, 20. His white blood cell (WBC) count was 16,000. There was weakness of the right superior and medial rectus muscle, of the left facial muscles, and bilateral papilledema. The Romberg test was positive. He was staggering to the left, and there was weakness of the left arm.

Otologic examination revealed a posterior marginal pars tensa perforation of the right tympanic membrane with ingrowth of squamous epithelium into the tympanic cavity. There was a cholesteatoma that extended into the attic and probably toward the antrum. Cochlear function studies showed a marked conductive hearing loss in that ear.

Trephine openings were made over the right temporal area, and pus was encountered that, when cultured, proved to be *S. aureus.* The patient died 5 days after admission.

Postmortem examination of the brain disclosed thickening, vascular injection, and a dark-blue discoloration of the dura over the right temporal and occipital lobes. No pus was encountered in the epidural and subdural space. The entire right temporal lobe was found to be the site of a dark, purplish-black, fluctuating mass from which engorged meningeal vessels radiated in all directions. Aspiration from the center of the mass revealed pus that, when cultured, proved to be *B. proteus.* Cross-sections of the brain exhibited a large abscess occupying most of the interior of the right temporal lobe, measuring about 4 cm in diameter. It was lined by a thick, gray exudate. A discolored, thickened, and firmly adherent dura covered the medial surface of the right petrous pyramid. Elevation of this dura exposed a large area of bone necrosis that extended from the arcuate eminence to the groove of the superior petrosal sinus and included the entire tegmental area.

Microscopic examination of the right temporal bone reveals an extensive middle ear cholesteatoma that had arisen from a large posterior marginal pars tensa perforation of the right tympanic membrane by ingrowth of squamous epithelium from the external canal (Fig. 12.52). It involved the entire middle ear and extended medially to the malleus and incus, eroding their medial surfaces, into the

attic, aditus, and antrum (Fig. 12.53). The aditus was completely blocked by keratinous debris. Osteitis with necrosis and resorption of bone had resulted in total destruction of the tegmen antri (Fig. 12.54) and allowed the infection to spread to the contents of the overlying middle cranial fossa, giving rise to a localized epidural and subdural abscess, circumscribed meningitis, and a large temporal lobe abscess (Figs. 12.55 and 12.56).

Case 3. Otogenic abscess of right cerebellar hemisphere (S. aureus) resulting from empyema of endolymphatic sac. History of persistent otorrhea following measles in childhood. Chronic right purulent tympanomastoiditis with cholesteatoma. Necrosis of annular ligament and round window membrane with labyrinthitis and empyema of endolymphatic sac. Rupture of empyema into subarachnoid space, giving rise to cerebellar abscess. Chronic osteitis and osteomyelitis of petrous pyramid with erosion of cochlear and vestibular capsule, fistulae into semicircular canals, erosion of cortical bone adjacent to middle and posterior cranial fossa, and epidural and subdural abscesses. Postoperative right radical mastoidectomy. Death from cerebritis and cerebral edema.

A 33-year-old man with chronic right otorrhea following measles in childhood, who was first examined at age 22 because of pains over the right side of his head but failed to return for 10 years, was seen. He complained of headaches and persistent aural discharge. He postponed a recommended right mastoidectomy for another year but was finally admitted after 2 months of increasingly severe pains over the right mastoid and temporal area.

On *admission,* his temperature was 99.4°F; pulse, 90; and respiration, 20. The otorrhea had ceased for the previous 3 days.

Otologic examination disclosed a partially destroyed right tympanic membrane and a middle ear filled with polypoid granulation tissue and cholesteatomatous debris. Cochlear function studies showed anacusis of the right ear. There was no spontaneous nystagmus or ataxia and no facial weakness or involvement of other cranial nerves. A right radical mastoidectomy was performed for the removal of a cholesteatoma with areas of osteitis in a sclerotic mastoid process. Malleus and incus had been destroyed. The stapes was deeply embedded in granulation tissue. As the patient appeared to improve, he was discharged after 1 week to be followed as an outpatient. Meanwhile, he continued to have severe diffuse and occipital headaches and pains over his right ear and eye. On the 14th postoperative day he became progressively weak and delirious and was readmitted the next day with nuchal rigidity. On that second admission his temperature was 100.4°F; pulse, 76; and respiration, 28. His WBC count was 21,520. The CSF pressure was greatly increased, and the fluid was clear, but it contained 410 polymorphonuclear cells. A subsequent culture grew *S. aureus.* The patient was comatose, his reflexes were hyperactive, the Bablinsky sign was positive, and the pupils were pinpointed and nonreactive. Death occurred a few hours after his second admission.

Postmortem examination disclosed a localized subdural empyema and meningitis over the posterior aspect of the right petrous pyramid, especially posterior to the porus of the internal auditory meatus, in the location of the endolymphatic sac. The empyema communicated through a sinus tract with an underlying right cerebellar abscess measuring $3 \times 2 \times 2$ cm, filled with greenish foul-smelling pus and located directly adjacent to the empyema. The dura covering the remainder of the petrous pyramid displayed several areas of bluish-green discoloration, indicating underlying focal bone necroses.

Microscopic examination of the right temporal bone revealed a chronic purulent tympanomastoiditis in a radical mastoid cavity with osteitis and residual cholesteatoma. The entire petrous pyramid was involved in an extensive osteitic and osteomyelitic process with multiple abscesses (Figs. 12.57–12.61). The inflammation had spread from the middle ear cleft to the cochlear and vestibular capsule along the nutrient vessels of Volkmann (Fig. 12.57). Some of these ab-

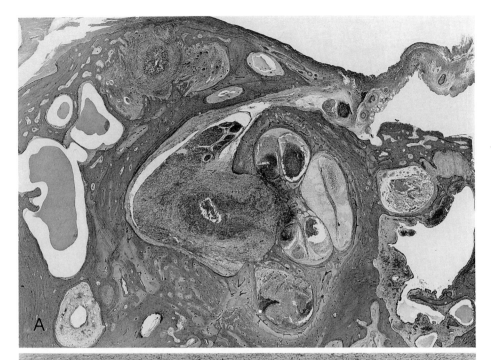

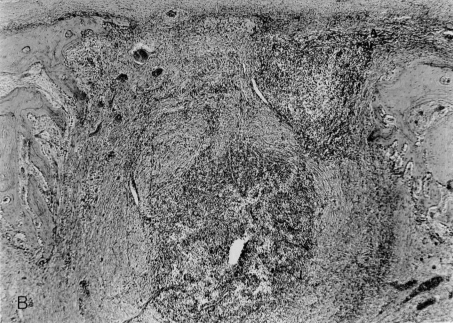

Figure 12.43. **A.** Vertical, posterior paramodular section through left temporal bone. The localized osteitis above the labyrinthine segment of the Fallopian canal has developed into an epidural abscess. (Hematoxylin and eosin, ×8.)

Figure 12.43. **B.** The cortical bone has been destroyed, but the overlying dura of the middle cranial fossa has remained intact. (×50.)

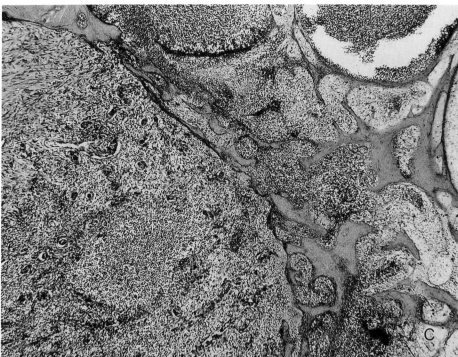

Figure 12.43.   C. The purulent exudate in the cochlea has extended from the basal and middle turn of the cochlea to the internal auditory canal along the perineural spaces. (×60.)

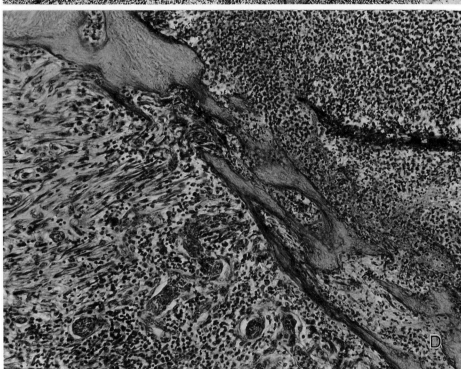

Figure 12.43.   D. The inflammatory exudate follows the cochlear nerve fibers through the neural canals in the modiolus and spiral foraminous tract. (×175.)

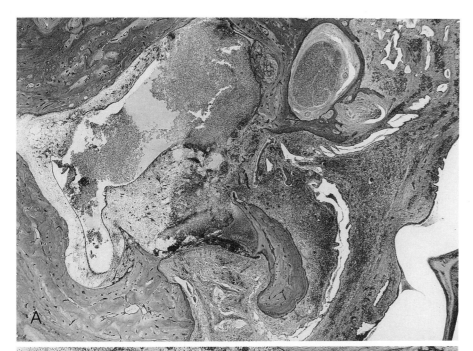

Figure 12.44. A. Vertical section through left temporal bone at level of oval and round windows. The purulent exudate from the middle ear has reached the perilymphatic and endolymphatic compartments of the vestibule across the vestibular and cochlear fenestrae. (Hematoxylin and eosin, ×13.)

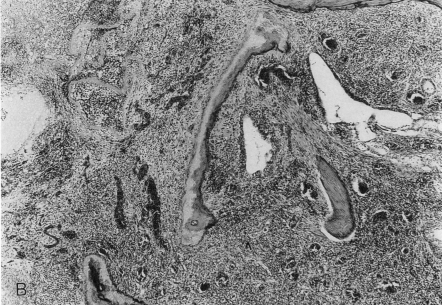

Figure 12.44. B. Necrosis of the annular ligament and round window membrane resulted in lateral dislocation of the stapes and allowed the spread of infection to the labyrinth. (×55.)

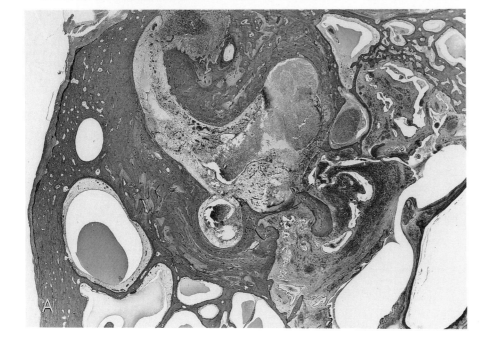

Figure 12.45. A. Vertical section through left temporal bone at level of ampullae of the three semicircular canals. An osteitic abscess near the subarcuate fossa has eroded the superior semicircular canal, and the inflammation has spread to the perilymphatic space of that canal. (Hematoxylin and eosin, ×7.)

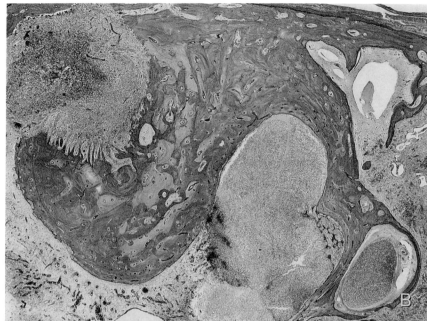

Figure 12.45.   B. In the osseous wall of the abscess that has eroded the superior semicircular canal, there is simultaneous occurrence of bone destruction and repair, side by side. (×15.)

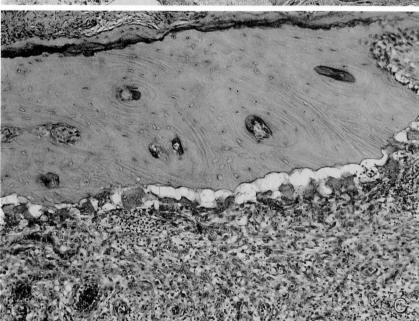

Figure 12.45.   C. In the superior wall, bone is being destroyed by numerous osteoclastic giant cells. (×125.)

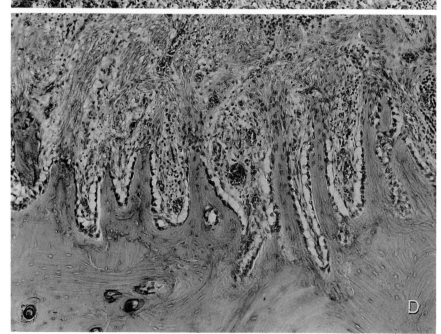

Figure 12.45.   D. In the inferior wall, new bone is being deposited by numerous osteoblasts rimming an irregular, jagged surface. (×125.)

13 Cholesteatomas of the Middle Ear

DEFINITION

The cholesteatoma represents an epidermoid inclusion cyst with an almost exclusive location in the middle ear cleft. Its characteristic feature is the capsule or matrix that consists of keratinizing stratified squamous epithelium. This epithelial lining continuously sheds keratohyalin lamellae in a concentric radial direction. The layers of desquamated keratin accumulate in an onionskin-like fashion and form the bulk of the cholesteatoma. The concentric lamellar structure creates an interference with the incident light that lends the surface its typical whitish mother-of-pearl sheen. Since the capsule of the cholesteatoma is very thin, it becomes delicate and friable. The term cholesteatoma is clearly a misnomer but shall be retained because of its long-established use in the literature.

CLASSIFICATION

Depending on the pathogenesis, cholesteatomas may be classified as follows:

1. Congenital cholesteatoma
2. Acquired cholesteatoma
   A. Cholesteatoma arising from a proliferation of an epidermal papilla of the external layer of the tympanic membrane or adjacent meatal skin
   B. Cholesteatoma arising from a localized retraction of the tympanic membrane with epithelial invagination
   C. Cholesteatoma arising from ingrowth of squamous epithelium of the tympanic membrane through a preexisting marginal or central pars tensa perforation of the drum
   D. Cholesteatoma arising from entrapment or implantation of squamous epithelium following trauma or a surgical procedure
   E. Cholesteatoma arising from squamous metaplasia of the middle ear mucosa

Most acquired cholesteatomas arise either from a proliferation of an epidermal papilla and immigration of squamous epithelium or from a localized retraction of the tympanic membrane and invagination of squamous epithelium. Depending on the site of origin in the tympanic membrane, each of these cholesteatomas may be further subdivided into pars flaccida (Shrapnell's membrane) or pars tensa papillary or retraction cholesteatomas.

Pathogenesis of Congenital Cholesteatoma

Congenital cholesteatomas are epidermoids that in all probability arise from aberrant epithelial remnants at the time of closure of the neural groove, between the third and fifth embry-

onic week (1, 2). Epidermoids are therefore considered blastomatous malformations, and their distribution along the neuraxis becomes readily understandable. Their location within the diploë of the skull, subarachoid space, ventricular system, etc. is well established (3). Most epidermoids, 30–40%, are encountered in the cerebellopontine angle (4–6). In the base of the skull the temporal bone is the most frequent site (7). They originate more often in the apical portion than in the middle or posterior portion of the petrous pyramid or in the mastoid process. The congenital cholesteatomas that originate in the temporal bone but outside the mesotympanum and epitympanum are purposely discussed in a separate chapter on epidermoids or congenital cholesteatomas (Chapter 30). Their size, local behavior, relationship to adjacent structures, clinical and radiologic features, and surgical implications are so different from the ones that arise in the middle ear that a treatment under individual headings has become necessary. In the middle ear cavity, congenital cholesteatomas may be encountered in the epitympanic or mesotympanic region. One conceivable example is the middle ear cholesteatoma behind an essentially normal tympanic membrane in a patient with no history of ear disease (Figs. 13.1 and 13.2). This presumably congenital lesion, however, must not be confused with an acquired cholesteatoma that developed from a proliferation of an epidermal papilla of the tympanic membrane and subsequently became separated from the undersurface of the tympanic membrane or that, in a rare instance, arose presumably from metaplasia of the middle ear mucosa.

Most congenital cholesteatomas of the middle ear are encountered in children. Unlike acquired cholesteatomas, they are not accompanied by infection unless they erode into the external auditory canal and become secondarily infected. Their local behavior and bone-eroding property are identical with other middle ear cholesteatomas.

In 1986, Michaels (7a) identified an ''epidermoid-like formation'' in the mucoperiosteum of the lateral wall of the developing middle ear. This structure is consistently located in the anterosuperior lateral wall of the tympanic cavity, anterior to the tympanic membrane. Michaels' structure is represented by one to three distinct formations of a thickened layer of stratified squamous cells that are obviously different from the surrounding low cuboidal and the tall pseudostratified or ciliated columnar epithelium. The assumption is that Michaels' structure develops at a certain time of epithelial transformation from the simple cuboidal to the ciliated columnar (respiratory) epithelium in that area of the middle ear. He had a specimen in which that structure showed evidence of a cellular differentiation to keratinocytes. These observations suggest that Michaels' structure may well represent a possible source for development of congenital cholesteatomas arising in the anterior superior quadrant of the middle ear cavity.

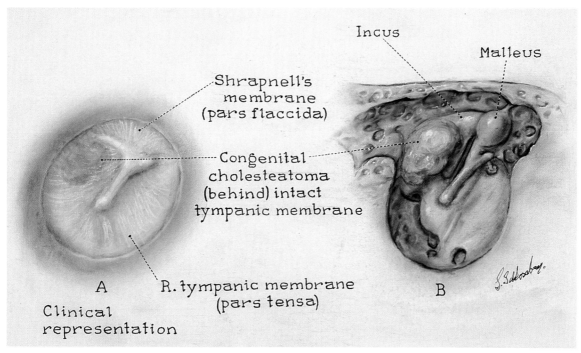

Figure 13.1.   A. Illustration of congenital cholesteatoma as recognized through intact tympanic membrane. **B.** The cholesteatoma occupies the posterior-inferior epitympanic and the upper mesotympanic space.

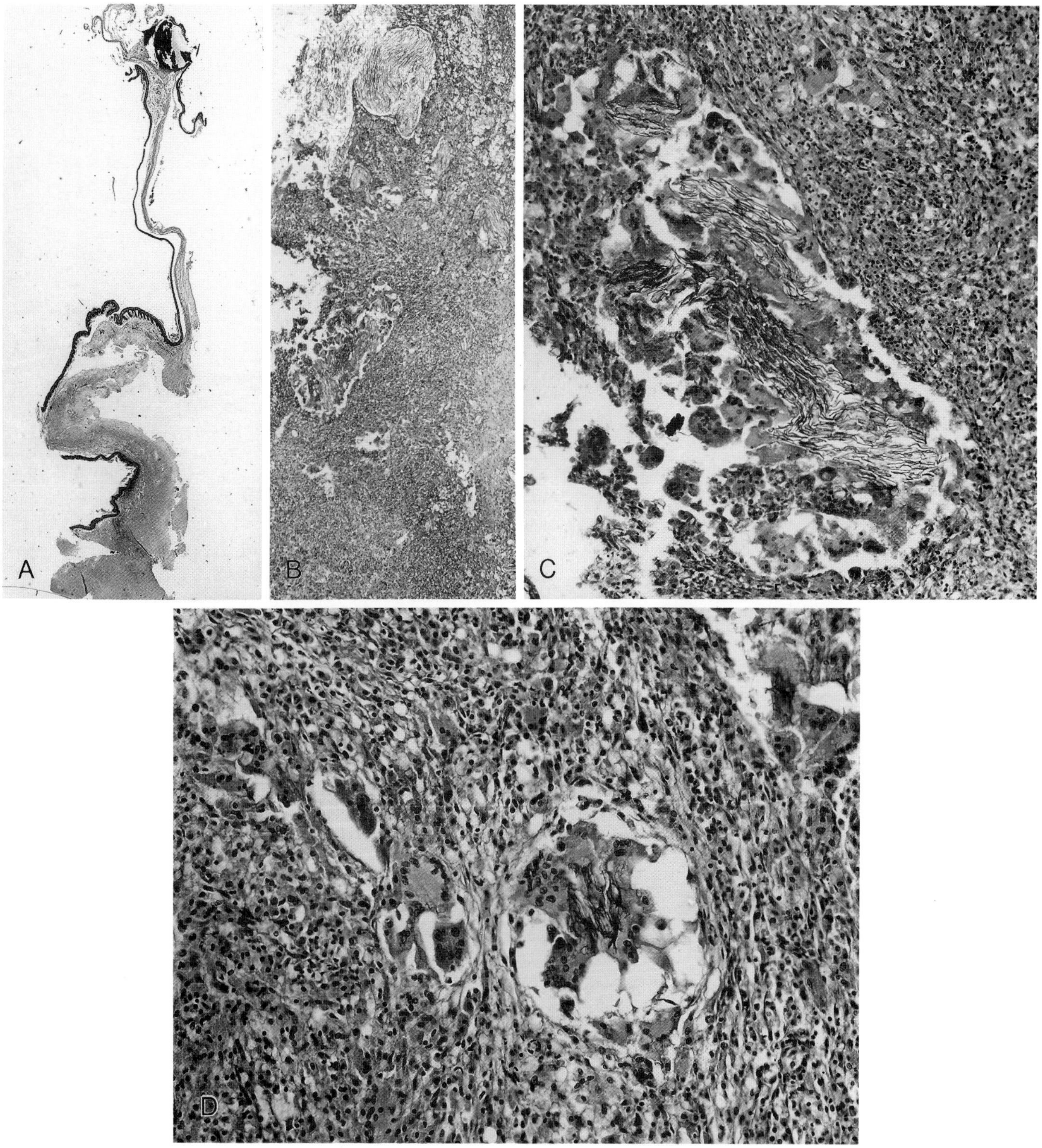

Figure 13.2. **A.** Vertical section through right tympanic membrane of a 12-year-old boy who at age 4 years developed progressive conductive hearing loss and at age 7 years presented with cholesteatoma behind an intact, partially fixed tympanic membrane, occupying the posterior middle ear space. There was no history of ear disease. Computed tomography (CT) disclosed a hypocellular right mastoid process and an extension of the soft tissue density in the posterior middle ear into the antrum and inferior periantral cells. At operation, the cholesteatoma extended into the upper mastoid process. Serial sections failed to show a connection be-

tween the matrix of the middle ear cholesteatoma and the squamous epithelium of the outer surface of the eardrum. However, granulation tissue occupies the space between the two. **B.** Granulation tissue surrounding the middle ear cholesteatoma reveals extensive foreign body reactions to islands of keratohyalin lamellae, indicating that some of the content of the cholesteatoma had previously leaked into the tympanic cavity. **C and D.** Clusters of keratohyalin lamellae surrounded by foreign body giant cells are scattered throughout the granulation tissue. (Hematoxylin and eosin, ×11.5, ×45, ×105, and ×210, respectively.)

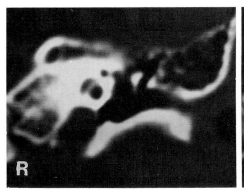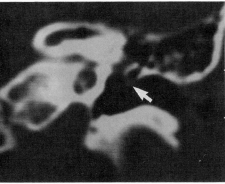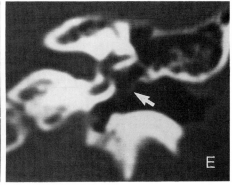

Figure 13.2. **E.** Serial, coronal CT scans of right temporal bone with a cholesteatoma in the middle ear cavity in a 11-year-old girl. The choles- teatoma developed behind an intact tympanic membrane in the absence of a history of previous external or middle ear disease.

Pathogenesis of Acquired Papillary Cholesteatoma

The acquired papillary cholesteatoma develops from a proliferation of an epidermal papilla of the intact tympanic membrane or adjacent meatal skin and immigration into the underlying submucosal connective or granulation tissue in the middle ear (Figs. 13.3 and 13.4). The predisposing factors for this mechanism are:

1. The inherent growth potential of the basal cells of that particular epidermis

2. The presence of submucosal connective or granulation tissue in the middle ear space and
3. A hypocellular pneumatization of the temporal bone

The causative factor is an inflammatory stimulus associated with a recurrent acute or chronic otitis media in childhood. This mechanism was first recognized around 1890 (8, 9), subsequently confirmed (10, 11), and later somewhat modified (12–14). In a rare instance, a chronic external otitis may also be responsible. There is evidence suggesting that inflammation may not always be the sole stimulus that can incite epidermal papillary immigration (Figs. 13.5–13.7) (15).

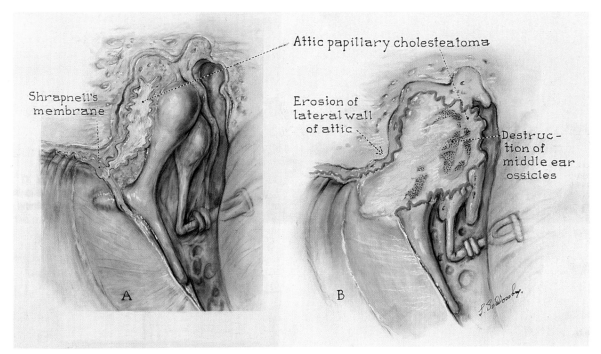

Figure 13.3. **A.** Illustration of early stage of an attic papillary cholesteatoma that evolved from proliferation of a papilla of keratinizing squamous epithelium lining the external surface of Shrapnell's membrane and from extension into the lateral recess of the attic. **B.** As it enlarges, it erodes the inferior lateral wall of the epitympanic recess and the adjacent surface of the malleus and incus.

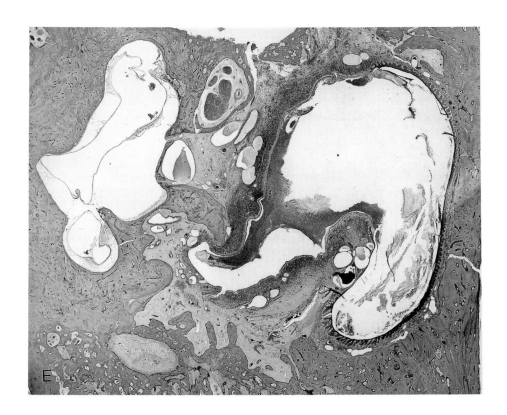

Figure 13.4. **E.** Vertical section through same temporal bone as in Figure 13.4*A* at center of oval window. The cholesteatoma totally destroyed the lateral wall of the epitympanum, malleus, incus, and stapedial arch. (Hematoxylin and eosin, ×10.)

Under normal circumstances, the epidermal papillae in the tympanic membrane and meatal skin are either very small or nonexistent. In the presence of a chronic inflammatory process in the middle ear and, on a rare occasion, in the external meatus, however, the squamous epithelium begins to proliferate and form elongated papillae (Figs. 13.8–13.10). These papillae tend to grow into the inflammatory connective and granulation tissue present in the middle ear on the undersurface of the tympanic membrane.

The underlying submucosal connective tissue in the middle ear is, by nature of its origin, either a persisting embryonic connective tissue (mesenchyme) or a secondary acquired, postinflammatory connective or granulation tissue. Persisting embryonic connective tissue is encountered among other locations, in the epitympanum and mesotympanum, in the latter primarily in the region of the oval and round windows. The secondary acquired connective tissue shares these locations in addition to others. Both types of connective tissue may obliterate areas of the epitympanic, mesotympanic, and hypotympanic space.

The immigration of the epidermal papilla into the middle ear is dependent on this underlying submucosal connective or granulation tissue, whereby the epidermoid cyst develops in the center of the deepest portion of the protruding papilla. As the stratum germinativum of the papilla differentiates into the stratum spinosum and stratum corneum, a central cleft forms in which the continuously exfoliating keratohyalin lamellae accumulate in an onionskin-like fashion. Thus originates an epidermoid inclusion cyst or the papillary cholesteatoma (Fig. 13.10). The stimulus for the papillary proliferation and epithelial immigration is the ongoing inflammation in the middle ear mucoperiosteum, connective tissue, and granulation tissue.

Once a tiny epidermoid cyst has formed, its further development may be in one of two directions, depending on the manner in which it expands. If the enlargement is in a medial direction, the cholesteatoma, while still attached to the undersurface of the drum by its papillary stalk, may remain asymptomatic and hardly detectable for a longer period of time. However, if the cyst enlarges laterally, which occurs more often, and perforates through the drum into the outer ear canal, the cholesteatoma becomes symptomatic and visible at an early stage. Further development is practically identical with one of the other acquired cholesteatomas in the same location.

The papillary cholesteatoma develops more frequently in the pars flaccida than in the pars tensa of the tympanic membrane. This may be related to the structure of Shrapnell's membrane, which lacks a central fibrous layer. Within the epitympanum, the cholesteatoma generally expands in the direction of least resistance toward the aditus and antrum, lateral, anterior, or medial and superior to the ossicular chain. Occasionally, it extends downward toward the mesotympanum and Eustachian tube. Most cholesteatomas present with a small, sometimes pinpoint perforation in Shrapnell's membrane and an extension already to or beyond the mastoid antrum at the initial clinical examination.

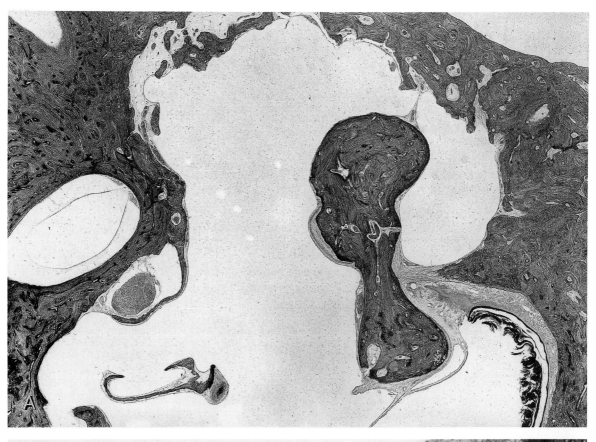

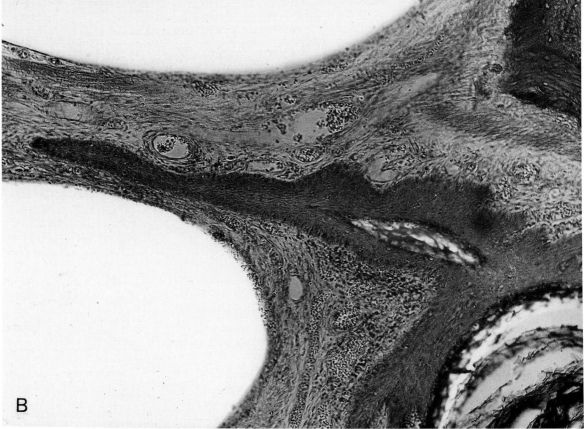

Figure 13.5. **A.** Vertical section through left temporal bone at level of head of malleus in a 41-year-old man. It shows the coniferous downgrowth of the epidermal lining in the anterior portion of Shrapnell's membrane, stimulated by nearby tumor cells associated with an external otitis. **B.** Ten sections posterior to that shown in Figure 13.5A. The sheath of keratiniz- ing squamous epithelium reveals a central cleft filled with keratinous ma- terial in a characteristic laminar arrangement. This beginning attic papillary cholesteatoma, which in all likelihood was incited by tumor cells, is actually developing within the epitympanic space, which itself is free from tumor or inflammation. (Hematoxylin and eosin, ×10 and ×100.)

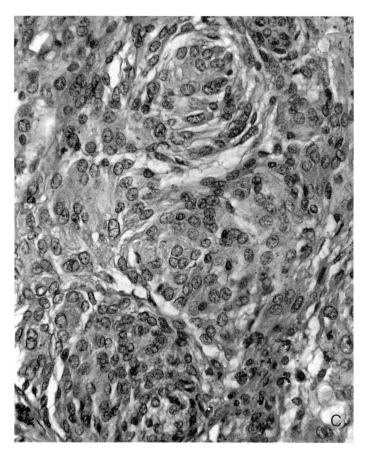

Figure 13.5.   C. The primary tumor is an endotheliomatous meningioma that originated from the right sphenoid ridge and invaded extensively the underlying and adjacent bones of the skull (floor of the right middle and anterior cranial fossa, entire right temporal bone, right parietal bone, sella turcica, and right sphenoid sinus). It also partially involved the left temporal bone.

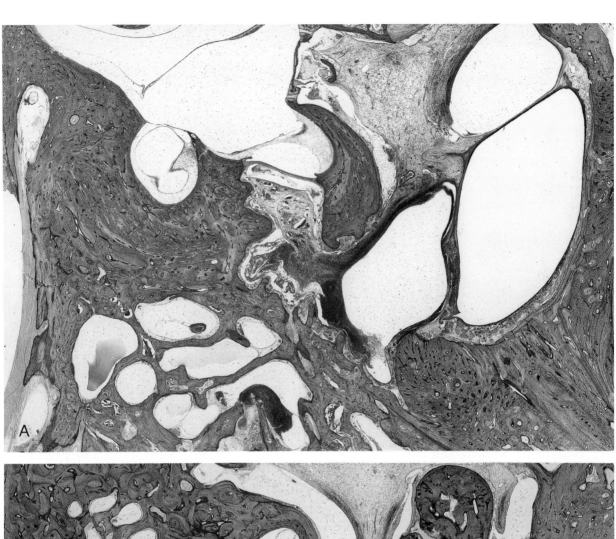

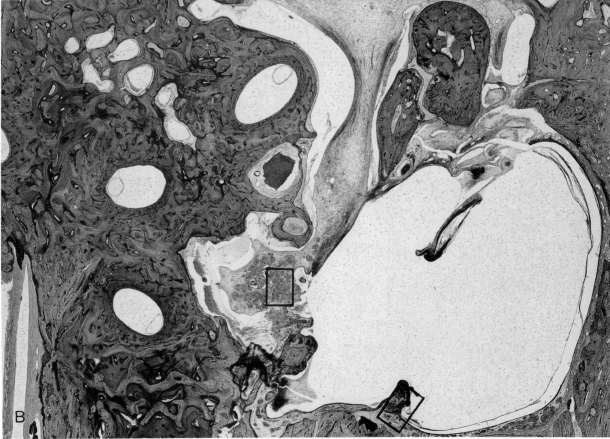

Figure 13.6. **A.** Vertical section through left temporal bone at level of oval and round windows of a 63-year-old man with carcinoma of the prostate that has widely metastasized to regional lymph nodes, lungs, pleura, vertebrae, ribs, and occipital, sphenoid, and left temporal bones. Chronic inflammatory granulation tissue and purulent exudate partially fill the middle ear cavity. **B.** Vertical section through same temporal bone as in *A* at level of incudomalleolar articulation. The chronic otitis media is associated with an inferior pars tensa tympanic membrane perforation. An epidermoid papilla from the outer surface of the remnant of the drum near the inferior annulus is seen protruding into underlying connective tissue. (Hematoxylin and eosin, ×100 and ×10, respectively.)

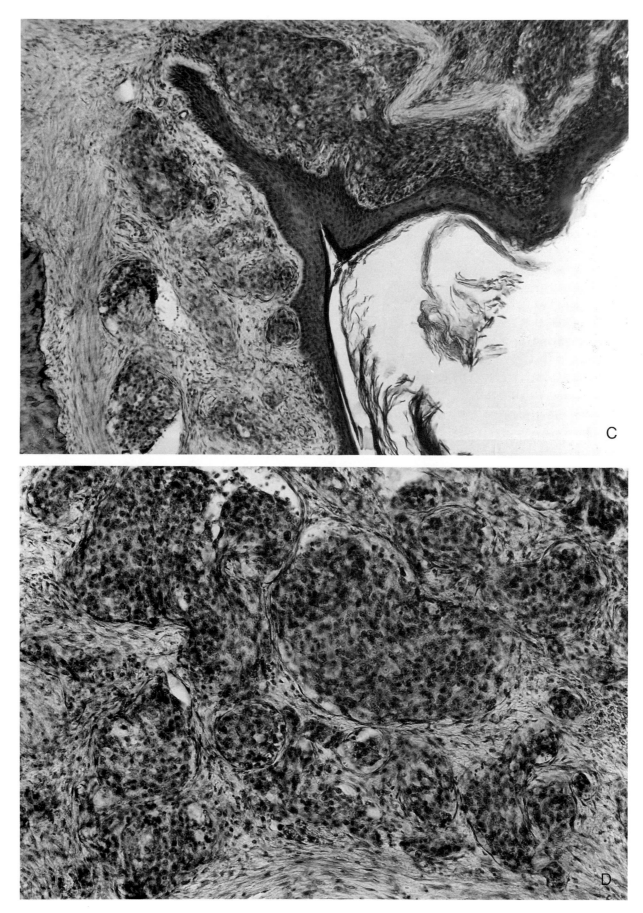

Figure 13.6.   C. This papilla is completely surrounded by a metastasis of the primary tumor. The ingrowth of the epidermoid papilla was stimulated by the underlying tumor and granulation tissue. **D.** The metastatic lesion reveals a moderate degree of anaplasia and variation in shape and staining of the cell nuclei. (Hematoxylin and eosin, ×150 and ×200, respectively.)

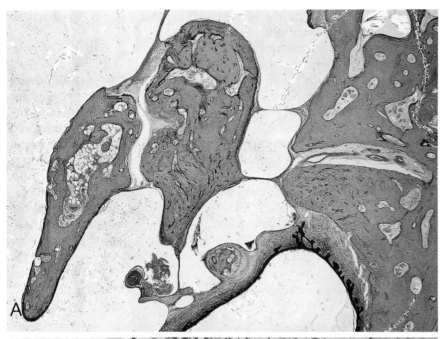

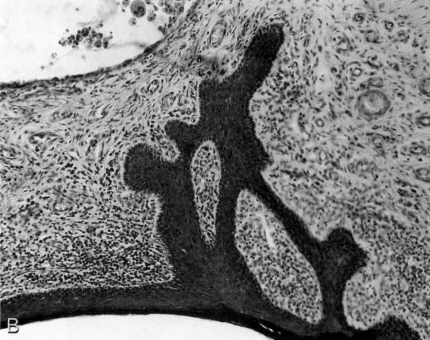

Figure 13.8.   A. Vertical section through left temporal bone at level of incudomalleolar articulation in a 31-year-old man with chronic external otitis and hyperplastic connective tissue in upper pars tensa and pars flaccida of tympanic membrane. (Hematoxylin and eosin, ×16.)

Figure 13.8.   B. The chronic external otitis induced the formation and proliferation of epidermal papillae in the squamous epithelium of Shrapnell's membrane and the adjacent meatal skin. These papillae aggressively infiltrate the underlying connective and inflammatory granulation tissue in the direction of Prussak's space. (×175.)

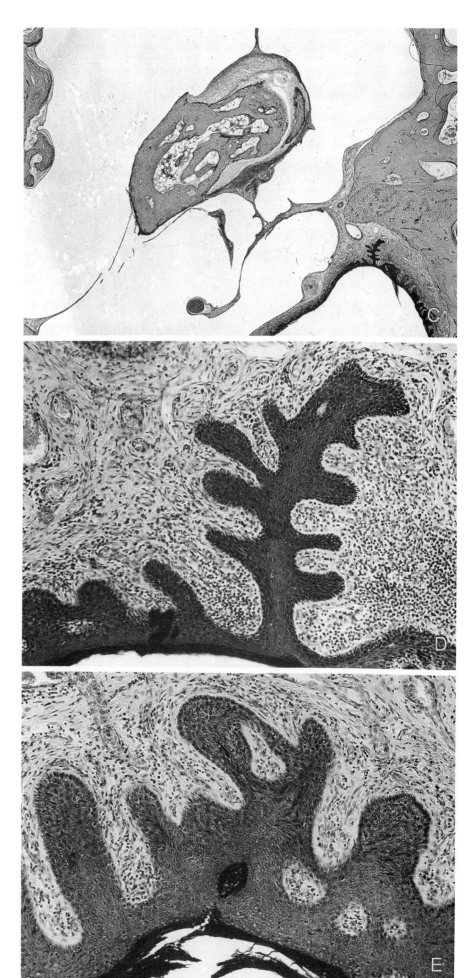

Figure 13.8. C and D. Vertical section through same temporal bone as in Figure 13.8A at level of incus. Several of the proliferating epidermal papillae that arise in the meatal skin near the superior annulus are deeply penetrating and invading the chronically inflamed underlying subcutaneous tissue. (Hematoxylin and eosin, ×16 and ×175, respectively.)

Figure 13.8. E. Several of these penetrating papillae include a central cleft filled with keratohyalin material that represents the beginning of an epidermoid inclusion cyst or cholesteatoma. (×175.)

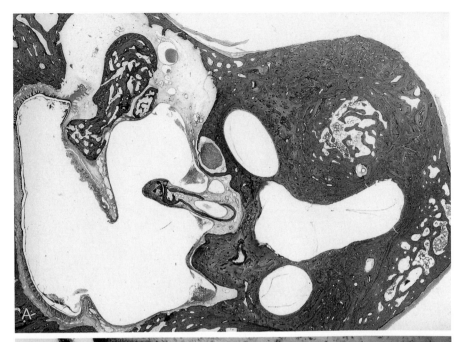

Figure 13.9. A. Vertical section through right temporal bone at level of posterior crus of the stapes of a 61-year-old woman with chronic perforative otitis media. A large central perforation occupies the inferior half of the tympanic membrane. The attic is completely obliterated by persisting mesenchyme. An epidermoid papilla from Shrapnell's membrane penetrates deeply into the underlying connective tissue in Prussak's space. (Hematoxylin and eosin, ×6½.)

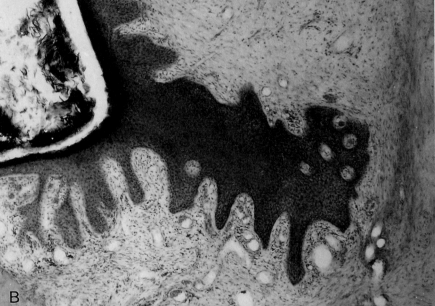

Figure 13.9. B. This large epidermoid papilla, which occupies most of Prussak's space, represents the initial stage of an attic papillary cholesteatoma. (×65.)

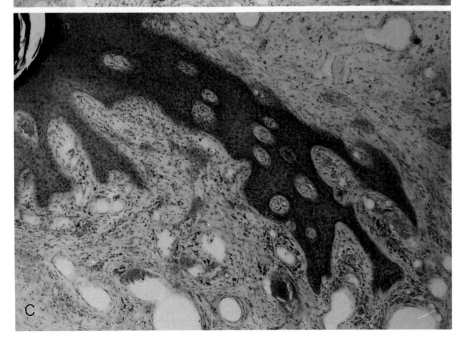

Figure 13.9. C. A more tangential section of the same epidermoid papilla as in Figure 13.9A displays the many finger-like radial extensions into a highly vascular surrounding connective tissue with round cell infiltrations. (×105.)

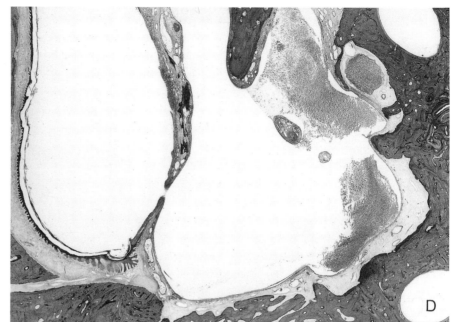

Figure 13.9.   D. The section just posterior to the oval window reveals proliferation of the epidermoid papillae at the inferior tympanic annulus. (×11½.)

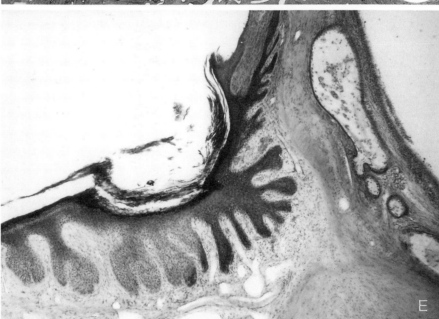

Figure 13.9.   E. Proliferation of the epidermoid papillae resulted in the beginning formation of an external cholesteatoma. (×70.)

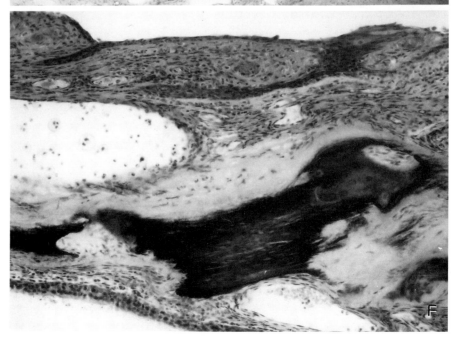

Figure 13.9.   F. The cross-section through the tympanic membrane discloses an area of metaplastic calcification and an ingrowth of squamous epithelium from the outer surface into the underlying connective tissue of the drum. (×250.)

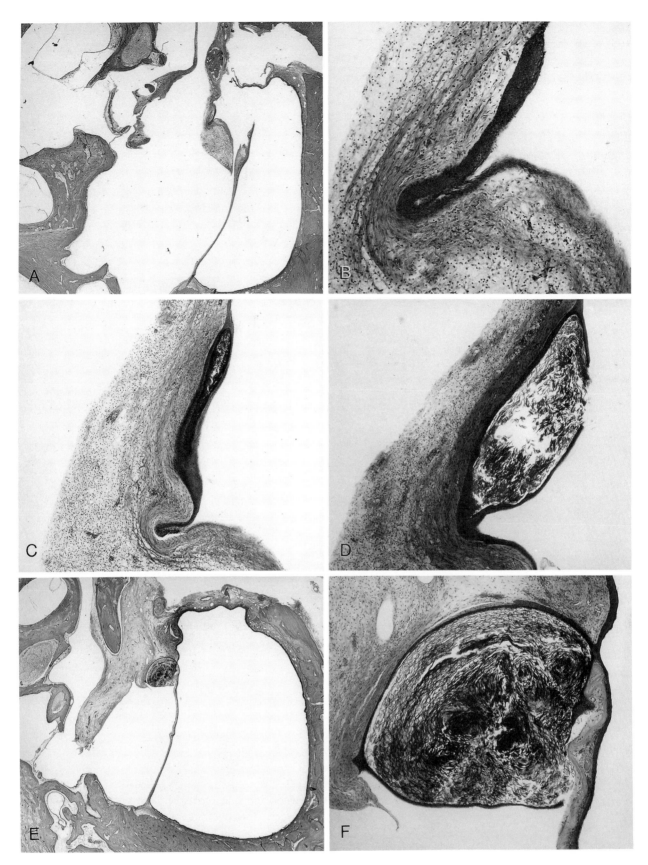

Figure 13.10. **A.** Vertical section through left temporal bone at level of round window in a 48-year-old man who died from systemic candidiasis 2 months after a motor vehicle accident that resulted in basilar skull fracture involving both temporal bones. The dislocation of the stapes, the separation of the bony fragments in the roof of the external meatus, and the tear in the eardrum are, in all likelihood, artifacts that occurred during the removal of the temporal bone. A circumscribed granuloma is encountered on the undersurface of the upper half of the pars tensa of the tympanic membrane. **B.** An epidermoid papilla that arose from the outer surface of

the drum has penetrated the underlying histiocytic granuloma. **C.** The epidermal papilla has begun to separate in the center. **D.** Continuous desquamation and accumulation of keratohyalin lamellae in the center of the papilla has given rise to an epidermoid inclusion cyst. **E.** This epidermoid cyst is developing within the underlying histiocytic granuloma that surrounds the handle of malleus. **F.** The epidermoid cyst or cholesteatoma is developing behind the drum in a middle ear cavity that lacks any evidence of acute or chronic inflammation. (Hematoxylin and eosin, ×9, ×10, ×60, ×120, ×9.5, and ×60, respectively.)

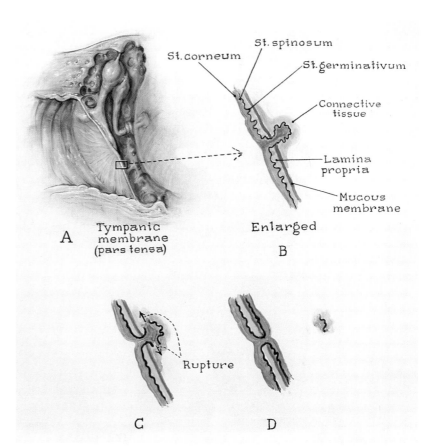

Figure 13.11. Schematic illustration of development of central pars tensa papillary cholesteatoma **(A)**. This cholesteatoma may remain intact and gradually expand within the middle ear **(B)**, or it may rupture during its evolution and give rise to a carpet-like spread of the cholesteatoma matrix covering the undersurface of the tympanic membrane **(C and D)**.

Pathogenesis of Acquired Retraction Cholesteatoma

Acquired retraction cholesteatoma arises from a localized retraction of the tympanic membrane with epithelial invagination (Fig. 13.13). The predisposing factors for this mechanism are: *(a)* a decrease in intratympanic pressure, *(b)* the presence of persistent submucosal embryonic or acquired connective or granulation tissue in the middle ear space, and *(c)* a hypocellular pneumatization of the temporal bone. The causative factor is a dysfunction of the Eustachian tube, leading to a chronic recurrent Eustachian salpingitis and otitis media.

It has long been established that a decrease in middle ear pressure can induce retraction of certain regions of the tympanic membrane, in either the pars flaccida, the pars tensa, or both (17). The site of retraction is determined by the locale of the negative pressure. A localized retraction of Shrapnell's membrane may result from a blockage of Prussak's space. A much more extensive or diffuse retraction of Shrapnell's membrane will develop, however, from a blockage of the communication between the mesotympanum and epitympanum around the malleus and incus, which separates the attic and antral space from the mesotympanum. Such an obstruction will give rise to negative pressure in the entire mastoid and epitympanic recess. Recurrent or chronic tubotympanic disease and the frequently following proliferation of submucosal connective and granulation tissue lead

initially to a medial retraction of the pars flaccida into Prussak's space and subsequently to adherence of that retraction pocket to the walls of that compartment (Fig. 13.14C and D). This skin-lined pocket may remain unchanged indefinitely as long as the superficial epidermal layers migrate outward into the external ear canal and the retraction pocket remains free from keratin (Fig. 13.14A). If keratin begins to accumulate within that pocket, however, a cholesteatoma develops that gradually increases in size as the desquamated material agglomerates (Fig. 13.14B, E, and F). This "dry" or "inactive" form of cholesteatoma may remain asymptomatic for sometime, as a minority of these lesions do. The majority, however, will slowly develop into "moist" or "active" cholesteatoma and, therefore, into a potentially dangerous form. This form of cholesteatoma is characterized by superinfection and osteoclastic bone resorption. The increasing collection of keratin causes a pressure necrosis of the matrix of the cholesteatoma and of the underlying endothelium of the middle ear. This exposes the cholesteatoma to the submucosal inflammatory granulation tissue. The once "dry" and asymptomatic cholesteatoma becomes superinfected and accompanied by a fetid, purulent discharge. Superinfection accelerates keratinization and desquamation and the growth of the cholesteatoma. Osteitis develops and leads to progressive resorption of adjacent bone. Rupture of the cholesteatoma sac at any stage of evolution may lead to a carpet-like spread of the matrix throughout the attic or entire middle ear.

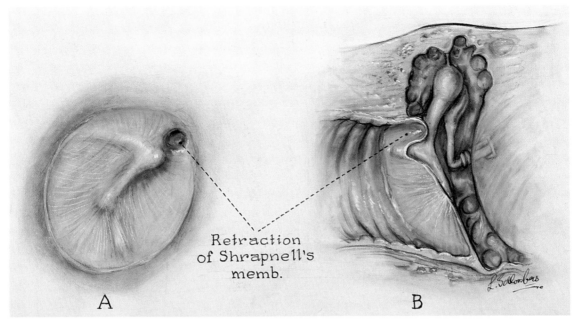

Figure 13.13. **A.** Illustration of most frequent site of retraction pocket in Shrapnell's membrane. **B.** This pocket extends medially into the superior recess of the tympanic cavity or Prussak's space. Prussak's space is bounded laterally by the pars flaccida and medially by the neck of the malleus. The floor of this recess is formed by the lateral process of the malleus.

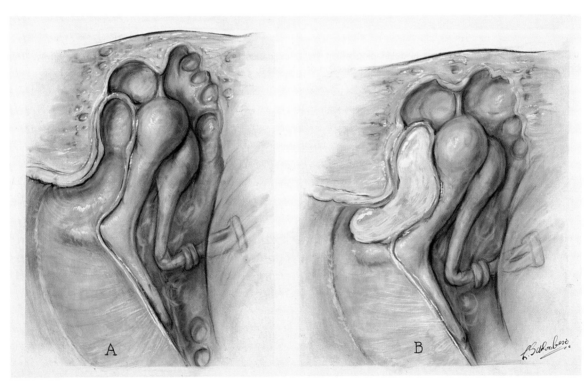

Figure 13.14. **A.** Illustration of empty, skin-lined retraction pocket in Shrapnell's membrane, which has become adherent to the walls of Prussak's space. **B.** The accumulation of keratin within that pocket leads to the development of the attic retraction cholesteatoma.

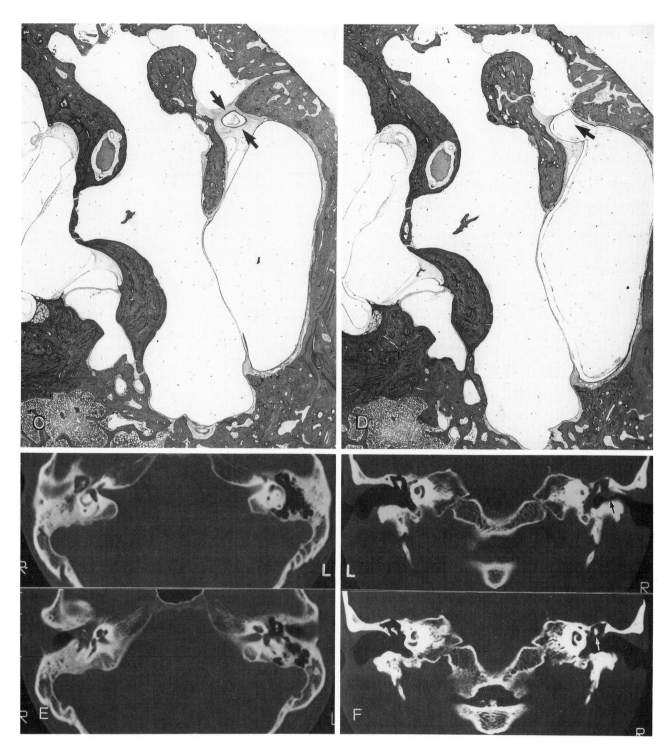

Figure 13.14.   C. Vertical section through left temporal bone at level of malleus with a retraction pocket of Shrapnell's membrane in a man *(arrows).* This pocket, being part of the pars flaccida, is lined by keratinizing squamous epithelium. **D.** This plane is further posterior and through the center of the pocket *(arrow),* has become firmly adherent to the neck of the malleus, and is, therefore, no longer reversible. As keratinous debris begins to accumulate within that retraction pocket, it becomes a "retraction pocket" cholesteatoma. (Hematoxylin and eosin, ×10 for *C* and *D*.) **E and F.** Serial axial **(E)** and coronal **(F)** CT scans of temporal bones with attic retraction cholesteatoma of right ear in a 43-year-old man. These scans reveal the soft tissue mass in the epitympanic recess *(arrows),* the reactive sclerosis of the mastoid process, the erosion of the lower lateral wall of the attic, and the medial displacement of the incus.

The pars flaccida retraction cholesteatoma arises generally just anterior or posterior to the short process of the malleus (Fig. 13.15A). It has the tendency to extend posteriorly toward the aditus and antrum along the lateral, medial, and superior aspect of malleus and incus (Fig. 13.15B). It can spread anteriorly under the head of the malleus toward the anterior epitympanum or the mesotympanum (Figs. 13.14B and 13.16) and inferiorly along the lateral or medial side of the body and long process of the incus (Fig. 13.17).

The local behavior of the attic retraction cholesteatoma is very similar to the one of the attic papillary cholesteatomas, with the difference being that the former generally produces a more extensive erosion and destruction of the lateral wall of the attic. This destruction may vary from a smaller defect to a much larger defect comparable to an atticoantrotomy created by nature, with exposure of a partially or subtotally destroyed malleus and incus (Figs. 13.17B and C and 13.18). An attic retraction cholesteatoma may extend inferiorly into the mesotympanum behind the pars tensa, giving its posterior-superior quadrant an opaque and whitish aspect and eventually leading to a second perforation in that area (Fig. 13.17D). Such simultaneous perforations in the pars flaccida and pars tensa are occasionally observed. Although the defect in Shrapnell's membrane may vary considerably, there is no correlation between its size and the actual extent of the underlying cholesteatoma. Eighty percent of attic retraction cholesteatomas with a small invagination or perforation are already extending into and beyond the mastoid antrum at the time of the initial clinical examination (18).

The pathogenesis of a pars tensa retraction cholesteatoma is practically identical with the one originating from the pars flaccida or Shrapnell's membrane. The predilective site is the posterior-superior quadrant (Fig. 13.19). In a rare instance the cholesteatoma may arise in the center or in another area (Fig. 13.19A). The posterior-superior pars tensa retraction cholesteatoma differs from the central form not only in location and frequency but also in its mode of development and sequels. Its relation to the adjacent bony canal wall predisposes it from the beginning to a development and expansion within the tympanic cavity. The constricted and unyielding opening toward the external ear canal therefore greatly determines its subsequent evolution. The retraction of the pars tensa leads in succession to atrophy of the drum and apposition and adherence to the long process of the incus and to its articulation with the stapes. Further retraction may proceed in two directions: anterior to the long crus of the incus, toward and sometimes underneath the malleus handle, and posterior to the longer process of the incus into the posterior epitympanic, facial, and tympanic recess. Occasionally, the two retraction pockets occur jointly (Fig. 13.20). Cholesteatomas in these retraction pockets have long been recognized (18). The further development of this cholesteatoma is in the direction of least resistance toward the antrum or toward the hypotympanum and tubal orifice (Fig. 13.20B). Increasing erosion of the adjacent posterior bony canal wall may, in a rare instance, result in a spontaneous radical mastoid cavity created by nature. On the other hand, a posterior-superior marginal pars tensa perforation may, in many instances, result from an outward perforation of an epitympanic cholesteatoma (19).

Central pars tensa retraction pockets have long been observed (20, 21). They are infrequent, however, and very rarely give rise to a cholesteatoma. They are frequently associated with an ipsilateral or contralateral retraction of Shrapnell's membrane (18, 22).

The differentiation between a cholesteatoma that has arisen from a localized retraction of the tympanic membrane and one that has originated from a papillary proliferation, may be difficult and, in an advanced stage, can only be assumed on clinical observations. The distinction becomes more reliable when a cholesteatoma is reviewed in serial sections of the temporal bone.

Of the two mechanisms involved in the development of an acquired cholesteatoma described above, epithelial papillary proliferation may be the prevalent one. It has also been observed that the two pathogenetic mechanisms may occur jointly (Fig. 13.21).

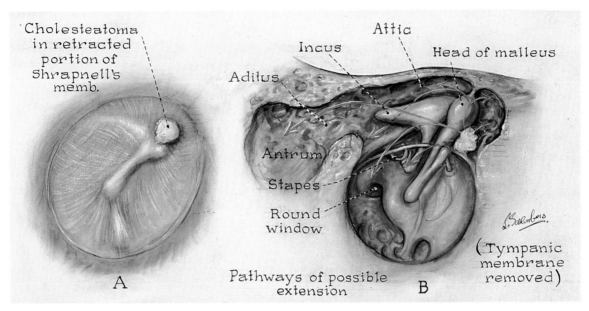

Figure 13.15.   Illustration, in lateral view, of directions in which the attic retraction cholesteatoma generally develops and of routes by which it reaches the aditus, antrum, and mesotympanum.

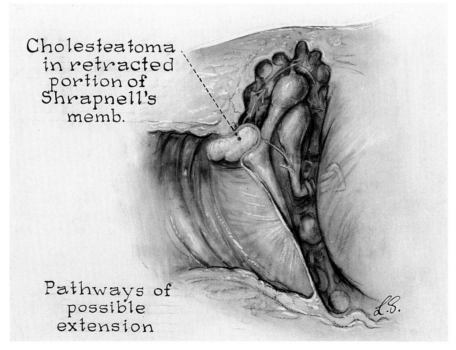

Figure 13.16.   Illustration, in coronal section, of directions in which the attic retraction cholesteatoma may expand within the anterior and superior region of the epitympanic recess.

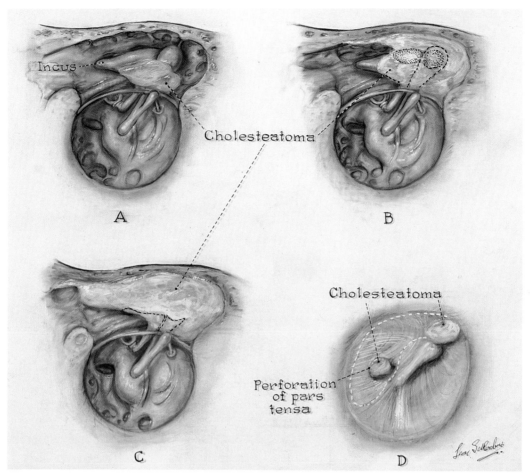

Figure 13.17. **A–C.** Illustration of gradual enlargement of attic retraction cholesteatoma and its effect on malleus and incus. **D.** Occasionally, a cho- lesteatoma may extend into the mesotympanum and eventually lead to a second perforation in the posterior-superior quadrant of the pars tensa.

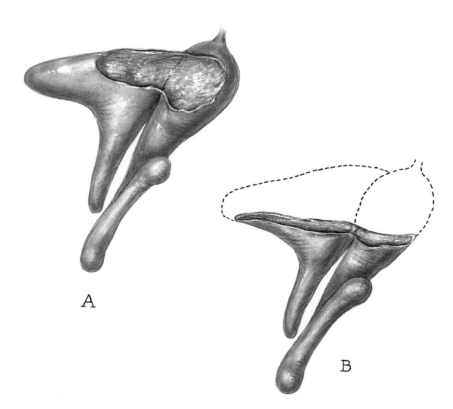

Figure 13.18. Illustration of manner in which the head of the malleus and the body of the incus are generally eroded by an attic retraction cholesteatoma.

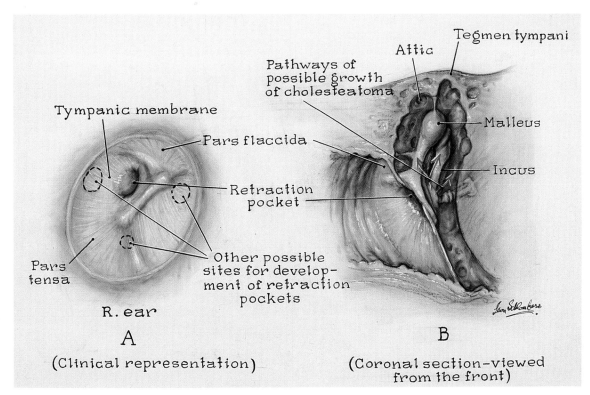

Figure 13.19.   A. Illustration of possible locations for development of retraction pockets in pars tensa. Progressive retraction of the posterior-superior quadrant of the drum may lead to invagination anterior and/or posterior to the long crus of the incus into the adjacent compartments of the epitympanic recess. **B.** *Arrows* indicate the directions in which a pars tensa retraction pocket cholesteatoma may expand.

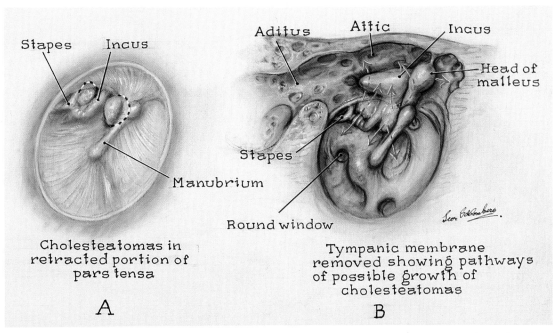

Figure 13.20.   A. Illustration of one of the most frequent locations of retraction pocket cholesteatoma in pars tensa of tympanic membrane. **B.** *Arrows* indicate the routes by which the posterior-superior pars tensa retraction pocket cholesteatoma generally reaches the aditus, antrum, and other areas of the tympanum.

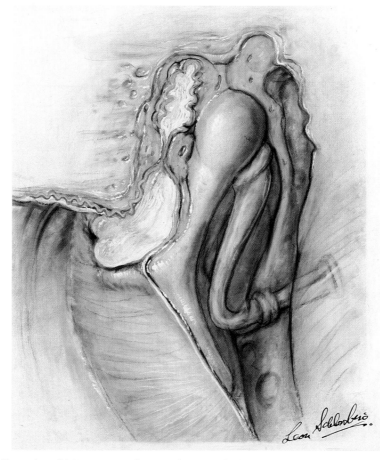

Figure 13.21. Illustration of infrequent coexistence of two mechanisms, attic retraction and papillary epithelial proliferation, in development of attic cholesteatoma.

Pathogenesis of Acquired Cholesteatoma Arising from Preexisting Marginal or Central Pars Tensa Tympanic Membrane Perforation

Another form of acquired cholesteatoma may arise from a marginal or central pars tensa tympanic membrane perforation that resulted from a necrotizing otitis media. The gradual extension of a localized inflammatory destruction in the peripheral region of the pars tensa eventually leads to necrosis of the tympanic annulus and to the development of a marginal perforation. This marginal perforation greatly facilitates the ingrowth of squamous epithelium from the external auditory canal into the middle ear cavity to resurface the denuded mucoperiosteum or bone (Figs. 13.22 and 13.23). Occasionally, squamous epithelium will invade the tympanic cavity through a central pars tensa perforation (Fig. 13.24). The continuing desquamation of keratohyalin lamellae within the middle ear and its concentric accumulation in an onionskin-like fashion lead to the formation of a cholesteatoma (Figs. 13.23 and 13.24). The local behavior of this cholesteatoma is identical with that of other acquired cholesteatomas.

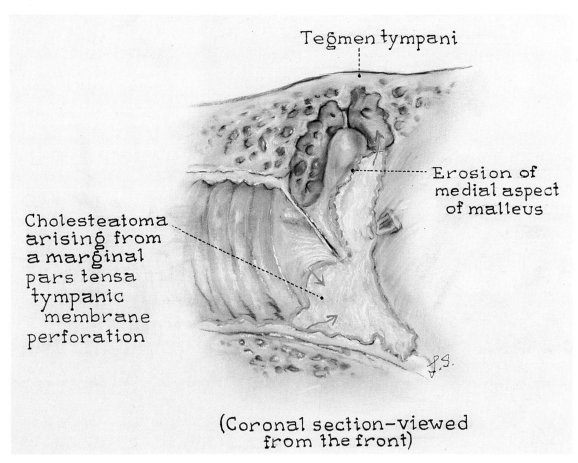

Figure 13.22.   Illustration of cholesteatoma that originates from ingrowth of squamous epithelium from the external auditory canal through a preexisting central or marginal pars tensa perforation to resurface the denuded submucosa and bone.

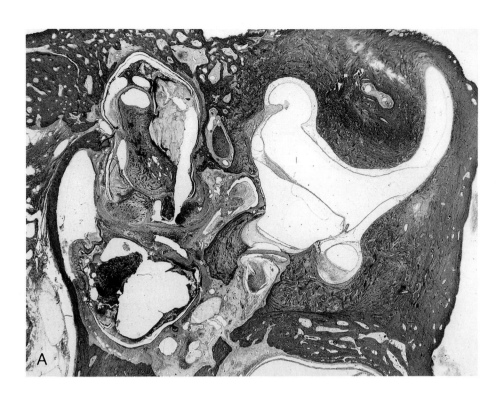

Figure 13.23.   A. Vertical section through right temporal bone at level of oval and round windows in a 16-year-old man with middle ear cholesteatoma. The cholesteatoma had arisen from ingrowth of squamous epithelium of the outer ear canal into the middle ear through a marginal inferior pars tensa perforation. (Hematoxylin and eosin, ×6.6.)

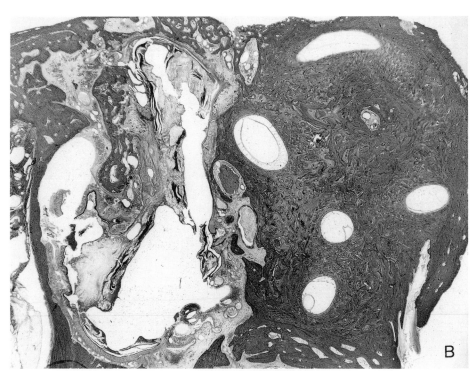

Figure 13.23.   B. Vertical section through right temporal bone at level of head of malleus. The cholesteatoma extends to the attic characteristically along the medial aspect of the malleus. (×6.6.)

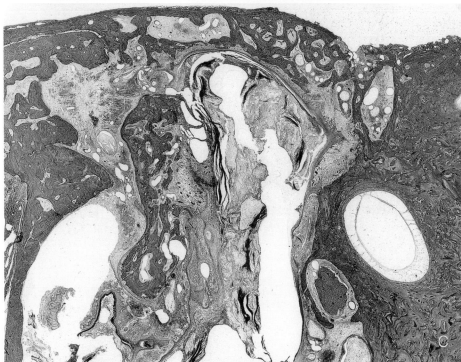

Figure 13.23.   C. The cholesteatoma caused a substantial erosion of the malleus head. (×10.7.)

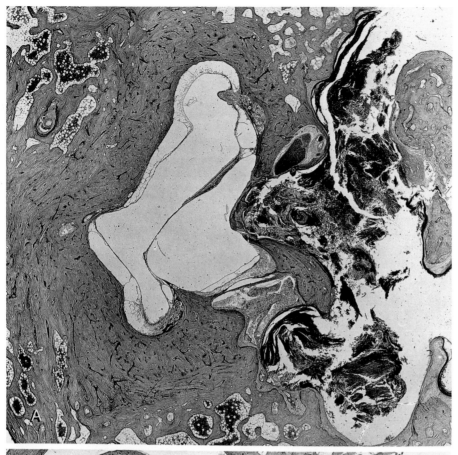

Figure 13.24. **A.** Vertical section through left temporal bone at level of malleus in a 86-year-old woman with acquired cholesteatoma. The cholesteatoma originated from an inferior central pars tensa perforation of the tympanic membrane. The perforation led to ingrowth of squamous epithelium from the outer surface of the drum into the middle ear. The cholesteatoma protrudes deeply into the oval and round window niches. (Hematoxylin and eosin, ×12.)

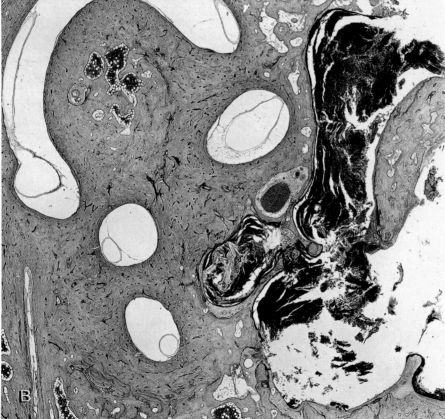

Figure 13.24. **B.** Vertical section through same temporal bone as in Figure 13.24A at level of incus. The cholesteatoma that extends to the attic, typically along the medial aspect of the ossicular chain, also occupies the tympanic and facial recess. (×12.)

Pathogenesis of Acquired Cholesteatoma Originating from Entrapment or Implantation of Squamous Epithelium

Another form of acquired cholesteatoma arises from entrapment of squamous epithelium within the tympanic bone, mastoid process, or middle ear cleft. This may result from a fracture, a bullet injury, some other mechanism of direct trauma, or a surgical procedure (Fig. 13.25). The responsible bone fracture is usually part of a laterobasal skull fracture that originates in either the parietal or the occipital region of the calvaria. This fracture runs along the posterior-superior wall of the external auditory canal, disrupts the annulus tympanicus at about 11 o'clock, and continues in the tegmental bone in the direction of the Eustachian tube. Occasionally, it extends with a ramification into the opposite (ipsilateral) anterior canal wall. In some instances, the tympanic ring and the annulus may become involved in a more complicated fracture, i.e., as part of a communuted fracture of the temporal bone. During the course of such a fracture, as the bony fragments are separated, squamous epithelium from the meatal skin or tympanic membrane may become entrapped and subsequently give rise to a so-called traumatic cholesteatoma. Such traumatic cholesteatomas have been observed repeatedly in the tympanic bone, mastoid process, and middle ear (23, 24). In a bullet or other form of direct injury, the mechanism leading to entrapment of squamous epithelium is identical. Similarly, a cholesteatoma may arise from iatrogenic displacement of squamous epithelium during a surgical procedure. Whereas such cholesteatomas are rarely seen after myringotomies, they are more often encountered following tympanoplasties. The iatrogenic cholesteatoma that develops in association with a long-standing middle ear ventilation tube results from in growth of squamous epithelium through the pars tensa perforation along the tube.

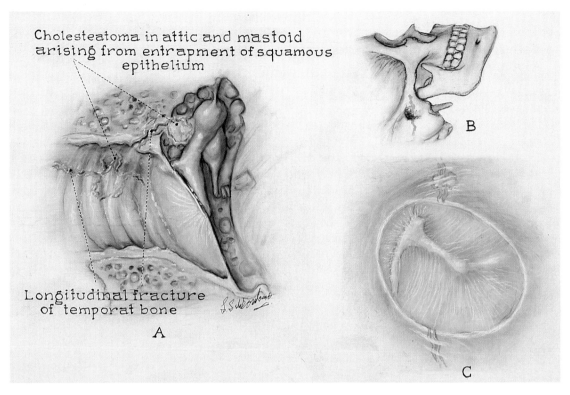

Figure 13.25. Illustration of rare traumatic cholesteatoma observed in canal wall, mastoid, and middle ear cleft. It arises from entrapment of squamous epithelium of the outer ear canal and tympanic membrane. The entrapment may occur during a longitudinal or comminuted fracture of the temporal bone or some other direct injury to the ear.

Pathogenesis of Acquired Cholesteatoma Arising from Squamous Metaplasia

Another, in all likelihood, very rare form of a presumably acquired cholesteatoma may arise from squamous metaplasia of the tympanic epithelium. It is a well-established fact that the respiratory epithelium of the nose, trachea, and bronchi may undergo localized squamous metaplasia, i.e., in atrophic rhinitis, tracheitis, and bronchiectasis. This is a response to long-standing irritation from a chronic inflammation. The question arises whether, and to what extent, such epithelial metaplasia can also develop in the middle ear mucosa in the presence of a chronic otitis media with an intact or perforated tympanic membrane. Under normal circumstances, the middle ear mucosa consists of a thin layer of fibrous tissue covered by an endothelium formed by flat cuboidal or low columnar cells. Ciliated columnar epithelium is usually encountered in the Eustachian tube and adjacent to its tympanic orifice over the anterior promontory. In chronic otitis media the flat cuboidal epithelium undergoes a reversible transformation to a papillary ciliated columnar endothelium with abundant goblet cells. At present, it is not known how often this common transition from a cuboidal to a ciliary columnar epithe-lium can proceed further to a stratified squamous epithelium under such circumstances. Our collection includes a temporal bone from a patient with a middle ear cholesteatoma in which the transition from a ciliated columnar epithelium of the middle ear to a stratified squamous epithelium can be followed (Fig. 13.26). This squamous epithelium then becomes the matrix of the cho-lesteatoma. In addition, there are several independent islands of stratified squamous epithelium completely surrounded by ciliated columnar epithelium (Fig. 13.26*D* and *E*). Since these islands have no connection with the matrix of the cholesteatoma, they represent areas of localized epithelial metaplasia as a response to the chronic middle ear disease. Another temporal bone, from a 12-year-old boy, shows a circumscribed area of keratinizing squamous epithelium surrounded by middle ear mucosa. This area is located on the anterolateral wall of the tympanic cavity (Fig. 13.27*A*). This island of squamous epithelium has already given rise to a small epidermoid inclusion cyst (Fig. 13.27*C*). It obviously developed in the absence of any recognizable inflam-matory process. These two examples of inflammatory and idio-pathic squamous metaplasia represent, in all likelihood, rare mechanisms involved in the development of an acquired choles-teatoma.

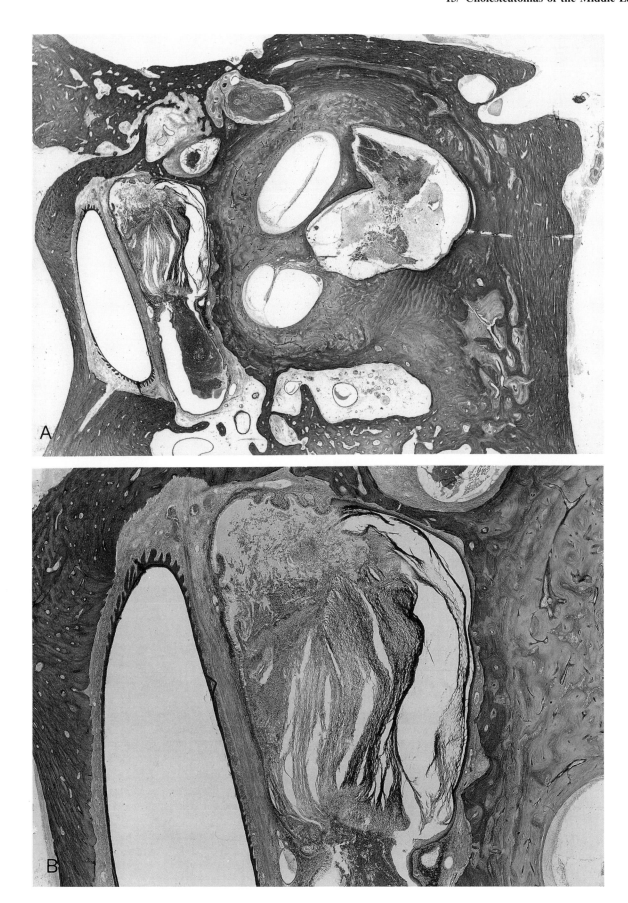

Figure 13.26.   A. Vertical section through right temporal bone at level of geniculate ganglion of a 38-year-old woman with posterior marginal pars tensa perforation and subsequently acquired middle ear cholesteatoma. **B.** Marginal zone of cholesteatoma. (Hematoxylin and eosin, ×9 and ×25, respectively.)

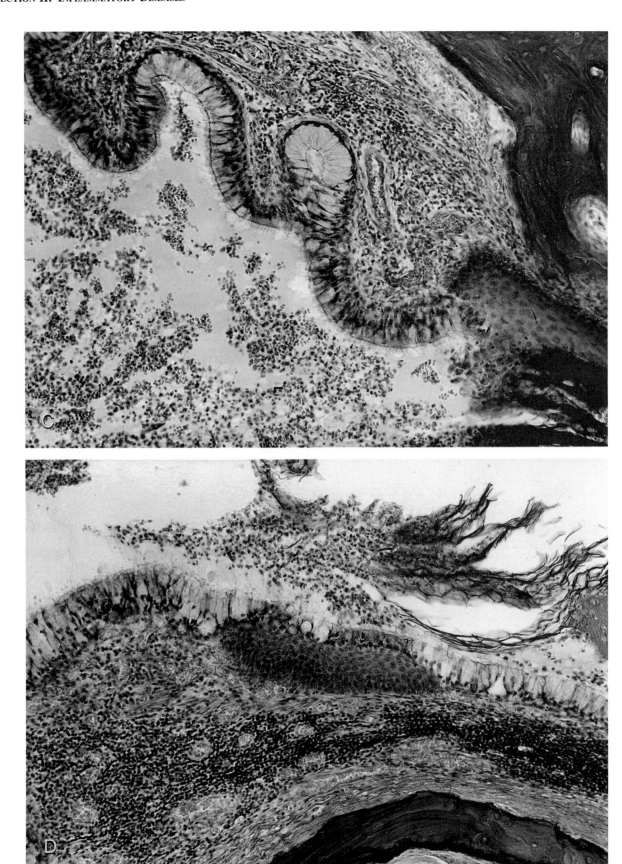

Figure 13.26. C. Transition from the squamous epithelium, constituting the matrix of the cholesteatoma, to the ciliated columnar epithelium with goblet cells can be seen. **D and E.** Several independent islands of stratified squamous epithelium are encountered in the middle of the ciliated columnar epithelium lining the anterior middle ear mucosa. These islands have no connection with the matrix of the cholesteatoma. They represent localized epithelial metaplasia incited by the chronic inflammatory process. It is possible that such islands of squamous epithelium may give rise to a cholesteatoma. (Hematoxylin and eosin, ×200 for each.)

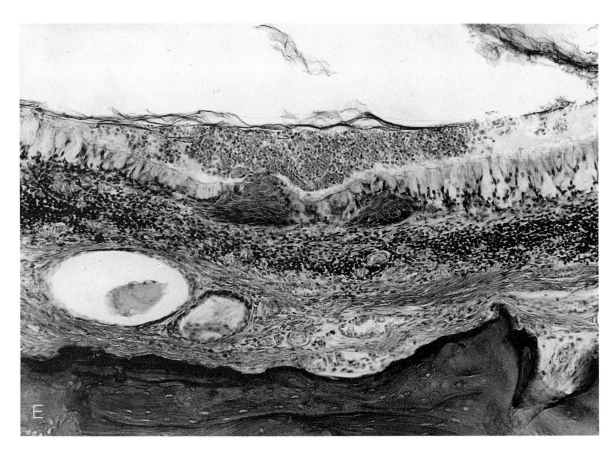

Figure 13.26.   E.

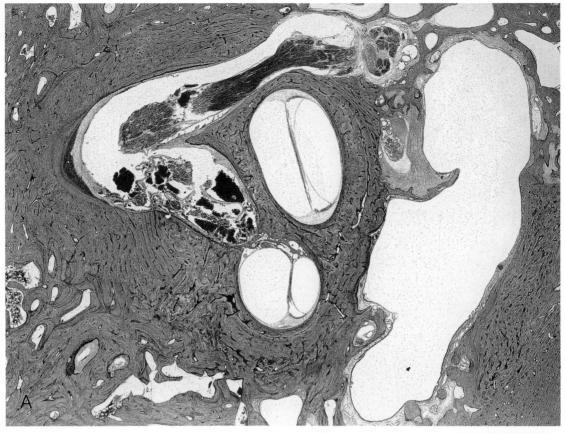

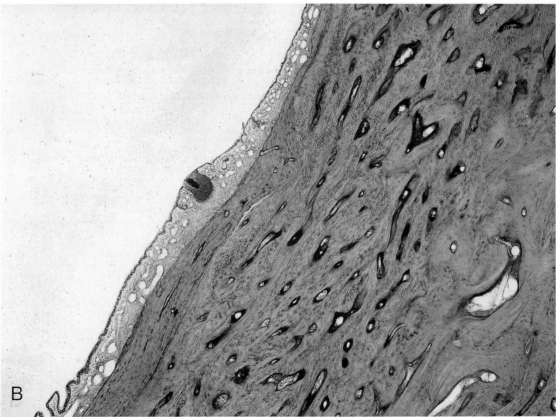

Figure 13.27. **A.** Vertical section through left temporal bone at level of geniculate ganglion in a 12-year-old boy. It shows the site of an island of keratinizing squamous epithelium in the middle ear mucosa lining the lat- eral wall of the mesotympanum. **B.** The cholesteatoma is located just an- terior to the annulus tympanicus. (Hematoxylin and eosin, ×10 and ×50, respectively.)

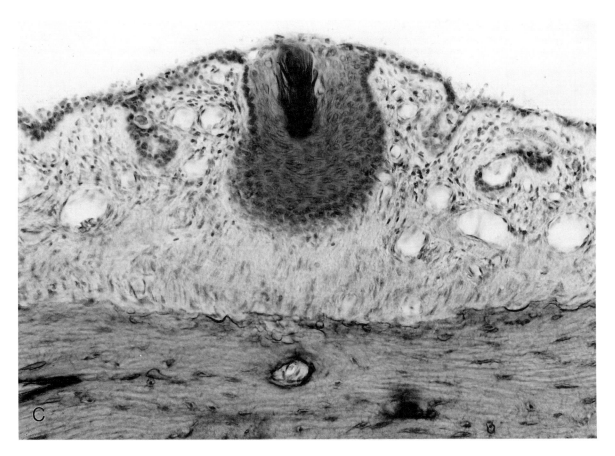

Figure 13.27. C. This tiny cholesteatoma is developing from a localized squamous metaplasia of the middle ear mucoperiosteum in the absence of any recognizable stimulus. (×300.)

LOCAL BEHAVIOR

The pressure exerted by the continuing accumulation of keratinous debris and the associated inflammation in the surrounding tissues cause a slowly progressive erosion of the surrounding bone. Depending on location and extent of the cholesteatoma, the erosion may involve the lateral wall of the attic (Figs. 13.3B, 13.4, and 13.28), the middle ear ossicles (Figs. 13.17B and C, 13.18, and 13.23B and C), the tegmental bone over the attic and antrum (Fig. 13.29C), and the mastoid cortex. Less frequently, it may involve the wall of the lateral sinus and jugular bulb, the vestibular and cochlear capsules, and the Fallopian canal (Figs. 13.30 and 13.31). The erosion may eventually expose the periosteum of the mastoid process, the dura of the middle and posterior cranial fossa, the lateral sinus, the lumen of the lateral or other semicircular canals, and the facial nerve (Figs. 13.29 and 13.31). The subsequent spread of the infection to these underlying structures leads to the well-recognized local and distal complications. They are discussed in the chapter on complications from acute and chronic tympanomastoiditis (Chapter 12). In a very rare instance, a cholesteatoma can invade the inner ear directly through the oval or round window and through the basal turn of the cochlea (Figs. 13.30 and 13.31).

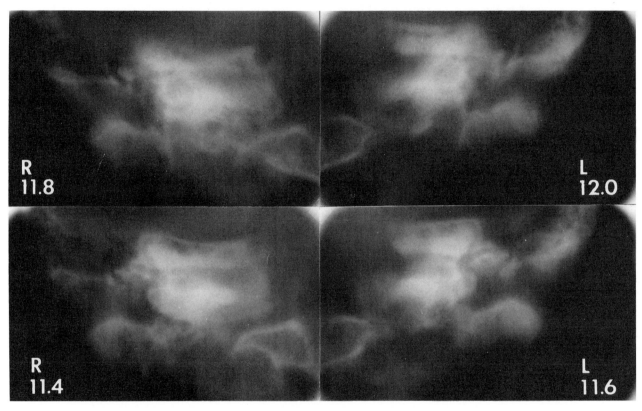

Figure 13.28.   Anteroposterior (AP) multidirectional tomograms of both temporal bones of a 15-year-old boy with a right attic cholesteatoma that has produced characteristic erosion of the lower lateral wall of the attic.

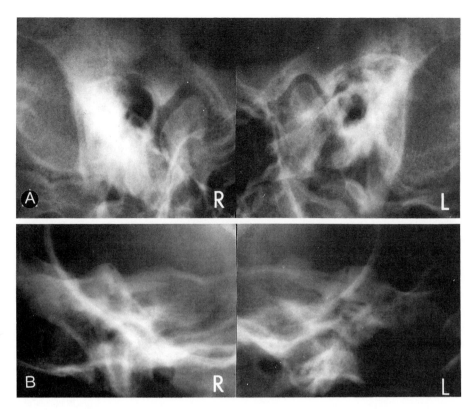

Figure 13.29. Lateral (Schüller) **(A)** and longitudinal (Stenvers) **(B)** projections of both temporal bones of a 27-year-old man with acquired right middle ear cholesteatoma extending into upper mastoid process. The right Stenvers view demonstrated the osteolytic process involving the antrum and periantral area, surrounded by a sclerotic margin, and the destruction of the lateral semicircular canal.

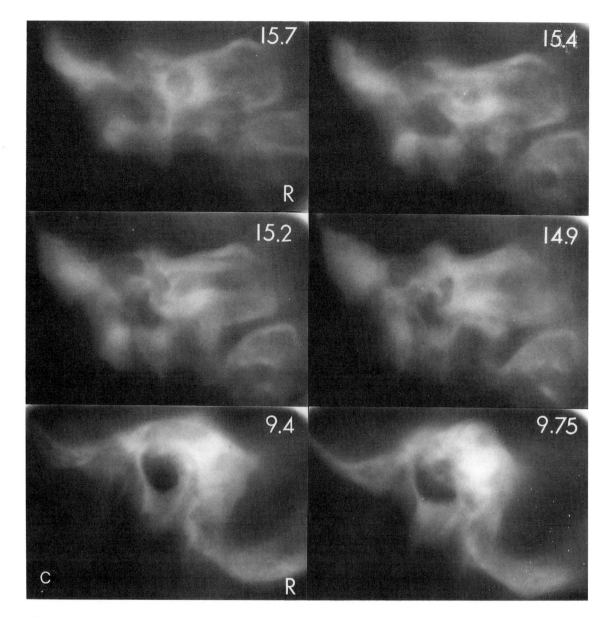

Figure 13.29.   C. AP and lateral multidirectional tomograms of right temporal bone. Destruction of the malleus and incus *(9.4)*, of the tegmental bone *(15.7)*, and of the lateral semicircular canal and the resulting labyrinthine fistula *(15.2)* are clearly recognized.

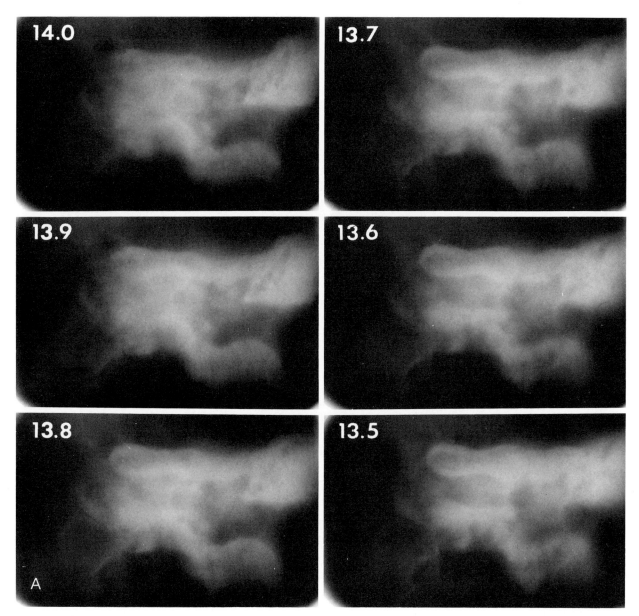

Figure 13.30. Serial AP multidirectional tomograms of left temporal bone of a 61-year-old man who at the age of 5 years had a foreign body (pea) removed from his left ear canal. This procedure had left him with a traumatic, anterior-inferior marginal pars tensa tympanic membrane perforation. The perforation led to the development of a chronic tympanomastoiditis and an acquired cholesteatoma. This cholesteatoma had destroyed most of the cochlear capsule and the entire lateral portion of the vestibular capsule, allowing massive invasion of the vestibule **(A).** The patient was first seen during a diffuse otogenic meningitis following labyrinthitis and osteitis of the otic capsule. At operation, the cholesteatoma had invaded the ampulated end of the lateral semicircular canal, creating a large fistula. It invaded the superior semicircular canal just above its ampulla. Almost the entire promontory had been destroyed by invasion of the cholesteatoma into the vestibule, which it occupied completely **(B).** The entire tympanic segment and the superior segment of the vertical portion of the Fallopian canal were completely destroyed, leaving the facial nerve circumferentially embedded in cholesteatomatous debris (Fig. 13.31). In spite of this, the patient never had any impairment of facial nerve function. Postoperative recovery was uneventful.

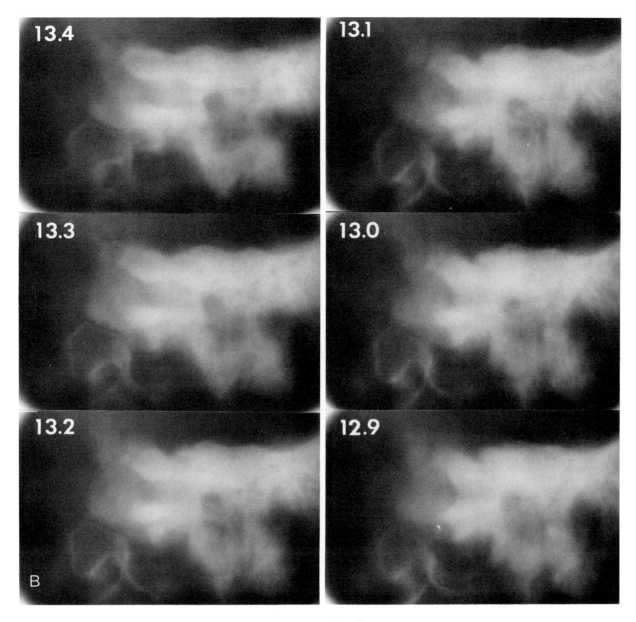

Figure 13.30.   B.

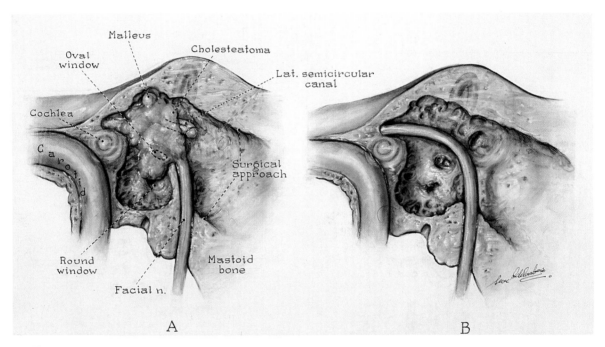

Figure 13.31. Illustration of rare form of middle ear cholesteatoma that directly invaded the cochlea, vestibule, and semicircular canals, destroyed vast areas of the inner ear capsule, and led to otogenic meningitis.

RADIOLOGIC MANIFESTATIONS

Computed axial and coronal tomograms (and formerly polycyclic anteroposterior (AP) and lateral tomograms) of the temporal bone are adequate in most instances to identify complications from a cholesteatoma. The epitympanic recess is the area most frequently involved. Erosion of the inferior lateral wall of the attic, the so-called "attic spur," is usually associated with a perforation in Shrapnell's membrane (Fig. 13.28). A discontinuity in the tegmen of the epitympanum or antrum may indicate a destruction (Fig. 13.29C). Erosion of the medial wall of the attic and aditus with destruction of the lateral wall of the horizontal semicircular canal near its ampulla may suggest the presence of a labyrinthine fistula (Fig. 13.29B and C). The enlargement of the aditus and antrum, the absence of the periantral cells, and occasionally a more clearly defined sclerotic margin of the bony defect may indicate an extension of the cholesteatoma into and beyond the mastoid antrum (Fig. 13.29B and C (15.2)). Malleus and incus are often partially and totally destroyed, and absence of the long process of the incus is a common observation. In chronic otitis media with osteitis, the differentiation between the presence or absence of a cholesteatoma is often impossible. The density of a cholesteatoma and an inflammatory granulation tissue and the destruction of adjacent bony structures may be identical. However, the erosion of the lateral wall of the attic and ossicles signifies in most instances the action of a cholesteatoma (Fig. 13.28). Polycyclic tomograms in the AP and lateral projections of the temporal bone may provide valuable information in situations where the Fallopian canal is involved. In summary, these studies may strongly suggest but cannot rule out the presence of a cholesteatoma. The definitive diagnosis is made almost exclusively during the otologic examination with the microscope.

Case Report

Case 1. *Giant cholesteatoma with total destruction of right mastoid process. Erosion through mastoid cortex, tegmen tympani and tegmen antri, sinus plate, vertical segment of Fallopian canal, lateral semicircular canal, and posterior wall of external auditory canal. Subperiosteal abscess, epidural abscesses involving dura of middle and posterior cranial fossa and lateral sinus. Wide exposure of facial nerve and lateral membranous semicircular canal. Fourteen-year history of chronic purulent right otorrhea. Maximal conductive hearing loss of right ear.*

A 23-year-old male immigrant from Afghanistan with a history of chronic recurrent right otitis media since the age of 9 years, following right aspiration myringotomy with placement of a middle ear ventilation tube in childhood and repeated removal of right aural polyps, was seen. During the past few months prior to admission, he developed increasing right otorrhea, otalgia, vertigo, and unsteadiness.

Otologic examination revealed a mass of polypoid granulation tissue protruding from the right outer ear canal, surrounded by creamy purulent exudate. There was marked postauricular inflammatory swelling and tenderness that on palpation and pressure on the tragus produced a "compression nystagmus" (positive fistula symptom). The cochlear function studies showed a maximal conductive hearing loss on the right but a discrimination score of 100%.

Computed tomography (CT) of the temporal bones revealed a large expansile soft tissue mass involving the right mastoid bone, middle ear, and external auditory canal (Fig. 13.32A). It showed erosion of the lateral aspect of the lateral semicircular canal and displacement of the dura overlying the right sigmoid sinus without evidence of transdural extension. The soft tissue mass was impinging on the vertical segment of the facial canal.

Magnetic resonance imaging (MRI) disclosed a 3.0-cm, well-defined, benign-appearing, ring-enhancing mass centered in the right temporal bone, involving the entire mastoid process, external auditory canal, and middle ear cavity (Fig. 13.32B). There was minimal dural enhancement along the inferior margin of the right temporal lobe but no evidence of intracranial extension.

At *operation,* a large cholesteatoma was encountered that occupied the entire mastoid process. It had caused widespread destruction of the mastoid cortex, tegmental bone, sinus plate, and posterior external auditory canal wall. The dura of the middle and posterior fossa and of the lateral sinus was covered with inflammatory granulation tissue. An extensive erosion of the lateral aspect of the horizontal semicircular canal had resulted in wide exposure of the membranous canal. The vertical segment of the Fallopian canal had been destroyed, exposing the nerve in a length of about 1.5–2 cm, leaving the sheath intact. The cholesteatoma, which had destroyed malleus, incus, and the stapedial superstructure, had extended into the root of the zygoma. Postoperatively, contrary to expectations, hearing was noticeably improved.

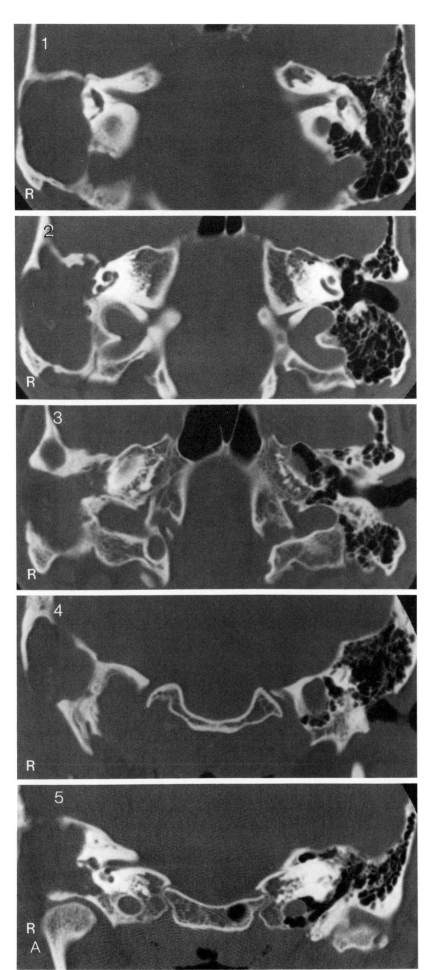

Figure 13.32.   A. Axial CT scan of the right temporal bone reveals a very extensive, well-demarcated, benign-appearing soft tissue mass occupying the entire mastoid process, root of the zygoma, middle ear cavity, and external auditory canal. It has destroyed the posterior wall of the external ear canal *(1)*, eroded the lateral portion of the descending Fallopian canal and displaced the dura of the sigmoid sinus medially *(2)*, eroded the lateral aspect of the horizontal semicircular canal *(3)*, and destroyed the mastoid cortex *(2* and *3)*. Coronal CT scans disclose the destruction of the tegmental bone and lateral mastoid cortex and the erosion of the lateral semicircular canal *(4* and *5)*.

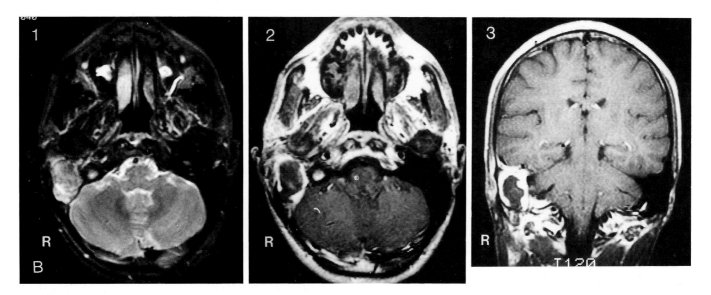

Figure 13.32.   B. Axial and coronal MRI scans demonstrate the ring-enhancing mass occupying the entire mastoid bone (1, 2). The margins are well defined, and the overall appearance is that of a benign lesion. There is minimal dural enhancement along the inferior surface of the right temporal lobe (3) but no sign of intracranial extension.

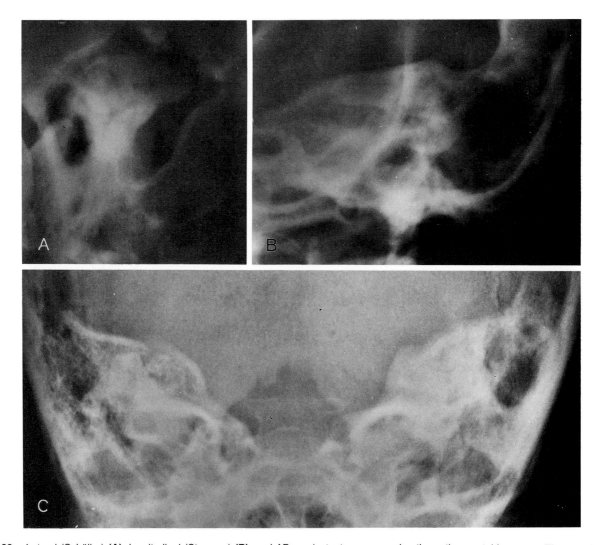

Figure 13.33. Lateral (Schüller) **(A),** longitudinal (Stenvers) **(B),** and AP (occipital) **(C)** views of left temporal bone of a man with a giant-size cho- lesteatoma occupying the entire mastoid process. The margins of the cav- ity are characteristically scalloped out and sclerotic.

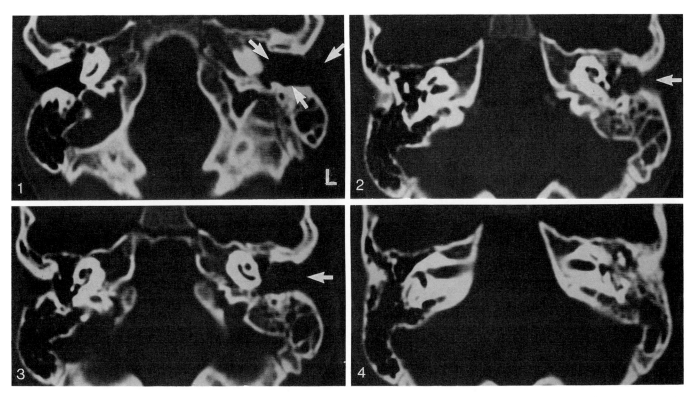

Figure 13.34. Serial axial CT scans of the temporal bones of a 5-year-old girl with progressive conductive hearing loss in the left ear and cholesteatoma in the left external auditory canal. Developing in the posterior meatal skin and gradually increasing in size, it assumed the form of a polypoid soft tissue mass covered by squamous epithelium that finally completely occluded the external meatus *(arrows) (1–3).* It had displaced the intact tympanic membrane medially and given rise to a chronic inflammatory edema of the mucosa throughout the middle ear cleft *(2–4).*

References

1. Bostroem E. Über die pialen Epidermoide, Dermoide und Lipome und duralen Dermoide. Zentralb Pathol 1897;8:1–98.
2. Rubinstein LG. Tumors of the central nervous system. In: Atlas of tumor pathology, Fascicle 6. Washington, DC: Armed Forces Institute of Pathology, 1972:288–292.
3. Scholz F. Einige Bemerkungen über das meningeale Cholesteatom im Anschluss an einen Fall von Cholesteatom des Ventrikels. Virchows. Arch Path Anat 1855;8:371.
4. Mahoney W. Die Epidermoide des Zentralnervensystems. Z Neurol 1936;155:416–471.
5. Thomalske G, Kienow-Rieg I, Mohr G. Critical obsevations concerning the diagnosis and clinical features in 100 cases of tumors in the cerebellopontine region. Adv Neurosurg 1973ᵏ(V):252–259.
6. Fromm H, Huf H, Schaefer M. Operations and results in 102 tumors of the cerebellopontine angle. Adv Neurosurg 1973;I (V):260–261.
7. Nager GT. Epidermoids (congenital cholesteatomas) involving the temporal bone. In: Cholesteatoma and mastoid surgery. Proceedings of the 2nd International Conference, Tel Aviv, Israel, March 22–27, 1981. Amsterdam: Kugler Publications, 1982:41–59.
7a. Michaels L. An epidermoid formation in the developing middle ear; possible source of cholesteatoma. J. Otolaryngol 1986;15:169.
8. Habermann J. Zur Entstehung des Cholesteatoms des Mittelohres. Arch Ohren-Nasen-Kehlkopfheilkd 1889;27:42–50.
9. Habermann J. Cholesteatomentstehung. In: Schwartze's Handbuch der Ohrenheilkunde. Leipzig: FCW Vogel, 1892;I:255.
10. Politzer A. Die desquamativen Prozesse und die Cholesteatombildung, etc. In: Lehrbuch der Ohrenheilkunde. Stuttgart: F Enke, 1901.
11. Lange E. Über die Entstehung der Mittelohrcholesteatome. Z Hals-Nasen-Ohrenheilkd 1925;11:250–271.
12. Tumarkin A. Pre-epidermosis. J Laryngol Otol 1961;75:487–500.
13. McGuckin F. Nonmalignant destructive ear disease. Panel on Selection of Technic for Chronic Draining Ear. Arch Otolaryngol 1963;78:358–363.
14. Rüedi L. Pathogenesis and surgical treatment of the middle ear cholesteatoma. Acta Otolaryngol Suppl (Stockh) 1978;361:1–45.
15. Nager GT. Theories on the origin of attic retraction cholesteatomas. In: Shambaugh GE Jr, ed. Fifth Internation Workshop on Middle Ear Microsurgery and Fluctuant Hearing Loss. Northwestern University Medical School, Chicago, Illinois, February 29–March 5, 1976. Huntsville, Alabama: Strode Publications, 1976.
16. Kupper. Cholesteatom des Trommelfells. Arch Ohren-Nasen-Kehlkopfheilkd 1876;11:6.
17. Bezold F. Cholesteatom, Perforation der Membrana flaccida Shrapnelli und Tubenverschluss, eine ätiologische Studie. Z Ohren Heilkd 1890;20:5–28.
18. Schwarz M. Das Cholesteatom im Gehörgang und im Mittelohr. Zwangslose Abhandlungen aus dem Gebiete der Hals-Nasen-Ohrenheilkunde, Heft 8. Stuttgart: Gerog Thieme, 1966.
19. Rüedi L. Cholesteatomas of the attic. J Laryngol Otol 1958;72:592–609.
20. Whittmaack K. Die Cholesteatomeiterung und die falsche Cholesteatombildung. In: Henke F, Lubarsch O, eds. Handbuch der speziellen pathologischen Anatomie und Histologie, Bd XII: Gehörorgan. Berlin: Julius Springer, 1962.
21. Steurer O. Zur Pathogenese der Mittelohrcholesteatome. Z Hals-Nasen-Ohrenheilkd 1929;24:402–415.
22. Beickert P. Hernienartige Entstehung und Entwicklung von Cholesteatomen. Z Laryngol 1957;36:154.
23. Escher F. Traumatische Cholesteatome. Pract Otol-Rhino-Laryngol (Basel) 1954;16:32.
24. Escher F. Traumatische Mittelohrcholesteatome. Acta Otolaryngol (Stockh) 1959;50:47.

14/ Granulomatous Diseases of Known and Unknown Etiology

Part 1
Tuberculosis

Tuberculosis, once the prevalent cause of death among the younger age group during the 18th and 19th centuries, has been progressively declining in all civilized countries. By 1985, the incidence of new cases had dropped to 9 in 100,000 for the United States (1). The extent of otolaryngologic manifestations of the disease, involving the oral cavity, neck, larynx, and ear, once common complications of cavitary and disseminated tuberculosis, has declined accordingly. To gain a clear understanding of the pathogenesis of middle ear tuberculosis, it is helpful to review briefly the pathology of the disease in general.

The organism almost exclusively involved in human tuberculosis today is *Mycobacterium tuberculosis*. The infection is usually transmitted from person to person by inhalation. During expectoration, verbal communication, singing, and laughing, droplets of respiratory secretions containing the organism are disseminated in the room air, where they remain suspended and are inhaled. The source is usually an adult with cavitary pulmonary disease (1). Ingestion of the *Mycobacterium bovis* organism is no longer a frequent mode of infection as in the days of unpasteurized milk and widespread tuberculous mastitis in cattle. In those days, tuberculosis of the tonsils and small intestines accounted for about 20% of all human tuberculous infections (2). Transplacental infection of the fetus is very rare and occurs only during a miliary dissemination of tuberculosis in the mother. Another rare pathway of infection is inoculation through a skin lesion in a laboratory technician or pathologist (2). The primary response to the tubercle bacillus in the nonsensitized individual is a pneumonitis at the site of deposition of the inhaled organism and the subsequent development of a granuloma. The extent of the exudative response varies with the number and virulence of the organisms and the host's resistance and immune response. Initially, polymorphonuclear leukocytes and mononuclear phagocytes engulf the organisms. As the tubercle bacilli proliferate within the cells, the turnover of the mononuclear phagocytes increases. The monocytes aggregate in close spherical formations and assume the form of epithelioid cells. A characteristic feature of the tuberculous granuloma is the appearance of multinucleated giant cells with their nuclei dispersed evenly or in a peripheral ring. The change to a granulomatous tissue reaction occurs concurrently with the host's acquisition of delayed sensitivity. The granuloma then becomes surrounded by lymphoctyes, plasma cells, fibroblasts, and capillaries (Figs. 14.1.1A and 14.1.2B and C). Depending on the immune response, the granuloma may become surrounded by a fibrous capsule, may undergo calcification and become quiescent, or may enlarge by coalescence with satellite lesions and undergo central necrosis and liquefaction, known as caseation (Fig. 14.1.3B and C) (2). The process of encapsulation prevents further canalicular and lymphohematogenous dissemination, while the organisms gradually lose their viability. The primary infection generally heals, as evidenced by a residual calcified parenchymal scar associated with calcifications in the draining hilar lymph node, which together are recognized as the primary or Ghon's focus (1, 2). Next follows a period of latency during which the organisms remain dormant but still alive. In a small group of previously infected individuals with a positive tuberculin skin test, reactivation may occur. It is by this mechanism of endogenous reinfection that tuberculosis of the lungs and in extrapulmonary locations generally develops in the adult (2). This form of postprimary tuberculosis usually manifests itself as a circumscribed lobular pneumonia in the subapical region of one or both upper lobes. This apical pneumonitis may resolve or may develop into granulomas with central necrosis and peripheral fibrous encapsulation and then eventually heal and calcify; or the original lobular pneumonia may undergo caseation and liquefaction, erode a bronchus, and give rise to a tuberculous cavity. Aspiration of the infected exudate may lead to new foci of acinous penumonia in other areas of the lung, to a caseous pneumonia, and to additional cavitation. Erosion of a bronchial or pulmonary artery within such cavities will lead to hemoptysis and even to lethal hemorrhages (2). As an expanding necrotizing penumonitis reaches the pleura, bronchopleural fistula and a tuberculous empyema may develop. A generalized or miliary tuberculosis usually results from hematogenous dissemination of the organisms of a pulmonary or extrapulmonary lesion. Death generally results from pulmonary insufficiency or general septicemia in the event of miliary tuberculosis.

An exogenous postprimary reinfection is also recognized. It may be documented by the identification of bacilli with a different phage type or a different drug sensitivity pattern than that of the primary infection (2).

In some instances, the primary lung lesion undergoes progressive colliquation necrosis with bronchogenic dissemination to other areas of the lungs. More often, dissemination occurs when a draining caseous lymph node erodes a bronchus and gives rise to a tuberculous pneumonia with cavitation. Finally, erosion of a blood vessel opens the pathway for a hematogenous spread and establishment of numerous small foci in many organs, a form of the disease recognized as miliary tuberculosis (1).

By the end of the 1950s, along with the decline of tuberculosis in general, the incidence of tuberculosis as a cause of middle ear infection had dropped to about 0.05% (3). Whereas this is true for civilized countries, it does not apply to underdeveloped nations where the disease is still frequently encountered. Recent reports from certain areas in Africa indicate that a high percentage (up to 40%) of patients afflicted with the acquired immune deficiency syndrome are dying from tuberculosis. It is therefore advisable to remain familiar with the otolaryngologic manifestations of this disease.

The middle ear may become involved at any stage of a tuberculous infection. It may be the site of a primary or a post-primary tuberculosis. The existence of a primary infection has been documented in the past by clinical and postmortem examinations and by observing the conversion of a previously negative tuberculin skin test (4–6, 7). The primary tuberculous otitis media is regularly associated with tuberculous lymphadenitis involving the regional periauricular and, occasionally, the ipsilateral cervical lymph nodes. The portal of entry is the nasopharyngeal lymphoid tissue or the middle ear cleft whereby the organisms reach the middle ear along the Eustachian tube. The primary complex may heal, or it may remain active and the infection subsequently spread to bone, to the inner ear, or (via the bloodstream) to the meninges (8). The primary infection is practically no longer observed in the United States and is encountered in developing countries exclusively in newborns and infants.

The postprimary or secondary tuberculous middle ear infection originates in the mucoperiosteum. It usually results from a hematogenous dissemination from the lung or from a draining lymph node associated with the primary complex. The simultaneous presence of tuberculomas in the middle ear mucosa and the bone marrow is proof that the spread had occurred via the bloodstream. The canalicular pathway, whereby the tubercle bacilli from coughed-up secretions enter the middle ear through the Eustachian tube, probably is of far lesser significance. Depending on the concentration and virulence of the organisms and the host's resistance and immunity, the postprimary infection may assume a predominantly productive or exudative form. The exudative form generally predominates (8). The productive form is characterized by the presence of noncaseous tuberculomas and by the proliferation of polypoid tuberculous granulation tissue (Figs. 14.1.1B and 14.1.2B and C) (5, 6, 8). The more frequent exudative form is distinguished by ulceration, caseation, and widespread necrosis of the mucoperiosteum and bone (Figs. 14.1.3B and C and 14.1.4) (7). The destructive osteitis primarily affects the middle ear ossicles, the Fallopian canal, and the medial wall of the middle cavity (Fig. 14.1.9). Extension to the petrous apex and carotid canal may lead to erosion of the internal carotid artery and involvement of cranial nerves V and VI (8). Necrosis of the mastoid cortex may result in the development of one or several fistula tracts, accompanied by abscesses in the postauricular area, medial to the sternocleidal muscle, and along the parapharyngeal space. Destruction of the mucoperiosteum will deprive the underlying bone of its blood supply, and consequently, the affected bone becomes necrotic and eventually sequestrated. In the preantibiotic area, sequestration of the petrous bone occasionally led to necrosis of the entire otic capsule (7–10). Necrosis of the lateral sinus and jugular bulb may give rise to septicemia, and destruction of the annular ligament and round window membrane can lead to tuberculous labyrinthitis and meningitis. The tympanic membrane often becomes involved in multiple tuberculomas that are located either in the submucosa or, occasionally, in the subcutis (Fig. 14.1.6). As these focal lesions undergo colliquation necrosis, they lead to multiple, irregularly shaped perforations and, ultimately, to total destruction of the eardrum. The diagnosis of middle ear tuberculosis is established by identification of the organisms in secretions and cultures and by histologic examination of the tuberculous granulation tissue.

Case Reports

Case 1. *Bilateral tuberculous tympanomastoiditis with tubercles in the mucosa of the Eustachian tube, mucoperiosteum of the middle ear and mastoid, tympanic membrane, subarachnoid space along cranial nerves VII and VIII, and bone marrow. Pulmonary tuberculosis with primary complex in the right middle lobe. Bronchial erosion by caseous lymph node of Ghon's focus with widespread pulmonary dissemination. Caseous peribronchial, peritracheal, and cervical lymphadenitis. Tuberculous tonsillitis. Tuberculous enteritis. Disseminated tubercles in liver, spleen, kidneys, adrenals, and pleura. Tuberculous pachymeningitis and leptomeningitis.*

A 4-month-old male infant was seen. Examination of the temporal bones revealed dissemination of predominantly productive tubercles in the mucosa of the Eustachian tube, tensor tympani muscle (Figs. 14.1.1 and 14.1.2), mucoperiosteum of the middle ear cleft (Figs. 14.1.4 and 14.1.5), mastoid, tympanic membrane (Fig. 14.1.6), bone marrow, and subdural and subarachnoid space along cranial nerves VII and VIII (Fig. 14.1.3). Bilateral tympanomastoiditis with central tympanic membrane perforations was noted.

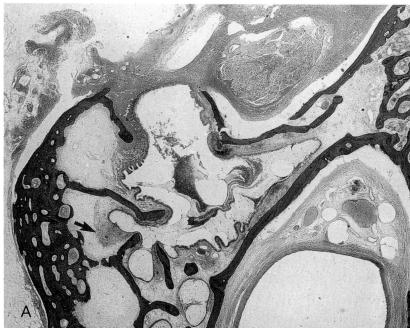

Figure 14.1.1.   A. Vertical section through right temporal bone near tympanic orifice of Eustachian tube, below tensor tympani muscle, and to the left of the carotid artery of a 4-month-old male infant with bilateral exudative tuberculous otitis media associated with miliary tuberculosis and tuberculous meningitis. It shows a tubercle in the mucosa of the floor of the Eustachian tube *(arrow)*. (Hematoxylin and eosin, ×18.)

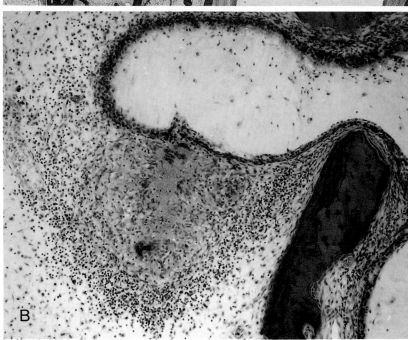

Figure 14.1.1.   B. The tuberculous granuloma is located in the submucosa of the Eustachian tube. Several multinucleated giant cells are recognized. (×130.)

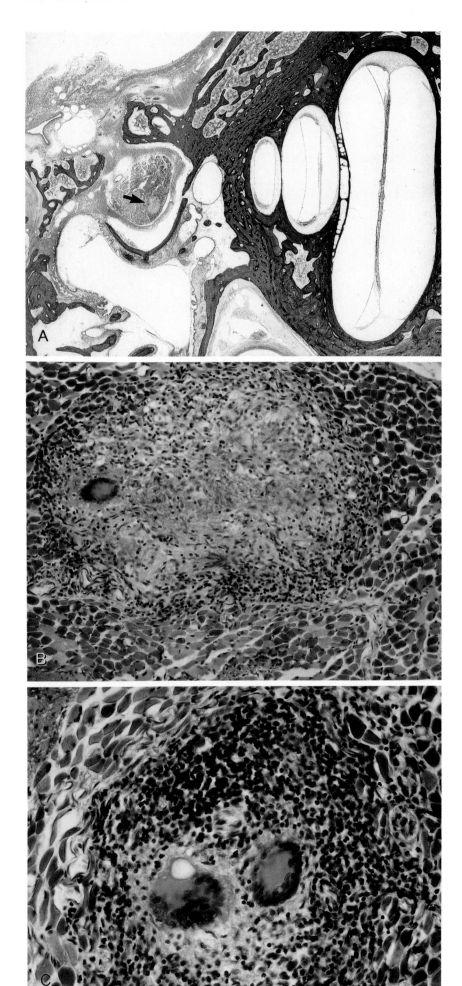

Figure 14.1.2. A. Vertical, anterior paramodiolar section through right temporal bone of the same patient as in Figure 14.1.1. It shows a miliary tubercle in the tensor tympani muscle *(arrow).* (Hematoxylin and eosin, ×12.)

Figure 14.1.2. B. The tubercle consists of an aggregation of densely packed epithelioid histiocytes with a necrotic center, surrounded by lymphocytes, plasma cells, monocytes, fibroblasts, and capillaries. The presence of a multinucleated giant cell is a characteristic feature of the tuberculous granuloma. (×220.)

Figure 14.1.2. C. Another section of the same granuloma as in *A* and *B* shows two giant cells, each with a different nuclear pattern. (×360.)

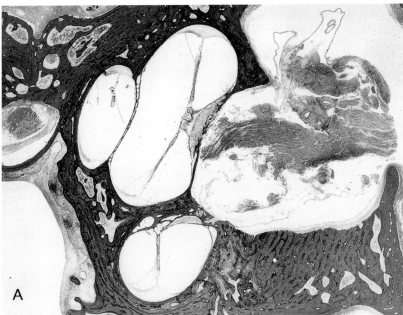

Figure 14.1.3. A. Vertical, anterior paramodiolar section through right temporal bone of the same patient as in Figure 14.1.1. The subarachnoid space of the internal auditory canal reveals evidence of a tuberculous leptomeningitis. (Hematoxylin and eosin, ×10.)

Figure 14.1.3. B and C. The cochlear, vestibular, and facial nerves are covered by multiple tuberculous granulomas. (×140.)

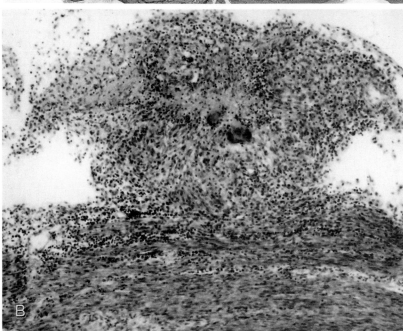

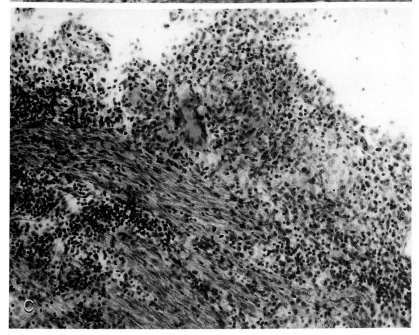

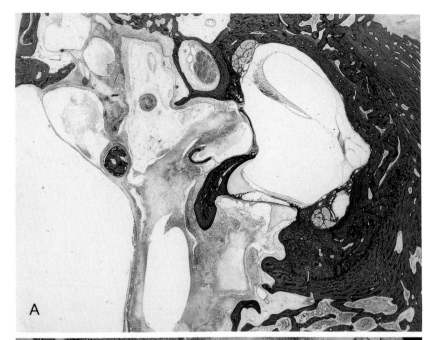

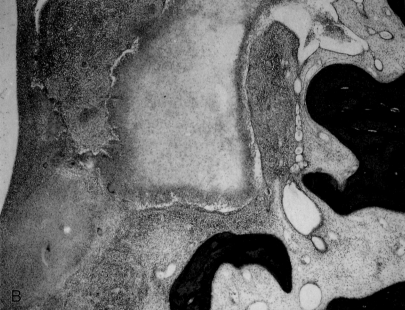

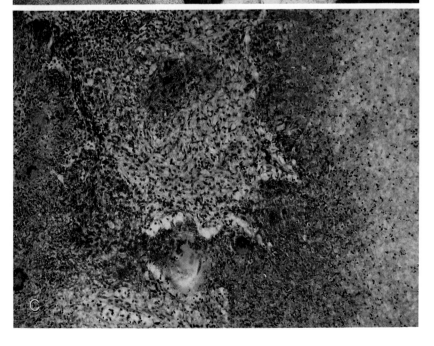

Figure 14.1.4. **A.** Vertical section through right temporal bone at level of oval and round windows of the same patient as in Figure 14.1.1. The middle ear is occupied by an inflammatory exudate. The mucoperiosteum discloses an inflammatory edema with numerous tubercles. (Hematoxylin and eosin, ×8.)

Figure 14.1.4. **B.** The mucoperiosteum within the round window niche includes multiple tubercles. (×40.)

Figure 14.1.4. **C.** Tuberculous granulomas with and without central necrosis (caseation) are recognized side by side. (×130.)

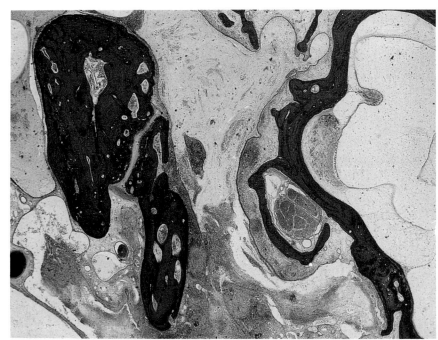

Figure 14.1.5. Vertical section through right temporal bone at level of incudomalleolar articulation of the same patient as in Figure 14.1.1. The mesotympanum and epitympanum are occupied by tuberculous granulation tissue in which productive and exudative tubercles, areas of recent hemorrhages, and multiple small cholesterol granulomas can be recognized. (Hematoxylin and eosin, ×10.)

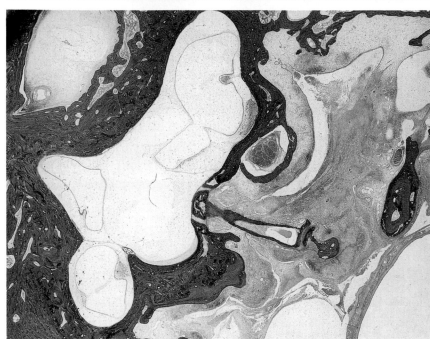

Figure 14.1.6. Vertical section through left temporal bone near posterior end of stapes footplate. The incudostapedial articulation and the posterior crus of the stapes are deeply embedded in tuberculous granulation tissue. (Hematoxylin and eosin, ×9.)

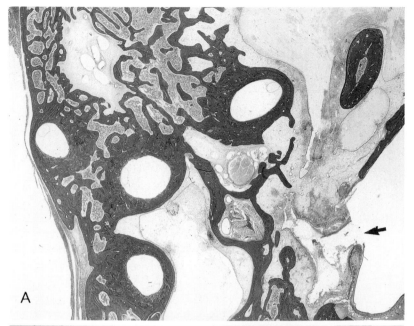

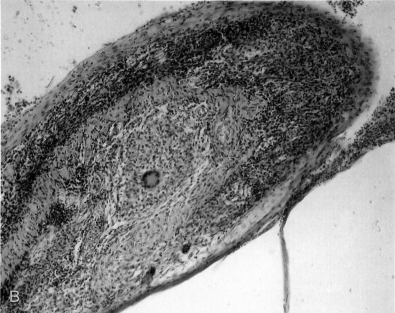

Figure 14.1.7.   A. Vertical section through left temporal bone at level of short process of incus of the same patient as in Figure 14.1.1. The tympanic membrane reveals a posterior-inferior marginal perforation *(arrow)*. A tubercle is recognized in the lower margin of the eardrum. (Hematoxylin and eosin, ×10.)

Figure 14.1.7.   B. The tubercle is situated in the outer epithelial layer of the tympanic membrane. (×126.)

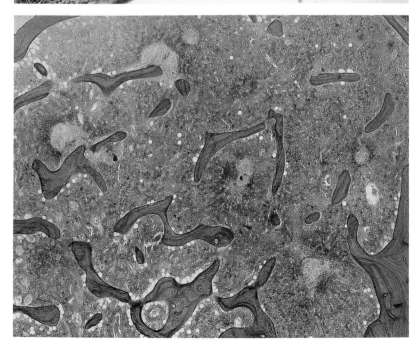

Figure 14.1.8. Vertical section through right petrous apex of the same patient as in Figure 14.1.1. Numerous miliary tubercles are disseminated throughout the hematopoietic marrow. (Hematoxylin and eosin, ×16.)

Case 2. *Chronic necrotizing tuberculous tympanomastoiditis and osteitis of right temporal bones. Beginning labyrinthitis secondary to necrosis of annular ligament and round window membrane. Early meningitis localized to internal auditory canal. Destruction of right tympanic membrane, malleus, incus, chorda tympani, and tensor tympani muscle. Bilateral, advanced, exudative pulmonary tuberculosis with cavitation. Ulcerative tuberculous laryngitis, tracheitis, and enterocolitis. Hematogenous dissemination to liver.*

A 52-year-old man 1 year prior to death developed rapidly progressive bilateral exudative pulmonary tuberculosis with cavitation. Eight weeks prior to death, he developed painless, creamy otorrhea from his right ear with profuse foul-smelling discharge and progressive loss of hearing in the right ear. Several samples from middle ear secretions were positive for tubercle bacilli. The right facial nerve was intact. There was no history of ear infections or impaired hearing.

Examination of the right temporal bone reveals a subtotal destruction of the tympanic membrane (Fig. 14.1.9C), extensive, complete necrosis of the mucoperiosteum of the middle ear (Fig. 14.1.9C),

multifocal osteitis involving walls of the middle ear cavity (Fig. 14.1.9A and B), Fallopian canal, and tegmen, and destruction of the malleus, incus, and tensor tympani muscle. Necrosis of the annular ligament and round window membrane allowed spread of infection to the perilymphatic and endolymphatic space of the cochlear and vestibular labyrinth (Fig. 14.1.9C and D). The subarachnoid space of the internal auditory canal contained numerous mononuclear cells, and there are a few caseous tubercles in the bone marrow (Fig. 14.1.10A and B).

Case 3. *Hematogenous dissemination of tubercles throughout the bone marrow of both temporal bones and meninges. Bilateral calcified cervical and paratracheal lymph nodes. Miliary tuberculosis. Tuberculous leptomeningitis.*

Examination of the temporal bones of a 3-year-old boy revealed dissemination of tubercles limited to the hematopoietic marrow, the middle ear mucoperiosteum, and the subarachnoid space of the internal auditory canal (Fig. 14.1.10A and B).

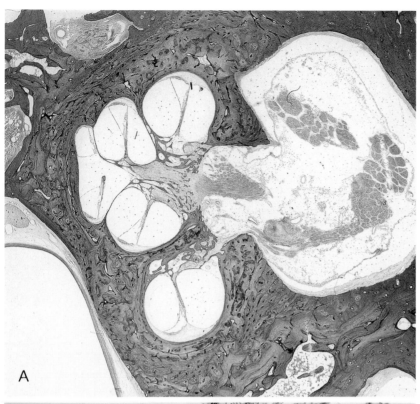

Figure 14.1.10. A. Vertical midmodiolar section through right petrous pyramid of a 3-year-old boy who died from tuberculous meningitis. (Hematoxylin and eosin, ×15.)

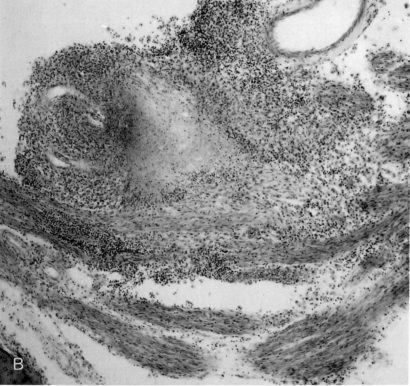

Figure 14.1.10. B. An exudative tuberculous, granulomatous process involves the cochlear nerve that supplies the lower basal turn of the cochlea. (×110.)

References

1. Wolinsky E. Tuberculosis. In: Wyngaarden JB, Smith LH, eds. Cecil textbook of medicine. 18th ed. Vol 2: Infectious diseases. Philadelphia: WB Saunders, Chap 302, 1988:1682–1693.
2. Kuhn C III, Askin FB. Lung and mediastinum. In: Kissane JM, ed. Anderson's pathology. 8th ed. St Louis: CV Mosby, Chap 22, 1985;I:852–859.
3. Jeans AL, Friedman I. Tuberculosis of the middle ear. Tubercle 1960;41:109.
4. Zarfl M. Das Mittelohr als Sitz der tuberkulösen Primärherde. Wien Med Wochenschr 1924:1113.
5. Zarfl M. Über primäre Mittelohrtuberkulose beim Säugling. Virchows Arch Pathol Anat 1927;266:274.
6. Kleinschmidt H, Schürmann P. Primäre Mittelohrtuberkulose im frühen Säuglingsalter. Monatsschrift Kinderheilkd 1928;40:193.
7. Theissing G. Beitrag zur Pathologie und Klinik der Mittelohrtuberkulose. Z Laryng Rhinol 1955;34:807.
8. Wittmaack K. Die entzündlichen Erkrangungsprozesse des Gehörorganes. In: Henke F, Lubarsch O, eds. Handbuch der speziellen pathologischen Anatomie und Histologie. Berlin: Julius Springer Verlag, 1926;12:258–271.
9. Schätzle W, Haubrich J. Tuberkulose. In: Schätzle W, Haubrich J, eds. Pathologie des Ohres. Berlin: Springer Verlag, 1975;9:98–101.
10. Theissing G. Die Labyrinth- und Felsenbeintuberkulose und ihre therapeutische Beinflussbarkeit. Arch Ohren-Nasen-Kehlkopfheilkd 1959;175:530.

Part 2
Syphilis

Syphilis is a systemic subacute or chronic infectious disease caused by *Treponema pallidum*. It is transmitted by sexual contact. If it is not treated, its course is characterized by sequential clinical stages and years of asymptomatic latency. The organism may enter the body through an intact mucosa or an epithelial abrasion to reach the regional lymph nodes within hours and to disseminate rapidly throughout the body. The local reaction is a focal obliterative endarteritis characterized by an increase of adventitia cells, endothelial proliferation, and the presence of an inflammatory cuff around the affected vessel with lymphocytes, plasma cells, and monocytes predominating. After an incubation period that averages about 3 weeks but may vary from 1 to 13 weeks, a red papule appears on the inoculation site. This papule gradually undergoes necrosis to form a flat, clean-based, painless ulceration with elevated, indurated margins, surrounded by a red areola. This primary syphilitic lesion, known as a chancre, is accompanied by a painless unilateral or bilateral regional lymphadenopathy. The primary chancre occurs on the penis, anus, or rectum of the male and on the vulva, cervix, or perineum of the female. Extragenital locations include the lips, tongue, buccal mucosa, tonsils, pharynx, nipples, fingers, and occasionally other areas (1). This primary lesion heals within 2–6 weeks, leaving a faint scar behind, and 6–12 weeks later, the disease process proceeds to the second stage. This second stage of the disease is characterized by the appearance of a mucocutaneous rash. The majority of patients display cutaneous or mucocutaneous lesions that vary in appearance but have certain characteristic features. Their distribution is widespread and symmetric. They are more marked on the flexor and volar surfaces of the body, especially on the palms and soles, and have a pink or dusk-red color. The rash generally occurs in crops, and it may be macular, populous, pustulous, or squamous but hardly ever vesicular or bullous. There is a tendency toward confluence and

induration. The lesions are most florid after 3–4 months, and they eventually heal without a scar but in some instances with a residual hyperpigmentation or hypopigmentation. The mucous membranes may exhibit circular patches that are grayish-white with a red areola. These patches are mostly encountered in the oral cavity on the palate, pharynx, larynx, and glans penis or on the vulva, in the anal canal, and in the rectum. At the mucocutaneous junctions or in moist areas of the skin, the papules become hypertrophic and flat, with a dull pink or gray color, and are recognized as condylomata lata. They are extremely infectious lesions. About 50% of patients with secondary syphilis have generalized lymphadenopathy, and about 10% have eye lesions (uveitis) and involvement of bones, joints, visceral organs, and meninges. At this stage, some patients develop an acute syphilitic meningitis with nuchal rigidity, headaches, cranial nerve involvement, deafness, and papilledema (1, 2). The latency stage begins as the clinical signs of the first attack of secondary syphilis subside. This stage has been divided into an early latent stage, less than 1 year after infection, and a late latent stage, longer than 1 year after infection. Most relapses of secondary syphilis occur during the first year, but when the skin lesions recur, they tend to be unilateral, fewer in number, occasionally solitary, more infiltrated, and longer in duration. They are a reflection of an increasing host immunity. Lesions affecting the eye and central nervous system may also recur. The late latent stage may last a few years or for the rest of the patient's life. About one-third of untreated patients eventually develop late or tertiary syphilis (1). Tertiary syphilis may be divided into (a) benign tertiary syphilis of skin, bone, and viscera, (b) cardiovascular syphilis, and (c) neurosyphilis (2).

The lesions of benign tertiary syphilis usually develop within 3–10 years of infection. They have almost disappeared in the antibiotic area. The pathognomonic lesion is the gumma, a chronic localized or diffuse granuloma with central necrosis and fibrosis affecting skin, soft tissues, viscera, and bone. They may involve the nasal septum, palate, pharynx, and larynx. They may occur almost anywhere, causing tissue destruction and a perforation. Diffuse gummatous lesions may affect the tongue and lead to chronic interstitial glossitis. Tertiary syphilis of bone may give rise to periosteitis with new bone formation or destructive osteitis (1, 2).

Cardiovascular syphilis may result in (a) an aneurysm of the thoracic artery, (b) stretching of the ring of the aortic valve, which produces aortic insufficiency, and (c) narrowing of the coronary artery as a result of obliterative endarteritis of the vasa vasorum. Similar changes may occur in other large vessels.

NEUROSYPHILIS

Involvement of the central nervous system takes place during the secondary or the latent stage of the disease within the first 2 or 3 years after the initial infection. The beginning of the process may be asymptomatic, but the cerebrospinal fluid (CSF) may already show some abnormalities. Asymptomatic neurosyphilis, in general, precedes symptomatic disease. It is encountered in about 15% of cases of latent syphilis, 12% of cases of cardiovascular syphilis, and 5% of cases of benign tertiary syphilis (2). About 5% of untreated patients will eventually develop neurosyphilis. Neurosyphilis may be subdivided into (a) asymptomatic neurosyphilis, (b) meningovascular syphilis, (c) tabes dorsalis, and (d) general paresis (1).

Asymptomatic Neurosyphilis

Asymptomatic neurosyphilis is diagnosed in the absence of neurologic disease and in the presence of a positive Veneral Disease Research Laboratory (VDRL) test of the CSF, which generally shows an increase in total protein and a lymphocytic pleocytosis. Asymptomatic neurosyphilis usually precedes symptomatic neurosyphilis and is observed in 15% of patients diagnosed as having latent syphilis.

Meningovascular Syphilis

Meningovascular syphilis results from an acute or subacute aseptic meningitis that often involves the base of the brain and leads to unilateral or bilateral cranial nerve palsies. It may develop anytime after the primary stage but usually manifests itself within the first year following infection. It coincides in about 10% of cases with the rash of secondary syphilis. Abnormalities of the pupil, the Argyll Robertson pupil, occur almost exclusively in neurosyphilis. As the cerebral cortex is primarily affected, it is characterized by impairment of mental functions, headaches, dizziness, blurred vision, nuchal rigidity, papilledema, seizures, aphasia, and monoplegia and hemiplegia (1, 2). In the initial stage of meningovascular syphilis, a patchy or diffuse, cloudy grayish exudate may be encountered within the leptomeninges primarily at the base of the brain and less frequently along the blood vessels over the cerebral convexities. It consists primarily of lymphocytes, plasma cells, and large mononuclear cells that tend to concentrate in the adventitia and perivascular area. In about 5% of patients the disease begins with an acute, severe meningitis. In such instances, the exudate is more abundant and, besides the usual round cells, contains neutrophils. As the exudate becomes organized, it forms patches or extensive areas of fibrosis. Involvement of the smaller arteries is a significant aspect of leptomeningeal infection whereby inflammatory cells infiltrate the media, separate the muscle fibers, split the internal elastic lamina, and incite a reactive intimal hyperplasia and endothelial hypertrophy (3). These vascular changes may lead to numerous ischemic infarcts of various sizes.

Tabes Dorsalis

Tabes dorsalis is a gradually progressive degenerative disease that involves the posterior columns and posterior roots of the spinal cord. It results in progressive loss of tendon reflexes, impairment of vibration and sensation of joint position, absence of deep pain sensation, ataxia, unsteadiness, and paresthesias. The painless disorganization of the joints involved, with abnormal range of movement, may result in Charcot's arthropathy. The loss of bladder sensation leads to retention of urine, incontinence, and chronic infection. The initial and very characteristic symptoms are the sudden and severe painful lightning crises that may involve the legs, perineum, larynx, and other areas, recurring at regular intervals. The Argyll Robertson pupils are generally present. There may be primary optic nerve atrophy, and the face may display the common sad-looking tabetic facial expression. The Romberg sign is positive (1, 2). The cause of tabes dorsalis continues to remain obscure. No spirochetes have so far been demonstrated in the posterior columns and nerve roots. The onset of the disease is slow and usually begins 20–30 years after the initial infection. On examination, the spinal cord and the posterior columns are smaller than normal, and axons and myelinated sheets are lacking in the affected tracts (3). The serum fluorescent treponemal antibody absorption (FTA-ABS) test is nearly always positive. Hearing may be impaired in the tabes dorsalis, and the loss is sensorineural in origin. The audiograms fail to show common tracing patterns (4). About 10% of all patients with tertiary syphilis and about 40% of all patients with clinical neurosyphilis are thought to have evidence of tabes dorsalis. The CSF generally reveals a lymphoid pleocytosis, an elevated protein, and a weakly positive serologic test for syphilis (STS) (1).

General Paresis (Dementia Paralytica)

General paresis is another form of neurosyphilis. It is characterized by a slowly progressive impairment of cortical function. Onset is insidious and manifested by behavior changes, forgetfulness, and fatigability. This may be followed by deterioration of memory and judgment, delusions with lack of insight, deterioration of the patient's hygiene and grooming, emotional instability, convulsions, aphasia, or transient hemiparesis (1, 2). On physical examination, the patient may exhibit a tremor of the mouth, tongue, outstretched hands, and body. In taboparesis the posterior columns are also affected. The CSF frequently exhibits a lymphoid pleocytosis and an increase in total proteins. The VDRL test is usually reactive in serum and CSF.

Examination of the brain reveals a patchy diffuse thickening of the leptomeninges and cortical atrophy, usually most prominent over the frontal lobes. The meningeal exudate is accompanied by vasculitis. The cerebral lesions are more concentrated in the cortex and central gray matter than in the white matter (3). Their intensity corresponds to the degree of the overlying meningeal involvement. The walls of the vessels are greatly thickened, and their lumina are constricted as a result of endothelial hypertrophy and hyperplasia. The vessels are surrounded by lymphocytes, plasma cells, and, occasionally, large mononuclear cells. There is ongoing degeneration and loss of neural elements with proliferation of microglia. The resulting scars resemble microscopic infarcts, leading to disseminated localized cortical atrophy, and there is characteristic cortical disorganization of the normal upper cortical layers. The presence of iron pigment in macrophages and walls of cortical blood vessels is diagnostic for general paresis. Spirochetes may be found singly or in clusters about the blood vessels in the cortex (Fig. 14.2.1) (3).

CONGENITAL SYPHILIS

The incidence of congenital syphilis in the United States among newborns and infants under 1 year of age is estimated to be about 100/yr (1). Untreated maternal syphilis may be transmitted to the unborn at least during the first 5 years after the mother's infection. The manifestations resemble secondary syphilis in the adult, except that the rash may be vesicular or bullous. There may be rhinitis, hepatosplenomegaly, anemia, jaundice, and pseudoparalysis resulting from painful osteochondritis (1). Later, the congenital syphilis may remain latent and asymptomatic. Cochlear nerve deafness and interstitial keratitis may develop, however. Periosteitis may give rise to frontal bossing,

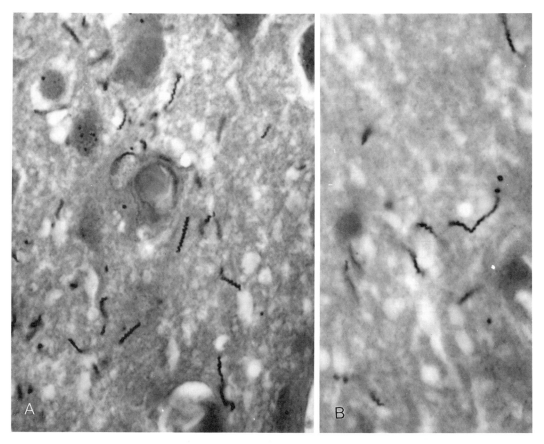

Figure 14.2.1.   Spirochetes *(Treponema pallidum)* in the section of the brain of a man with general paresis (dementia paralytica). The spirochetes are tightly coiled, regularly spiraling organisms 6–15 mm in length that move with a distinct rhythm. (Silver impregnation, ×1600 and ×2000, respectively.)

saddle-nose deformity, underdevelopment of the maxilla, and anterior bowing of the tibiae. The permanent dentition may show the characteristic abnormalities known as Hutchinson's teeth (1). The diagnosis of congenital syphilis, as that of primary acquired syphilis, is established by identification of the organism *Treponema pallidum* in dark-field examination.

SYPHILIS OF THE EAR

Involvement of the ear and temporal bone occurs almost exclusively in the second and third stages of the disease. Primary syphilis, sporadically reported before the turn of the century (4–6), practically no longer exists. The lesion may be on the auricle, in the crease, or in the periauricular area. It is associated with a painful infra-auricular, submandibular, or parotid lymphadenopathy (6). It results from inoculation through an epithelial abrasion. During the second stage, maculopapillary lesions may occasionally be observed *(a)* on the anterior external auditory canal wall near the entrance and *(b)* in the postauricular crease. These flat, broad-based condylomata lata are grayish-pink and covered by a greasy exudate (4, 6). Their healing may result in scarring and stenosis of the external auditory canal. At times, the periauricular lymph nodes may participate in the generalized lymphadenopathy of stage 2. During the early phase of that stage, the eighth nerve may become involved in the perivascular and endovascular inflammatory process so characteristic for syphilis. These vascular lesions are presumed to affect the intramedullary segment of the nerve, since there is no correlation between the impairment of nerve function and the abnormalities in the CSF. Not rarely can a mucoperiosteitis of the middle ear be proven to be syphilitic in origin by identification of spirochetes in the exudate (6).

Any part of the temporal bone, middle ear ossicles, membranous labyrinth, and neural structures may become affected during the benign tertiary stage of the disease (7). However, it is extremely rare for a gumma to involve the auricle. Such a lesion can partially destroy the pinna and result in a sharply define punched-out lesion involving skin, soft tissues, cartilage, and bone. The middle ear ossicles may become involved in a granulomatous osteitis by one gumma or several small gummas (8). Similarly, the mastoid process, middle ear, otic capsule, and petrous pyramid may become involved by a gumma, as reported in the earlier literature (6, 7). Today, this lesion is practically no longer encountered.

Syphilis affects the inner ear more often than the middle or outer ear. The neural impairment is probably more often the result of a meningeal infection than a direct involvement of the cochlear nerve and organ of Corti by the spirochetes and their toxins (4, 6). The presence of spirochetes in the cochlear nerve and spiral ganglion has been well documented histologically (9–15). Two kinds of morphologic changes have been recognized: *(a)* predominantly inflammatory, and *(b)* predominantly degenerative in nature. Inflammatory changes and their sequels have been observed in the perilymph compartments where a wide meshed network of connective tissue and new bone formation have been recognized (6). Lymphocytic round cell infiltrations have been encountered in the cochlear nerve and spiral ganglion

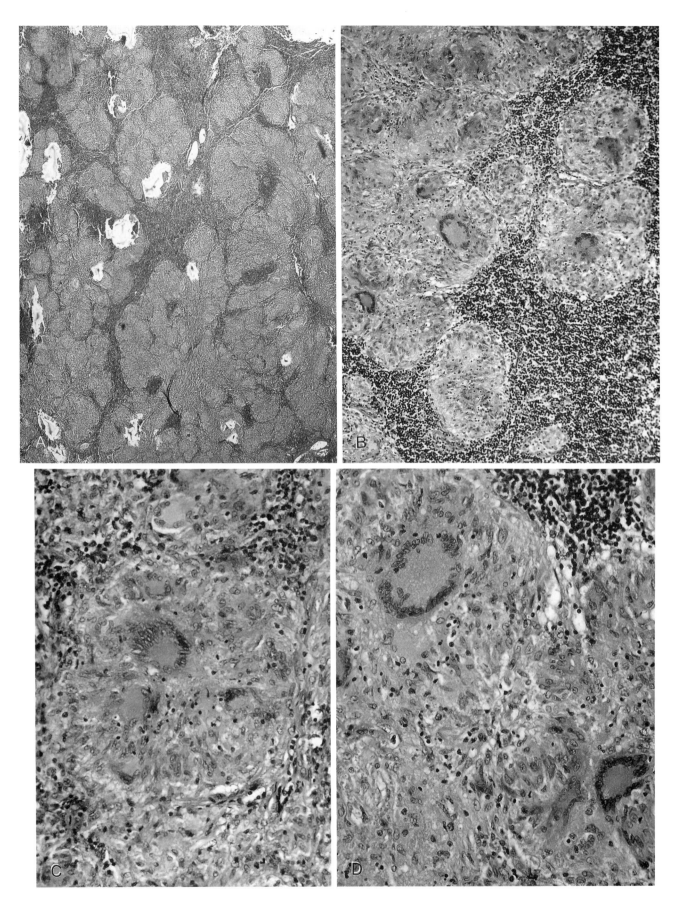

Figure 14.3.1. **A.** Biopsy from the lymph node of an adult patient with sarcoidosis. The nodular lesion consists of a conglomerate of granulomas. (Hematoxylin and eosin, ×26.) **B.** Sheets of lymphocytes, monocytes, and phagocytes surround the granulomas. (×70.) **C and D.** The noncaseating granulomas in sarcoidosis consist of compact nodules of epithelioid cells with a few lymphocytes, monocytes, and macrophages. Some granulomas display evidence of an early formation of a fibrous capsule. The multinucleated giant cells are of the foreign body or Langhans' type. (×230 and ×220, respectively.)

References

1. Kuhn C III, Askin FB. Sarcoidosis. In: Kissane JM, ed. Anderson's pathology. 8th ed. Vol I: Lung and mediastinum. St Louis: CV Mosby, Chap 22, 1985;I:889–892.
2. Franburg BL. Sarcoidosis. In: Cecil textbook of medicine. 18th ed. Vol 1: Respiratory diseases. Philadelphia: WB Saunders, Chap 7, 1988:451–457.
3. Prockof LD. Sarcoidosis. In: Rowland EL, ed. Merritt's textbook of neurology. 8th ed. Philadelphia: Lea & Febiger, 1989:149–152.

Part 4
Eosinophilic Langhans' Cell Granulomatosis

Eosinophilic Langhans' cell granulomatosis is a distinct, idiopathic disorder characterized by proliferation and infiltration of tissues by histiocytes and eosinophils. The proliferating cell that appears to be fundamentally responsible for the clinical manifestations is the Langhans' cell. The accumulation of eosinophils may represent a secondary phenomenon (1). The Langhans' cell belongs to the category of cells known as histiocytes. Histiocytes are mobile macrophages of connective tissue derived from blood monocytes originating in the bone marrow. The histiocytic cell series represents a progressive maturation from the monoblast and promonocyte in the bone marrow to the circulating monocyte in the blood, which enters the tissues and differentiates into a particular type of histiocyte (1). The local behavior and the effect of the active proliferation and infiltration of histiocytes on adjacent tissue are responsible for the various clinical manifestations of Langhans' cell granulomatosis.

UNIFOCAL LANGHANS' CELL (EOSINOPHILIC) GRANULOMATOSIS

Clinical Manifestations

Unifocal Langhans' cell granulomatosis is characterized most often by a solitary lesion, occasionally by several osteolytic lesions, and usually by a lack of soft tissue involvement. The most frequent presentation is a single destructive process in a flat or long bone—in a child often in the calvaria, femur, or humerus and in the adult frequently in a rib. The lesions are generally purely lytic, but a combination of lytic and blastic lesions may be observed (1). Their predilection for the skull, mandible, ribs, vertebrae, pelvis, and femur remains unexplained. The granuloma originates within the bone marrow as a proliferation of histiocytes. The defect in the bone is clearly delineated. Some lesions have a tendency to develop rapidly and break through the cortex of the affected bone. At that stage they may cause swelling and pain; occasionally, however, they may remain asymptomatic. In patients under the age of 20 years, granulomas are usually encountered with equal frequency in the flat and long bones. In patients over the age of 20 years, the flat bones are more frequently involved. Involvement of a vertebral body may result in compression, destruction, and collapse of a vertebra, giving rise to an angular deformity of the spine and spinal cord and to nerve root compression (2, 3). Disruption of the teeth and a spontaneous fracture may be observed with involvement of the mandible. Involvement of the temporal bone occurs quite frequently, and it is regularly associated with middle and external ear infection. Occasionally, a lesion may be discovered incidentally during a radiologic evaluation for unrelated problems. Unifocal granulomas rarely involve the salivary glands, lymph nodes, and thymus (1). The disease affects primarily younger children, but infants, older children, adults, and older individuals may occasionally also become afflicted (2). Males are affected more often than females, and the disease has a predilection for the white race.

Diagnosis

A bone scan will determine that the disease is limited to a single lesion. It will identify new osteolytic lesions that may develop over time. The diagnosis is established by an open biopsy revealing a proliferation of well-differentiated histiocytes with an eosinophilic cytoplasm interspersed with eosinophils. The identification of the X-body, a cytoplasmic inclusion, and the S-100, a cytoplasmic protein, provides further confirmations (1).

MULTIFOCAL LANGHANS' CELL (EOSINOPHILIC) GRANULOMATOSIS

Clinical Manifestations

Multiple Langhans' cell granulomatosis is characterized by the involvment of bone, viscera, and soft tissue. Osteolytic lesions may be encountered in many parts of the skeleton, but the bones of the calvaria, skull base, and mandible and the long bones of the upper extremities are more frequently affected. The temporoparietal region is the area of predilection. Solitary and multiple lesions are observed. A lesion originating in the spongiosa of the calvaria may perforate through the external table, or it may destroy the inner table first, infiltrate the dura, spread epidurally and subdurally, and invade the adjacent substance of the brain. In the radiograph the erosions are usually well demarcated, with clear-cut scalloped margins and complete loss of trabecular structure. The osteolytic defects, therefore, have been compared to "punched-out" defects or the "moth-eaten" holes in a piece of flannel. Their size may vary from barely detectable defects to vast irregular "geographic" areas (Figs. 14.4.1 and 14.4.2). Extensive involvement of the occipital bone can result in platybasia with indentation of the floor of the posterior cranial foss and distortion of the foramen magnum and the foramina of exit of the cranial nerves (2). If the sella turcica has been encroached upon, disturbance of pituitary function may result. Compression of the pituitary gland by histiocytic granulomas arising from the dura and by infiltration of its posterior lobe, pituitary stalk, or hypothalamus can give rise to diabetes insipidus (2, 3). Within the orbital bones the defects are more frequently localized in the superior and lateral walls. When the process extends into or develops in the periorbital soft tissue, exophthalmos may develop. Protrusion of the bulb may be unilateral or bilateral. It should be remembered, however, that only a minority of patients manifest the complete triad of Hand-Schüller-Christian's disease, namely calvarial defects, exophthalmos, and diabetes insipidus (2). Hand-Schüller-Christian disease should, therefore, be considered as a variant of multifocal Langhans' cell granulomatosis (4). Invasion of the temporal bone occurs rather frequently and often bilaterally. Usually, it is

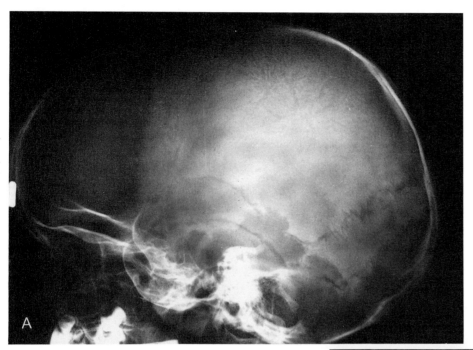

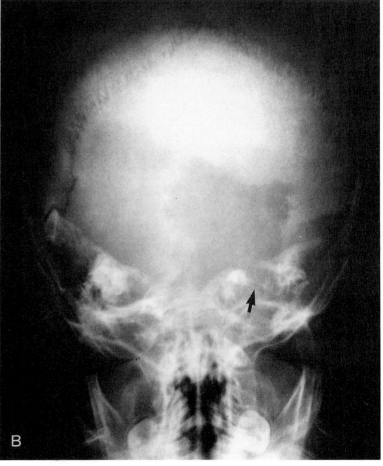

Figure 14.4.1. Left lateral **(A)** and occipital **(B)** views of the skull of a 4-year-old child with multifocal Langhans' cell granulomatosis involving the calvaria, temporal bones, orbits, sinuses, mandible, pelvis and femur. It was associated with the triad of skull masses, diabetes insipidus, and exophthalmos and with otitis, hearing loss, and skin lesions. **A.** An extensive "geographic" osteolytic process involves the left temporal and occipital bone, resulting in secondary invagination of the skull base. **B.** A large osteolytic lesion in the left petrous pyramid has eroded the cochlear capsule and the floor of the internal auditory canal *(arrow).*

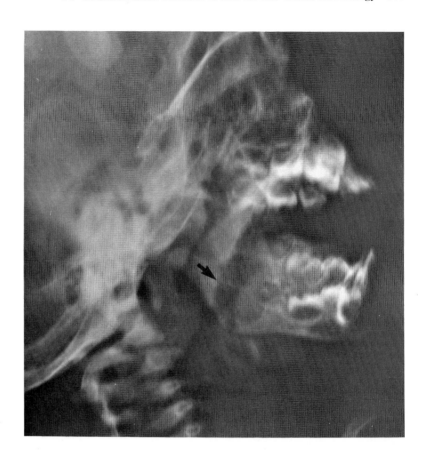

Figure 14.4.2. Lateral view of the skull reveals an ovoid, clearly demarcated osteolytic lesion involving the right angle of the mandible *(arrow)*.

associated with symptoms of chronic purulent middle and external ear disease and impairment of hearing. Involvement of the bony structure of the paranasal sinuses may produce symptoms of sinusitis. The course and duration of the cranial lesions may vary. Some disappear within a few weeks, others persist for many years in spite of therapy. Also, while some lesions heal, new ones may appear simultaneously in other areas of the skull. Areas of bone rarefaction are frequently encountered within the mandible where they often arise in the tooth-bearing portions. As the granuloma expands, the teeth become surrounded from all sides, and the crowns from unerupted and erupted teeth give the radiographic appearance of "floating in the air." Gradually, a large number of deciduous and permanent teeth are exfoliated. In addition to the skull and mandible, osteolytic granulomas are encountered in the pelvis, long bones, vertebrae, ribs, clavicles, scapulae, and bones of the hands and feet. In the pelvis the most common sites are: *(a)* in the ileum, just above the acetabulum and adjacent to the sacroiliac joint, and *(b)* in the ischiopubic rami (2, 5). In the long bones the foci are usually located in the epiphyseal rather than the diaphyseal portion of the shaft (5). Skeletal lesions, however, should no longer be considered a condition sine qua non for the diagnosis of multifocal granulomatosis. They can be absent, or if they develop, they may not become manifest until granulomas in extraskeletal sites are already well established (2).

Skin lesions are among the frequent clinical manifestations of the disease and may involve the scalp, face, neck, shoulders, trunk, groin, perineum, and extremities. Papular cutaneous eruptions resembling seborrheic dermatitis or xanthomas are the usual expression of histiocytic granulomas in the skin (2, 5). The location of the infiltrates is usually in the papillary layer of the dermis, adjacent to the epidermis.

Ulcerative lesions in the gingiva, palate, and elsewhere in the oral cavity are the local manifestations, and many may be among the initial expressions of multifocal granulomatosis (2, 3, 5). These ulcers are often painful and bleed, and the gums become swollen and spongy. Microscopic examination of these lesions reveals a proliferation of histiocytes and infiltration of eosinophils and other inflammatory cells associated with superficial ulceration and superinfection. There appears to be no correlation between the ulcerative lesions of the gingiva and the radiologic destruction in the maxilla or mandible. These granulomatous mucosal lesions may usher in the disease for some time before the full-blown clinical picture has developed (2).

Histiocytic granulomas with eosinophilic infiltration may be found in the lungs, heart, walls of the larger arteries and veins of the extremities, lymph nodes, thymus, thyroid, spleen, liver, pancreas, kidney, bladder, prostate, vagina, jejunum, ilium, colon, and the adipose tissue surrounding the viscera (2, 3, 5, 6).

Neurologic manifestations are very unusual. In one instance, the disease caused involvement of cranial nerves V, VII, VIII, and IX; in another, it caused blindness and increased intracranial pressure.

Involvement of the temporal bone is a frequent occurrence, and it is often bilateral. Numerous instances have been reported (7–17). It is commonly associated with intractable external otitis, superinfection of the middle ear, and evidence of an osteolytic process. The instance of involvement of the temporal bone is about 38% (15). Auditory and vestibular symptoms may be observed in about 12% of cases (17). The osteolytic process may be very small and asymptomatic, or it may be very extensive and involve any portion of the temporal bone. As it involves the cochlear and vestibular capsule, it may cause loss of cochlear, vestibular, and facial nerve function (16). By eroding the bony wall, the granuloma may present in the external auditory canal.

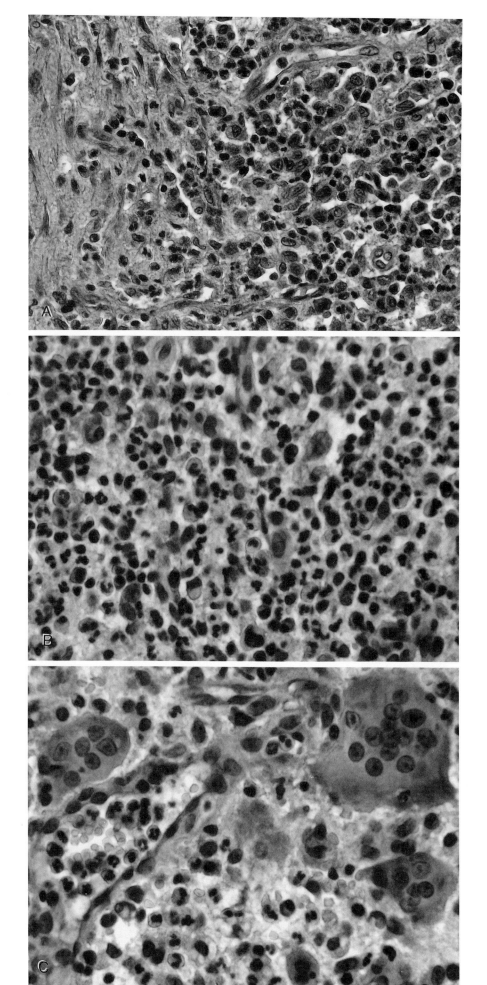

Figure 14.4.3 A. An area of fibrous connective tissue adjacent to a proliferation of histiocytes with eosinophils and lymphocytes from biopsy of an osteolytic lesion in the right mandible. (Hematoxylin and eosin, ×500.)

Figure 14.4.3. B. An area of diffuse proliferation of histiocytes from the same biopsy as in A with a larger number of eosinophils, lymphocytes, and some plasma cells than those seen in A. (×750.)

Figure 14.4.3. C. Multinucleated giant cells that have originated by fusion of several histiocytes, from the same biopsy as in A, are encountered in many areas. (×750.)

In a rare instance, involvement of the temporal bone may be the initial clinical symptom.

Case Report

Case 1. A 15-month-old infant was seen who since the age of 3 months had been treated for intractable seborrheic eczema of the scalp and inguinal area and bilateral external otitis that had remained refractory to all forms of local therapy. At 8 months he developed a firm, tender swelling over the right mandible, which corresponded radiographically to a 2-cm, sharply defined, "punched-out" osteolytic defect (Fig. 14.4.2) in the angle of the jaw and on biopsy was diagnosed as eosinophilic granuloma (Fig. 14.4.3). He was treated with local radiation to the mandible and a course of nitrogen mustard. During the next few months the infant developed multiple osteolytic lesions in the calvaria (Fig. 14.4.4), manifested by swelling and tenderness. At 12 months, osteolytic lesions of varying size were detected in the left iliac crest and just above the left acetabulum, in the left ischium, and in the left femoral neck (Fig. 14.4.5). Therapy during that time included methotrexate and local radiation to the various osteolytic lesions of the skeleton. At 14 months the infant was exposed to measles and received preventive γ-globulin. In spite of this, 3 weeks later the infant developed conjunctivitis, cough, typical Koplik's spots on the buccal mucosa, and a spreading maculopapular cutaneous rash over the scalp and entire body. The patient was readmitted because of difficulties with breathing. On admission a chest radiograph disclosed a diffuse dissemination of miliary lesions throughout both lung fields, which is consistent with far-advanced reticuloendotheliosis of the lungs, and areas of pneumonitis in the right middle and lower lobe.

Otologic examination revealed bilateral purulent external otitis and thickened, pale tympanic membranes. When a specimen was cultured, *Proteus mirabilis* and *Pseudomonas* grew. Hearing was reduced bilaterally. A localized cutaneous swelling was noted over the squamous portion of the right temporal bone. It corresponded radiographically to an underlying osteolytic defect (Fig. 14.4.6). A skin biopsy from the right inguinal area showed evidence of histiocytosis. Treatment included penicillin, chloramphenicol, methotrexate, cytoxin, prednisone, and digitalis.

Ten days after admission, the patient developed a bilateral spon-

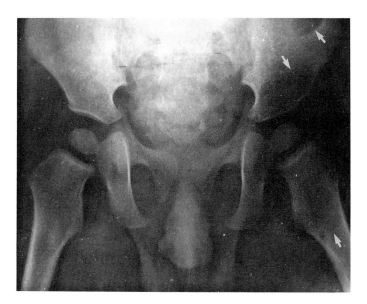

Figure 14.4.5. Anteroposterior view of the pelvis displays two large osteolytic lesions in the left ileum, with one located in the iliac crest and the other located just above the acetabulum *(arrows)*. A third lesion involves the left femoral neck *(arrows)*.

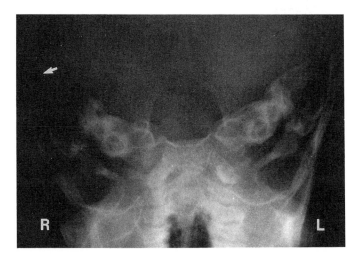

Figure 14.4.6. Occipital view of the skull displays a sharply delineated osteolytic process in the squamous portion of the right temporal bone *(arrow)*.

taneous pneumothorax with rapidly progressive respiratory distress. In spite of surgical intervention, he never recovered.

Postmortem examination revealed that the only persistent lesions consistent with the diagnosis of multifocal Langhans' cell granulomatosis were the ones involving the skeletal system. No histologic infiltrations or granulomas were encountered in the visceral organs or cervical, thoracic, abdominal, or peripheral lymph nodes. Microscopic examination of the lungs disclosed evidence of lobular hemorrhagic pneumonia, characterized by the occurrence of marked squamous metaplasia of bronchial and alveolar epithelial linings, and the presence of giant cells morphologically resembling those described by Warthin and Finkeldey. Based on the history of exposure to and clinical findings of rubella and the histologic examination of the lung sections, the pathologist concluded that the most reasonable cause for the lobular pneumonia was a disseminated measles infection.

Microscopic examination of the temporal bones revealed two basic tissue abnormalities in both temporal bones: *(a)* a proliferation of histiocytes in the dermis of the external auditory canal, in the submucosa of the Eustachian tube (Fig. 14.4.7), middle ear cavity

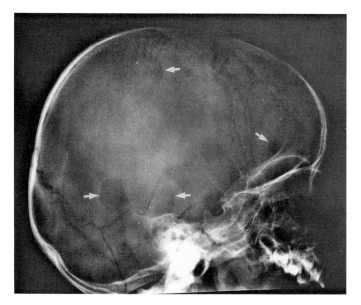

Figure 14.4.4. Right lateral view of the skull demonstrates multiple, distinctly marginated lytic lesions in the lower parietal area, squamous portion of the temporal bone, frontal region, and high parietal area near the vertex *(arrows)*.

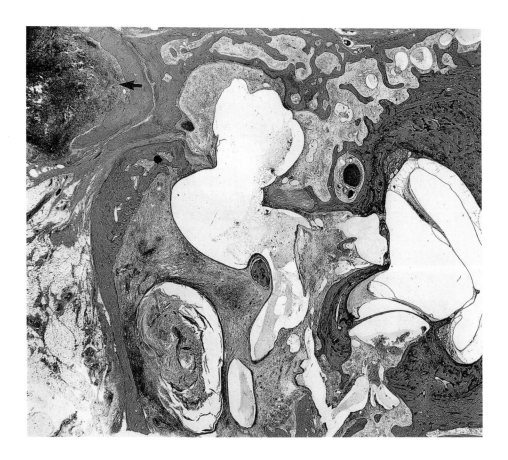

Figure 14.4.8. Vertical section through right temporal bone at level of oval and round windows. It demonstrates the thickening of the middle ear mucoperiosteum that led to the occlusion of the oval and round windows and the marked widening of the tympanic membrane caused by the diffuse histiocytic infiltration. A large osteolytic lesion involves the base of the squamous portion of the temporal bone *(arrow)*. The diffuse, subacute, ulcerative external otitis resulted in near-total obliteration of the external canal with exudate and cellular debris. (Hematoxylin and eosin, ×8.)

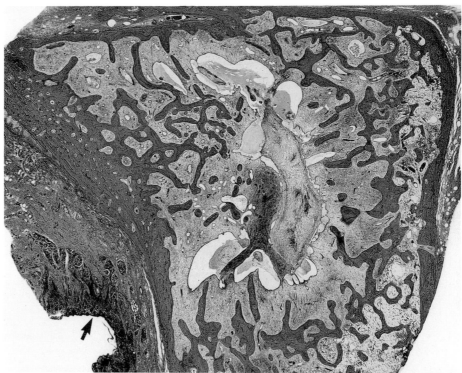

Figure 14.4.9. Vertical section through right temporal bone at entrance of antrum. It shows the histiocytic infiltration throughout the periantral cells and marrow spaces and the massive proliferation of histiocytes in the skin lining the adjacent external auditory canal *(arrow).* (Hematoxylin and eosin, 6½.)

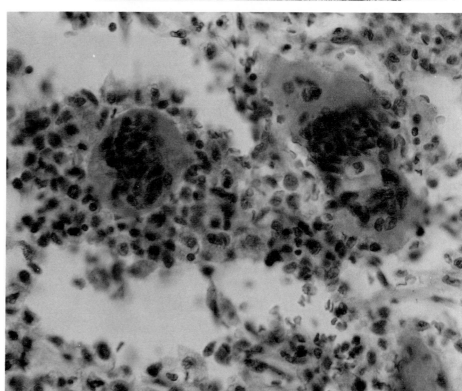

Figure 14.4.10. Multinucleated giant cells are encountered throughout areas of histiocytic proliferation. (Hematoxylin and eosin, ×500.)

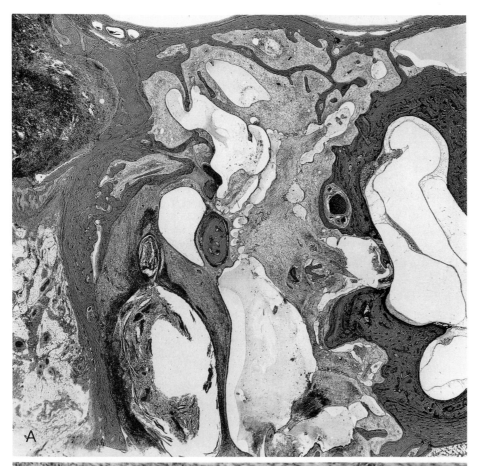

Figure 4.4.11. A. Vertical section through right temporal bone near posterior end of stapes footplate. A small epidermoid inclusion cyst has developed in the markedly thickened Shrapnell's membrane as a result of a deeply penetrating epidermoid papilla. (Hematoxylin and eosin, ×8.)

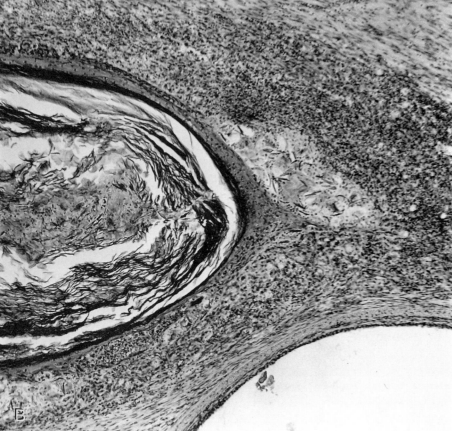

Figure 14.4.11. B. The epidermoid inclusion cyst is surrounded by a dense infiltration of histiocytes and inflammatory cells. (×100.)

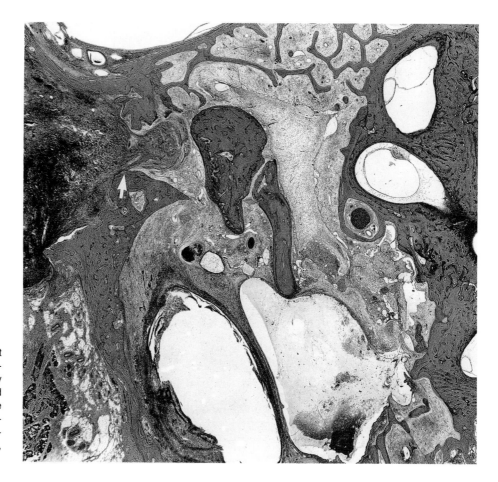

Figure 14.4.12. Vertical section through right temporal bone at level of incudomalleolar articulation. The attic is completely obliterated by histiocytic infiltrations of the mucoperiosteum and persistent embryonic connective tissue. The lateral wall of the attic has been partially destroyed by a large osteolytic lesion in the adjacent squama *(arrow).* (Hematoxylin and eosin, ×8.)

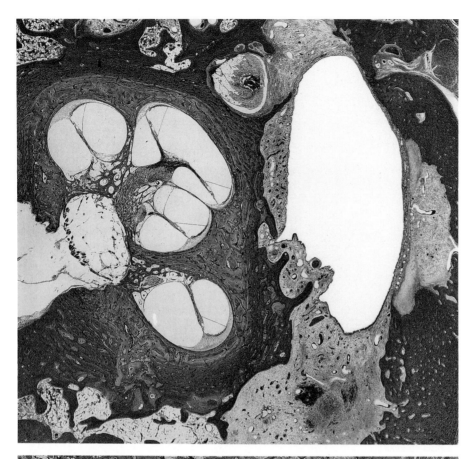

Figure 14.4.14. Vertical midmodiolar section through left temporal bone. The histopathologic changes are identical with those in the opposite right temporal bone. The mucoperiosteum outlining the tympanic cavity, the persisting embryonic connective tissue in the adjacent marrow spaces, and the subepithelial connective tissue in the external auditory canal display massive localized and diffuse histiocytic and inflammatory infiltrations. Extensive epithelial ulcerations resulted in leakage of inflammatory exudate into the middle ear and outer ear canal. (Hematoxylin and eosin, ×10.)

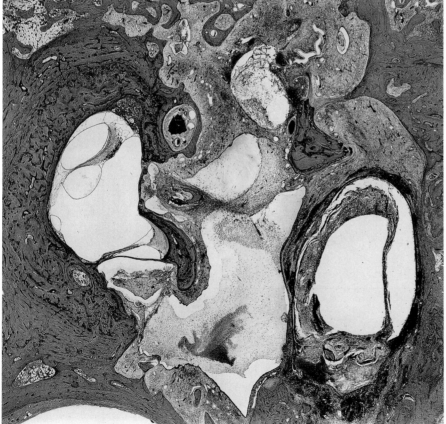

Figure 14.4.15. Vertical section through left temporal bone at level of oval and round windows with external auditory canal. An extensive osteolytic granuloma has eroded the bony floor of the external meatus adjacent to the tympanic annulus. It widely infiltrates the overlying meatal skin and causes a diffuse, ulcerating inflammatory external otitis. (Hematoxylin and eosin, ×8.)

References

1. Groopman IE. Langenhans cell (eosinophilic) granulomatosis. In: Wyngaarden JB, Smith LH, eds. Cecil textbook of medicine. 18th ed. Vol 1: Hematologic diseases. Philadelphia, WB Saunders, Chap 161, 1988:1011–1024.

2. Lichtenstein L. Histiocytosis X (eosinophilic granuloma of bone, Letterer-Siwe disease, and Schüller-Christian disease). J Bone Joint Surg 1964;46A:76–90.

3. Oberman HA. Idiopathic histiocytosis. A clinicopathologic study of 40 cases and review of the literature on eosinophilic granuloma of bone, Hand-Schüller-Christian disease and Letterer-Siwe disease. Pediatrics 1961;28:307–327.

4. Lieberman PH, et al. A reappraisal of eosinophilic granuloma of bone, Hand-Schüller-Christian syndrome and Letterer-Siwe syndrome. Medicine 1969;48:375.

5. Avery ME, McAfee JG, Guild HG. The course and prognosis of reticuloendotheliosis (eosinophilic granuloma, Schüller-Christian disease and Letterer-Siwe disease). Am J Med 1957;22:636–652.

6. Avioli LV, Lasersohn JT, Laproseti JM. Histiocytosis X (Schüller-Christian disease): a clinicopathological survey, review of ten patients and the results of prednisone therapy. Medicine 1963;42:119–147.

7. Greifenstein A. Die Mitbeteiligung des Gehörgans, der Nebenhöhlen und der Kiefer bei der Schüller-Christian' schen Krankheit nebst einer neuen eigenen Beobachtung. Arch Ohren-Nasen-Kehlkopfheilkd 1932;132:337–357.

8. Lederer F, Panchet H, Fabricant ND. Aural manifestations of lipoid granulomatosis. Arch Otolaryngol 1935;21:27–40.

9. Shea J. Xanthomatosis (Schüller-Christian disease): a report of a case with radiosensitive pathology in mastoid. Laryngoscope 1938;48:589–598.

10. Rosenwasser H. Lipoid granulomatosis (Hand-Schüller-Christian disease) involving the middle ear and temporal bone. Arch Otolaryngol 1940;32:1045.

11. Osborne R, Freis E, Levin A. Eosinophilic granuloma of bone presenting neurologic signs and symptoms. Arch Neurol Psychol 1944;51:452.

12. Schuknecht H, Perlman H. Hand-Schüller-Christian disease and eosinophilic granuloma of the skull. Ann Otol Rhinol Laryngol 1948;57:643–676.

13. Beickert P, Weissenbecker L. Knochenzerstörende Prozesse an der Pyramide des Felsenbeines durch eosinophiles Granuloma mit Taubheit. Arch Ohren-Nasen-Kehlkopfheilkd 1951;148:489–596.

14. Chisolm J. Otorhinologic aspects of Hand-Schüller-Christian disease. Laryngoscope 1954;64:486.

15. Tos M. A survey of Hand-Schüller-Christian disease in otolaryngology. Acta Oto-Laryngol 1966;62:217.

16. Tos M. Facial palsy in Hand-Schüller-Christian disease. Arch Otolaryngol 1969;90:563.

17. Hudson W, Kenan P. Otologic manifestations of histiocytosis X. Laryngoscope 1969;79:678.

Part 5
Actinomycosis

Actinomycosis is a chronic suppurative granulomatous bacterial infection that if left untreated tends to extend to adjacent tissues, forming abscesses and sinus tracts that drain pus and grains or "sulfur granules" that represent organized aggregates of filamentous bacteria. The disease occurs worldwide; males are affected three times as often as females. The principal etiologic agent in humans is *Actinomyces israelii*, an anaerobic, Gram-positive, filamentous bacterium normally present in the oral flora.

The "sulfur granules" are commonly found in the crypts of normal tonsils in the absence of inflammatory reaction. Among the four clinical forms (cervicofacial, thoracic, abdominal, and disseminated), the cervicofacial form is the most common. It is most often seen in men. The prevalent portal of entry and predisposing factors are a break in the integrity of the oral mucosa for the organism and the regularly accompanying group of anaerobic bacteria and the presence of devitalized tissue essential for their anaerobic growth. Dental caries, periodontal disease, dental extraction, and musosal lacerations are the main predisposing factors of the cervicofacial form (1, 2).

The cervicofacial form generally begins as a localized, flat, woody-hard induration, with or without pain, under the oral mucosa or the skin of the neck or as a subperiosteal swelling of the mandible or parotid region. Subsequently, areas of colliquation appear and develop into sinus tracts and fistulae with a discharge that contains the characteristic rounded or spherical, usually yellowish granules up to 1 mm in diameter. Direct extension can lead to involvement of the cheek and neck, salivary glands, tongue, pharynx, and larynx. Spread to the periosteum may give rise to osteomyelitis of the mandible, cervical spine, and skull base with subsequent involvement of the meninges and brain.

Actinomycosis of the temporal bone is a rare complication. It may develop directly or indirectly. The primary route is very uncommon; the middle ear becomes involved through the Eustachian tube or the external auditory canal across a tympanic membrane perforation. More often, the temporal bone and middle ear become affected indirectly from a primary disease process in the epipharynx, parapharyngeal or retromaxillary space, or the paravertebral soft tissue, which results in an extension to the petrous or tympanic bone (3).

The diagnosis is based on the clinical symptoms and manifestations, the radiographic observations, and the demonstrations of the organism in sputum, secretions, and biopsy specimens.

Untreated, the disease slowly progresses. The cervicofacial form has the most favorable prognosis. Most patients with this disease respond to medical treatment. Because of the extensive induration and the poorly vascularized fibrosis, the response is slow, and treatment must be continued for weeks and occasionally for many months. The initial treatment includes penicillin G with at least 12 million units/day i.v. Small abscesses should be aspirated, and large ones should be drained. Extensive and repeated surgical procedures may be required.

References

1. Drutz DG. Actinomycosis. In: Wyngaarden JB, Smith LH, eds. Cecil textbook of medicine. 18th ed. Vol 2: Infectious diseases. Philadelphia: WB Saunders, Chap 297, 1988:1673–1674.

2. Richtsmeier WJ, Johns MJ. Actinomycosis of the head and neck. Crit Rev Clin Lab Sci 1979;II:175–179.

3. Theissing G, Kittel G. Aktinomykose des Ohres und des Schläfenbeins. In: Berendes J, Link R, Zöllner F, eds. Hals-Nasen-Ohrenheilkunde in Praxis und Klinik. 2nd ed. Vol 6: Ohr II. Stuttgart: G Thieme, 1980;6:16–20.

15/ Neoplasms and Other Lesions of the External Ear

CHONDRODERMATITIS NODULARIS CHRONICA HELICIS

DEFINITION

Chondrodermatitis nodularis chronica helicis (also known as Winkler's disease, painful nodular growth of the ear, and chondrodermatitis helicis) is a benign but painful lesion of unknown etiology, occurring mainly on the superior helix of the auricle; it affects mainly the elderly population, particularly men. The lesions are most frequently unilateral, and proper therapeutic approaches will usually cure the disease.

FREQUENCY AND AGE

The Armed Forces Institute of Pathology (AFIP) Otolaryngic Tumor Registry (OTR) contains only 6 patients recorded from 1976 through 1985. These were all men with an age range of 55–80 years and an average age of onset of 68 years. The reason for the small number of cases is that this particular pathologic entity is usually diagnosed by the dermatopathologist and is consequently recorded in *their* tumor registry. Shuman and Helwig (1) from the dermatopathology department of the AFIP reported on 100 patients. Two were black, and the remainder were white. The age range was 20–74 years, and all were men. The majority were in the 30–60-year range. Sixty patients had their lesion on the right, while 33 had their lesion on the left, and 7 had bilateral lesions. Ninety percent were single lesions and confined to one ear, and 10% were single on both ears or multiple on one or both ears. The anatomical location in the series revealed 85 patients with nodules limited to the outer margin of the helix. Seventy-three of these were in the region of the crown angle or top surface of the helix. Six patients revealed an antihelix location; 3 were on the tragus, 2 were on the concha, and 1 was on the antitragus. The 50 patients presented by Metzger and Goodman (2) ranged from 29 to 96 years, with 82% being over 50 years of age. Thirty-five patients were men, and 15 were women. The lesions were distributed equally between the right and left side. The lesion was identified by site in 34 patients, with 25 being on the helix and 12 of these being on the superior helix. Eight patients had antihelical lesions, and 5 of these were female. Fifty percent of the female patients had lesions other than on the helix.

ETIOLOGY

The cause of this disorder remains unknown (1). It may somehow be related to the anatomy of the ear. The skin of the auricle, particularly over the anterior or lateral surface, is tightly stretched over the underlying cartilage. Circulation in this area is poor because of the thin subcutaneous layer, particularly in men, that exists between cartilage and skin. This results in a compromised blood supply with increased vascular demands from the perichondrium and cartilage. The resulting ischemia is thought to cause the lesion and the pain that is so clinically impressive. Of interest anatomically is the notation that the female does have a thicker layer of fat in the subcutaneous layer between the cartilage and skin of the auricle than does the male. Perhaps the disease is related to an external traumatic event. Frostbite or prolonged exposure to pressure could initiate the cycle of pathology. Some investigators have suggested advancing age, with its attendant degenerative and vasular changes of the skin, to be a predisposing cause. Patients and investigators have blamed such factors as sleeping on the ear, wearing tightfitting headgear (such as a nuns' habit), ear injury, frostbite, and sunburn.

CLINICAL AND GROSS FINDINGS

The most characteristic symptom associated with the nodule is pain or tenderness (1). This is generally present at the beginning, described as stabbing or piercing in quality, and prompts the patient to seek medical advice. Occasionally, there is a latent period before the pain is felt; or the symptom is very slight or even absent, and the crusted nodule itself attracts the patient's attention. The pain is mainly initiated on pressure, although in some cases it occurs spontaneously or is associated with climatic change. The discomfort is either paroxysmal or continuous and persists from a few minutes to several hours. Some patients gain temporary relief by removing the central crust.

The clinical fully developed lesion (Figs. 15.1 and 15.2) is a relatively small, firm, well-defined nodule varying 3–18 mm in diameter, with an average of 7 mm except in the rare patient in whom the lesion may be 2–3 cm in greatest diameter. The nodule is generally raised several millimeters above the surrounding skin surface and is convex, round to ovoid, with a dome-shaped or slightly flattened surface (Figs. 15.2 and 15.3). The color often differs only slightly from normal skin but is usually grayish-white or translucent. After a time, a bluish or reddish-brown discoloration appears as a result of concomitant capillary dilation. A hyperemic zone of inflammatory redness often surrounds the periphery. An adherent scale or crust usually covers the summit, and its removal discloses a small central depression or ulcer.

The condition appears spontaneously and, as a rule, reaches its maximal size within a relatively short time unless it is altered by trauma or secondary infection. The disease mostly follows a very protracted course, sometimes lasting for years (3 weeks to 13 years in the series of Shuman and Helwig (1)). Rarely, there is evidence of spontaneous regression or complete disappearance of the nodule. Most spontaneous disappearances of the nodule were associated with subsequent recurrence.

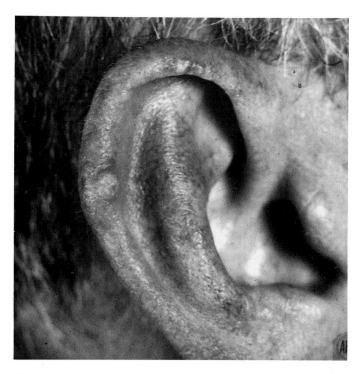

Figure 15.1. Typical clinical presentation of chondrodermatitis nodularis chronica helicis on the helix of an elderly man.

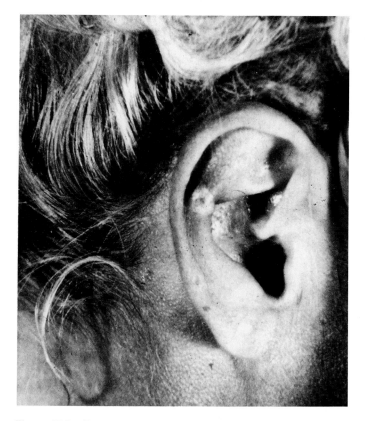

Figure 15.2. The patient is a 45-year-old nun with a recent development of chondrodermatitis nodularis chronica helicis on her antihelix.

MICROSCOPIC FINDINGS

The biologic aspects of the lesions are highly characteristic. There is a cytologically benign nodular hyperplasia (pseudoepithelial hyperplasia) of the epidermis that is centrally depressed or ulcerated and is topped by a hyperkeratotic and

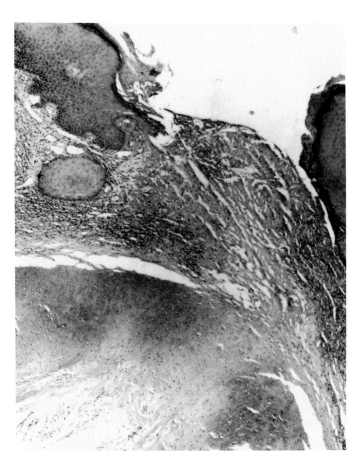

Figure 15.3. Histologic section of ulcerated lesion of chondrodermatitis nodularis chronica helicis. Note involvement of the perichondrium and cartilage by granulation tissue at the bed of the ulcer as well as the adjacent surface pseudoepitheliomatous hyperplasia. (Hematoxylin and eosin, ×63.)

parakeratotic scale. At the base of the ulcer or in the upper dermis, there is edema, homogenization, and fibrinoid necrosis of the dermal collagen and proliferation of a highly vascularized granulation tissue (Fig. 15.3). This reactive histology partially replaces the altered dermis along with an admixture of an inflammatory infiltrate of varying amounts, usually small, composed mainly of lymphocytes and plasma cells. There is commonly a perichondritis with or without degeneration of the auricular cartilage. The cartilage may be altered, indicated by changes in the basophilic chondroid matrix, with edema of the interstitial ground substance and chondrocytes. There may be focal disappearance of the cartilage cells and loss of homogeneity and orientation in the cartilage structure, with subsequent smudging and hyalinization of the auricular cartilage. Malignant dyskeratosis, such as keratinization of individual cells, clumping of nuclei, and frequent mitoses suggestive of senile keratosis and squamous cell carcinoma, are notably absent (1).

Barker et al. (3) believed there were both clinical and microscopic differences between the helix lesion and the antihelix lesion. They described the helix morphology as such, as was presented above, but the antihelix nodule, they believed, revealed the primary histologic change located in the cutis. The blood vessels were dilated, and their walls were thickened. The epidermis was thinned without hyperkeratosis. The cartilage and perichondrium might be involved with minimal inflammatory changes. The antihelix nodules were more likely to occur in the female and, by history, were supposedly precipitated by pressure or injury. Pain was minimal throughout its course. The antihelical lesions gradually resolved without treatment according to their findings.

DIFFERENTIAL DIAGNOSIS

The experience of Metzger and Goodman (2) is typical of the clinical differential diagnostic difficulty. In 43 of their 50 cases where a clinical diagnosis was recorded, only 5 were correctly identified as chondrodermatitis nodularis chronica helicis. Basal cell carcinoma was diagnosed in 25; squamous cell carcinoma, in 3; nonspecified carcinoma, in 4; and a variety of benign entities, in the rest, so that 80% of their 43 patients were given clinically proven malignant or premalignant diagnosis. Even on microscopic examination, malignant diagnoses such as basal cell carcinoma, squamous cell carcinoma, or malignant or premalignant keratoses were often mistakenly made (1).

TREATMENT AND PROGNOSIS

Various treatment modalities have been advocated in the past, including x-ray therapy, radium implant, injection with procaine hydrochloride, cryotherapy, fulguration, topical antibiotic therapy, and curettage (4). All have been abandoned because of high recurrence rates. Currently, two treatment modalities seem most appropriate. In those patients in whom a diagnosis of chondrodermatitis nodularis chronica helicis is made, a trial of intralesional steroid injections is carried out. A 50% success rate with intralesional steroid injections has been reportedly (2). Those lesions that persist or recur after intralesional steroid injections should be excised. A surgical technique that allows good visualization of the damaged cartilage, contouring of adjacent healthy cartilage, and good cosmesis is recommended. This surgical treatment is considered the most effective, as it removes the lesion entirely, relieves pain by transecting the sensory nerves, and reduces the amount of projecting helical cartilage.

IDIOPATHIC CYSTIC CHONDROMALACIA

DEFINITION

Idiopathic cystic chondromalacia (also known as pseudocyst, endochondral pseudocyst, and seroma) is a benign cystic mass, mainly unilateral, of the auricular cartilage that is of unknown etiology and occurs predominantly in men. The most effective therapeutic approach has been partial resection of the anterior wall of cystic structure together with postsurgical pressure dressings.

FREQUENCY AND AGE

Heffner and Hyams (cited in Ref. 3) recorded 23 patients with an age range of 16–73 years. Two were female. Eleven were white, and 1 was black; no race information was furnished on 11 patients. Five patients had bilateral lesions that were not known to be simultaneous in onset. Choi et al. (5) from Hong Kong reviewed the cases of 31 patients with the disease with an age range of 26–65 years and a mean age of onset of 43.8 years. Twenty-eight patients were men, and 3 were women. All were Chinese, with the men being laborers from a low socioeconomic class. In the AFIP OTR for the years 1976–1985, there were 35 patients included. Thirty-three patients were male, and 2 were

female. Their ages ranged from 4 to 73 years, with an average age of onset of 37 years. The majority of these patients (two-thirds) were in the 20–60-year group.

CLINICAL FINDINGS AND ETIOLOGY

These cysts occur within the auricular cartilage as a swelling in the upper half of the ear (Fig. 15.4), usually in the area of the scaphoid or triangular fossae. The swellings are usually painless and nontender, although slight pain and mild inflammatory signs can occur. Ulceration is absent. The cystic lesions are slightly fluctuant. If the tumor has been present for many months, it can become firm, suggesting a fibroma or a chondroma. Serous fluid can be aspirated in the untreated lesion and is sometimes viscous, having been described as like "olive oil." The fluid usually reaccumulated rapidly if further therapeutic methods were not undertaken.

There is seldom a history of trauma, and the definite cause of the cystic lesion is not known. Choi et al. (5) obtained a history of repeated minor trauma to the ear in a substantial number of their patients. Their Chinese patients were also in the habit of sleeping on hard pillows. There is no explanation of the premise that the entity occurs more in the Chinese. Since the race question is not followed in the AFIP OTR, it is not known whether this predominance in the Chinese is real or not.

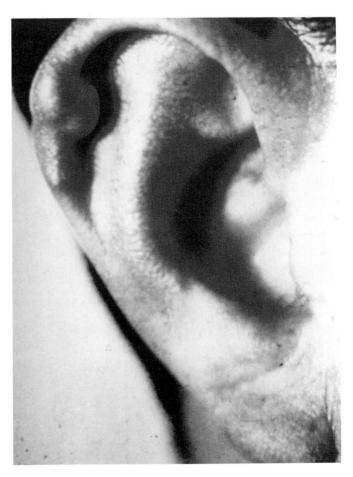

Figure 15.4. Young man with slowly enlarging, painless soft cystic nodule involving the helix of the ear. The lesion was an idiopathic cystic chondromalacia.

HISTOGENESIS

The primary stage of development of the lesion is thought to be an overproduction of glycosaminoglycans engendered by repeated minor trauma to the ear cartilage (5).

GROSS AND MICROSCOPIC FINDINGS

The excised portion of the cyst wall is usually a piece of cartilage 1–2 mm thick. The inner surface is partly smooth and partly rough, with or without a brownish material attached (5). The basic pathologic process appeared to be a dissolution or degenerative change that produced a cavity within the central area of the auricular cartilage (3). The cavity formation can expand to the outer margins of the cartilage. Occasionally, there were multiple cystic areas within the affected cartilage. In most cases, the cavity had progressed to the point of a long split or cleft in the center of the cartilage (Fig. 15.5). Granulation tissue was present in most lesions, and it was usually located along an edge of the cleft, although it occasionally filled a portion of the cavity. Apparently in those lesions of particularly longer duration, there was some suggestion of cartilage proliferation. These proliferating areas of cartilage did contain atypical but definitely not malignant chondrocytes. Histochemistry did not have any appreciable advantage in the diagnosis. Electron microscopy revealed numerous necrotic chondrocytes and their remains in the cartilaginous wall of the pseudocyst. A large amount of matrical lipidic debris derived from necrotic chondrocytes was also present. Electron microscopy also disclosed findings similar to those seen in deeply fibrillated, crumbling osteoarthrotic cartilage. The few viable chondrocytes present showed no noteworthy change, and there was no increase in the number of lysosomes (5). Despite a thorough search, no infectious agent (virus or bacterium) was detected in any of the specimens studied.

DIFFERENTIAL DIAGNOSIS

The most frequent misdiagnosis was relapsing polychondritis, followed by epidermoid inclusion cyst, chondrodermatitis nodularis chronica helicis, cauliflower ear, hemangioma, low-grade angiosarcoma, chondroma, and low-grade chondrosarcoma. Heffner and Hyams (cited in Ref. 3) have included a chart comparing the differential histologic features of the more common differential diagnostic problems of the relapsing polychondritis and the idiopathic cystic chondromalacia.

TREATMENT AND PROGNOSIS

Various forms of treatment of pseudocyst have been suggested in the past. Aspiration of the fluid in the pseudocyst can be successful, but unless the cystic space becomes completely obliterated postoperatively, fluid buildup often recurs rapidly.

Excision of the entire cartilaginous cyst may result in a floppy ear. Excision of the anterior wall and use of a contour pressure dressing are the standard methods recommended (5). The goal of the operation is to remove the pseudocyst and to prevent excessive thickening of the auricle while maintaining an acceptable framework. The posterior wall of the cyst is maintained intact to provide support to the auricle. This surgical approach has provided a 90% satisfactory cosmetic result (5).

ANGIOLYMPHOID HYPERPLASIA WITH EOSINOPHILIA

DEFINITION

Angiolymphoid hyperplasia with eosinophilia (also known as Kimura's disease, atypical pyogenic granuloma, subcutaneous angiolymphoid hyperplasia with eosinophilia, pseudo-atypical granuloma, papular angioplasia, dermal angiolymphoid hyperplasia, and inflammatory angiomatous nodules of the face and scalp) is a rare, benign, inflammatory vascular lesion of unknown etiology, occurring in a young to middle-aged adult who will present with one or more cutaneous and/or subcutaneous pruritic nodules occurring about the ears, scalp, forehead, and temples (Fig. 15.6). The pathology is characterized by a proliferation of atypical blood vessels lined by plump, vacuolated endothelial cells lying in a stroma heavily infiltrated with lymphocytes and eosinophils. Excision is the most frequent form of therapy and will usually obtain a cure (6). Rosai et al. (7) suggested this entity be included as part of the "histiocytoid hemangioma" group, which includes many types of vascular lesions of the skin, intravascular atypical proliferations, and others.

INCIDENCE, FREQUENCY, AGE, AND SEX

The disease is considered a rare pathologic entity. It is mostly investigated and published in the dermatopathology literature, but it is important that the otolaryngologist be aware of the disease because he or she will most likely be one of the first specialists to see the patient and to instigate therapy. The AFIP

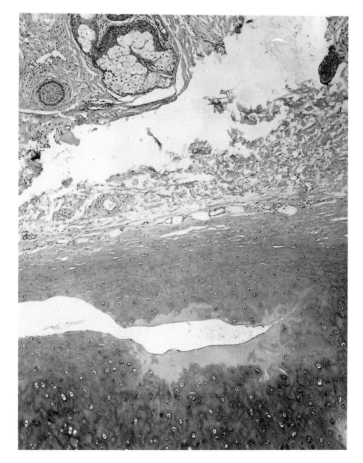

Figure 15.5. Histologic section of idiopathic cystic chondromalacia. The cystic space involves the auricular cartilage without the reactive cellular element. (Hematoxylin and eosin, ×63.)

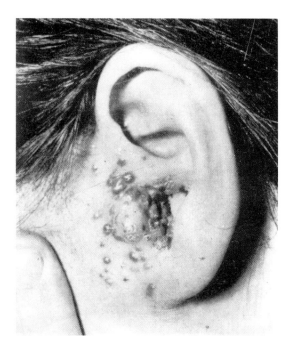

Figure 15.6. Benign angiomatous nodules of external ear of a young woman. They are raised, skin-covered, purple, firm papules.

OTR contained only 12 patients during the 1976–1985 period. Their ages ranged from 23 to 58 years, with an average age of onset of 36 years. Six were men, and the lesions were described as involving the external ear, external auditory canal, and peri-auricular tissue. Barnes et al. (6) presented 12 patients, 6 of whom were female. Their ages were between 14 and 68 years, with an average of 38.5 years. There have now been at least 240 examples of angiolymphoid hyperplasia with eosinophilia reported in the literature; 167 of these were from China and Japan, and 73 were from the United States and the United Kingdom. The disease has occurred in patients as young as 1 year of age and as old as 79 years of age. In over half of the patients, there were multiple lesions (usually 2–6), but up to 20 occurred in one patient, and these were generally synchronous (6).

CLINICAL FINDINGS

In the series of Barnes et al (6), symptoms lasted 2 months to 6 years with a mean of 23 months. Ten patients presented with a solitary lesion, while 2 had multiple lesions. Sites of involvement included the auricle, posterior auricular sulcus, external auditory canal or meatus, scalp, temple, forehead, and thigh. The patients complained of one or more of the following symptoms: increase in size of tumor, pruritus, bleeding usually after minor trauma, and pain, especially upon pressure and stenosis of the external auditory meatus. Occasionally, a patient will present with an asymptomatic mass. Although the lesions center about the head, there are some reported extrafacial involvements either with or without facial involvement. The breast, axilla, chest, trunk, arm, hand, thigh, gluteal, cubital, and inguinal regions, urinary bladder, prostate, the bones of the femur, tibia, and skull, and the periosteum of the pubic bone have all been implicated as sites (6). Analysis of cases of angiolymphoid hyperplasia with eosinophilia occurring in the United States and the United Kingdom reveals some clinical dissimilarities when these cases are compared with those from China and Japan. In the United States and United Kingdom, there is a predominance of female pa-

tients. The lesions average less than 2 cm, and peripheral eosinophilia and regional adenopathy are unusual. Extrafacial lesions are also rare. In China and Japan, there is an 85% male predominance, peripheral eosinophilia is frequent, and to a greater degree, regional adenopathy is common, and extrafacial tumors are not unusual. Some investigators have suggested that the Chinese and Japanese disease be considered as Kimura's disease in contrast to the angiolymphoid hyperplasia with eosinophilia designated in the United States and United Kingdom.

CLINICAL APPEARANCE AND GROSS FINDINGS

The tumors were generally sessile and slightly raised with either a smooth or a nodular surface. Their colors varied from deep red to skin colored, and their greatest dimension averaged 1.2 cm (0.4–4.0 cm) (Fig. 15.6) (6). Some exhibited superficial excoriations probably secondary to scratching. The tumors were either soft or firm, depending on the vascular-to-stroma ratio. In a patient of Barnes et al. (6), the tumor was associated with palpable, firm, nontender, freely movable, right posterior cervical and supraclavicular lymph nodes measuring up to 1.6 cm in greatest dimension. None of their patients were believed to have a peripheral eosinophilia.

On gross dissection the lesions presented as either a circumscribed or a poorly defined area of pink-white, gray-pink, tan-pink, or tan-brown discoloration limited to the dermis, subcutis, or both. Focal areas of hemorrhage were sometimes noted. The consistency varied from that of the surrounding tissue to moderate firmness.

MICROSCOPIC FINDINGS

All lesions should reveal, in varying degrees, the diagnostic morphology that is considered pathognomonic for angiolymphoid hyperplasia with eosinophilia, which is: proliferation of blood vessels that are lined by atypical, frequently vacuolated endothelial cells; tissue eosinophilia; and diffuse and/or nodular collections of lymphocytes (Figs. 15.7–15.9). In the series of Barnes et al. (6), the tumor was confined to the dermis in 5 and to the subcutis in 1. In 6 patients, both dermis and subcutis were involved, and in 1 of these patients, adjacent skeletal muscle was involved.

On scanning microscopy the tumors were either poorly defined, blending into the surrounding normal tissue, or were circumscribed and demarcated from surrounding normal tissue by a zone of collagen. Collections of lymphocytes with or without germinal centers frequently lined tumor margins (Fig. 15.7).

A distinguishing and sometimes misinterpreted feature is the proliferation of abnormal blood vessels, often observed in the central and superficial portions of the tumor. They can range in size from capillaries, venules, and arterioles to small and medium-sized arteries and veins (Figs. 15.8 and 15.9). Arteries and veins can sometimes become difficult to differentiate. The possibility of lymphatics being included among the vessels cannot be excluded on histology. These atypical vessels within the tumefaction are always lined with plump endothelial cells that are arranged one or two layers thick; and these cells contain pink cytoplasm and enlarged hyperchromatic nuclei with one or more irregular blue-to-pink nucleoli. The shape of these cells varies from round to spindled, and they occasionally project into the lumen, with their long axis perpendicular to the vessel wall. Many

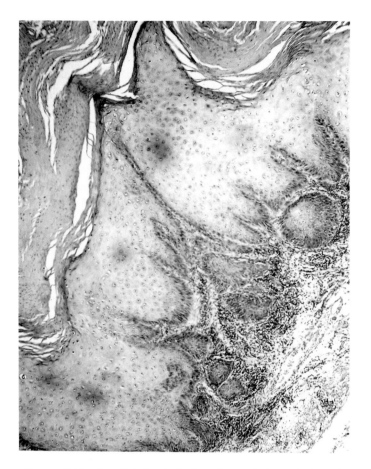

Figure 15.10. In actinic keratosis, there is usually hyperplasia and surface hyperkeratosis of the epidermis. The basal portions of the epidermis will contain foci of dysplastic squamous epithelium that does not violate the basal cell membrane. (Hematoxylin and eosin, ×63.)

cally suggest the actinic keratosis, except for the history of radiation exposure. *Bowen's disease,* which represents a squamous cell carcinoma in situ involving the entire thickness of the epidermis, the *intradermal epithelioma of Jadassohn,* which is a lesion of the skin in which interwoven bands of considerably thickened and mildly papillomatous epidermis surround irregular nests of atypical epithelial cells, and *xeroderma pigmentosum,* a lesion of the epidermis with areas of mild hyperkeratosis, acanthosis, atrophy or proliferation of rete ridges, and focal hyperpigmentation of the basal layer with release of melanin into the dermis where severe chronic inflammation is noted are all considered premalignant skin entities, and although they have not been reported in the medical literature as favoring the skin of the external ear, there is no reason why they may not do so.

Where the histology of a biopsy of the external ear, particularly of the external auditory canal, leaves doubt as to whether the histologic diagnosis is solar keratosis or squamous cell carcinoma, the experienced surgeon will favor complete removal of the lesion rather than merely rely on clinical observation. The habit of observation is commendable on skin lesions that can readily be observed, such as on the external auricle. In the external ear canal, however, if a malignancy is overlooked or underdiagnosed, because of its recurrent aggressive behavior it will usually undergo a silent clinical extension into the middle or inner ear and, possibly, to the cranial cavity and could then be beyond therapeutic help.

SEBORRHEIC KERATOSIS

Seborrheic keratosis (also known as seborrheic verruca, benign epithelioma, and basal cell papilloma) is a common, benign, pigmented skin growth that is related to tumors that have intraepidermal basal cell proliferation (11). These tumors appear primarily on the body and arms and secondarily on the face, neck, and external ear (12). Supposedly, they begin to occur in the fifth decade of life (13). The AFIP OTR listed 8 patients with seborrheic keratosis of the external ear. Seven were men. Their ages ranged from 21 to 58 years, with an average age of onset of 38 years. Seven of these patients had external auditory canal tumors, and 1 patient had a lesion apparently on the external auricle.

Clinically, the most common appearance of seborrheic keratosis on the skin surface is that of a sharply demarcated, oval, verrucous plaque "stuck" on the normal skin. The tumors average 1 cm in diameter, and they appear early as a light yellow area, increase in size, and become more deeply pigmented, usually turning brown. The lesion may be covered by a thin, greasy scale that can be rubbed off (12,13).

The essential histologic feature of seborrheic keratosis is a thickened epidermis secondary to an accumulation of immature keratinocytes between the basal layer and the surface (Figs. 15.11 and 15.12). The microscopic examination also reveals that the tumor protrudes above the horizontal plane of the skin and rests

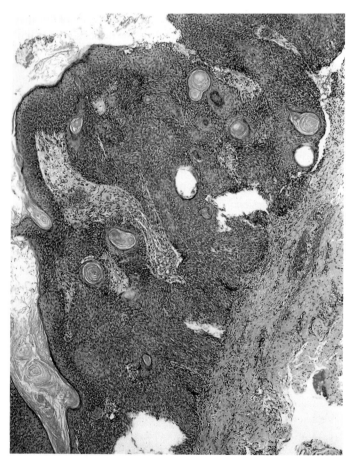

Figure 15.11. This low-power histologic section of seborrheic keratosis reveals the thickened epidermis resulting from accumulation of the keratinocytes and protrusion of the tumor above the plane of the skin surface. (Hematoxylin and eosin, ×25.)

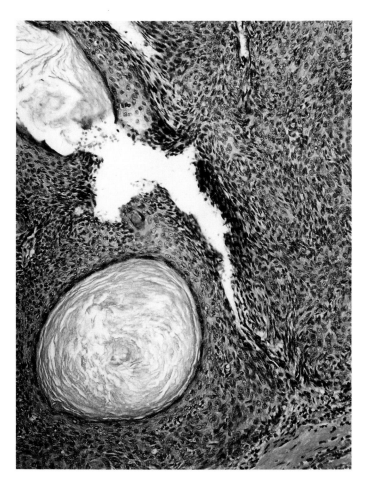

Figure 15.12. Higher magnification of the same seborrheic keratosis as in Figure 15.11 emphasizes the compact arrangement of the uniform tumor cells and the occlusion of a keratin whorl within the tumor mass. (Hematoxylin and eosin, ×160.)

on the dermis (Fig. 15.11). It grows up, instead of down, and does not penetrate into the dermis. This thickened epithelium contains invaginations from the surface that produce keratin tunnels (horn cysts). Bacterial infection within the keratin tunnels can produce edema and an inflammatory infiltrate. Inflammation appears to stimulate maturation of the keratinocytes and increases the number of mitoses and thus resembles *activated seborrheic verruca,* which can be mistaken for a malignant condition by the inexperienced pathologist (12–14). The malignant transformation of seborrheic keratoses is recorded (13), but this must be an exceedingly rare occurrence. The main histologic types according to the dermatopathologists are the solid, papillomatous (acanthotic, verrucous), and reticulated varieties (14). Other than histologic differences, these types do not apparently affect the benign behavior of the tumor.

When the seborrheic keratosis occurs in the external auditory canal, the typical clinical appearance cannot·be appreciated, and only after an adequate biopsy can the diagnosis be made by a competent pathologist. Incidentally, the sudden appearance of multiple seborrheic keratoses may herald the presence of a visceral carcinoma or other malignant condition (Leser-Trélat sign (13). In several patients from the AFIP OTR with seborrheic keratosis of the external auditory canal, there was at least one episode of recurrence of the canal tumor following supposedly complete surgical removal. None of the patients had invasion

into surrounding vital areas, but the recurrence and necessary repeat surgery caused them considerable morbidity. One has to assume that the treatment of choice is surgical removal regardless of the anatomical location. The possibility of tumor left behind in the external auditory canal can lead to a recurrence and increased morbidity for the patient.

SEBACEOUS NEOPLASMS

Sebaceous neoplasms of the skin are considered somewhat rare in the body generally and even scarcer in the external ear. Rulon and Helwig (15) have reported on 95 patients with a single cutaneous sebaceous neoplasm involving the skin throughout the body (except for the eyelid area); only 3 were from the ear, although lesions of the head and neck, particularly of the external nose and cheek, accounted for 60% of the lesions in their patients. There were only 3 reports in the medical literature of patients with sebaceous neoplasia of the external ear canal (16–18). Supposedly, the neoplasm will involve the areas of greatest sebaceous gland concentration, and in the head and neck, the cheek, external nose, and eyelid are quite well known for the presence of these glands. The eyelid does become involved with primary sebaceous neoplasms, apparently much more commonly than other skin areas, perhaps because of the excessive number of sebaceous glands in that anatomical area (glands of Zeis, Meibomian glands along with hair follicles, caruncle and eyebrow glands). In addition to the patients of Rulon and Helwig (15) mentioned above, there were an additional 88 patients with only eyelid sebaceous tumors contained in the AFIP Ophthalmic Tumor Registry up to the mid-1960s (19).

Rulon and Helwig (15) classified the sebaceous tumors into sebaceous adenoma, basal cell carcinoma with sebaceous differentiation, and sebaceous carcinoma. This classification concurs essentially with other dermatopathology texts. These were 46 patients with sebaceous adenoma, and 75% had head and neck lesions, but only 1 patient presented with an ear canal tumor. The male-to-female ratio was 2.5:1, and 1 patient was black. Clinically, the sebaceous adenoma occurs as a smooth, elevated, often slightly pedunculated, firm to soft and even friable solitary tumor, with most being less than 0.5 cm in diameter, although the range could be from 0.1 to 9.0 cm (15). They may be tan, skin colored, or pink to red and on section will be yellow and, less often, gray. Signs and symptoms include bleeding, particularly following trauma, rarely ulceration, slow to rapid growth, and occasionally pain, particularly on pressure. Microscopically, the lesion frequently replaces the surface epithelium, and with tumor compressing surrounding fibrous tissue, there may appear to be a capsule. The tumor lobules occupy the dermis and are composed of tumor cells that tend to duplicate the progression from the small generative cell at the periphery of the lobules, through maturing sebaceous cells with increasing amounts of finely divided lipid within the cytoplasm, to central areas of holocrine necrobiosis (Figs. 15.13 and 15.14). Slight pleomorphism of the cells and nuclei is sometimes present, and mitotic figures are occasionally seen. The stroma may contain chronic inflammatory cells including lymphocytes, plasma cells, and histiocytes.

This atypia makes the differentiation from sebaceous carcinoma difficult. Of the 6 cases reported by Rulon and Helwig (15), there was 1 case of an external auditory canal lesion. Of

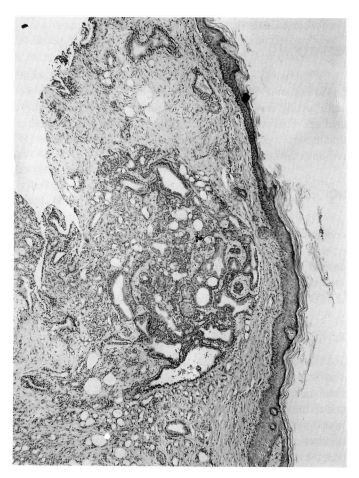

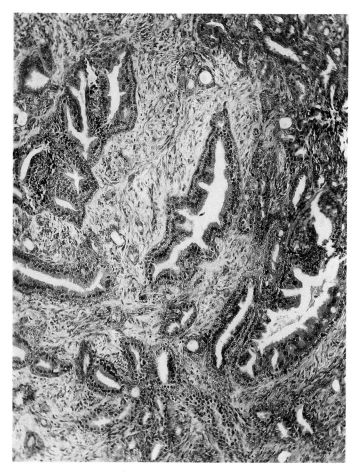

Figure 15.26. This microscopic presentation emphasizes primarily the usual demarcation of a ceruminal adenoma from surrounding tissue. No capsule is seen. The adenomatous morphology is well differentiated, resembling the makeup of a normal ceruminal gland. (Hematoxylin and eosin, ×125.)

Figure 15.27. Note the close resemblance of the adenoma to the normal ceruminal gland. The neoplasm reveals a double-layered gland pattern, with the inner layer demonstrating secretory activity. The outer layer of myoepithelial cells is more prominent than in the normal gland. (Hematoxylin and eosin, ×160.)

eccrine gland tumors. PAS-positive, diastase-resistant granules were demonstrated in the neoplasm of this tumor.

NATURAL HISTORY

The histologic classification of ceruminal gland tumors is definitely correlated with prognosis and morbidity. In the low-grade or benign tumors, the only reported complication is the rare recurrence of the tumor following inadequate surgical removal. Occasionally, the adenoma or its recurrence may spread to involve the middle ear space.

DIFFERENTIAL DIAGNOSIS

Adenocarcinomatous metastases from regional and distal sites must be ruled out. The adenoma of the middle ear may spread through a perforated eardrum and may be mistaken for a ceruminal tumor. Jugulotympanic paraganglioma and basal cell carcinomas may also pose histologic and clinical differential diagnostic problems, particularly if they spread to involve the external auditory canal.

TREATMENT

Surgical removal is recommended, to prevent recurrence.

Ceruminous Gland Adenocarcinoma

DEFINITION

Ceruminous gland adenocarcinoma (also known as hidradenocarcinoma, malignant ceruminoma, and ceruminal adenocarcinoma or carcinoma) is characterized by origin in mainly the outer, cartilaginous half of the external auditory canal from the ceruminous glands of the anatomical area. The micromorphology will indicate an epithelial, glandular pattern of varying anaplasia that may resemble the histology of the ceruminous gland. The histology is definitely malignant when compared with the cytology of the ceruminous gland adenoma. This neoplasm is capable of rapid, aggressive local growth and may rarely metastasize to regional and distal sites. Fatalities result from invasion into adjacent vital areas such as the cranial cavity, especially when initial surgery of the neoplasm is inadequate.

INCIDENCE

Thirty-three patients recorded in the AFIP OTR had the ceruminous gland adenocarcinoma. Nineteen were men, and their ages ranged from 26 to 71 years of age, with an average age of onset of 50 years.

CLINICAL AND GROSS FINDINGS

The most commonly described symptom is a feeling of blockage in the external auditory canal (37). Decreased hearing is related to the size of the mass. Pain is a likely symptom. An external otitis may accompany the prediagnosis symptomatology. The physical findings have been those of a nodule or a mass in the ear canal. Erosion of surrounding bone and other tissue structures may exist. Radiographs, especially polytomograms, may be of help in delineating an invasive process.

The overlying skin surface is likely to reveal an ulceration. The tumors are generally firm but can reveal a cystic consistency. The cut surface can suggest a juicy, resilient tissue with a whitish scirrhous irregular tumor outline, with the more aggressive or neglected neoplasms revealing infiltration into surrounding tissues including bone.

MICROSCOPIC FINDINGS

The ceruminous gland adenocarcinoma will reveal loss of demarcation from surrounding tissue with infiltration into adjacent tissues. The overall pattern of the micromorphology is of an adenocarcinoma in varying states of differentiation (Fig. 15.28), with the more anaplastic portions concentrating at the ulcerated surface of the skin (40). The neoplastic cells usually have no uniform architecture but grow in irregular strands and clumps with little intervening corium (Fig. 15.29). The tumor cells may

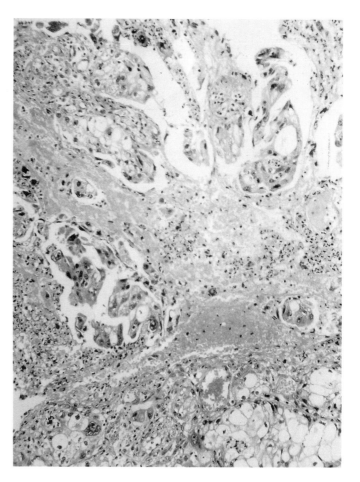

Figure 15.29. Anaplastic ceruminal gland adenocarcinoma of external ear. The cytology does not support the double-layered cell morphology of the ceruminal gland adenoma. (Hematoxylin and eosin, ×160.)

be large and polyhedral with finely granular, foamy, or reticulated cytoplasm that tends to be neutrophilic. The nuclei are moderate to large, with mitotic figures being present, some of which are atypical (Fig. 15.30). Some parts of the neoplasm may appear more differentiated cytologically. In some neoplasms, these areas may be impossible to tell from normal ceruminal glands. Fine fat droplets and iron-positive granules may be demonstrated histochemically. Dehner and Chen (38) have divided the ceruminous gland adenocarcinoma into a low-grade and a high-grade type. They believed that the low-grade adenocarcinomas approached a suggestive apocrine histology, whereas the high-grade type did not. They mentioned the demonstration of mucin throughout their adenocarcinoma spectrum.

DIFFERENTIAL DIAGNOSIS

The most important neoplastic entity that must be considered in the differential diagnosis is metastasizing adenocarcinoma from a regional or distal site (possibly undetected). It may require time and money to perform an extensive search for a distant primary, but from a humanitarian and medical-legal standpoint, the peace of mind that this extensive search will provide is worth the costs.

TREATMENT AND NATURAL HISTORY

An initial aggressive surgical procedure is advocated. This is based on a review of the literature with regard to the results

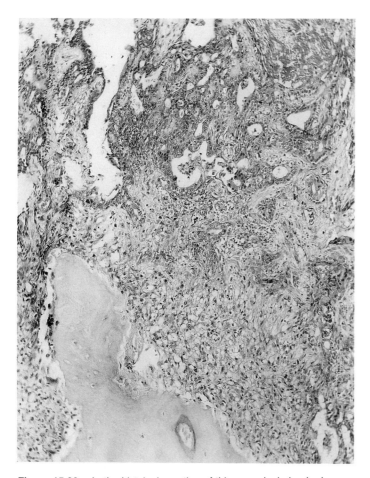

Figure 15.28. In the histologic section of this ceruminal gland adenocarcinoma, there is an area that suggests a ceruminal glandular pattern, but the remaining areas of the neoplasm reveal a transformation into a pleomorphic malignant cellular infiltrate that is destroying adjacent cartilage. (Hematoxylin and eosin, ×63.)

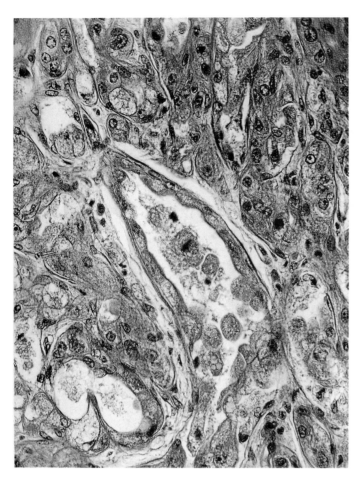

Figure 15.30. Higher magnification of ceruminal gland adenocarcinoma with no hint of cytology suggesting a normal ceruminal gland. (Hematoxylin and eosin, ×250.)

of "lesser" therapeutic approaches. With a postoperative follow-up of at least 5 years, when only a local excision and/or radical mastoidectomy was done, even with postoperative irradiation, there were few cases without recurrence (37). With such "lesser" operative approaches, there were recurrences usually within months, but some tumors recurred as long as 7 years later. Subsequent therapy for these recurrences usually consisted of either further radiotherapy or limited surgical procedures. These inadequately treated cases illustrate the unpredictable and usually aggressive, unrelenting, deceptive biologic behavior of the ceruminous gland adenocarcinoma. The behavior supports an initial radical operative procedure whether the neoplasm can be confined to the membranous area alone or involves the bony canal. The surgical procedure should consist of a wide en bloc excision of the entire ear canal, surrounding bone, associated cartilage, mastoid, middle ear, parotid and all contingent muscle, lymphatic, and nerve structures with, it is hoped, preservation of the facial nerve. For those tumors involving the middle ear and temporal bone with or without facial nerve involvement, the recommended treatment is a subtotal temporal bone resection with modifications and nerve grafting. It may be necessary to include removal of the dura and the ascending ramus of the mandible and to perform an upper neck dissection, especially if there is suspicion or evidence of lymph node metastasis. These surgical procedures should be followed by irradiation therapy (37). Metastases to regional or distal nodes or sites are rare in the experience of the AFIP OTR as well as in medical literature case reports of ceruminous gland adenocarcinomas. There was only one incidence of a patient with ceruminous gland adenocarcinoma from the AFIP OTR in which a known metastasis occurred in the regional anatomical area, although there were several deaths in AFIP OTR patients that resulted from the local aggressiveness of the neoplasm.

A case of *extramammary Paget's disease* of the external canal in association with ceruminous gland adenocarcinoma is presented by Fligiel and Kaneko (41). Supposedly, extramammary Paget's disease is not uncommonly seen in regions where apocrine glands are prevalent, with or without underlying apocrine gland carcinoma, but such occurrence in the external auditory canal has rarely been reported.

Ceruminous Gland Mixed Tumors

DEFINITION

Ceruminous gland mixed tumor (also known as pleomorphic adenoma and chondroid syringoma) is a circumscribed tumor believed to arise from the ceruminous glands and is characterized microscopically by a pleomorphic or "mixed" appearance, with a clearly recognizable epithelial tissue element being intermingled with mucoid-, myxoid-, or chondroid-appearing tissue (42). They histologically resemble the mixed tumor or pleomorphic adenoma of salivary gland origin.

HISTOGENESIS

There are discussion and disagreement in the medical literature concerning the origin of these tumors. Some investigators have suggested that these external auditory canal mixed tumors are extensions from the adjacent parotid salivary gland. One of the authors (V.J.H.) has not seen anatomical or histologic evidence to support such origin. Goldenberg and Block (43) believed that the tumor arose from the ectopic parotid salivary gland and listed several ways that such tissue could reach the external auditory canal. Again, one of the authors (V.J.H.) has never noted an ectopic salivary gland rest in this anatomical area. Only one reference to a salivary gland choristoma occurring in the external auditory canal has been found in the medical literature (44). We favor the origin of the mixed tumor to be from the external auditory canal ceruminous gland. Mixed tumors have been described arising from skin adnexa throughout the body (45). There is also the case report of a rare mixed tumor arising in the auricle (27); supposedly, it originated from the eccrine sweat glands of the anatomical area and may be referred to as a chondroid syringoma.

INCIDENCE

According to Hicks (37), there have been 5 cases in the literature of the ceruminous gland mixed tumor of the external auditory canal. The AFIP OTR lists 16 patients with this diagnosis, ranging in age from 42 through 84 years, with an average age of onset of 59 years. In other published series, ages ranged from 27 to 79 years, with an average age of onset of 57 years. There was a male-to-female ratio of 2:1 in the AFIP OTR material, while in Hicks' series (37) 4 of 5 patients were female.

CLINICAL AND GROSS FINDINGS

The signs and symptoms of a mixed tumor of the external auditory canal are similar to those of the benign ceruminous adenoma. Usually, they present as a slow-growing mass, a sensation of obstruction or blockage, and possibly an external otitis secondary to canal obstruction (37). The mass may be sessile or polypoid, is usually skin-covered with no surface ulceration, and fluctuant, movable, and not fixed to underlying connective tissue. Pain on manipulation of the external ear can be quite severe (46).

MICROSCOPIC FINDINGS

The neoplasm is demarcated from surrounding tissue but fails to develop a capsule. The biphasic histology so familiar in the mixed tumors of salivary gland origin is present (Figs. 15.31 and 15.32). The epithelial cells are arranged in tubular formations and, as they extend as attenuated strands into the stroma, often become elongated or stellate. In the tubular epithelial formations the inner layer of cells disclosed the doming characteristic of ceruminal glands (Fig. 15.33). The stroma is fibrocellular or hyaline and sometimes assumes a myxoid or chondroid appearance (Figs. 15.31 and 15.32). Occasionally, one can note the pattern of a typical ceruminal gland adenoma in one area and the biophasic features of a mixed salivary type tumor elsewhere.

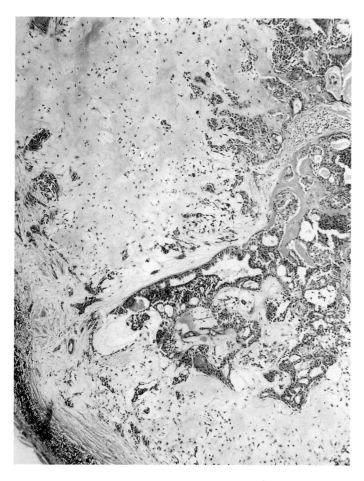

Figure 15.31. Microscopic view of a mixed tumor of ceruminal gland origin depicts a prominent pseudochondromatous matrix and a tubular epithelial element characteristic of a mixed tumor of salivary gland origin. (Hematoxylin and eosin, ×25.)

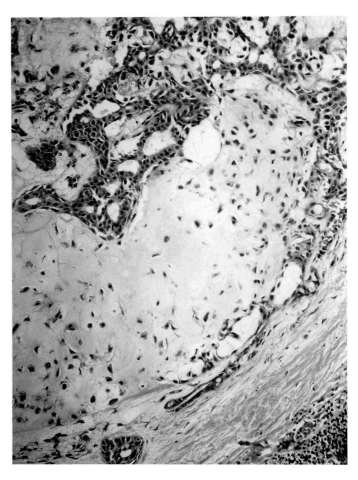

Figure 15.32. Higher microscopic view of a mixed tumor of ceruminal gland origin reveals the pseudochondromatous stroma with gland structures that can occasionally demonstrate apocrine secretion with cytoplasmic droplets within the lumen. (Hematoxylin and eosin, ×160.)

DIFFERENTIAL DIAGNOSIS

With the diagnosis of a mixed tumor or pleomorphic adenoma of the external auditory canal, the obligation to rule out origin from the adjacent parotid gland is a necessity, but this has not been a particular problem in the experience of one of the authors (V.J.H.).

NATURAL HISTORY AND TREATMENT

Most mixed tumors in all anatomical areas behave in a benign fashion. Recurrences usually depend on the adequacy of the surgical removal. The first operation for this benign external auditory canal neoplasm, whether adenoma or mixed tumor, is critical. Unless there are surgical margins completely free of tumor, a patient may be destined for a lifetime of recurrences.

Syringocystadenoma Papilliferum

DEFINITION

Syringocystadenoma papilliferum is a skin lesion that most commonly occurs on the scalp or the face near the age of puberty in a sebaceous nevus present since birth. In about one-fourth of the cases, however, it arises on the trunk or thigh during adolescence or adult life without a preexisting lesion (33).

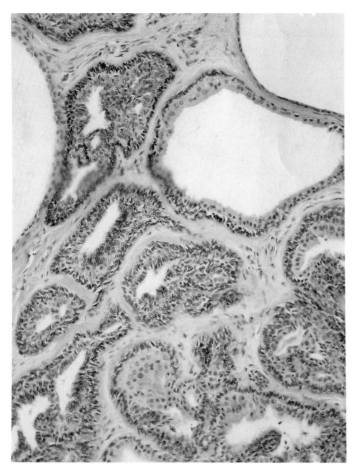

Figure 15.33. The apocrine character of the glandular element in this portion of a ceruminal gland mixed tumor is evident. (Hematoxylin and eosin, ×115.)

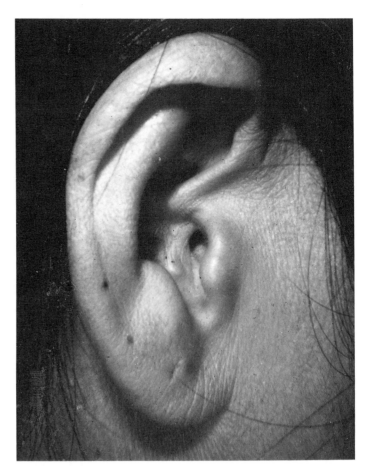

Figure 15.34. Clinical photograph of syringocystadenoma papilliferum in concha area of the external auricle of a 17-year-old woman. The lesion was essentially asymptomatic, with the patient complaining of only an occasional itching and soreness connected with the tumor.

Apparently, the rare case occurring in the external ear area (Fig. 15.34) fits into this latter group because of the rarity of the preexisting sebaceous nevus in this anatomical area.

INCIDENCE AND CLINICAL AND GROSS FINDINGS

Of the 6 patients contained in the AFIP OTR from 1976 through 1985, 2 were men and 4 were women, with ages ranging from 22 to 75 years and an average age of onset of 47 years. Clinically and grossly, the lesion consists most commonly of a fleshy nodule or plaque (Fig. 15.35) that may have a papillary, hyperkeratotic surface (33).

MICROSCOPY AND HISTOGENESIS

The epidermis may reveal varying degrees of papillomatosis. Usually one but possibly several cystic invaginations extend downward from the epidermis (Fig. 15.35). Portions of the cystic, papillary invaginations may be lined by squamous, keratinizing, or cuboidal to columnar epithelium, while in other areas the papillary projections are lined by glandular epithelium, often consisting of two rows of cells (Fig. 15.36). These latter cells, on their luminal surface, will reveal active "decapitation" secretion, supporting the claim that the neoplasm is derived from the glands when in the external auditory canal.

TREATMENT

Complete surgical removal should be curative. The adjacent skin area should be inspected for the association with a sebaceous nevus, with removal of this essentially benign tumor (47).

Cysts of the external auditory canal will include the cholesteatoma of the canal and the reduplication cysts of the first branchial cleft, all of which are discussed in Chapter 10, Part 4, of this volume. The AFIP OTR contains a report of a rare 1 or 2-cm cyst that formed in the external auditory canal from an apparent dilatation of a ceruminous gland. The cause of the obstructed gland or duct could be due to an external otitis.

Adenoid Cystic Carcinoma

DEFINITION

Adenoid cystic carcinoma (also known as adenocystic carcinoma and cylindroma) is an infiltrative malignant tumor having mainly a characteristic cribriform histologic appearance, with a minority of the neoplasms having a tubular or solid epithelial micromorphology. The cells of the neoplasm are described as two types: duct-lining cells and cells of myoepithelial type (42). The former can be arranged as small duct-like structures, and

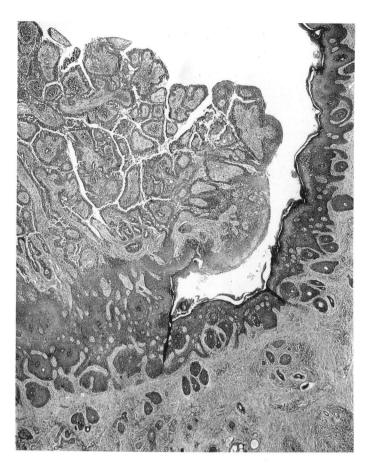

Figure 15.35. Scanning microscopic view of syringocystadenoma papilliferum with cystic invagination from skin surface and papillomatous projections from cyst wall. (Hematoxylin and eosin, ×25.)

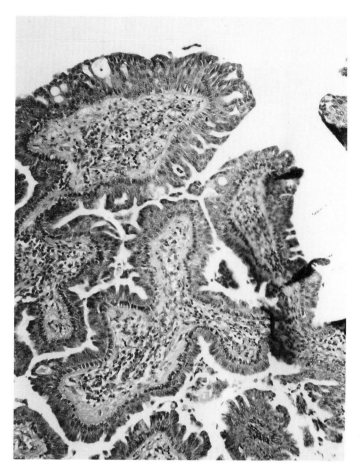

Figure 15.36. Higher magnification of the same syringocystadenoma papilliferum as in Figure 15.35 in which a portion of the papillary invagination is covered by a glandular epithelium formed of a double row of cells resembling apocrine ceruminal gland cell lining. (Hematoxylin and eosin, ×160.)

the latter may form larger masses of myoepithelial cells disposed around cystic spaces to give a cribriform or lace-like pattern.

The term "cylindroma" used to designate this particular neoplasm is to be condemned. The cylindroma, in dermatopathology tests (14), is considered a benign neoplastic cell proliferation formed from skin adenexa, most often in the scalp. The histology of the cylindroma at first glance may resemble an adenoid cystic carcinoma, but on closer inspection the experienced pathologist will recognize the histologic difference.

INCIDENCE

There were 44 patients with the diagnosis of adenoid cystic carcinoma of the external auditory canal among 160 patients with apparent ceruminal gland external auditory canal tumors listed in the AFIP OTR. Among 25 patients that were additions to the OTR during the period of 1976–1985, 16 were men. Their ages varied from 16 through 80 years, with an average age of onset of 54 years. In the excellent article by Perzin et al. (48), 7 of 16 patients were women. The ages in their series ranged from 20 to 72 years, with an average age of onset of 41 years.

CLINICAL FEATURES

According to Perzin et al. (48), the majority of patients complained of pain in the ear, often of several years duration. Three patients had a history of an ear canal "cyst" or "pimple" that had been incised or drained. The nature of these cysts is not clear, although the possibility exists that ceruminous glands had

been obstructed by an invasive adenoid cystic carcinoma and had become secondarily dilated or infected. More than half of the patients will have a history of otitis externa before the neoplasm is recognized as the true cause of the canal disease. Facial nerve paralysis may be an initial symptom.

Physical examination in the majority of patients will reveal a localized mass or nodule within the ear canal (48). Occasionally, some patients reveal an external canal that is narrowed by circumferential swellings, and a clinically unsuspected tumor is identified only when biopsy tissue is examined histologically. The radiographic studies, when performed early in the disease or symptomatology, usually reveal no bone abnormalities. In advanced cases of the neoplasm, bone destruction is often found in the mastoid and temporal regions. The mass may present clinically as a polyp, ulceration, granulation tissue, or simply a subepithelial swelling.

DIAGNOSIS

The biopsy is an extermely important part of the diagnostic procedure. An excisional biopsy is recommended. Aspiration biopsy and frozen section techniques are not believed reliable (37), owing to the histologic variation of these neoplasms and the possibility of getting a nonrepresentative section of tissue. The surgical specimen may have irregular, somewhat fragmented borders, especially in areas of osseous tissue. Because of this, Perzin

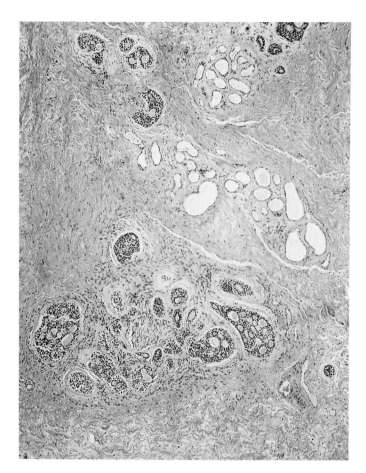

Figure 15.37. Adenoid cystic carcinoma clinically and histologically supporting origin from the ceruminal gland, revealing the typical cribriform morphology. Normal ceruminal glands are also seen. (Hematoxylin and eosin, ×25.)

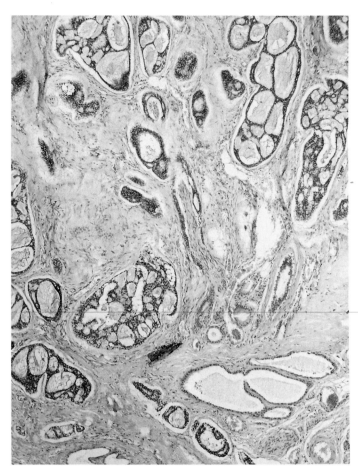

Figure 15.38. Higher magnification of the same adenoid cystic carcinoma as in Figure 15.37 in which perineural space invasion by neoplasm is noted. (Hematoxylin and eosin, ×63.)

et al. (48) recommended applying India ink to the fixed resection specimen so that the resected edge may be readily identified in the histologic specimen.

MICROSCOPIC FINDINGS

The major histologic pattern is that of a small, hyperchromatic nucleated cell, with little anaplasia, that is arranged in cribriform, cord-like, glandular, and basaloid patterns (Figs. 15.37–15.39). Some neoplasms will reveal a tubular histologic pattern containing a single layer of tumor cells. The type of morphology that supposedly carries the poorest prognosis is the solid cellular growth with a basaloid cellular appearance. Mucin-positive material can be found in the cribriform or tubular-type neoplastic formation, or the lumen can be filled with hyalinized eosinophilic material. The adenoid cystic carcinoma has a propensity for invasion of perineural and lymphatic spaces.

DIFFERENTIAL DIAGNOSIS

Histologically, adenoid cystic carcinoma can be incorrectly diagnosed as a basal cell carcinoma or a mixed tumor. Usually, the latter diagnosis is made in the aftermath of too small a biopsy specimen. The former diagnosis is difficult to rule out when the cribriform pattern is seen in an otherwise typical basal cell carcinoma. These basal cell neoplasms have been termed "adenoid cystic basal cell carcinoma" with the same local behavior of the typical nodular basal cell carcinoma. The possible origin of the adenoid cystic carcinoma arising primarily in the parotid

major salivary gland must be considered, and if such is the case, then a different therapeutic approach is needed.

PROGNOSTIC FACTORS

The following clinical situations were associated with a worse prognosis: extension to the parotid salivary gland, bone involvement, solid histologic tumor cell pattern, perineural invasion, and recurrent neoplastic disease at the resection site (48).

TREATMENT

For adenoid cystic carcinoma of the external auditory canal, whether it be confined to membranous tissue alone or involve the bony canal, the procedure advocated is that of a wide radical surgical resection. This is especially true when a histologic examination of previous surgically removed specimens demonstrates tumor at or near the lines of the surgical excision, or the preoperative assessment reveals advanced disease, or the tumor has recurred after a more limited resection. In the experience of one of the authors (V.J.H.), the extent of aggressiveness of the adenoid cystic carcinoma is underestimated at the preoperative clinical assessment, at the surgical resection, and often at the gross pathology examination of the specimen. The operative specimen should include those anatomical structures that have been mentioned previously in the surgical treatment of the ceruminous gland adenocarcinoma. The involvement by neoplasm of the middle ear or temporal bone with or without involvement of the facial nerve would entail a subtotal temporal bone resection. All

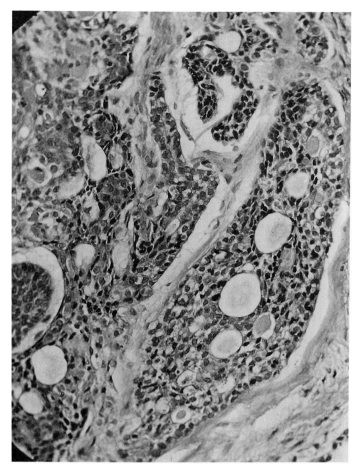

Figure 15.39. The cribriform and solid pattern areas are demonstrated in this adenoid cystic carcinoma of the external auditory canal. (Hematoxylin and eosin, ×200.)

surgical procedures are then followed by irradiation (37). Most authorities have agreed that the adenoid cystic carcinoma cannot be cured by radiation therapy, but it is difficult to prove that radiation therapy does not help prolong survival. It has definitely been successful in the palliation of pain and other symptoms.

NATURAL HISTORY

In a series of 16 patients (48), 7 had no evidence of recurrence following surgical resection (2–16 years following initial therapy), 2 were living with recurrent, unresectable tumor (15 and 16 years following initial treatment), 5 had died of the disease (3–20 years following therapy), 1 died of other causes, and 1 was lost to follow-up. Some patients died of tumor after a prolonged clinical course with multiple recurrences. Death was usually caused by intracranial extension by the tumor or by pulmonary metastases.

Mucoepidermoid Carcinoma

DEFINITION

Mucoepidermoid carcinoma is a tumor characterized by the presence of squamous cells, mucus-secreting cells, and cells of intermediate type (42).

There is the occasional report of a primary mucoepidermoid carcinoma of the external canal appearing in the medical literature (49), but these instances may well represent a ceruminous gland adenocarcinoma with prominent mucin production or,

possibly, the rare presentation of a primary parotid gland neoplasm in the external auditory canal (30). Gallager et al. (50) and Helwig (51) have reported primary mucoepidermoid carcinoma occurring in the skin, in both cases involving the foot. Pulec (49) has published two cases that were diagnosed as mucoepidermoid carcinomas of the external ear and has suggested their possible origin from the ceruminous glands. The AFIP OTR lists 2 patients with this diagnosis.

CLINICAL FINDINGS

Pulec's cases consisted of a 28- and a 58-year-old woman, while the AFIP OTR patients were a 29-year-old woman and a 22-year-old man. The female patient from the AFIP OTR appears to have been the same patient reported by Pulec. The main symptomatology was that of the presence of a mass and the sensation of blockage of the ear. The clinical description was only that of a pedunculated and pea-size mass.

MICROSCOPIC FINDINGS

A striking feature of the AFIP OTR cases was the presence of abundant material, present within glandular lumina and also occurring as intracellular globules, that gave a positive reaction to the PAS and mucicarmine histochemical stains. Beneath the epidermis there were ducts filled with secretion and lined by cuboidal or flat epithelium. Deeper, the tumor assumed a more solid aspect with a relative reduction in the amount of stroma (Figs. 15.40 and 15.41). Glandular spaces containing mucus were

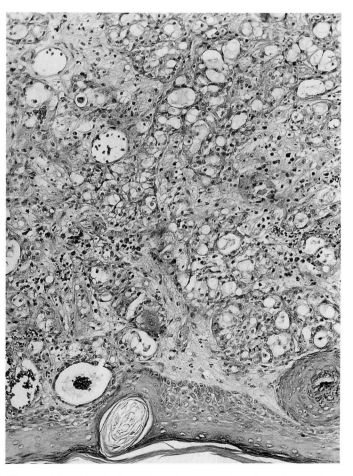

Figure 15.40. Histologic section of mucoepidermoid carcinoma of the external ear demonstrates a glandular architecture with prominent mucus production. (Hematoxylin and eosin, ×160.)

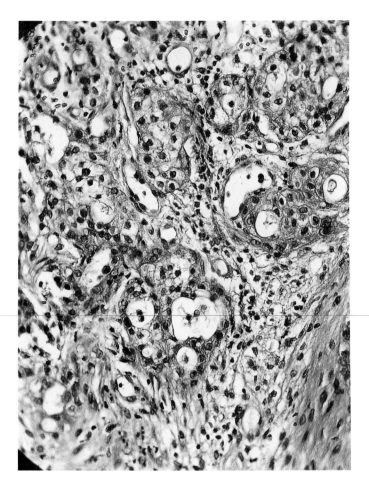

Figure 15.41. Higher histologic magnification of the same mucoepidermoid carcinoma as in Figure 15.40 supports a glandular morphology, with mucus-producing cells admixed with groups of epidermoid cells, qualifying the neoplasm as a mucoepidermoid carcinoma. (Hematoxylin and eosin, ×200.)

surrounded by clumps of cells, polyhedral-shaped with large nuclei and rarefied cytoplasm. Epidermoid features such as intercellular bridges or pearls were not demonstrated with light microscopy.

THERAPY AND PROGNOSIS

Pulec (49) stated that local excision of the mucoepidermoid carcinoma of the external auditory canal was inadequate. The histology tended to be of a low-grade differentiation, but he favored wide resection to include the external canal, radical mastoidectomy, excision of the mandibular condyle, and total parotidectomy with preservation of the facial nerve. The small number of patients prevents a decent estimation of the percentage of cures, but one of Pulec's patients has survived 6 years without recurrence.

NONCERUMINOUS GLAND ADENOMATOUS NEOPLASMS OF THE EXTERNAL EAR— ECCRINE CYLINDROMA

The benign eccrine cylindroma considered most likely to arise from sweat gland adnexa usually presents on the scalp but can occur on the face and neck. The neoplasm is typically a 0.5–1.5-cm smooth, firm, pink to red, hairless nodule in the skin. Scalp tumors have been referred to as turban tumors. They seldom ulcerate and are rarely painful. Females are affected twice as often as males. The onset is customarily in early adult life but may occur in childhood or adolescence.

The microscopic examination reveals well-circumscribed islands of epithelial cells arranged in a mosaic pattern invested by a narrow band of hyaline material and separated from one another by thin bonds of stroma (Fig. 15.42). The epithelial cells are of two types. One is large with a moderate amount of cytoplasm and a vesicular nucleus, and the other is a small cell with little cytoplasm and a compact nucleus. The smaller cells tend to palisade at the periphery of the nests, and the larger, centrally located cells surround duct-like spaces filled with eosinophilic hyaline material (Fig. 15.43). It is this material that surrounds the individual epithelial islands, forming a thick wall that is so characteristic of these tumors. The collection of intracellular acidic mucopolysaccharide substance can resemble the cribriform pattern of the adenoid cystic carcinoma.

The authors prefer that the designation of cylindroma be directed at this benign, usually safely surgically treated neoplasm and not connected with the adenoid cystic carcinoma, as has been the case in the past.

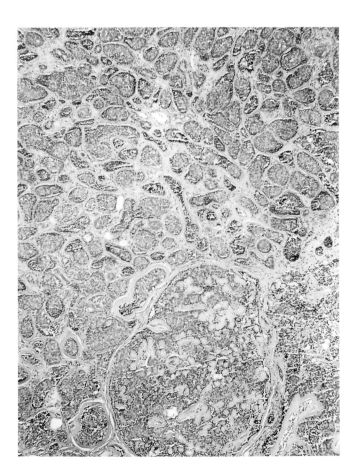

Figure 15.42. Histologic section of an eccrine cylindroma reveals circumscribed islands of epithelial cells arranged in a mosaic pattern invested by bands of hyaline material. (Hematoxylin and eosin, ×60.)

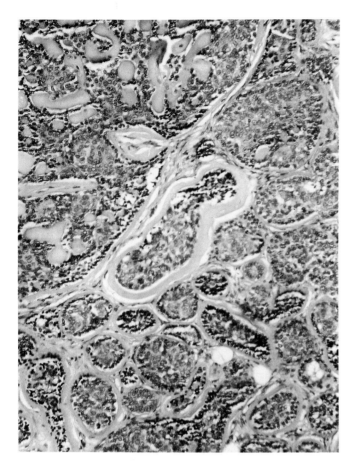

Figure 15.43. Higher magnification of the same neoplasm as in Figure 15.42 reveals a smaller cell tending to palisade at the periphery of the cell nests while the centrally located larger cells surround duct-like spaces filled with an eosinophilic mucopolysaccharide material. This latter feature can resemble the cribriform pattern of the adenoid cystic carcinoma. (Hematoxylin and eosin, ×160.)

References

1. Shuman R, Helwig EB. Chondrodermatitis helicis. Am J Clin Pathol 1954;24:126–144.
2. Metzger SA, Goodman ML. Chondrodermatitis helicis: a clinical re-evaluation and pathological review. Laryngoscope 1976;86:1402–1412.
3. Barker LP, Young AW, Sachs W. Chondrodermatitis of the ears. A differential study of nodules of the helix and antihelix. Arch Dermatol 1960;81:15–25.
4. Cannon CR. Bilateral chondrodermatitis helicis: case presentation and literature review. Am J Otol 1985;6:164–166.
5. Choi S, Lam K, Chan K, Ghadially FN, Ng AS. Enchondral pseudocyst of the auricle in Chinese. Arch Otolaryngol 1984;110:792–796.
6. Barnes L, Koss W, Nieland ML. Angiolymphoid hyperplasia with eosinophilia: a disease that may be confused with malignancy. Head Neck Surg 1980;2:425–434.
7. Rosai J, Gold J, Landry R. The histiocytoid hemangiomas. Hum Pathol 1979;10:707–730.
8. Suster S. Single case report: nodular angiolymphoid hyperplasia with eosinophilia. Am J Clin Pathol 1987;88:236–239.
9. Thompson JW, Colman M, Williamson C, Ward PH. Angiolymphoid hyperplasia with eosinophilia of the external ear canal. Arch Otolaryngol 1981;107:316–319.
10. Graham JH, Johnson WC, Helwig EB. Dermal pathology. Hagerstown, Maryland: Harper & Row, 1972.
11. Lund HZ. Tumors of the skin. In: Atlas of tumor pathology. 1st series, Fascicle 2. Washington, DC: Armed Forces Institute of Pathology, 1957.
12. Deutsch HJ. Tumor of the ear canal. Seborrheic keratosis. Arch Otolaryngol 1970;91:80–81.
13. Lambert PR, Fechner RE, Hatcher CP. Seborrheic keratosis of the ear canal. Otolaryngol Head Neck Surg 1987;96:198–201.
14. Mehregan AH. Pinkus' guide to dermatohistopathology. 4th ed. Norwalk, Connecticut: Appleton-Century-Crofts, 1986.
15. Rulon DB, Helwig EB. Cutaneous sebaceous neoplasms. Cancer 1974;33:82–102.
16. Batsakis JG, Littler ER, Leahy MS. Sebaceous cell lesions of the head and neck. Arch Otolaryngol 1972;95:151–157.
17. Doble HP II, Snyder G, Carpenter RJ III. Sebaceous cell carcinoma of the external auditory canal. Otolaryngol Head Neck Surg 1981;89:685–688.
18. Toppozada HH. A review on sebaceous adenoma with report of a case in the external auditory meatus. J Laryngol Otol 1963;77:970–973.
19. Boniuk M, Zimmerman LE. Sebaceous carcinoma of the eyelid, eyebrow, caruncle and orbit. Tr Am Acad Ophthalmol Otol 1968;72:619–642.
20. Krausen AS, Ansel DG, Mays BR. Pilomatrixoma masquerading as a parotid mass. Laryngoscope 1974;84:528–535.
21. Forbis R Jr, Helwig EB. Pilomatrixoma (calcified epithelioma). Arch Dermatol 1961;83:608–618.
22. Cazers JS, Okum MR, Pearson H. Pigmented calcifying epithelioma. Review and presentation of a case with unusual features. Arch Dermatol 1974;110:773–774.
23. Lopansri S, Mihm MC. Pilomatrix carcinoma or calcifying epitheliocarcinoma of Malherbe. A case report and review of literature. Cancer 1980;45:2368–2373.
24. Sasaki CT, Yue A, Enriques R. Giant calcifying epithelioma. Arch Otolaryngol 1976;102:753–755.
25. Harper PS. Calcifying epithelioma of Malherbe. Association with myotonic muscular dystrophy. Arch Dermatol 1972;106:41–44.
26. Patterson HC. Facial keratoacanthoma. Otolaryngol Head Neck Surg 1983;91:263–270.
27. Senturia BH, Marcus MD, Lucente FE. Diseases of the external ear. An otologic-dermatologic manual. 2nd ed. New York: Grune & Stratton, 1980.
28. Zehekson AS, Lynch FW. Electron microscopy of virus-like particles in keratoacanthoma. J Invest Dermatol 1961;37:79–83.
29. Ghadially FN. Keratoacanthoma. In: Fitzpatrick TB, et al, eds. Dermatology in general medicine. New York: McGraw-Hill, 1971.
30. Hyams VJ, Batsakis JG, Michaels L. Tumors of the upper respiratory tract and ear. In: Atlas of tumor pathology. 2nd series, Fascicle 25. Washington, DC: Armed Forces Institute of Pathology, 1988.
31. Johnstone JM, Lennox B, Watson AJ. Five cases of hidradenoma of the external auditory meatus: so-called ceruminoma. J Pathol Bacteriol 1957;73:421–427.
32. Cankar V, Crowley H. Tumors of ceruminous glands: a clinicopathological study of seven cases. Cancer 1964;17:67–75.
33. Lever WF, Schaumburg-Lever G. Histopathology of the skin. 5th ed. Philadelphia: JB Lippincott, 1975.
34. Welti CV, Pardo V, Millar M, Derdson K. Tumors of ceruminous glands. Cancer 1972;29:1169.
35. Main T, Lim D. The human external auditory canal secretory system. An ultrastructural study. Laryngoscope 1976;85:1164.
36. Habib MA. Ceruminoma in association with other sweat gland tumours. J Laryngol Otol 1981;95:415–420.
37. Hicks, GW. Tumors arising from the glandular structures of the external auditory canal. Laryngoscope 1983;93:326–340.
38. Dehner LP, Chen KTK. Primary tumors of the external and middle ear. Benign and malignant glandular neoplasms. Arch Otolaryngol 1980;106:13–19.
39. Neldner KH. Ceruminoma. Arch Dermatol 1968;98:344–348.
40. Warren S, Gates O. Carcinoma of ceruminous gland. Am J Pathol 1941;22:821–829.
41. Fligiel Z, Kaneko M. Extramammary Paget's disease of the external ear canal in association with ceruminous gland carcinoma. A case report. Cancer 1975;36:1072–1076.
42. Thackray AC. Histological typing of salivary gland tumors. Int Histol Classif Tumors No 7, 1972.
43. Goldenberg RA, Block BL. Pleomorphic adenoma manifesting as aural polyp. Arch Otolaryngol 1980;106:440–441.
44. Braun GA, Lowry LD, Meyers A. Bilateral choristomas of the external auditory canals. Arch Otolaryngol 1978;104:467–468.

45. Stout AP, Gorman JG. Mixed tumors of the skin of the salivary gland type. Cancer 1959;12:537–543.
46. Smith HW, Duarte I. Mixed tumors of the external auditory canal. Arch Otolaryngol 1962;75:28–33.
47. Helwig EB, Hackney VC. Syringoadenoma papilliferum. Arch Dermatol 1955;71:361.
48. Perzin KH, Gullane P, Conley J. Adenoid cystic carcinoma involving the external auditory canal. A clincopathologic study of 16 cases. Cancer 1982;50:2873–2883.
49. Pulec JL. Glandular tumors of the external auditory canal. Laryngoscope 1977;87:1601–1612.
50. Gallager MD, Miller GV, Grampa G. Primary mucoepidermoid carcinoma of the skin. Report of a case. Cancer 1959;12:286–288.
51. Helwig EB. Seminar on skin neoplasms and dermatoses. In: Proceedings of the American Society of Clinical Pathologists. Washington, DC, September 11, 1954. Washington, DC: American Society of Clinical Pathologists, 1955.

16/ Adenomatous Neoplasms of the Middle Ear Space

Adenomatous neoplasms, benign and malignant, arising in the middle ear cleft do not form an appreciable percentage of neoplasia of the temporal bone, but of the 521 patients listed in the Armed Forces Institute of Pathology (AFIP) Otolaryngic Tumor Registry (OTR) (1945–1985) as possessing primary middle ear neoplasms, 188 had adenomatous growths. This latter group included essentially an entity that is considered an adenoma of the middle ear mucosa. There were also a lesser number of primary histologic and clinical adenocarcinomas and some that were metastatic from regional and distal primary sites.

There is confusion as to the histologic and clinical classification of adenomatous neoplasia arising in the temporal bone, particularly when involving a specialized and perplexing area such as the middle ear. These problems are enumerated in an excellent publication on the middle ear adenomas by Mills and Fechner (1). The first adenomatous neoplasm discussed below is an adenoma of the middle ear. Although troublesome aspects of this entity are detailed in the discussion, there is disagreement as to whether this entity should be considered a simple adenoma, a carcinoid tumor, or an adenocarcinoma. This middle ear adenoma, as well as the primary adenocarcinoma of the middle ear, is a unique topic that is relatively new to the medical literature.

Early medical literature considered all adenomatous neoplasms originating in the temporal bone as adenocarcinomas, and it was not until 1976 that two articles were published that suggested that benign-behaving adenomas could arise from the middle ear area (2, 3). Since these publications, there have been numerous reports of an acceptance of the existence of the middle ear mucosal adenoma (4–10). However, other terminologies have been utilized in recent publications, such as carcinoid tumor, ceruminous gland adenoma, monomorphic adenoma, and middle ear adenocarcinoma, that portray tumors histologically identical with the middle ear mucosal adenoma.

As suggested above, there is also an adenomatous neoplasm listed in the AFIP OTR that qualifies both clinically and histologically as an adenocarcinoma, although it occurred much less frequently than the middle ear adenoma. The neoplastic entity, adenocarcinoma of the middle ear, is discussed later in detail.

MIDDLE EAR ADENOMA

Definition

Middle ear adenoma (also known as adenocarcinoma, carcinoid tumor, monomorphic adenoma, and ceruminous gland adenoma of the middle ear), is a benign neoplasm originating in the middle ear, probably from middle ear mucosa, and is a variably encapsulated, avascular, fleshy gross tumefaction capable of filling the middle ear cleft from the Eustachian tube to the mastoid cells. In most patients, however, there is no radiologic, clinical, or histologic evidence of aggression. Metastases have not been reported.

Incidence

In the years 1976–1985, there were 116 patients with the diagnosis of middle ear adenoma added to the AFIP OTR. There were 74 males to 42 females. The ages ranged from 5 to 80 years, with an average age of onset of 40 years, but three-quarters of the neoplasms occurred in patients in the second through the fourth decade. Two patients were mentioned as having involvement of the temporal bone, 8 were listed as having the external auditory canal as the site of the tumor, and 106 were noted to have only middle ear tumor.

Clinical Presentation

Mills and Fechner (1) listed the presenting symptoms in a series of 28 patients, in order of decreasing frequency, as decreased hearing, tinnitus, asymptomatic, fullness and/or mass, pain, facial weakness, vertigo, and drainage. In this group, patients experienced these symptoms for 3 months to 10 years. Most had been symptomatic for over a year at diagnosis (median duration 4.5 years). In 21 patients there was at least one radiologic procedure documented (1). In none of these patients was bony erosion described, and in 6 patients only, nonspecific changes included sclerotic or cloudy mastoid air cells. The left side was involved in 18 patients, and the right side was involved in 12 patients. Clinical examination of the involved ear would reveal a clean, normal external auditory canal and an intact drum in three-quarters of the patients. Those examinations that did reveal a perforated tympanic membrane did occasionally display a protrusion of neoplasm through the drum defect. At operation, the neoplasm was described as a variably encapsulated, lobulated, avascular, rubbery gray-tan to pinkish-white to yellow tumor. Some middle ear adenomas were more diffuse and appeared as a thick layer of "granulation tissue" coating the middle ear contents. The tumor mass could fill the mesotympanum with possible extension to the attic, additus, antrum, and surrounding mastoid air spaces or to and into the Eustachian tube. In the rare case, one of the authors (V.J.H.) has noted tumor present in the external auditory canal that supported spread from the middle ear around the annulus of an intact drum. Hagan et al. (4) recorded that the tumor resisted fragmentation during biopsy, its tenacious character contrasted with the friable cholesteatoma, its resiliency contrasted with the gritty carcinoma, and its avascularity contrasted with the hemorrhagic occipital-temporal paraganglioma.

Mills and Fechner (1) noted one case of erosion of bone by tumor, and such was questioned in one other case. The middle ear neoplasms that were designated as carcinoid tumors (11–14) did present the essentially same signs, symptoms, and operative findings as the so-called middle ear adenomas.

A number of case reports have designated a middle ear neoplasm as a ceruminous gland adenoma (15) or adenocarcinoma (16) or as a simple adenocarcinoma of middle ear origin. Some of these neoplasms would occasionally reveal bone destruction and some local aggression, but most behaved very blandly, very much like the middle ear adenoma described above.

Light Microscopic Findings

According to Mills and Fechner (1), the middle ear adenoma formed histologically diverse patterns, both from tumor to tumor and within the same lesion. It was impossible to identify a capsule on the histologic specimens because the tissue was divided at surgery and the minute pieces submitted for histology could not be oriented as to the presence of a capsule (Fig. 16.1). The neoplasms were mainly composed of cytologically similar cells. They were columnar to cuboidal or slightly rounded and closely resembled normal middle ear epithelium (Fig. 16.2). The tumor cells were best seen in areas where they were arranged in sheets. Although most were slightly ovoid, a few were round, and occasionally their contour was markedly irregular. Regardless of the shape of the cell, nearly all had a maximum width of 14–16 μm.

The cytoplasm of most cells was eosinophilic and finely granular to powdery, with a minority having small vacuoles lo-

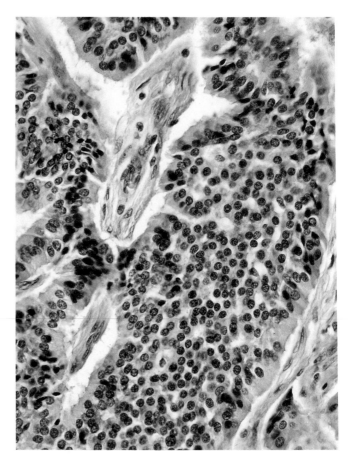

Figure 16.2. Magnification showing the uniformity of neoplastic cells and the formation of glandular architecture. The tumor cells resemble the normal middle ear mucosal cell. (Hematoxylin and eosin, ×160.)

cated in the periphery. Rarely, the entire cytoplasm was finely vacuolated. Lipofuscin was rarely seen within the cytoplasm.

The nucleus was typically round to ovoid, occupying 30–60% of the cell volume (Fig. 16.3). It was usually eccentric and occasionally appeared to bulge beyond the cell membrane. This nuclear eccentricity resembled a plasma cell, and sheets of such tumor cells were occasionally mistaken for a plasmacytoma. However, the nuclei had an evenly distributed chromatin that ranged from light powdery to dark, coarsely staining granules and not the "wheel spoke" chromatin arrangement that characterizes plasma cells. Rarely, a small, single nucleolus was recognizable. Mitosis was not found.

In some foci, the epithelium formed solid sheets of closely packed cells with a few arterioles, venules, and capillaries as the only other element (Fig. 16.4). In some middle ear adenomas there were irregular strands of tumor cells intermixed with fibrous tissue that suggested a crushing artifact (Fig. 16.5). The cell groups were tightly bunched, crowded, and compressed to a dark irregular nucleus and little if any visible cytoplasm.

The stroma throughout all tumors varied from loose to myxomatous, to edematous fibrous tissue, to sparsely cellular, densely collagenized areas. Usually, the fibrous tissue contained scattered individual tumor cell nests (Fig. 16.6). There was great variation in the vascularity of the desmoplastic areas.

Well-formed glandular formations were prominently seen, and many lumina contained an amorphous secretory product. "Back-to-back" arrangements were common (Figs. 16.7 and 16.8). Some glands were simple tubular structures lined by a

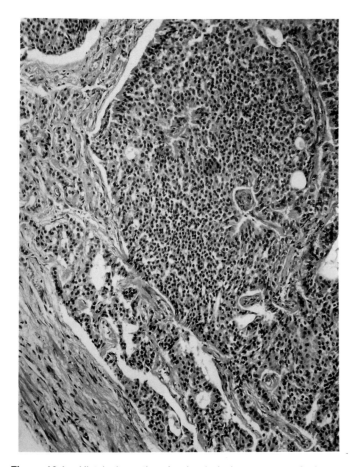

Figure 16.1. Histologic section showing typical appearance of adenoma of middle ear mucosa, with areas of sheets of small uniform cells alternating with foci of definite glandular structures. (Hematoxylin and eosin, ×63.)

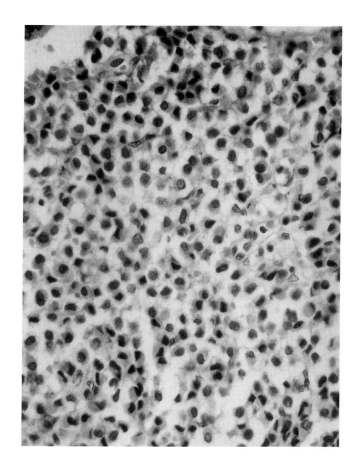

Figure 16.3. Histologic section of typical round to ovoid cell of middle ear adenoma, with a nucleus occupying the greater portion of the cell volume. The cells are arranged in a sheet-like pattern and, along with some nuclear eccentricity, resemble plasma cells. (Hematoxylin and eosin, ×160.)

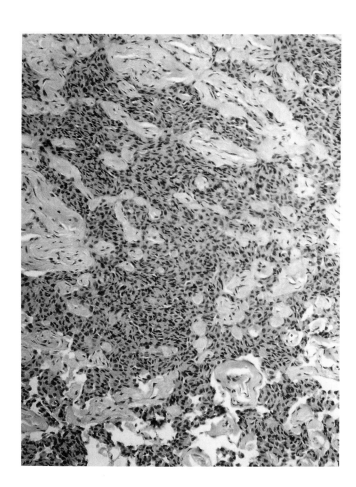

Figure 16.4. In this microscopic view of a middle ear adenoma, the tumor cells form solid sheets of closely packed cells, with the intervening stroma containing vascular and peripheral nerve structures. (Hematoxylin and eosin, ×63.)

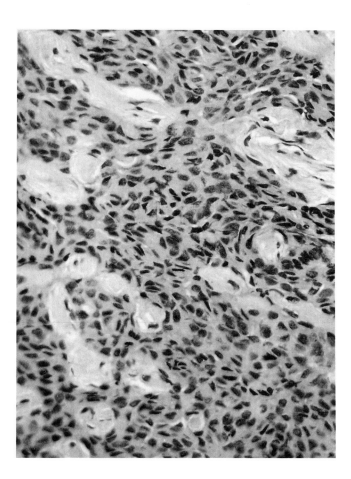

Figure 16.5. Higher magnification of the same adenoma as in Figure 16.4 supports compression of the tumor and suggests the so-called "crush artifact." (Hematoxylin and eosin, ×160.)

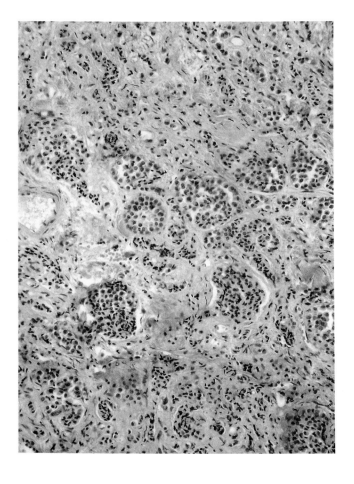

Figure 16.6. Microphoto emphasizing the sparsely cellular stromal element with scattered individual tumor cell rests. (Hematoxylin and eosin, ×63.)

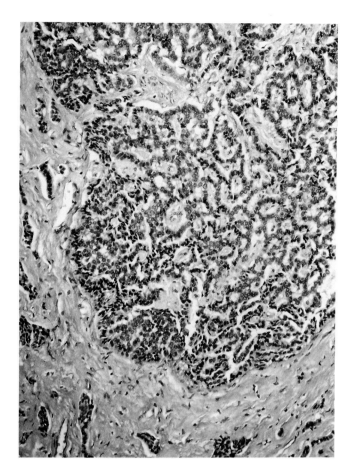

Figure 16.7. Adenomatous arrangement of tumor cells is prominent in this middle ear adenoma with a prominent "back-to-back" glandular component. (Hematoxylin and eosin, ×63.)

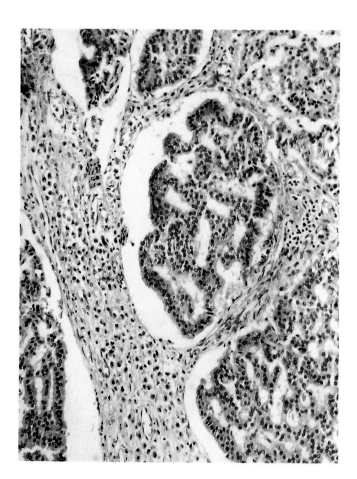

Figure 16.8. Higher magnification of the glandular tumor arrangement found in Figure 16.7 suggests some luminal secretion that can stain positive for mucin. (Hematoxylin and eosin, ×160.)

single layer of cells and separated by fibrous tissue. Lumen formation could also occur within solid sheets of cells. One pattern consisted of trabecular cords of tumor formed by single to multiple layers of cells (Fig. 16.9).

Mills and Fechner (1) noted tumor growing immediately beneath the outer squamous lining of the tympanic membrane and extending around the membrane beneath the skin of the external auditory canal. This confirms the previous clinical notation of the neoplasm growing from the middle ear around the annulus of drum into the external canal. They noted one instance of microscopic invasion of bone in the region of the facial nerve. One of the authors (V.J.H.) has also noted fragments of histologically benign keratinizing stratified squamous epithelium among tumor tissue, usually suggesting that it is a surface covering. Of interest is the finding that these particular tumors accompanied a drum perforation together with a history of bone erosion or facial nerve weakness. These findings support the occurrence of a middle ear cholesteatoma forming among the tumor mass and being responsible for the local aggressive impression. A rare middle ear adenoma will reveal an area of middle ear mucosa transposing into neoplasms (Fig. 16.10), which supports the contention that middle ear lining cells are the origin of the middle ear adenoma (2).

Argyrophilic granules were noted in some tumors when the Grimelius technique was utilized (Fig. 16.11) (1). When the Churukian-Schenk technique was used, the granules were not as prominent. Mills and Fechner (1) utilized the immunoperoxidase staining techniques to demonstrate lysozyme in all tumors tested. Most examiners have readily demonstrated mucin in the glandular lumen, on the luminal surface of the tumor cells, and occasionally in the fibrous stroma, and some have noted it within the tumor cell cytoplasm. Murphy et al. (11) also demonstrated argyrophilic granules, but the Fontana-Masson stain (for melanin and argentaffin), ferric ferricyanide (for iron), and periodic acid-Schiff (PAS) stain, with and without diastase digestion, were negative. Stanley et al. (12) using a battery of immunoperoxide stains found a tumor that stained positive for cytokeratin and pancreatic polypeptide but was negative for lysozyme, prolactin, calcitonin, serotonin, neuron-specific enolase, glial and neural filaments, S100 protein, and other enzymes. Those investigators who utilized formaldehyde-induced fluorescence on the tumor obtained positive results.

Three patients in the AFIP OTR presented with all the signs and symptoms, including the operative findings, of the middle ear adenoma, but on histologic examination there was a papillomatous proliferation consisting of cytologically benign epidermoid cells admixed with tall columnar cells that suggested middle ear mucosal origin (Figs. 16.12 and 16.13). There was even a suggestion of an "inversion"-type papilloma into the underlying stroma, much as is seen in the sinonasal cavity papillomas. These three patients all had a benign clinical course following surgery, with no recurrences or other complications.

Electron Microscopy Findings

The ultrastructural descriptions varied among different reports. Only a small portion of the tumors were so examined. Hyams and Michaels (2) found the tumor composed of acini of cells in one or two rows. A basal lamina delimited the deep aspect of the lining cells. In the tumor cell cytoplasm, in addi-

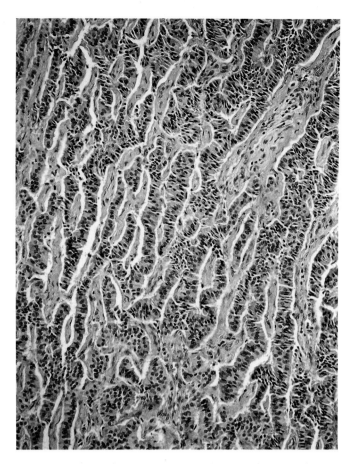

Figure 16.9. Prominent trabecular architecture of a middle ear adenoma. (Hematoxylin and eosin, × 160.)

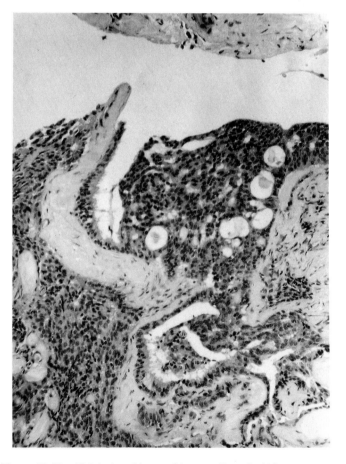

Figure 16.10. Histologic evidence of transposition of middle ear mucosa into neoplasm, a rare finding. (Hematoxylin and eosin, × 160.)

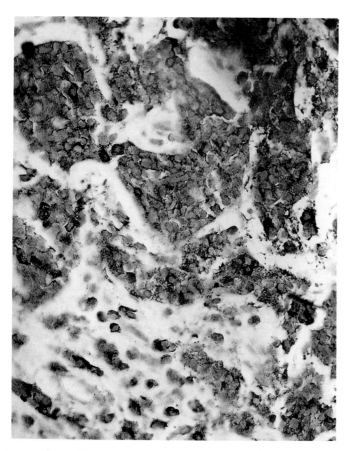

Figure 16.11. Special stained section showing argyrophilic granules within tumor cell cytoplasm. (Grimelius stain, ×250.)

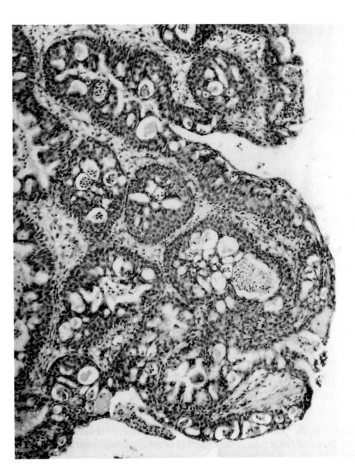

Figure 16.13. Higher magnification of the rare benign squamous cell middle ear tumor seen in Figure 16.12 supports an admixture of the squamous cell element with a secretory-type epithelium. (Hematoxylin and eosin, ×160.)

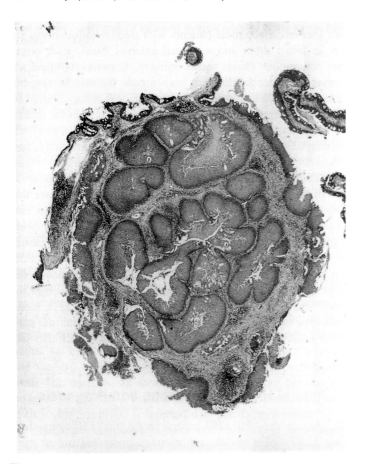

Figure 16.12. Rare form of benign middle ear tumor consisting of benign cytologic-appearing squamous cell epithelium. There is also a suggestion of "inversion" of the neoplasm into underlying stroma. (Hematoxylin and eosin, ×25.)

tion to mitochondria, rough endoplasmic reticulum and large electron-dense non-membrane-bound granules were present. A rare intracytoplasmic "myelin figure" was identified. From the luminal cell surface, microvilli were delineated. Desmosomes were present at points of contact. The stroma revealed only bundles of collagen fibers. Hyams and Michaels (2) were also able to demonstrate intracytoplasmic membrane-limited dense granules (greater than 300 nm in diameter) on other tumors (Figs. 16.14 and 16.15). These were in a separate group of cells, other than the surface cells, that revealed the microvilli. Light and dark cells were seen, and perinuclear microfilaments were noted, but the latter were not considered characteristic of myoepithelial cells. Kochilas et al. (10) noted some cells exhibiting large cytoplasmic projections into the lumen that were considered cilia-like.

The *carcinoid* controversy is confusing. Four papers (11–14) refer to these middle ear adenomatous tumors as carcinoid tumors. There is nothing in the clinical history that would separate these patients from those discussed earlier with middle ear adenoma. One patient was tested for urine 5-hydroxyindoleacetic acid, and the results were normal (11). There was nothing different in the operative findings. The presentation of the microscopy of these published cases is identical with that noted in the middle ear adenoma. The histochemistry has, with the positive Grimelius stain and formaldehyde-induced fluorescent studies for catecholamines, supported the idea of a carcinoid-type cell. Even more supportive of the idea that these are carcinoid tumors is the

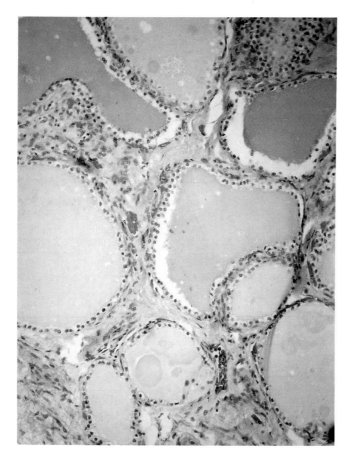

Figure 17.5. Histologic section of primary papillary cystadenocarcinoma of the temporal bone emphasizes particularly its resemblance to a thyroid neoplasm, including even the colloid and scalloping appearance. (Hematoxylin and eosin, ×160.)

tain mucin. The immunoperoxidase studies for the thyroglobulin antibody have been negative. The stroma is variable and usually consists of hyalinized connective tissue. The neoplasm and its stroma can be found replacing the osseous tissue of temporal bone.

Histogenesis

We would assume that these papillary cystadenocarcinomas of the middle ear arise from the middle ear mucosa, although we have not histologically noted the neoplasm arising from such epithelium. Some investigators have noted an aberrant papillary structure in the vestibular end of the cochlear duct, sometimes occurring in conjunction with Ménière's disease, so that Schuknecht (5) wondered if such a structure represented an aberrant choroid plexus and raised the question as to whether this structure could be the cause of endolymphatic hydrops. Heffner (6) suggested that this papillary structure within the endolymph might be the etiology of the papillary cystadenocarcinoma.

Differential Diagnosis

This low-grade malignant neoplasm must first be differentiated from the benign adenoma of the middle ear. Overall, the middle ear adenoma is accompanied by all the symptoms, signs, and findings of a benign middle ear neoplasm. Rarely, the be-

nign adenoma will reveal minimal aggressive findings such as bone erosion or facial nerve involvement, and certainly such symptomatology is confusing, but if a middle ear adenomatous tumor is unmistakenly acting aggressively and destructively, it is obviously not the benign middle ear adenoma, regardless of any micromorphologic findings, and has to be considered and treated as a malignant neoplasm.

The possibility of a metastatic adenocarcinoma in the temporal bone must also be ruled out, as discussed in the differential diagnosis of the middle ear adenoma. Gobel et al. (2) believed that the occipital temporal paraganglioma (glomus tumor) could cause differential diagnostic problems, especially preoperatively. Angiography would be of help in this distinction.

Treatment

Combination therapy appears to be the treatment of choice of the presenters in the medical literature (1–4, 7). The extent of the surgical approach varied among operators. Some suggested a subtotal temporal bone removal, while others believed an operative plan for complete removal of the neoplasm was sufficient. Glasscock et al. (7) believed that the same surgical approach and technique that are followed in the surgical resection of large glomus jugulare tumors would be sufficient. All believed that the surgery should be followed by significant doses of radiotherapy.

Prognosis

Only 1 patient in the AFIP OTR died of this low-grade malignant neoplasm, and this patient was a middle-aged woman who had been confined to a mental institution because of psychotic symptoms. After her death, an autopsy provided the first clue that a papillary cystadenocarcinoma had involved the temporal bone with extension into the posterior cranial fossa and cerebellum. Review of the medical literature supports a 15–20% incidence of mortality from the papillary cystadenocarcinoma. Death was usually due to uncontrolled encroachment into adjacent vital structures, especially the cranial cavity. Most of the remaining patients were considered cured, as were those contained in the AFIP OTR. Those in the latter group were without symptoms of tumor for 2–10 years following surgical treatment. There was no metastatic disease detected in the cured group or in those who died from the neoplasm.

HIGH-GRADE (UNDIFFERENTIATED) ADENOCARCINOMA OR ADENOID CYSTIC CARCINOMA OF THE MIDDLE EAR

High-grade adenocarcinoma of the middle ear is a rare aggressive neoplasm considered to be poorly differentiated, i.e., not exhibiting the cystadenocarcinoma histologic features, and on occasion, it may micromorphologically suggest an adenoid cystic carcinoma (Figs. 17.6 and 17.7). The simultaneous occurrence of a rapid, aggressive, destructive clinical course is essential for this diagnosis. Metastasis to regional and distant sites may be expected. Metastasis to the middle ear from a regional or distal primary site must be ruled out if possible.

In the AFIP OTR, there were only 2 patients who fitted this description, i.e., presented with a highly aggressive, appar-

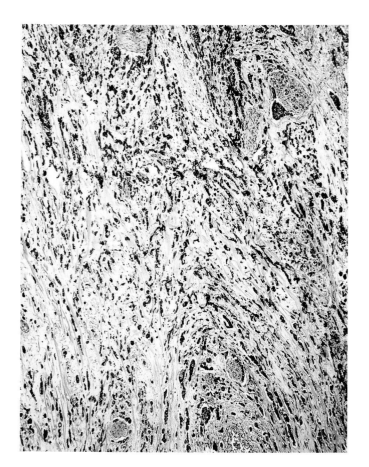

Figure 17.6. Histologic section of high-grade or anaplastic primary temporal bone adenocarcinoma from one of only two patients with this neoplasm who are listed in the AFIP OTR. (Hematoxylin and eosin, ×25.)

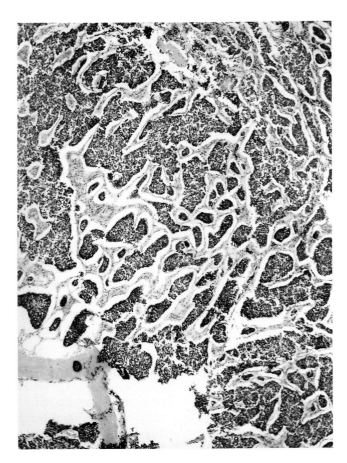

Figure 17.7. Histologic section of high-grade or anaplastic primary temporal bone adenocarcinoma from one of only two patients with this neoplasm who are listed in the AFIP OTR. (Hematoxylin and eosin, ×63.)

ently primary middle ear adenocarcinoma. These were 2 middle-aged men. Both patients underwent radical surgical procedures in addition to radiation therapy but succumbed to local and systemic metastatic neoplasms, one 6 months following initial surgery and the other 1½ years after diagnosis and treatment. Four papers in the medical literature were considered reports of adenoid cystic carcinoma involving the middle ear. In one report, the tumor was obviously, from accompanying illustrations, an adenoma of the middle ear. In the other three reports the illustrations could be considered histologically consistent with an adenoid cystic carcinoma.

Cannon and McLean (8) reported a 71-year-old woman with a 3–4-year history of right-sided tinnitus and decreased hearing with eventual right facial nerve involvement and other cranial nerve weakness. Radiographic examination confirmed middle ear and petrous apex bone destruction. At operation, a bluish mass was detected in the hypotympanum. Histology supported the finding of a focus of neoplasm that resembled adenoid cystic carcinoma. Another case report was of an adenoid cystic carcinoma involving the vertical portion of the facial nerve (9), but no further information was available as to a primary site. The histology of these neoplasms is discussed under the adenoid cystic adenocarcinoma of the ceruminous glands of the external auditory canal (Chapter 15).

Johnston and Strong (10) presented a case report of a primary mucoepidermoid carcinoma of the mastoid in a 79-year-old man whose chief complaint was of a tender swelling behind his ear for 2 months. At surgical exploration, a ''moth-eaten''

cortical defect was found with the mastoid filled with a firm, avascular tumor. The dura of the middle and posterior fossae was found to be studded with tumor nodules. Histology supported the finding of a neoplasm composed of epidermoid and glandular cancer tissue, with strong suggestions of mucin production by the latter. The designation as a high-grade mucoepidermoid carcinoma cannot be considered in error, although one wonders if this neoplasm could not be considered an adenosquamous cell carcinoma, since a squamous cell carcinoma retains its ability to produce mucus-producing neoplastic cells. Such multipotential mucosa is certainly present in the middle ear. The argument is academic. A follow-up history of this patient was not provided, but we would assume the prognosis was fatal.

Fortunately, involvement of the middle ear by a primary high-grade adenocarcinoma or adenoid cystic carcinoma is apparently rare, since they afford a poor prognosis regardless of the choice of therapy. Also, because of its rarity there has not been a consensus as to the best therapeutic approach.

References

1. Schüller DE, Conley JJ, Goodman JH, Clausen KP, Miller WJ. Primary adenocarcinoma of the middle ear. Otolaryngol Head Neck Surg 1983; 91:280–283.
2. Gobel, JA, Smith PG, Kemink JL, Graham MD. Primary adenocarcinoma of the temporal bone mimicking paragangliomas: radiographic and clinical recognition. Otolaryngol Head Neck Surg 1987;96:231–238.
3. Gulya AJ, Glasscock ME, Pensak ML. Primary adenocarcinoma of the

19/ Tumors and Lesions of the Melanogenic System—Pigmented Nevi and Malignant Melanoma

PIGMENTED NEVI

Pigmented nevi of various types and potentials may occur on the external ear, especially the pinna, but also in the external auditory canal. Their occurrence in the middle ear would be unusual. During embryonic life, the primitive melanoblast migrates from the neural crest to its ultimate resting place in the epidermis where, in its mature state, it supposedly becomes a functioning melanocyte. Apparently, migration and development may be altered or interrupted in some manner, resulting in abnormal developmental lesions such as the pigmented nevi. These nevi may be present at birth or may appear later in life and imply mainly a benign tumor unless specially qualified. Most of pigmented nevi discussed below can occur on the auricle and possibly in the external auditory canal, but the Armed Forces Institute of Pathology (AFIP) Otolaryngic Tumor Registry (OTR) contains only a few cases, since these skin entities are collected by the dermatopathology department of the AFIP or perhaps contributors do not feel a need for consultation because of their familiar-

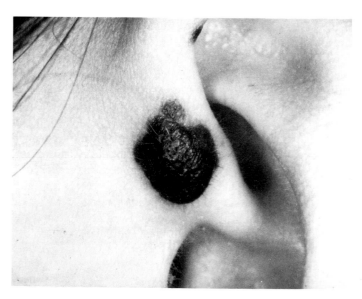

Figure 19.2. The intradermal nevus will most likely present clinically as a skin lesion with a dome-shaped or polypoid configuration and prominent pigmentation and surface hair.

ity with the entity. Pack et al. (1) stated that one rarely sees pigmented lesions on the external ear in comparison with the rest of the body.

The *ephelis* (plural: *ephelides*) is the common "freckle" that presents as a small macular area of pigmented skin, and the *lentigo* (plural: *lentigines*) is a pigmented skin lesion of various dimensions that can occur in the juvenile or can occur in the elderly as a "senile lentigo." These lesions are usually not included as true nevi.

The *junctional nevus* is a flat, macular, pigmented skin lesion devoid of hair (Fig. 19.1), which may present at birth or may appear at any age. Histologically, nests of nevus cells are found at the epidermal-dermal junction. In the *intradermal nevus* the nevus cells are confined entirely to the dermis; the overall lesion commonly assumes a dome-like, nodular, or a polypoid configuration and may be pigmented and hairy, with the latter being a particular clinical point of identification (Fig. 19.2). Histologically, although the nevus cells that may be multinucleated are virtually limited to the dermis, there may be a few cells found at the epidermal-dermal junction. The *compound nevus* is a small, possibly papillary pigmented and hairy tumor (Fig. 19.3) that histologically contains both junctional and intradermal nevus components.

The *blue nevus,* although not reported on the external ear, can involve the face and the preauricular ear skin and may be known as Mongolian spots or the nevus of Ota. They are generally flat, blue-black or brownish-black, and hairless. Micromorphologically, they are formed of elongated pigmented mel-

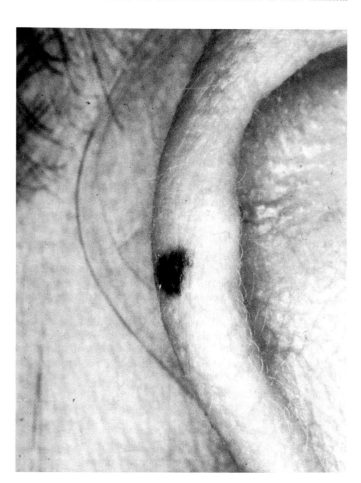

Figure 19.1. Clinical presentation of junctional nevus represented by a flat, macular, pigmented skin lesion.

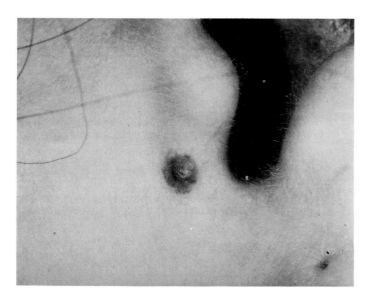

Figure 19.3. The compound nevus is usually a small, papular, pigmented skin surface tumor, possibly with surface hairs.

anocytes (Fig. 19.4) packed in groups that are generally parallel to the epidermis and may extend into the subcutaneous fat.

Epithelioid and/or spindle cell nevus (juvenile melanoma) occurs primarily in children and, although sometimes disturbing, microscopically exhibits an essentially benign biologic behavior. Clinically, it is a benign-appearing, lightly pigmented, dome-shaped lesion commonly occurring on the face but also occurring

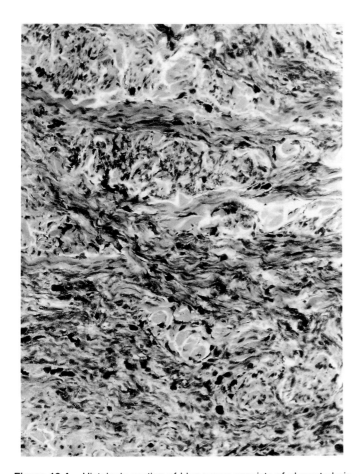

Figure 19.4. Histologic section of blue nevus consists of elongated pigmented melanocytes packed in groups that are generally parallel to the epidermis; the nevus quite often extends into the subcutaneous skin layer. (Hematoxylin and eosin, ×160.)

elsewhere. Histologically, it is a compound nevus that occasionally shows considerable junctional changes, and the tumor cells are elongated and/or rounded and epithelioid in appearance, with usually minimal or absent melanin pigment. Mitotic figures may be quite numerous. The epithelioid cells may reveal the presence of multinucleated cells resembling the Touton giant cell. This nevus is frequently confused histologically with malignant melanoma and, although not exclusively found in children, is an important diagnostic differentiation.

The *giant pigmented nevus, balloon cell nevus,* and *halo nevus* may rarely involve the external ear.

The *melanotic freckle* or *nevus of Hutchinson (lentigo maligna)* is considered a precancerous neoplasm (2) that in its most characteristic form occurs as a flat, pigmented macule on the cheek or preauricular area of an elderly person. There is no sex preference, although it occurs only in Caucasians. The lesion grows peripherally over a period of years and may attain an area of several centimeters. Histologically, there is an accumulation of mainly abnormal melanocytes along the lower border of the epidermis, and this accumulation is occasionally accompanied by similar cells throughout the whole thickness of the epidermis and possibly the outer layer of hair follicles. The melanoma that may develop from this lesion appears to be less aggressive than the usual nodular malignant melanoma, because of its lateral or horizontal spread.

Treatment

These benign nevi and precancerous lesions may require local complete surgical removal for the sake of cosmesis. When, however, the junctional, the compound, and rarely the blue nevus as well as the melanotic freckle (nevus of Hutchinson) clinically have a suspicious appearance with irritation and a suggestion of growth, they must be surgically removed for prophylaxis.

MALIGNANT MELANOMA

Definition

Malignant melanoma (also known as malignant nevocytoma, melanoblastoma, melanocarcinoma, melanocytoblastoma, melanoepithelioma, melanoma, melanosarcoma, nevocarcinoma, and nevocytoblastoma) is a malignant tumor apparently arising from epidermal melanocytes (or antecedents thereof). It histologically differentiates in a manner similar to that of the benign pigmented nevus, although to a more limited degree. The tumor is the malignant counterpart of the ordinary pigmented nevus (3).

Frequency, Incidence, and Age

Compared with other skin cancers, the incidence of malignant melanoma is low (4), but in the United States, fatalities resulting from malignant melanoma probably compare closely with those of other cancers of the skin. It forms approximately 1% of all malignant neoplasms in men and women and is the cause of death in 0.11% to 0.12% of patients brought to autopsy. Although the malignant melanoma is found in all races, it supposedly is less common in blacks, although some investigators dispute this latter claim. Malignant melanoma are rare in childhood, and the highest incidence is found in adults above 30 years of age.

On the external ear, Byers et al. (4) found the malignant melanoma comprising 7% of all melanomas arising in the head and neck region and 4% of all skin cancers of the ear. Pack et al. (1) found a 14.5% external ear location for all head and neck melanomas and a 6.7% external ear location for all melanomas treated at the Pack Clinic. Their youngest patient was 7 years of age, and their oldest was 81 years of age, with an average age of onset of 49.6 years. The majority of patients were in the fourth through seventh decades of life. The male-to-female ratio was 3:1. Pack et al. remarked that there was a definite ethnic characteristic in the majority of their patients in which reddish or blonde hair, fair skin, and hazel or blue eyes predominated.

The youngest patient in the series of Byers et al. (4) was 8 years old, and the oldest was 83 years old with a median age of 56 years for their series. Three-quarters were male, and 63% worked in outdoor occupations. There were no blacks in their series of malignant melanomas of the external ear. In the AFIP OTR there were 3 patients with external auricular malignant melanoma, 2 of whom were men, and the average age of onset was 65 years. Also, there were 3 patients with middle ear malignant melanoma, only 1 of whom strongly supported a primary origin (5). Two were known to be females, with only the age of 52 years recorded in one. Pack et al. (1) mentioned two cases of primary middle ear malignant melanoma.

Etiology and Histogenesis

Trauma, irritation, frostbite, x-ray, actinic rays, hereditary factors, and hormonal influence have all been raised as possible causes, but they are mostly speculative at this point (2). Malignant melanoma originates from melanocytes in the epidermis whether in normal skin, in lentigo, or in the epidermal component of a benign pigmented nevus.

Site

Sylven and Hamberger (6) listed only 4 of their 36 patients as having tumor in the central part on auricle, including the external auditory canal, concha, tragus, and antitragus. The remainder of their patients were listed as arising mainly on the periphery of the auricles and in the preauricular, infraauricular, and retroauricular areas. Pack et al. (1) listed 42 patients whose tumors originated from the auricle. They did mention 1 patient with a tumor occurring in the auditory canal. Byers et al. (4) listed only the auricle as the anatomical location for tumors in their 102 patients. The AFIP OTR has no malignant melanoma listed as occurring in the external auditory canal, either primary or metastatic. Three patients in the AFIP OTR had malignant melanoma occurring in the middle ear, and in only 1 patient in the series of McKenna et al. (5) was the tumor believed to be primary. Pack et al. (1), in their 42 patients, listed the helix as the site of auricular origin in 43%, the antihelix as the site of origin in 24%, the lobule and tragus as the site of origin in 7%, and the posterior part of the helix, posterior ear, and immediate preauricular region as the site of origin in 5% each; 1 patient each had tumor of the fossa of the helix and concha. Other series (4) listed a similar auricular distribution.

Clinical Findings

In the series of Pack et al. (1) approximately half of the patients reported a pigmented lesion present on the ear for less than a year. Eight patients reported a pigmented lesion that had been present for 1–5 years, and 14 believed that such a lesion had been present for more than 5 years prior to any change in its character. None of their patients reported the pigmented lesion as having been present since childhood.

On the basis of gross clinical appearance and behavior, malignant melanomas of the skin surfaces (Fig. 19.5) have been divided by Clark et al. (7) into three types: the flat, spreading lesions that has been designated as superficial spreading melanoma, the nodular lesions that have been designated as nodular melanoma, and those arising in the melanotic freckle of Hutchinson that have been designated as lentigo maligna melanoma. Donnellan et al. (8) in 119 patients with head and neck malignant melanoma revealed that 40 males and 19 females had the nodular type, 13 males and 10 females had the lentigo maligna melanoma, and 27 males and 10 females had the superficial spreading melanoma. In the series of Byers et al. (4) of 102 patients, 44 lesions were characterized as superficial spreading, and 31 were characterized as nodular. In this latter series, 9 patients with superficial spreading lesions and 13 patients with nodular lesions had clinically positive cervical nodes when first seen. In this same series, a total of 42 patients eventually developed clinical positive nodes. Fifteen patients had initial positive nodes in the preauricular area, 4 had them in the parotid area, and 14 had them in the jugulodigastric region. No patient presented or developed metastasis to lower jugular nodes.

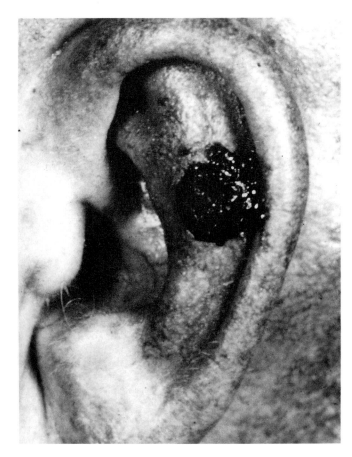

Figure 19.5. Clinical photograph of auricular malignant melanoma with superficial spreading, together with satellitosis.

In most instances, lesions appeared as brown or black flat spots (3) that remained static for variable periods of time, even decades, and during this time, they were considered as ordinary nevoid lentigines or flat pigmented nevi. In contrast, many lesions arose in what was considered normal skin and immediately progressively grew (nodular-type melanoma). Eventually, lesions that seemed static (superficial spreading or lentigo maligna) showed any or all of the following changes: peripheral enlargement, irregular intensification of color, focal loss of color, expansile growth, and degenerative and inflammatory changes such as ulceration, blistering, redness, and soreness. Amelanotic tumors were particularly confused with inflammatory ulcers and granuloma pyogenicum.

Microscopic Findings

Although the clinical history and gross observations may be strongly suggestive of malignant melanoma, the definitive diagnosis must be made histologically (2). The principal histologic criterion for the diagnosis is the presence of dermal invasion by atypical melanoma cells from the overlying epidermis (Fig. 19.6). Not until the atypical cells have actually invaded the dermis is the lesion diagnosed as malignant melanoma. Melanoma cells differ from benign nevus cells in several respects: The size and staining characteristics of nuclei and nucleoli vary, and mitotic figures are present and occasionally abnormal. The melanoma cells may lack cohesion. Atypical cells may progress upward through the epidermis to the surface, either individually or in small groups. The epidermis is frequently ulcerated, particularly in larger melanomas. Frank invasive malignant melanomas may or may not exhibit an accompanied inflammatory infiltrate. The individual melanoma cells may be spindled or polyhedral, large or small, and may have abundant or little cytoplasm. The nuclei may be hyperchromatic or vesicular, and the nucleoli may be prominent or small. The cells may be amelanotic or so heavily pigmented that the cytologic features cannot be visualized. All of these types of cells may be observed in one lesion.

Natural Behavior

There is no apparent correlation between cytologic types, histologic patterns, and biologic behavior. The histologic feature that can best be related to behavior and prognosis is said to be the depth of invasion or the thickness of the neoplasm. Generally, the larger the lesion, the worse the outcome; however, the lentigo maligna melanoma may occupy a large area of skin and show little invasion.

The methods whereby the microscopic depth of the invasion of cutaneous malignant melanoma into the dermis and subcutaneous tissue is measured were the Clark method for level I–V groups (7) and Breslow's measurement of actual tumor thickness in millimeters (9). There are many studies that have verified the relationship of depth of invasion and tumor thickness with prognosis and the recommended specific treatment (4, 8, 10, 11). Hansen and McCarten (11) have also noted prognostic implications in those patients with and without prominent lymphocyte infiltrations. Ulceration of cutaneous malignant melanoma was considered a bad prognostic sign in the study by Balch et al. (10).

There is also an obvious relationship to the clinical stage of the melanomas of the external ear. Clinical stage I occurs when there is no evidence of malignant melanoma of the head and neck spreading to the cervical nodes or distal sites. Clinical stage II occurs when there is metastatic spread of the malignant melanoma of the head and neck primary to the cervical lymph nodes. Clinical stage III occurs when there are distal metastases to distant organ sites. The spread of the malignant melanoma to cervical lymph nodes may initially involve the preauricular or upper jugular groups. Occasionally, the parotid nodes may become involved.

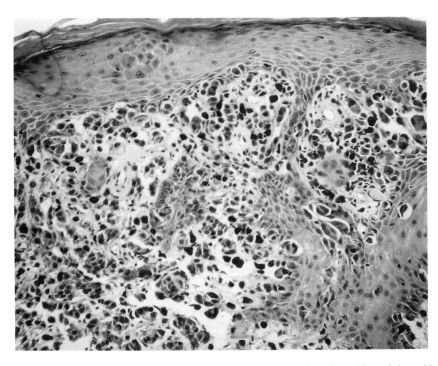

Figure 19.6. Histologic section reveals an early malignant melanoma of the external ear, consisting of nests of atypical pigmented melanoma cells arranged in nests at the epidermal-dermal junction and extending into the underlying dermis. (Hematoxylin and eosin, × 160.)

Treatment

Surgery is the main therapeutic avenue to effect a cure for malignant melanoma of the external ear. The extent of the operation and, particularly, the value of a neck dissection will depend on the clinical stage and the microscopic depth of dermal and subcutaneous invasion of the neoplasm.

The advantages of radiation therapy as the primary treatment for malignant melanomas of the head and neck has been championed by Harwood and Lawson (12).

Chemotherapy has not been advocated for the primary treatment modality of malignant melanoma of the external ear (4) but appears appropriate for poor-risk patients with thick lesions, nodal and/or distal metastasis, or both.

Prognosis

According to Byers et al. (4), the prognosis is not adversely affected by the sex, the level of invasion, the anatomic site of origin, the clinical appearance of the lesion, the type of treatment for the primary lesion, or the type of neck dissection (classic or functional). The status of the cervical nodes and the thickness of the lesion measured microscopically did directly affect survival. Hansen and McCarten (11) came to the conclusion that the thickness of the lesion and the degree of lymphocytic infiltrate were related to prognosis. Donnellan et al. (8) looking at 119 patients with head and neck malignant melanoma supported a significant correlation between the depth of dermal invasion and the type of melanoma. Prognosis for the superficial spreading melanoma or melanoma arising as premelanotic melanosis, or melanoma arising in Hutchinson's freckle, or lentigo maligna melanoma was much better than that for the nodular melanoma.

Pack et al. (1) believed, however, it was reasonable to state that 70% to 80% of small superficial melanomas of the external ear region would have a good prognosis. Infiltrative melanomas of the anatomical area and recurrent melanoma should produce a 30% salvage. In melanoma with gross metastasis or satellitosis, the cure rate was approximately 14%. Generally, the more peripherally the tumor was positioned on the ear, the better was the prognosis.

References

1. Pack GT, Conley J, Oropeza R. Melanoma of the external ear. Arch Otolaryngol 1970;92:106–113.
2. Graham JH, Johnson WC, Helwig EB. Dermal pathology. Hagerstown, Maryland: Harper & Row, 1972.
3. Lund HZ, Kraus JM. Melanotic tumors of the skin. In: Atlas of tumor pathology. Section 1, Fascicle 3. Washington, DC: Armed Forces Institute of Pathology, 1962.
4. Byers R, Smith JL, Russell N, Rosenbert V. Malignant melanoma of the external ear. Review of 102 cases. Am J Surg 1980;140:518–521.
5. McKenna EL, Holmes WF, Harwick R. Primary melanoma of the middle ear. Laryngoscope 1984;94:1459–1560.
6. Sylen B, Hamberger CA. Malignant melanoma of the external ear. Report of 36 cases treated between 1928 and 1944. Ann Otol Rhinol Laryngol 1950;59:631–647.
7. Clark WH, From L, Berandino EA. The histogenesis and biologic behavior of primary human malignant melanomas of the skin. Cancer Res 1969;29:705.
8. Donnellan MJ, Seemayer T, Huvos AG, Mike V, Strong EW. Clinicopathologic study of cutaneous melanoma of the head and neck. Am J Surg 1972;124:450–455.
9. Breslow A. Tumor thickness, level of invasion and node dissection in stage I cutaneous melanomas. Ann Surg 1975;182:572.
10. Balch CM, Wilkerson JA, Murad TM, Soon S-J, Ingalls AL, Maddox WA. The prognostic significance of ulceration of cutaneous melanoma. Cancer 1980;45:3012–3017.
11. Hansen MG, McCarten AB. Tumor thickness and lymphocytic infiltration in malignant melanoma of the head and neck. Am J Surg 1974;128:557–561.
12. Harwood AR, Lawson VG. Radiation therapy for melanomas of the head and neck. Head Neck Surg 1982;4:468–474.

20/ Squamous Cell Carcinomas

TEMPORAL BONE SQUAMOUS CELL CARCINOMA

Squamous cell carcinoma of the temporal bone can originate in the external ear (the auricle and/or the external auditory canal) or the middle ear cleft. It would be safe to say that the patients with squamous cell carcinomas arising on the skin of the auricle would have the best prognosis, while those with neoplasms arising in the middle ear cleft would have the worst prognosis. Patients with tumors arising from the epidermis of the external auditory canal would be expected to have a prognosis in between those for patients with tumors in the above two locations. Of course, prognosis depends on factors other than the anatomical location, such as the size and extension of the neoplasm, the length of time the lesion has grown before treatment, its histologic differentiation, and the presence of metastases either in the same region or distal to lymph nodes or extranodal tissue. The discussion below of squamous cell carcinoma of the temporal bone attempts to combine the information for both the external and the middle ear, but it is anticipated that in some facets they may necessarily be considered separately.

Definition

Temporal bone squamous cell carcinoma (also known as epidermoid carcinoma, prickle cell carcinoma, and spinocellular carcinoma) is a malignant neoplasm of skin, epidermis, or mucosal origin that in the best differentiated histology will mimic the cells and organization of the normal squamous cell epidermis or mucosa. These neoplasms are capable of invasion and metastasis.

Frequency, Incidence, and Age

Squamous cell carcinoma has been documented as the second most common type of skin cancer occurring on the auricle (1). It has accounted for about 10–15% of skin carcinomas, with basal cell carcinoma being the most common in this particular anatomic area (2), but Metcalf (3) has claimed that more than half of the carcinomas of the pinna are squamous cell carcinomas. He has also stated that carcinoma of the auricle represents 5% of all skin cancers and 25–33% of epidermoid carcinomas of the head. Crabtree et al. (4) has stated that external auditory canal malignancies ranged from 1 in 5,000 to 1 in 15,000 ear complaints. From the Armed Forces Institute of Pathology (AFIP) Otolaryngic Tumor Registry (OTR), squamous cell carcinomas of the external ear accounted for approximately 50% of all malignancies considered primary in this anatomical area. Michaels and Wells (5) have stated that squamous cell carcinoma was the most frequent malignant neoplasm in the middle ear. In a series of 40,000 patients with a diagnosis of chronic otitis media seen

during a 16-year period, only 28 cases of squamous cell carcinoma of the middle ear were diagnosed. Morton et al. (6) have cited a figure of 6 cases of middle ear cancer per 1 million population.

In 486 patients with squamous cell carcinoma of the external ear (auricle), the median age was 68 years, with the youngest age at onset being 16 years and the oldest being 98 years (1). More than 95% of the patients were white men, and 82% had a history of previous skin cancer. Shiffman (7) found, out of 52 patients with squamous cell carcinoma of the pinna, 50 men and 2 women whose ages ranged from 28 years through 96 years, with a mean age at onset of 73 years. Of the 154 patients in Metcalf's series (3), there were 134 males and 20 females, with an average age at onset of 68 years. In Lewis' patients with squamous cell carcinoma of the external auditory canal, there were 40 males and 65 females, with a median age at onset of 55 years (8). Of the 20 patients in the series of Johns and Headington (9), 90% were women, with an age range of 38–73 years and a median age at onset of 50 years. In the series of Kenyon et al. (10), there were 21 patients with squamous cell carcinoma of the middle ear, with an age range of 33–82 years and a mean age at onset of 62 years; 13 of these patients were women. In the series of Michaels and Wells (5), there were 8 patients with middle ear squamous cell carcinoma who ranged in age from 34 years to 85 years, with an average age at onset of 60 years and with no sex predominance.

Site

In Shiffman's series (7), 30 of 52 patients with squamous cell carcinoma of the pinna had neoplasm on the left side. The most common sites were the helix (27 patients), the medial aspect of the pinna (11 patients), the antihelix (6 patients), the triangular fossa and concha (3 patients each), and the lobule (2 patients). Of 486 patients in the series of Byers et al. (1), 53% had tumor on the rim of the helix, 19% had tumor on the antihelix and triangular fossa, 14% had tumor on the posterior pinna, 5% each had tumor on the lobule or concha, and 4% had tumor on the tragus. Information as to the anatomical area of the external auditory canal where the squamous cell carcinoma arose was difficult to obtain from the medical literature or the AFIP OTR. Johns and Headington (9) mentioned that half of the squamous cell carcinomas of the external canal in their series were confined to the canal itself. Goodwin and Jesse (11), reporting on 142 patients with malignant neoplasm involving the temporal bone with the majority of neoplasms being squamous cell carcinomas, found 76 patients with the tumor involving the conchal region of the pinna and/or the cartilaginous ear canal. Twenty-two patients had tumor involvement of the superficial portion of the temporal bone (from both the ear canal and the mastoid cortex), and 38 patients had tumor involvement of the deep structures of the temporal bone (middle ear, facial canal, base of skull, or mastoid air cells). In the reported series of squamous cell carci-

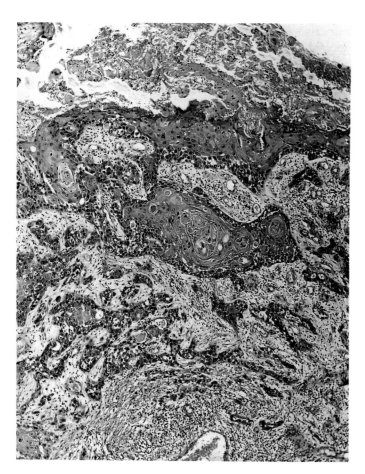

Figure 20.5. Higher magnification of an infiltrating squamous cell carcinoma arising in the external ear canal shows moderate differentiation. (Hematoxylin and eosin, ×63.)

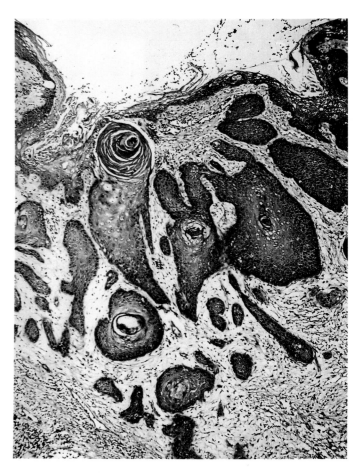

Figure 20.6. Histologic section of middle ear squamous cell carcinoma that had produced symptoms of chronic otic media. (Hematoxylin and eosin, ×63.)

Differential Diagnosis

The differential diagnostic problems mainly occur in the clinical identification of the squamous cell carcinoma of the temporal bone. The histology of squamous cell carcinoma, once the biopsy has been taken, is usually specific. There may be the rare occasion when the microscopic difference between squamous cell carcinoma, solar or actinic keratosis, basal cell carcinoma, and squamous cell papilloma may be difficult to differentiate. The smaller squamous cell carcinoma of the auricle may, in particular, be mistaken clinically for an actinic or solar keratosis and basal cell carcinoma. With squamous cell carcinoma of the external ear canal, the serious misdiagnosis that may be made is that of chronic external otitis. With squamous cell carcinoma of the middle ear cleft, the same mistake may also be made; i.e., the chronic drainage may be thought to be due to chronic otitis media. It is obvious that in the pathology of the external auditory canal and middle ear, failure to respond to treatment or the gradual or sudden development of additional signs and symptoms is a bad omen, and there is no substitute for an adequate biopsy specimen when there is any doubt.

Natural History and Metastases

In the case of squamous cell carcinoma of the external auricle, the neoplasm may spread and invade the local tissue, particularly in neglected patients, to present a hideous sight. In the investigation of 468 patients by Byers et al. (1), 6% pre-

sented with suspected nodal metastases. Within 24 months, another 6% developed positive nodes. The parotid lymph nodes were the most commonly involved, followed by jugulodigastric and upper posterior cervical, the midjugular and middle posterior cervical, the periauricular, and, rarely, the lower posterior cervical and lower jugular nodes. Distant metastases developed in only 1% of their patients.

In squamous cell carcinoma of the external auditory canal, there seems to be little to restrict spread of squamous cell carcinomas that arise in the cartilaginous portion of the canal, since the cartilaginous walls are easily infiltrated (15). Carcinomas arising in the bony canal are surrounded by dense bone that provides a more effective barrier to spread than does the cartilage. The tumor, therefore, progresses along the easier path, spreading along the main axis of the canal, and sooner or later may invade the middle ear or the cartilaginous portion of the canal. Metastases to lymph nodes take place slowly, with the periauricular group being involved first and the superficial and deep cervical nodes being involved later (16). In the series of Johns and Headington (8), 4 of 20 patients presented with lymph node metastases. Widespread distant metastases are rarely seen, since death occurs primarily from local extension to vital structures before such metastases develop (15).

Michaels and Wells (5) in their investigation of 28 fatal cases of squamous cell carcinoma of the middle ear believed that an important feature in each case was the penetration by tumor of the bone on the medial wall of the middle ear to infiltrate the carotid canal and of the thin layer of bone between the posterior mastoid air cells and the dura, with subsequent invasion along the dura and into the internal auditory meatus. In one of their cases the cochlea was infiltrated through these above-mentioned routes. Only one of their patients revealed metastasis to a cervical lymph node. Kenyon et al. (10) have pointed out the indication of regional invasiveness of squamous cell carcinoma of the middle ear as facial weakness, parotid infiltration, displaced pinna, and postaural fistula. Seven of the 21 patients in their series developed associated lymph node involvement.

Treatment and Prognosis

Byers et al. (1) used surgery to treat 99% of their 486 patients with squamous cell carcinoma of the auricle. The surgery consisted of wide excision with primary closure, wide excision with skin graft, wedge excision with primary closure, partial pinnectomy, and total pinnectomy. Less than 10% of the patients required a total excision of the pinna. Local recurrence developed in 14% of their patients. Local treatment failure was the cause of death in 2.5%. Five percent required a temporal bone resection as part of their local treatment, and the cancer recurred in 65% of these patients. The 2- and 5-year survival rates for patients with recurrences were 80% and 45%, respectively. Eleven of these patients underwent extensive local resection of the parotid gland, temporomandibular joint, and mandible, with recurrence of tumor in 6 patients. There was no statistically significant correlation between local regional failure or survival and age, sex, type of neck dissection (radical or modified), site of primary cancer, site of nodal metastases, or histologic finding. The histologic findings and the size and site of the primary tumor did not correlate with the initial presence or subsequent development of nodal metastases. There was no correlation between the incidence of nodal metastasis and the age of the patient. The overall 2- and 5-year survival rates in this series of 486 patients with no adverse criteria, such as positive regional lymph nodes or spread to the temporal bone, parotid gland, or temporomandibular joint, was 68% and 48%, respectively. Intercurrent disease was the cause of death in 35% and a second primary cancer was the cause of death in 27%, while the cause of death was unknown in 6%.

Of the 20 patients with squamous cell carcinoma of the external auditory canal in the series of Johns and Headington (9), radiotherapy alone was utilized in 3 patients (2 with early lesions and 1 with an advanced lesion), followed by recurrent neoplasm in all. Four patients with advanced lesions treated by radiotherapy followed by surgery were also radiation failures, for surgery was not done until recurrence was discovered. Three patients with early lesions treated by radiotherapy followed by surgery were alive without evidence of recurrent disease at the time of follow-up. One patient with an early lesion treated by surgery alone survived without recurrence of disease for 14 years. In summary, they were 10 patients living, with 3 having recurrent disease 3, 6, and 12 years after treatment and with 7 free of disease 3–13 years following diagnosis. Ten patients died of disease 1 month to 15 years following diagnosis. Lederman (17) reported that in a series of 40 patients, 8 of 31 (26%) were alive after 3 years, 6 of 25 (24%) were alive at 5 years, and 3 of 10 (30%) were alive after 10 years. He recommended radiotherapy follow radical surgery for advanced lesions.

Kenyon et al. (10) revealed that in a series of 21 patients with squamous cell carcinoma of the middle ear, 5 patients (1 with bilateral neoplasms) underwent standard radical mastoid surgery, and no patient underwent en bloc resection of the temporal bone. In an additional 5 patients, attempts at formal exploration were made but were abandoned when no major landmarks could be identified. In 6 patients, polyps or granulation were removed from the mastoid bowl, but no reexploration was performed. All patients then received radiotherapy. Two of the patients had additional treatment with fast electrons, and 4 patients with rapidly progressive disease had adjuvant chemotherapy with bleomycin and methotrexate given either alone or in combination. Twelve patients died as a result of their disease. From presentation to death they averaged 1.3 years and all had well-differentiated or moderately well differentiated tumors histologically. Five patients died during the follow-up period (mean survival 15.5 years) from causes other than their middle ear disease. Three patients who survived remain alive and well 2, 5, and 19 years following diagnosis. Of interest, those who died of intercurrent disease and the survivors all had what was considered to be a poorly differentiated squamous cell carcinoma arising primarily in the middle ear.

ADENOID SQUAMOUS CELL CARCINOMA (ADENOACANTHOMA)

Adenoid squamous cell carcinoma (adenoacanthoma) is a neoplasm of the skin that is considered a low-grade squamous cell carcinoma with a unique micromorphology. It occurs essentially on the head and neck, including the external ear. Of the 155 patients with adenoid squamous cell carcinoma in the series of Johnson and Helwig (18), 144 had tumors of the head and neck, and 34 had tumors of the external ear.

Clinically, approximately half of the lesions present as a nodular, round to oval, flesh-colored to pink, red, or brown raised tumors. The tumor elevation will be variable, with a few revealing rolled edges and/or a pearly appearance. Some patients are asymptomatic, but most complain of drainage, bleeding, itching, tenderness, and burning or stinging. In the series of Johnson and Helwig (18), most patients were Caucasian, and most were male, with only 3 females among the 155 patients. The prototypical patient is a blond-, red-, auburn-, or sandy-haired Caucasian with blue, gray, or green eyes and fair or ruddy skin. The ages of patients in the Johnson and Helwig series ranged from 20 to 84 years, with the sixth and seventh decades being the average age of occurrence. Median age was 57.7 years. The time from first symptoms to diagnosis would vary from 1 month to 34 years, with the median time of 1.2 years.

Of interest, 65 of the 155 patients with adenoid squamous cell carcinoma related a 20% instance of a family history of skin cancer, compared with 7% for patients with squamous cell carcinoma of the skin and 6% for patients with a skin keratoacanthoma (18). The geographic location of patients in the United States was heavily centered in the South. Of the 155 patients of Johnson and Helwig (18), 90 had additional skin tumors, which, in the order of decreasing frequency, were senile or solar keratosis, basal cell carcinoma, and squamous cell carcinoma. Twenty-eight patients had additional adenoid squamous carcinomas, and 28 patients had additional primary internal or extracutaneous cancers (lung, prostate, stomach, rectum, larynx, or other sites).

The histologic findings on low-power examination are usu-

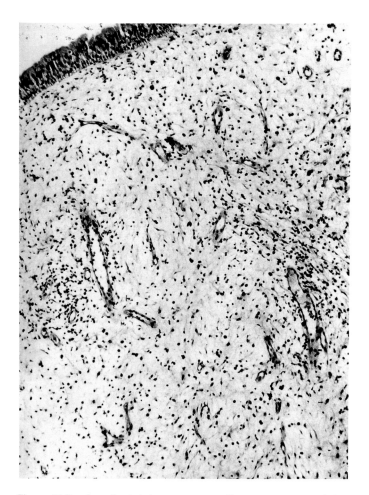

Figure 21.3. Juvenile rhabdomyosarcoma with myxomatous morphology that is sometimes confused with an inflammatory polyp of the anatomical area. (Hematoxylin and eosin, ×63.)

tures as the embryonal type. These polypoid-shaped tumors (Fig. 21.2), which usually grow into an open space such as the nasopharynx or sinus, have a more or less compact layer of small lymphocytic-like cells beneath the mucous membrane (the so-called cambium layer), below which the tumor has a loose, more sparse structure, and the cells have a more haphazard arrangement. The *alveolar rhabdomyosarcoma* consists of one or more layers of neoplastic cells arranged more or less in a trabecular pattern intermixed with vascular connective tissue (Fig. 21.7). The central part of the trabecula may appear empty (hence alveolar) or contain varying numbers of free-floating cells. Some of these cells may be large and multinucleated or round to oval or strap-like. Both longitudinal striations and cross-striations may be found in these cells (12). Alveolar rhabdomyosarcoma occurs more often in the older child (15 years old) (13) than in the younger child.

Special histochemical staining may be of help. The demonstration of cross-striations by the phosphotungstic acid-hematoxylin (PTAH) or the Masson's trichrome histochemical strain can be confirmatory. The demonstration of glycogen within the tumor cells via the periodic acid-Schiff (PAS) stain will also strengthen the diagnosis. Among the immunoperoxidase stains (PAP), the demonstration of a positive desmin and myoglobin is compatible with the diagnosis of rhabdomyosarcoma. Electron microscopy on specially prepared tumor tissue (glutaraldehyde fixed) will reveal features of the rhabdomyosarcoma that are diagnostic. Eccentric nuclei, abundant mitochondria, and cytoplasmic filaments are seen. Cytoplasmic material suggestive of

glycogen is observed in more developed tumor cells, and the Golgi apparatus is more prominent in less-differentiated cells. The development of alternately arranged thin and thick filaments with the formation of "Z bands" separates the rhabdomyosarcoma from other malignant mesenchymal tumors.

DIFFERENTIAL DIAGNOSES

Poorly differentiated round and spindle cell carcinomas, especially when occurring in children or young adults, constitute the most common problem in the differential diagnosis. Included in this group are neuroblastoma, neuroepithelioma, Ewing's sarcoma, poorly differentiated angiosarcoma, synovial sarcoma, malignant melanoma, granulocytic sarcoma, malignant lymphoma, and small cell carcinoma (11). Fetal rhabdomyoma and soft tissue Ewing's sarcoma must also be considered in the differential diagnosis.

TREATMENT

The recommended therapy for rhabdomyosarcoma of the head and neck (14) consists of a standard protocol of surgery when feasible, radiation to residual local and regional and metastatic disease, and adjuvant chemotherapy using vincristine, dactinomycin, and cyclophosphamide as subsequently outlined by the Intergroup Rhabdomyosarcoma Study II (15). Adriamycin would be included in some cases with metastatic disease (14). There has been some indecision as to whether a radical surgical procedure should be performed for extensive local disease or whether debulking of the neoplasm is all that is needed; and both

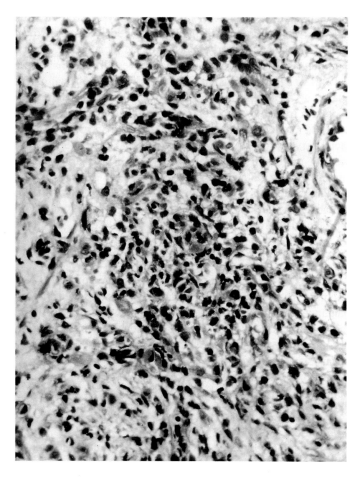

Figure 21.4. Higher magnification of the same neoplasm as in Figure 21.3 reveals the clustering of small round and spindle undifferentiated cells with varying amounts of cytoplasm. (Hematoxylin and eosin, ×160.)

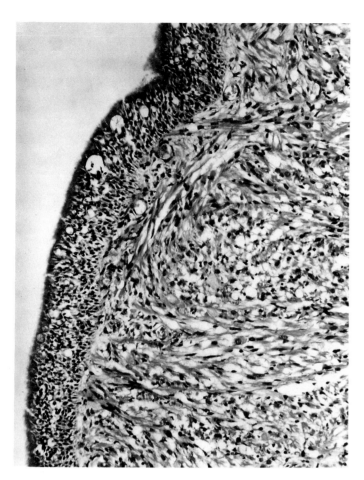

Figure 21.5. In this histologic presentation of a juvenile rhabdomyosarcoma, the derivation of neoplastic cells from muscle is more recognizable. (Hematoxylin and eosin, ×160.)

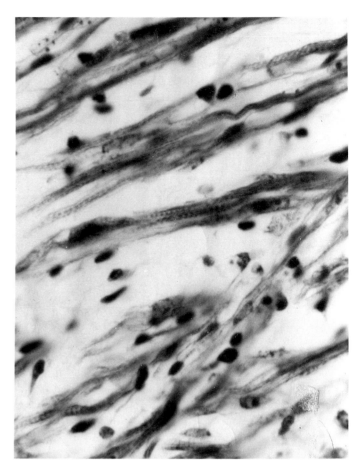

Figure 21.6. In the more differentiated juvenile rhabdomyosarcoma, cross-striations are occasionally noted. (Hematoxylin and eosin, ×230.)

procedures would be accompanied by radiation and a chemotherapy regimen (16). There are advocates for both types of surgical approaches, and the final choice has apparently not been made.

PROGNOSIS

The rhabdomyosarcoma is clinically grouped into four categories: group I—localized disease only and completely surgically resected; group II—localized disease only but microscopic residual disease following surgery; group III—localized disease but with gross residual disease following surgery; and group IV—metastatic disease present at onset. In 202 patients with rhabdomyosarcoma of the head and neck (17), 26% had tumors of the eye and orbit, 46% had tumors in parameningeal sites (nasopharynx, temporal bone (middle ear), paranasal sinuses, oropharynx, scalp, base of skull, and parotid), and 28% had tumors of the head and neck areas. Of the tumors in this series, histologically 78% were embryonal, 9% were alveolar, 10% were undifferentiated, and 3% were extraosseous Ewing's sarcoma. The actual 3-year survival rate calculated on 103 patients free of distant metastatic disease at diagnosis was 91% for those with eye and/or orbit primary tumors, 46% for those with parameningeal primary tumors, and 75% for those with other head and neck sites affected. In a study of rhabdomyosarcoma involvement systemically (18), the alveolar subtype had the highest proportion of distant metastases and the lowest occurrence of local progression from the primary site. Parameningeal tumors, irrespective of their histologic subtypes showed a high incidence

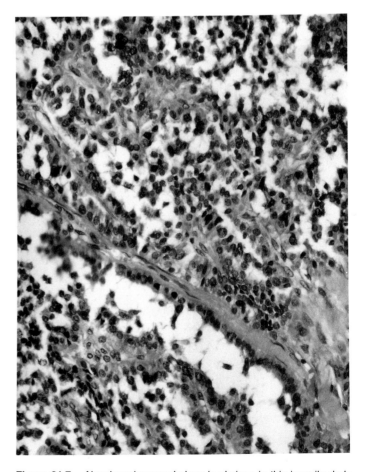

Figure 21.7. Alveolar micromorphology is obvious in this juvenile rhabdomyosarcoma. (Hematoxylin and eosin, ×160.)

of direct extension from the primary lesion, especially into the CNS. The lung was the most common site of metastasis at death, followed by the regional lymph node, bone, liver, and brain. Regional node involvement was observed more commonly in patients with lower extremity primary tumors and alveolar subtypes. Patients under the age of 1 year did not appear to have a worse prognosis than those over 1 year of age (14). In a series of 24 children with rhabdomyosarcoma of the temporal bone area following surgery plus radiation and chemotherapy, 9 of 19 patients who presented with localized sarcoma were free of disease at 2.2–6.5 years after diagnosis. One additional patient was alive with regional recurrence at 6.7 years. One died of other disease at 4.4 years after diagnosis without neoplasm present. The remaining 13 patients died of recurrent rhabdomyosarcoma at 5–25 months after diagnosis. The outcome was unfavorably influenced by meningeal and cranial cavity extension and facial nerve involvement (19). The prognostic picture appears governed by the following observations (15). Survival is directly related to the extent of the disease at diagnosis. Recurrent disease, whether locally, in adjacent nodes, or in distant metastatic sites, carries a poor prognosis. Complete surgical excision of primary lesions may improve survival in all head and neck rhabdomyosarcomas except orbital lesions. The survival of patients with head and neck rhabdomyosarcoma has reportedly improved since the institution of planned multimodal therapy but is still poor in those treated with surgical biopsy only, prior to radiation and chemotherapy (15).

Extraskeletal Ewing's Sarcoma

Extraskeletal Ewing's sarcoma is mentioned because it is quite often mistaken histologically and clinically for the juvenile rhabdomyosarcoma. The neoplasm, whether in bone or extraskeletally, is believed to be derived from primitive mesenchymal tissue that gives no hint of further differentiation. Patient ages vary from a year through the sixth decade, with approximately 70% of neoplasms occurring in patients under 20 years of age. These neoplasms are slightly more common in males and affect the paravertebral areas, lower extremities, and torso (11) rather than the head and neck, although Soule et al. (20) have reported some involvement of the latter area. No case of temporal bone involvement has been noted.

The gross appearance of this neoplasm will imitate the juvenile rhabdomyosarcoma with a gray-yellow or a gray-tan cut surface, often with large areas of necrosis, cyst formation, or hemorrhage. Microscopically, the pattern consists of solid, packed, lobulated formations with a striking uniformity and immature appearance to the cells and a paucity of mitotic figures (Fig. 21.8). The individual tumor cell will be rounded or ovoid, with a vesicular nucleus and a distinct nuclear membrane, finely divided chromatin, and frequently a single minute nucleolus. The cytoplasm is ill-defined, scanty, pale staining, and irregularly vacuolated as a result of intracellular storage of glycogen, which is rarely absent in the malignant neoplastic cells. The tumor is richly vascular, and occasionally, rosette-like structures will be seen as the tumor cells arrange around a vessel. The electron microscopic picture of Ewing's tumor reveals round or ovoid nuclei with multiple minute nucleoli along with a cytoplasm with few organelles, poorly developed Golgi apparatus, and abundant glycogen. The differential diagnosis includes the juvenile rhabdomyosarcoma, neuroblastoma, and malignant lymphoma.

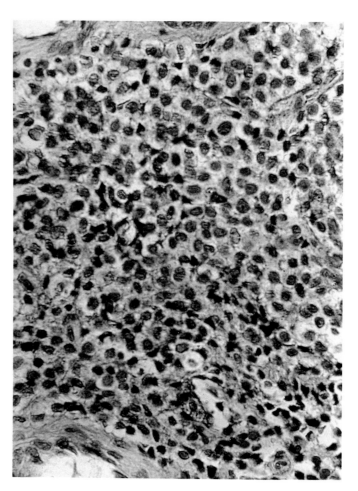

Figure 21.8. Histologic section of Ewing's soft tissue sarcoma showing a pattern of solid, packed, lobular formations of uniform and immature cells and rare mitotic activity. (Hematoxylin and eosin, ×160.)

Therapy is essentially the same as that for juvenile rhabdomyosarcoma, i.e., complete surgical excision if possible, followed by high radiation doses and sequential chemotherapy. In a follow-up of 35 patients, Enzinger and Weiss (11) reported that 22 died of the disease and 10 were alive without neoplasm.

Undifferentiated Sarcoma

In the publication by Naufel (1), 89 of the 211 patients reported had only the diagnosis of undifferentiated sarcoma, such as spindle cell, round cell, atypical, and anaplastic sarcoma. If possible, the sarcoma should be further classified, since such vague terminology is meaningless and conveys little information as to the nature and potential behavior of a given tumor. Moreover, these terms do not clearly distinguish between neoplasms and tumor-like reactive processes. With the help of immunoperoxidase and other histochemical stains and electron microscopy, there should be little excuse for not specifically classifying the sarcoma.

MYXOMA

The myxoma (also known as fibromyxoma) is a tumefaction that is well appreciated throughout the world, especially as occurring in the heart, soft tissues of the body, bone, and other anatomical areas and organs except for the temporal bone region. There is the rare reference over the past century to myxomas of the external ear (21). The AFIP OTR does contain listings of 16 patients with either a diagnosed myxoma or fibromyxoma of the temporal bone area that were entered between the years 1939 and 1986.

The myxoma is defined by Stout (22) as a true neoplasm of unknown genesis composed of stellate cells set in a loose mucoid stroma through which course very delicate reticulin fibers; its histology closely resembles primitive mesenchyme. When there is delineation of denser areas as a result of a thickening of the delicate connective tissue fibers and a lessening of the mucoid material, the term "fibromyxoma" has been utilized. It is not considered proper to add the suffix of sarcoma to these above terms, since the myxoma or fibromyxoma does not metastasize except in the rare case of cardiac myxomas. There may be portions of other malignant metastasizing neoplasms that appear myxomatous in part, such as the liposarcoma, fibrosarcoma, chondrosarcoma, malignant peripheral nerve neoplasms, and mesenchymoma, but these are not myxomas and should be considered under the designation of their most prominent malignant tissue element.

In the AFIP OTR, information on 11 of the 15 patients noted revealed 8 males, with ages ranging from 7 to 56 years of age and an average age at onset of 27 years. Six patients were considered to have external canal tumors, while 2 were listed as having tumor in the middle ear, and 3 were listed as having tumor in the mastoid. The time from initiation of a myxoma until diagnosis throughout the body varies from 2 weeks to 37 years, with an average of 4 years (22). There are no descriptions of myxomas of the temporal bone except for one of the external ear (21) and the illustration in the color atlas by Becker et al. (22) of external canal myxoma. These and the descriptions of myxomas of other anatomical areas support a yellow to brownish gelatinous to lipomatous semitransparent friable tumefaction that on its exposed surfaces may support a capsule, although in adjacent tissue there is usually gross evidence of infiltration. The histology is that of a benign-appearing micromorphology but often with an infiltrating mixture of small inconspicuous round, spindle, or stellate cells within a matrix containing abundant mucoid material, chiefly hyaluronic acid, a loose meshwork of reticulin and collagen fibrils, and scant vascularity (2). There may be focal formations of denser areas as a result of thickening of the delicate connective tissue fibers. The resemblance of these areas to fibromas has led to the term of fibromyxoma. In spite of the benign histologic appearance when myxomas grow into bone, they develop in the marrow, expand the cortex, destroy bone by aseptic pressure necrosis, and produce a deformity of the bone that radiologically may be mistaken for osteitis fibrosa, giant cell tumor, or fibrous dysplasia and, in the jaws, for ameloblastoma or a paradental epithelial cyst (22).

Although the myxoma or fibromyxoma does not metastasize, it can easily infiltrate adjacent tissue, including bone. At this point the best therapy would seem to be complete surgical removal, or repeated recurrence or more serious invasiveness will be the outcome. Use of radiotherapy has been reported with some success (2). Chemotherapy has not yet been evaluated in the treatment of myxoma.

NODULAR FASCIITIS

Nodular fasciitis (also known as pseudosarcomatous fibromatosis and pseudosarcomatous fasciitis) is a benign and proba-

bly reactive fibroblastic growth extending as a solitary nodule from the superficial fascia into the subcutaneous fat or, less frequently, into the subjacent muscle. Diagnostic confusion as to its being a sarcoma is possible because of its cellularity, its mitotic activity, its richly mucoid stroma, and its rapid growth. It tends to occur in young adults, mainly on the upper extremity, the trunk, and the neck region (2). It has not been particularly noted to occur in the external ear according to a medical literature survey, but the AFIP OTR lists 10 patients in the 1976–1985 period with involvement of the external ear area by nodular fasciitis. Three are listed as having nodular fasciitis on the external ear; 3, as having it in the external auditory canal; 3, as having it in the para-auricular area; and 1, as having it on the pinna. In the study by Dahl and Jarlstedt (24) on 18 patients with head and neck nodular fasciitis, 6 patients, according to information of the anatomical location of the patient's lesions, had tumors that would be considered para-auricular in location.

The ages of patients in the AFIP OTR were from 12 through 67 years, with the average age at onset of 33 years. Most were in the second and third decades. Seven were males. In a series of 114 patients with nodular fasciitis, Bernstein and Lattes (25) recorded the youngest as 17 months and the oldest as 74 years. The majority of their patients were in the second through fifth decades of life. There was no sex predominance, and 15% of their patients had head and neck tumors.

Clinically, the patients have a history of a rapidly growing lesion, and usually surgical removal is done close to the time of first notation. The lesion is mostly solitary and is found in the subcutaneous tissue. It may vary from 1 to 5 cm in diameter. It is attached to fascia, and the overlying skin is freely movable (26). There may be a history of trauma to the site or pain and tenderness accompanying the tumor. Pathologically, the gross features are typically a 2-cm, tan to grayish-white appearance with a slimy, nodular to soft gelatinous consistency, often suggesting circumscription. Grossly, the tumor cannot be differentiated from other soft tissue neoplasms. Microscopically, the tumor reveals a proliferation of fibroblasts of varying shapes. Proliferating thin, elongated, S-formed or wavy cells mixed with plumper, cytoplasmic, elongated cells are seen (Figs. 21.9 and 21.10) (1). Nuclei vary from elongated with pointed ends to oval with delicate clumped chromatin and nucleoli. These spindle cells are arranged focally as compact bundles with possibly a storiform pattern discerned. Micromorphologically, a capsule is not noted, and often the tumor gives the impression of invading adjacent muscle. The vascularity is prominent, and extravasated red blood cells and chronic and even acute inflammatory cells including mast cells may be seen. Multinucleated reactive giant cells as well as reactive vascular endothelial proliferation may also be noted. Mitotic figures may be as prominent as 1 mitosis per high-powered histologic field (25). Nodular fasciitis has been classified mainly on the anatomical and gross appearance into a subcutaneous, an intramuscular, and a fascial type (11).

Under a differential diagnosis, hardly any other soft tissue lesion has caused as many problems and difficulties in diagnosis (11). Mistaken diagnoses of fibrosarcoma, fibromatosis, fibrous histiocytoma, neurilemmoma, and possibly others have caused many instances of unnecessary surgical procedures. The nodular fasciitis does not recur following surgical removal (25); in fact, portions of the lesion left behind at surgical removal will usually atrophy and disappear (27). Bernstein and Lattes (25) presented 18 patients who, they believed, had nodular fasciitis on the orig-

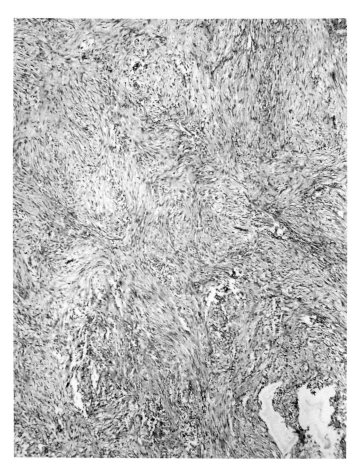

Figure 21.9. Microscopic view of nodular fasciitis reveals a pattern of proliferating fibroblasts arranged in a so-called "storiform" pattern. (Hematoxylin and eosin, ×63.)

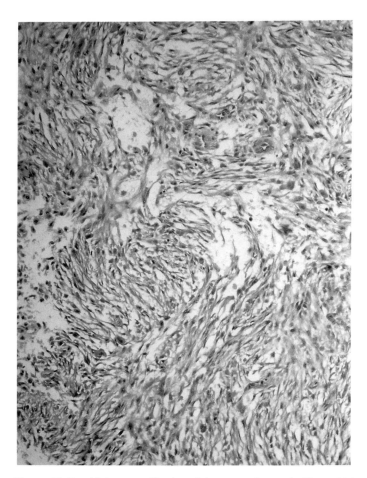

Figure 21.10. Higher magnification of the same view as in Figure 21.9 demonstrates the spindle cells with their "whorl-like" (storiform) pattern. Multinucleated giant cells may be seen. (Hematoxylin and eosin, ×160.)

inal surgical removal, while on recurrence of the lesion the diagnoses were changed to entities such as fibrosarcoma, fibrohistiocytoma, lipomatous and perineural sheath neoplasms, and fibromatosis.

Therapy has been local surgical excision of the lesion. After such a therapeutic procedure, if there is a recurrence or if suspicion of local extension or metastasis occurs, the possibility of a mistaken diagnosis of nodular fasciitis must be considered.

FIBROMATOSIS

Fibromatosis (also known as aggressive fibromatosis, extra-abdominal desmoids, and juvenile fibromatosis) is defined as an infiltrating fibroblastic proliferation revealing none of the histologic features of an inflammatory response and none of the features of an unequivocal neoplasm (28). In other words, the histology reminds one of scar tissue that continues to grow. This tumor may occur anywhere and to any extent. It may be fatal or relatively harmless. It has been encountered in patients from fetal life to old age (12).

This pathologic entity does not apparently involve the external ear with any regularity, although the head and neck may account for 9.5–25% of neoplasms in some series of patients (29, 30). The AFIP OTR does not contain a case. Morioka et al. (31) did publish the case of a 19-month-old child with a posterior aural lesion that was adherent to the conchal cartilage. Apparently, only an excisional biopsy was done at the time of di-

agnosis, and 30 days later the recurrence of a mass occurred in the vicinity of the previous surgery. Complete surgical removal was then accomplished with apparent success for at least 4 years postoperatively.

Conley et al. (30) presented a series of 40 patients with head and neck fibromatosis. In this series there was no sexual preference. Twenty-five percent of patients were under the age of 15 years, and the most common area of tumor involvement was the neck (40%). Etiology was undetermined, with no significant history of previous trauma or radiation to the areas of involvement. Clinically, the picture was that of muscle and fibroadipose tissue being replaced by or infiltrated with a fibrous tissue of varying cellularity. The lesion was either single, diffuse, or multifocal. Histologically, fibroblasts are well differentiated, uniform in size, and often devoid of any mitotic activity (Figs. 21.11 and 21.12). They imitated a fibrosarcoma in their ability to infiltrate but not to metastasize. Conley et al. (30) believed that it was imperative to carry out an adequate operation for the tumor by proper preoperative planning and understanding of the characteristics of biologic growth of the disease. Excessive mutilation, organ compromise, and high morbidity were prudently excluded from the operative plan. In the series of 40 patients of Conley et al. (30), there was a 47% local recurrence of tumor postoperatively. Fifteen percent of the patients are living with persistent disease, but there were no deaths from local invasion, and there was no evidence of lymphatic or vascular metastasis. Irradiation therapy was recommended in inoperable cases (31).

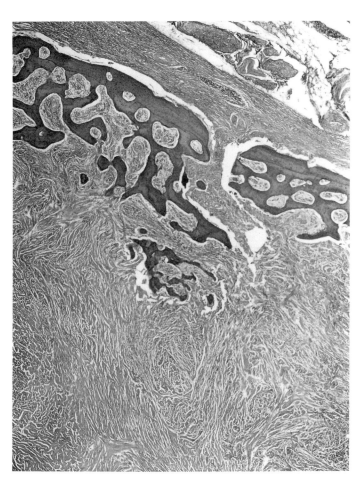

Figure 21.11. Histologic section of aggressive fibromatosis demonstrates the local invasive characteristics of the neoplasm into adjacent temporal bone. (Hematoxylin and eosin, ×63.)

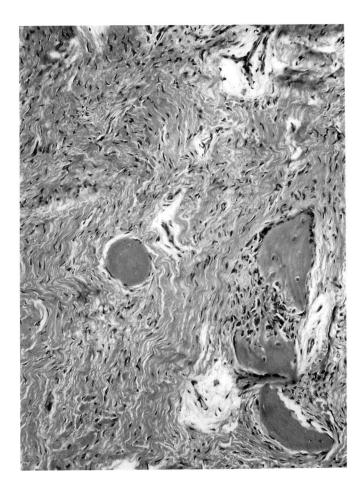

Figure 21.12. Higher magnification of the same view as in Figure 21.11 emphasizes the well-differentiated, uniform, and nonmitotic appearance of the fibroblastic tumor cell. (Hematoxylin and eosin, ×160.)

A similar clinical and partly histologic entity has been designated by Wold and Weiland (32) as "tumefactive fibroinflammatory lesion of the head and neck," which according to the authors has a similar histologic appearance to Riedel's thyroiditis, sclerosing mediastinitis, and retroperitoneal fibrosis. There were 7 patients in their series who had tumors of the sinonasal tract, parotid gland, orbit, and external auditory canal. Five of the patients were women whose ages ranged from 33 to 74 years, with a mean age at onset of 48 years. The lesion usually presented as a tumor mass and was characterized histologically by an admixture of mature fibrous tissue and an inflammatory infiltrate of lymphocytes and scattered polymorphonuclear leukocytes. Treatment had been surgical excision, but 2 of 6 patients required additional irradiation because of recurrent disease. Five of the six patients (32) were surviving 14 to 49 months following diagnosis. One patient died at 64 months, apparently from tumor.

FIBROMA

Pure benign neoplasms of the fibroblast are rare in any part of the body, and there is some doubt whether such an entity exists. "Fibroma" has been incorrectly applied, but without danger, to certain pedunculated lesions of the skin, which are either malformations or, more likely, hyperplastic proliferations to some form of injury or inflammation. *Dermatofibroma* (sclerosing hemangioma) is a benign skin-covered fibromatous tumor

occupying the dermis and subcutaneous tissue. In keeping with the original statement regarding fibromas, this particular one is questionable as to its genesis being neoplastic or traumatic. Others consider it in the histiocytic group of tumors. There are 10 patients in the AFIP OTR from 1940 through 1985 with this diagnosis of an external ear tumor. Clinically, it presents as a 0.5–1.0-cm round but occasionally flat, slightly raised, well-circumscribed, firm lesion that is nonulcerated, skin-covered, and slightly red, but it may appear yellowish-brown as a result of lipid content or bluish-black, reflecting the presence of hemosiderin. Histologically, there is a well-demarcated but nonencapsulated tumor containing largely fibroblasts, with spindle-shaped nuclei arranged in parallel intertwining and anastomosing bands suggesting a storiform pattern. The young lesions containing prominent endothelial cells and histiocytic-appearing cells that are difficult to differentiate from histiocytes (31). The older lesions with their hemosiderin and older vasculature have been popularly referred to as sclerosing angiomas. The information concerning the patients contained in the AFIP OTR was incomplete, but the patients were listed as 6–38 years of age. There was no sex differentiation. All were treated with complete surgical removal, with no recurrences.

DERMATOFIBROSARCOMA PROTUBERANS

Dermatofibrosarcoma protuberans is a slowly growing, locally aggressive, rarely metastasizing, malignant mesenchymal

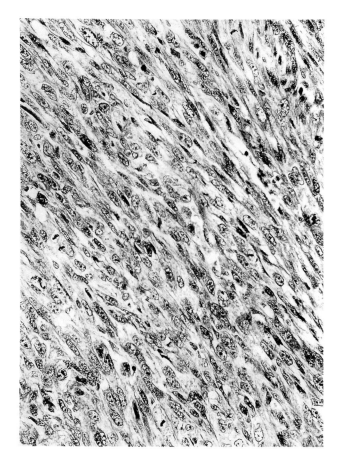

Figure 21.16. In this histologic section of a fibrosarcoma of the temporal bone area, the cellularity and anaplasia of the neoplastic fibrocytes would qualify it as a high-grade fibrosarcoma. (Hematoxylin and eosin, ×150.)

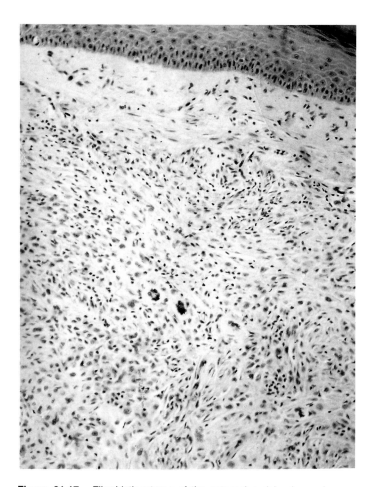

Figure 21.17. Fibrohistiocytoma of the external auricle shows demarcation, and, together with the histiocytes, prominent multinucleated giant cells (Touton cells) are noted. (Hematoxylin and eosin, ×63.)

were females. In the series of Blitzer et al. (38), the mean age was 43 years but with a 3:1 male-to-female predominance. In the AFIP OTR, there were 25 patients with external ear involvement, either of the auricle or of the external auditory canal. One was listed as having involvement of the middle ear.

Clinically, the tumefaction could be a large mass, but mostly it occurs as a single nodule or ulcer averaging 2 cm in diameter. Grossly, there is a yellow tint to the tumor mass. The histology reveals tumor cells that have elongated, spindle-shaped nuclei with the appearance of fibroblasts or fibrocytes (Figs. 21.17 and 21.18). These cells often produce a storiform architectural pattern. The cells may also be found in a more fascicular pattern, with myxoid areas identified. In addition, more rounded cells, often containing fine vacuoles in their cytoplasm and having the features of histiocytes, may be seen (Fig. 21.20). Multinucleated giant cells (Touton giant cells) often with a foamy cytoplasm may be found (Figs. 21.19 and 21.20). As mentioned above, the proportion of fibroblast-like and histiocyte-like components varies greatly, and some tumors may be composed predominantly of one or the other. The micromorphology varies as to differentiation and anaplasia. They can display a strictly benign histology or exhibit overtly malignant micromorphologic features. Histologically, anaplasia of stromal cells, extensive cellular pleomorphism, atypical mitoses, and diffuse often-intense neutrophilic infiltrate unassociated with necrosis have been proposed as criteria for malignancy, although some investigators have thought these findings lack a strict correlation with biological behavior (12). When Fretzin and Helwig (37) listed their 140 patients with a typical fibroxanthoma of the skin, no tumor had

metastasized, and only 9 lesions recurred following surgical removal. The term *atypical fibrohistiocytoma* may suggest to others a possibility of aggressive behavior, and complete surgical removal is needed to protect against complications. There are two features that seem to be most associated with an aggressive nature, i.e., infiltrative margins and tumor size over 6 cm (12).

As to treatment, the histiocytomas of the head and neck represent a spectrum of disease. The majority are benign, but recurrence is frequent. Therefore, the initial approach to these tumors should be an aggressive, wide, local excision (36). Radiotherapy appears to have very limited efficacy with this entity and should be preserved for those that are inoperable. Prognosis among the 32 tumors investigated by Blitzer et al. (38) revealed a 22% metastatic rate.

KELOID

A keloid is defined as a benign tumor occurring as a response to the formation of a scar from trauma or irritation in certain predisposed persons, usually of the black race, that is quite common on the external auricle, particularly the lobe. These tumors are usually instigated by the habit of piercing the ears for earring insertion. Histologically, they reveal an actively growing collagenous tissue (39).

Cheng (39) discussed a series of 40 patients with 60 keloid tumors, with each patient presenting at least 1 on the external

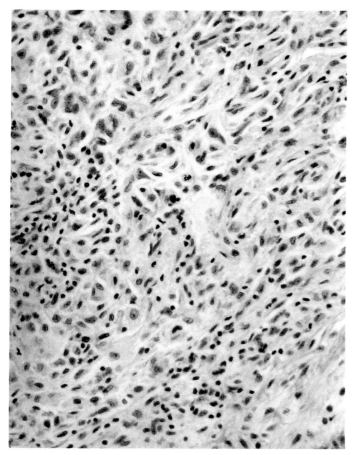

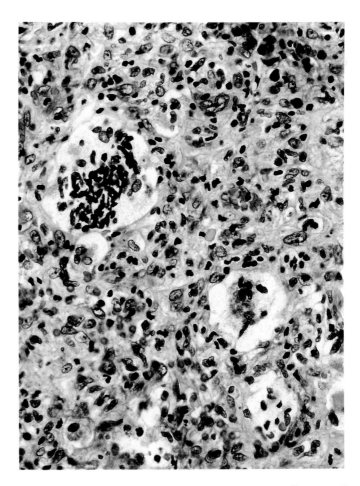

Figure 21.18. Higher magnification of the same view as in Figure 21.17 emphasizes the histiocytic nature of the main tumor cell. (Hematoxylin and eosin, ×160.)

Figure 21.20. Higher magnification of the same view as in Figure 21.19 reveals the prominent multinucleated giant cell (Touton cell) that can be found in the fibrohistiocytoma. (Hematoxylin and eosin, ×160.)

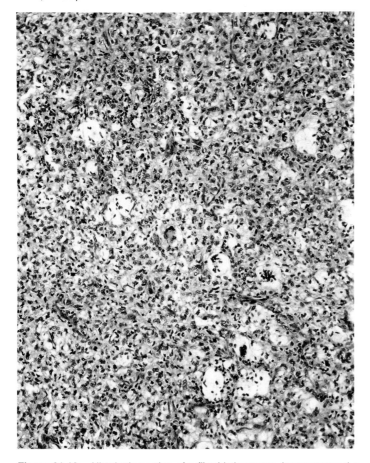

auricle. Only 1 male was included in the group. The ages of these patients ranged from 11 to 29 years, with an average age at onset of 16 years. All were black. All external auricular keloids followed ear-piercing procedures, except in the male who had lacerating trauma to the external ear. Keloids developed within 2–48 months after ear piercing, with an average time of 7 months. From presentation to treatment averaged 2 years. Sizes ranged from 0.5 to 5 cm in diameter, with an average of about 1.5 cm. Most tumors were on the posterior aspect of the earlobe, with some few on the anterior and posterior aspect of the external ear; 1 patient had only an anterior surface tumor. Patients with one or more extra-auricular keloid tumors had their additional tumor or tumors usually on the chest wall and upper extremities. There may be some symptoms such as itching, pain, or paresthesias associated with the keloid. Malignant transformation has been reported (39).

Grossly, the external auricular keloids are readily diagnosed as a progressive growth of a shiny, smooth hard mass (Fig. 21.21). The lesion may be pedunculated at the point where the skin is pierced. The skin overlying the tumor is taut (39). Microscopically, the overlying epidermis is unremarkable, but the dermis and subcutaneous tissue contain a collection of moderately demarcated bundles of multisized hyalinized collagenous fibers intermixed with fibroblasts (Fig. 21.22). Adnexa are atrophic (12). The keloids must be differentiated clinically and histologically from the hypertrophic scar, sarcoid, scleroderma, paraffinoma, and the lesion of Ehlers-Danlos syndrome.

Figure 21.19. Histologic section of a fibrohistiocytoma demonstrates the fibrohistiocytic nature of the tumor cells. (Hematoxylin and eosin, ×63.)

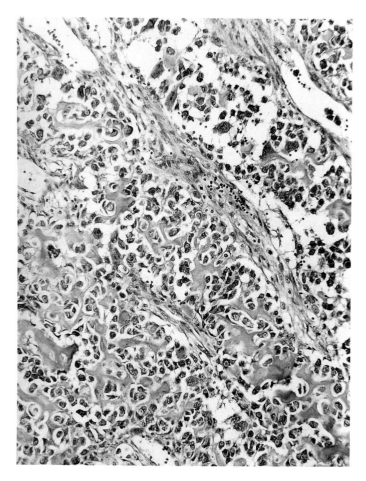

Figure 21.29. Higher magnification of the same view as in Figure 21.28 emphasizes the more uniform appearance of the neoplasm, with the osteoblastic cells being quite variable but not malignant. (Hematoxylin and eosin, ×160.)

There are several case reports of the ossifying fibroma involving the facial and skull bones (49–52).

In presenting the clinical, gross, radiologic, histologic, therapeutic, and prognostic findings, there will be a comparison of the findings of ossifying fibroma with those of fibrous dysplasia, which is, of course, the disease entity most confused with ossifying fibroma. One must remember that the differences are always not as "black and white" as they are presented here but many times will be "shades of grey."

Patients with ossifying fibroma are 15–70 years of age, with more than half being between 20 and 40 years. Fibrous dysplasia will usually present before the patient is 20 years old, and there is no sex preference in fibrous dysplasia, while in ossifying fibroma 84% of patients are female (46). It has long been the idea that ossifying fibroma is a true benign neoplasm, while fibrous dysplasia was a developmental bone maturation defect with osseous metaplasia. Wells and Fechner (46) have disagreed with this idea and believe that fibrous dysplasia is a true neoplasm. The ossifying fibroma is usually slow growing but may be more aggressive in younger patients (49). Fibrous dysplasia is potentially progressive. The radiologic appearance of ossifying fibroma is a monostotic, rarely multiple, well-demarcated lesion with decreased density and an eggshell appearance. There is poor demarcation in the fibrous dysplasia with a ground-glass appearance to the lesion. Incidentally, there is also the so-called polyostotic fibrous dysplasia that is accompanied by sexual precocity in the female (Albright's syndrome). Histologically, the

ossifying fibroma reveals woven and lamellar bone with osteoblastic rimming (Figs. 21.30 and 21.31). There are smooth borders of the tumor and parallel birefringence with polarized light. The fibrous dysplasia will contain essentially woven bone, with no osteoblastic rimming and no feathery irregular borders. There is random birefringence with polarized light. One must remember again that there is somewhat of an overlap in the micromorphologic features of each tumor. Surgically, the ossifying fibroma is considered easily enucleated, whereas the fibrous dysplasia is difficult to remove and will occasionally recur following removal.

Two types of tumors appear somewhat related to the ossifying fibroma in histology and clinical behavior. One is the cemento-ossifying fibroma, which is a small (1–4-cm) lesion with sharp radiographic margins that is described as an ossifying fibroma located near a tooth, usually in the mandible. The second type of tumor that appears somewhat related to the ossifying fibroma contrasts with the above type by tending to be larger than 4 cm and having an irregular radiographic contour. These tumors are concentrated in the maxilla and periorbital bony area and occur in young patients. To reflect the histology or clinical behavior, these latter neoplasms have been termed aggressive or active ossifying fibroma, juvenile ossifying fibroma, psammomatoid ossifying fibroma, and cementifying fibroma (46). Patient ages have ranged from 4 months to 52 years, with most patients being teenagers. The clinical course is one of slow progression over several years, resulting in a variety of visual complaints and possibly nasal obstruction and proptosis. Histologi-

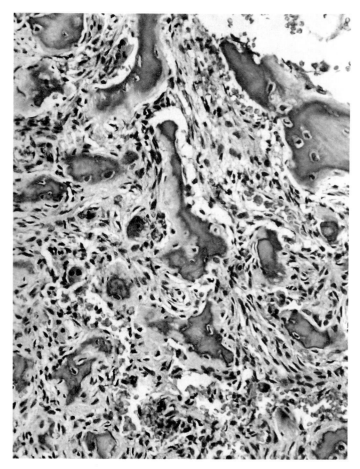

Figure 21.30. Higher magnification of the same view as in Figure 21.29 exhibits the peculiar cementum-like spicules of bone seen in the aggressive ossifying fibroma. (Hematoxylin and eosin, ×250.)

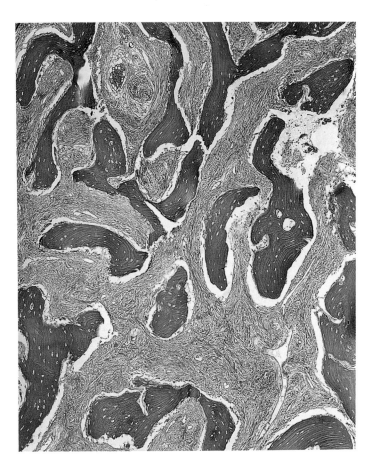

Figure 21.31. Ossifying fibroma revealing a benign fibro-osseous histology consisting of woven and lamellar bone. (Hematoxylin and eosin, ×25.)

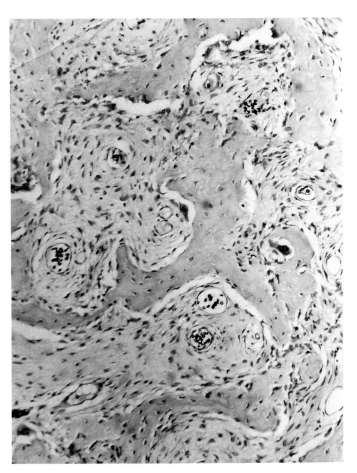

Figure 21.32. Higher magnification of the same view as in Figure 21.31 shows the prominent rimming of osteoblastic-like cells around the bony matrix. (Hematoxylin and eosin, ×160.)

cally, there are irregular trabeculae of bone, either isolated from one another or interconnected (Fig. 21.32). The mineralized spherules noted may contain osteoblasts (Fig. 21.33). This somewhat aggressive form of ossifying fibroma is best seen as a variant of ossifying fibroma with characteristic clinical features in terms of anatomic location, age, and progressive growth (46). In the differential diagnosis, desmoplastic fibroma, giant cell granuloma, and aneurysmal bone cyst can all form bone and cause diagnostic difficulties. Reactive new bone and fibrous tissue that can be seen in osteomyelitis may also result in confusion in diagnosis with the fibro-osseous neoplastic spectrum.

Therapy for the ossifying fibroma is enucleation, which apparently is readily accomplished (49), whereas the removal of fibrous dysplasia can be difficult. Recurrence of tumor is not unusual following treatment for fibrous dysplasia, but the so-called aggressive or ossifying fibroma can also require multiple surgical procedures in an attempt to cure the disease. In patients with fibrous dysplasia, especially those treated by irradiation or radium, there is the occasional development of a fibrosarcoma or osteosarcoma (50, 51). This will usually occur 10 years or more following treatment. No malignant transformation in the ossifying fibroma group has been reported; the aggressive or juvenile type, however, may cause encroachment into adjacent vital areas with possible death.

GIANT CELL TUMORS

Under the term *giant cell tumors,* particularly those that will involve the temporal bone, there is confusion and sometimes difficulty in communicating the definite type of giant cell

tumor present, i.e., whether it is a true giant cell tumor (a neoplasm) that is capable of local aggression and metastasis as well as a possible fatal outcome or whether it belongs to that group of giant cell tumors of bone that are considered in the category of reactive, chemical, congenital, or tumorous abnormalities such as the giant cell granuloma, brown tumor of hyperparathyroidism, cherubism, or the aneurysmal bone cyst. From the experience gained from the literature and the patients listed in the AFIP OTR, most giant cell tumors involving the temporal bone area are not in the true neoplastic classification (true giant cell tumor) but are more likely the so-called giant cell granuloma, brown tumor of hyperparathyroidism, or, rarely, an aneurysmal bone cyst. Unfortunately, most of the medical articles that dwell on the subject do not elaborate on the diagnosis of "giant cell tumor." Some discussion is in order to differentiate the types of giant cell tumors that commonly involve the bones, particularly those of the craniofacial skull area.

True Giant Cell Tumor of Bone

True giant cell tumor of bone (also known as osteoclastoma and myelogenic giant cell tumor) is utilized to emphasize that this neoplastic entity of bone is a true neoplasm. The AFIP fascicle on bone tumors (41) and the WHO "International Histological Classification of Bone Tumours" (44) have relied on the simple designation of "giant cell tumor." This neoplasm is defined as developing within bone and apparently arises from the mesenchymal cells of the connective tissue framework (51). It

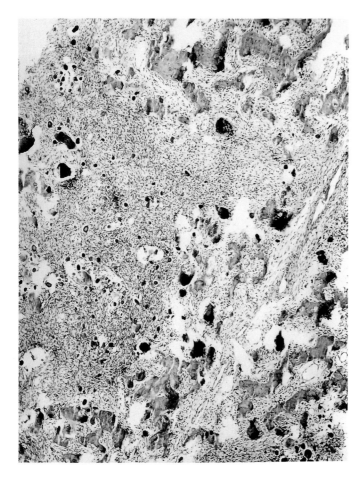

Figure 21.33. The so-called aggressive ossifying fibroma is characterized particularly by an irregular trabeculae of bone. (Hematoxylin and eosin, ×25.)

comprises about 4% of all bone tumors (29). The neoplasm is rare before the age of 20 years or after the age of 55 years. It appears to be predominant in women.

The true giant cell tumor of bone almost invariably arises primarily from the epiphysis and secondarily from the metaphysis of the long bones. There were 5 patients with skull tumors that, because of the presenters' experience with large collections of bone neoplasms, are accepted as true giant cell tumors of bone (53, 54). There are several articles in the literature in which giant cell tumor involving the temporal bone is discussed, but based on the information available it is difficult to consider these as true giant cell tumors of bone. There is 1 patient listed in the AFIP OTR who fulfills all the criteria for a diagnosis of true giant cell of the temporal bone. The other 9 patients in the AFIP OTR with the diagnosis of giant cell tumor of the temporal bone may have the nonneoplastic variety.

The radiologic findings are apparently not specific for the diagnosis. Grossly, the tumors reveal irregular sharp borders that extend into surrounding tissue. The cut surfaces show vascular grayish-red tissue with liquefied zones of necrosis, flecks of yellow, and areas of trabeculation extending across cystic cavities. Brown areas of hemorrhage may be seen (41). Histologically, the basic microscopic pattern of a true giant cell tumor is that of a moderately vascularized stroma associated with rather plump spindle-shaped or ovoid cells regularly interspersed with giant cells. The latter have multiple nuclei sometimes numbering 50–100. There are areas of scarring, cyst formation, hemorrhage, foam cells, and possibly osteoid tissue. Cartilage is apparently

not seen in the neoplasm, and new bone formation is conspicuously absent (41). The neoplasms can be histologically graded from well to poorly differentiated, and this grading can be related to prognosis. It is estimated that 15–30% of cases of true giant cell neoplasm of bone will probably have a malignant behavior by virtue of metastases, recurrence, and local invasion. Some are malignant from the start, and others convert from benign to malignant behavior. The histology will support the malignant behavior by revealing a stroma that consists of a fibrosarcomatous micromorphology and giant cells that reveal anaplastic histology (Figs. 21.34 and 21.35).

Treatment of the well-defined neoplasm consists of local resection with, it is hoped, complete removal of the neoplasm without mutilation. This rather than curettage is recommended because with this latter approach there is a 50–60% recurrence rate (41). When surgical excision is not possible, well-planned radiation therapy may be useful; this treatment has also been advocated for tumors not completely eradicated by surgery. Radiation, however, does increase the risk of inducing a malignant change in the neoplasm and always the possibility of developing a later irradiation fibrosarcoma. The differential diagnoses of the true giant cell tumor must include the giant cell reparative granuloma, brown tumor of hyperparathyroidism, aneurysmal bone cyst, and the chondroblastoma. Those lesions mentioned in the differential diagnoses are all associated with a favorable prognosis, and such factors as their location in a bone, their predilection for certain bones, their characteristic age distribution, their associated chemical findings, and their radiographic aspects are

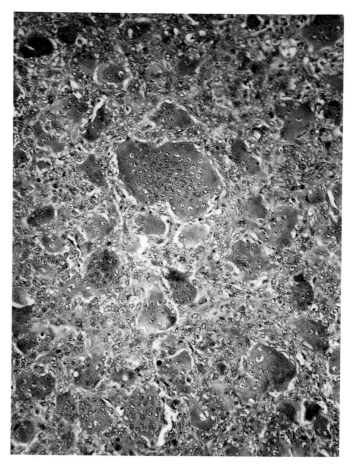

Figure 21.34. Histology of true giant cell tumor of bone with numerous large multinucleated giant cells with the intervening plump spindle to ovoid stromal cells. (Hematoxylin and eosin, ×160.)

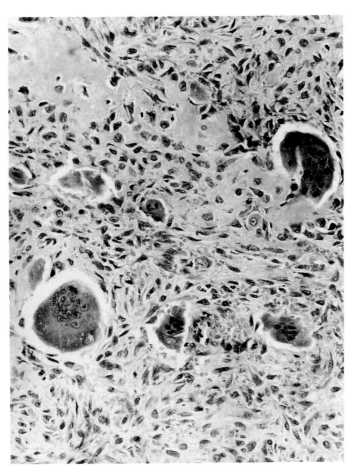

Figure 21.35. Histology of malignant true giant cell of bone with obvious dysplasia and atypia of the giant cell element. (Hematoxylin and eosin, ×250.)

all useful aids in the purely histologic identification of their true nature (41).

Central Giant Cell Reparative Granuloma

Central giant cell reparative granuloma is more regarded as a reactive tumefaction than a true neoplasm. It does mimic the histology and gross presentation of the bona fide true giant cell neoplasm of bone. It is best to attempt to discourage association with the true giant cell neoplasms, however, simply because this central giant cell reparative granuloma has a benign course, requires less extensive treatment, and has an excellent prognosis. Nine of the 10 patients in the AFIP OTR with the diagnosis of a giant cell neoplasm involving the temporal bone actually had what is believed to be a central giant cell reparative granuloma. The reported cases of giant cell tumor of the temporal bone area in the literature also appear to be mainly the central giant cell reparative granuloma. Only 2 of 9 patients reported to have giant cell tumor involving the temporal bone in the literature reviewed by Hirshl and Katz (55) were believed to have a true giant cell tumor of bone.

Although not a common lesion, this central giant cell reparative granuloma is the most common tumor composed of giant cells that is seen in the bones of the head and neck. It has a preference for females, and the patients are most often between 10 and 25 years of age. It is mainly seen in the jaws, more often in the mandible than in the maxilla. Symptoms depend on the

location and aggressiveness of the tumor. Local swelling, pain, tenderness, anesthesia, headache, diplopia, and epistaxis have all been noted (56). In the temporal bone area, a hearing loss appears to be the first sign of the tumor. Then the lesion may narrow the external auditory canal or the middle ear cleft. Radiographically, the lesion appears as a roundish or oval area of increased radiolucency that is sometimes faintly trabeculated. It thins and expands the cortex but does not perforate the cortex of the affected bone. The x-ray picture is somewhat nondescript and does not, in itself, permit a definitive preoperative diagnosis (57). When surgically entered, the lesion consists of a variable amount of soft, spongy, reddish, friable tissue. The histologic picture consists of a fairly loose vascular stroma composed of small, spindle-shaped cells and much hemorrhagic extravasation. The multinuclear giant cells present are sparse, small, and unevenly distributed and are often clumped in areas of hemorrhage (Fig. 21.36). There are occasional edema and even cystification. Between microscopic lobules of tumor, here and there some delicate trabeculae of newly formed osteoid or bone can be seen (57). This central giant cell reparative granuloma of bone is a benign lesion that yields to curettage, after which the lesion is usually obliterated. Occasionally, the curettage has to be repeated subsequently, but if a lesion thought to represent a giant cell reparative granuloma has recurred, the investigator must make sure that the patient is not suffering from hyperparathyroidism and that the jaw lesion in question does not represent an expression of the brown tumor of hyperparathyroidism (57). Cytologically, it is difficult and sometimes impossible to distinguish be-

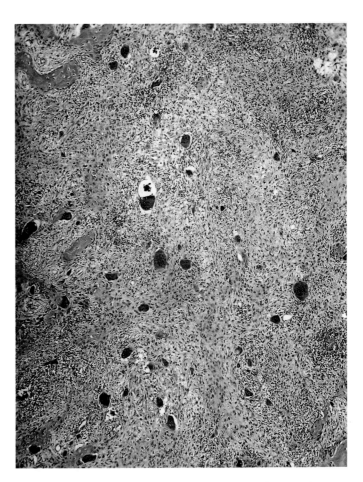

Figure 21.36. Histology of central giant cell reparative granuloma reveals a loose vascular stroma with sparse, small, multinucleated giant cells.

tween the central reparative giant cell granuloma that has developed in a skull bone as a solitary lesion unrelated to hyperparathyroidism and the brown tumor of hyperthyroidism. This problem has led to the recommendation that in any giant cell tumor of the bone an investigation of the serum calcium and phosphorus is a necessity to rule the hyperparathyroid-related tumor. Fechner et al. (58) described an extraordinary growth of a giant cell reparative granuloma during pregnancy. In spite of an aggressive growth in the area of the nasal fossa and left antral area and of incomplete removal of the neoplasm in the area of optic chiasma prepartum, following the birth of the child the patient has remained well for 11 years with no additional therapy.

An important differential consideration is the bona fide giant cell tumor of bone. This lesion rarely appears before the age of 20 years, with most patients being between 25 and 40 years of age. It rarely involves the skull bones, as its principal site is in the end of either a long bone of the limbs or a trunk bone. Histologically, the true giant cell tumor reveals large numbers of giant cells distributed more or less evenly throughout the tissue field, and these giant cells are set in a rather cellular stroma of spindled or polyhedral cells. Clinically, it tends toward clinical aggressiveness, with curettage. Metastases are not unusual (57).

Aneurysmal Bone Cyst, Cherubism, and Peripheral Reparative Giant Cell Tumor

The *aneurysmal bone cyst* is much less of a differential diagnostic problem, particularly regarding morbidity. It is a benign, usually solitary expansile lesion of bone most often occurring in the metaphysis of long bones and in vertebrae and flat bones (Fig. 21.37). Three percent of the lesions occur in the skull (41). There is the rare report of an aneurysmal bone cyst occurring in the temporal bone (59). Blood-filled spaces impart a multicystic appearance, and histologically, solid areas with spindled stroma, osteoid, and multinucleated giant cells are characteristically seen (41). There is indecision as to the origin of this tumor. Some believe it represents an alteration or a different manifestation of such entities as giant cell tumors, chondroblastomas, hemangiomas, and other fibro-osseous tumors. Regardless of its genesis, it is benign, and if it is confused with the central reparative granuloma, the therapy for both is curettement, with good prognoses for both. *Cherubism,* even though it can histologically be confused with the central reparative granuloma of bone, occurs in the jaws of young persons, mainly in the mandible, and should not cause confusion on an anatomical basis alone. The so-called *peripheral reparative giant cell tumor* also mimics the histology of the central variety in bone but is found most often as an exophytic soft tissue tumor of the oral cavity and, in the experience of one of the authors (V.J.H.), sometimes presents in the nasal cavity.

Ewing's Sarcoma of Bone

Ewing's sarcoma of bone is discussed separately from the Ewing's soft tissue sarcoma described earlier in this chapter. Both have the same histologic findings, but the Ewing's soft tissue sarcoma occurs in competition with the juvenile rhabdomyosarcoma in its anatomical area of presentation and gross appearance and, hence, is discussed in the section on sarcomas of the tem-

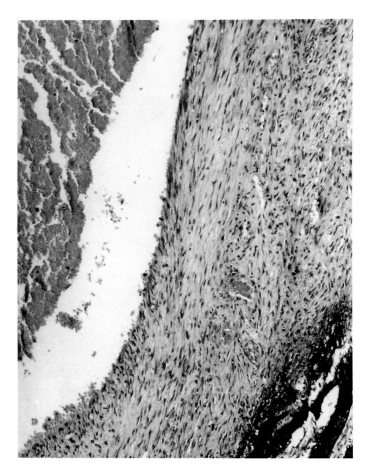

Figure 21.37. Wall of a so-called aneurysmal bone cyst with the compact fibrous wall that quite often will contain multinucleated giant cells. (Hematoxylin and eosin, ×63.)

poral bone area. The Ewing's sarcoma of bone, however, begins as an intraosseous, glycogen-containing, small, round cell malignant tumor cell and occurs most frequently in patients in the second and third decades (60). It accounts for 4–10% of all malignant bone neoplasms, and involvement of the skull, craniofacial bones, and particularly the jaws accounts for 1–10% of all Ewing's sarcomas of bone.

Arafat et al. (60) presented 17 patients with Ewing's sarcoma of the jaw who were listed in the AFIP tumor registry. A search of this same registry and the medical literature did not reveal a case of temporal bone involvement by Ewing's sarcoma. It would seem that the temporal bone is susceptible to such involvement. In the 17 patients mentioned in the study of jaw neoplasms by Arafat et al. (60), ages ranged from 2 to 38 years, with a mean age at onset of 16 years. Eight patients were male. Swelling was the most common symptom, while pain was next in frequency, followed by paresthesia. Reported systemic findings included albuminuria and secondary anemia. The radiographic findings reported were consistent with osteomyelitis, eosinophilic granuloma, bone cysts, osteosarcoma, or metastatic neoplasm. The possibility of the so-called "onionskin" appearance in the periosteal area of the long bones may be of help in the differential diagnosis of neoplasms in those areas. The biopsy specimen is most important with the lack of definite radiologic, gross, and other clinical findings. Histopathologically, the tumor consists of small, round cells with large hyperchromatic nuclei, few nucleoli, and distinct nuclear membranes. A rosette-like cell pattern is not unusual. Mitotic figures are common. The neoplasm is usually fairly vascular with hemorrhage and necrosis (60).

The differential diagnoses that must be considered are intraosseous neuroblastoma and the non-Hodgkin's reticulum cell sarcoma or lymphoma.

The therapy has consisted of local surgical resection, radiation therapy, and chemotherapy. Encouraging results have also been obtained with the use of multitherapy protocols employing combinations of the above-mentioned therapeutic entities. In spite of these encouraging developments, the 5-year cure rate is under 10% in most reported series (60).

LYMPHOMATOUS NEOPLASTIC INVOLVEMENT OF THE TEMPORAL BONE

The term *lymphoma* as used here indicates a neoplasia of lymphoreticular tissue and its cellular derivatives, including non-Hodgkin's lymphoma (lymphosarcoma), Hodgkin's lymphoma, leukemia, and plasmacytic neoplasia that involve the temporal bone. We do not intend to discuss in detail the different classifications of lymphoma, particularly the non-Hodgkin's lymphoma, which can be quite involved, confusing, and difficult even in the most experienced and learned hands.

Non-Hodgkin's Lymphoma

Non-Hodgkin's lymphoma can be defined as a primary malignant neoplasm of lymphoreticular tissue that is composed of primitive reticular cells, their histiocytic or lymphocytic derivatives, or combinations of these cell types (61). This definition also fits Hodgkin's disease, but this discussion includes only the non-Hodgkin's lymphoma. Hodgkin's disease is presented below.

As mentioned above, it is not our intention to discuss the complicated as well as controversial classifications utilized and proposed for non-Hodgkin's lymphoma. One of the authors (V.J.H.) has relied on the Rappaport classification (61, 62) and believes that it provides a classification that is easily understood and correlates well with the severity as well as the projected prognosis of the disease. It can also facilitate the ability of the pathologist to transmit the type and degree of lymphomatous pathology to the clinician in an understandable language. The so-called "New Working Formulation of Non-Hodgkin's Lymphomas" utilizes a classification that divides the neoplasm into low-grade, intermediate-grade, and high-grade malignancies (63). The remaining classifications will usually make use of the immunologic phenotype of the malignant lymphocytic cell, such as a B, T, or miscellaneous lymphocytic type (62). All classifications should convey to the clinician the prognostic outlook of the non-Hodgkin's lymphoma with regard to the patient.

In the AFIP OTR there were only 3 patients listed with non-Hodgkin's lymphoma involving the temporal bone area, 1 with lymphoma involving the external ear and 2 with lymphoma of the middle ear space. No further information was available. Paparella and ElFiky (64) described 6 patients with non-Hodgkin's lymphoma (lymphosarcoma and reticulosarcoma) in which the temporal bone was removed at autopsy and examined. The main pathology was generally systemic, but all the temporal bones revealed varying amounts of hemorrhage and neoplastic infiltrates within the varying marrow spaces as well as in most middle ears and Eustachian tubes with some revealing tumor involvement of the cochlea, vestibule, and facial nerve. Takehara et al. (65) reported 1 patient with a systemic poorly differentiated non-Hodgkin's lymphoma in which there was marked tumor cell involvement, not only of the lateral part of the cartilaginous portion of the Eustachian tube but also of the anterior part of the temporal bone. A serous middle ear effusion without accompanying neoplasm was noted and believed to be due to Eustachian tube obstruction secondary to the effects of the neoplastic infiltration of the peri-Eustachian tube area.

Midline Malignant Reticulosis

Midline malignant reticulosis is known as polymorphic reticulosis and, erroneously, as the nonspecific entity "lethal midline granuloma." It is defined as a rare, progressive, destructive lesion usually involving initially the midpalate and/or the nasal septum and, if not responsive to therapy, the facial area with a hideously appearing ulcerative lesion (64). Although the temporal bone has not been singled out as being involved with the midline malignant reticulosis, it is difficult to believe that the ear has escaped, with the neoplastic process being quite prominent in the pharyngeal area. Perhaps the dramatic presentation and the appearance of the disease in the upper respiratory tract cause the temporal bone involvement to be overlooked. The disease process is considered by most to be a mixed non-Hodgkin's lymphoma and requires the same treatment as a localized lymphoma, which consists of therapeutic doses of irradiation.

Hodgkin's Disease

In the AFIP OTR there is no patient of record with Hodgkin's disease involving the temporal bone. In the series of Paparella and ElFiky (64), there were 2 patients with systemic Hodgkin's disease with autopsy examination of the temporal bones revealing marked involvement of marrow by tumor, 1 with thickened middle ear and mastoid lining and a serous nonneoplastic fluid effusion. Neither patient had a clinical history of otologic symptoms!

VASCULAR NEOPLASMS OF THE TEMPORAL BONE

Vascular neoplasia (excluding the extra-adrenal paragangliomas and the angiolymphoid hyperplasia with eosinophilia) is not a prominent pathologic entity in the temporal bone area. Of approximately 3000 patients with temporal bone neoplasia contained in the AFIP OTR between 1940 and 1985, there were only 23 patients listed with a vascular tumor or neoplasm in this specific anatomical area. Only 4 of these patients were diagnosed with a malignant vascular process. In spite of the low incidence of vascular neoplasia in the temporal bone, the blood vessels of the temporal bone are subject to the same types of vascular pathology as are vessels of similar size and structure elsewhere in the body. These conditions include calcium plaques, atheromas, aneurysms, tortuosity, congestion, stasis, obliterative arteritis, and sympathetic constriction (66).

The pathologic and cytology classification of the various vascular neoplastic entities can be somewhat involved, and one wonders if an organization of these tumors into a benign and malignant category would not be sufficient. In the discussion below, the benign vascular neoplasms of the temporal bone area as well as the malignant counterparts are discussed separately, and Kaposi's sarcoma is also considered a separate subject because of the recent interest in this particular disease.

Benign Vascular Neoplasms

A difficulty in dealing with benign vascular neoplasia, particularly in the head and neck area, is the determination of whether the tumor is to be considered a congenital vascular malformation or a true benign neoplasm. This is especially difficult in the pediatric patient and less of a problem with the older patient. It probably makes little difference in determining whether or not intradermal capillary hemangiomas of the young, such as the "salmon patch, port-wine stain, spider hemangioma, strawberry mark," are congenital, but in the case of an arteriovenous fistula or cirsoid angioma, there may be a need to utilize special therapeutic procedures. Persky (67) has mentioned the observation that 73% of these benign vascular lesions are present at birth and 85% are present before the first year of life. Miller (68) reported on 55 patients who up to 1949 had hemangiomas of the ear and mastoid process. He has considered them as hamartomatous hemangiomas and divided them into capillary and cavernous types. He mentioned the rare occurrence of a sclerosing hemangioma in the temporal bone area that apparently is synonymous with the granuloma pyogenicum. In the AFIP OTR (1940–1986) were listed 18 patients with benign vascular tumors of the temporal bone area. There were 7 patients with vascular malformations, 5 with hemangiomas, 2 with lymphangiomas, and 1 each (among the remaining 4 patients) with granuloma pyogenicum, intravascular hemangioma, angiokeratoma, or vascular leiomyoma. Patients in Miller's group (68) had an age range of 3–78 years, with 2 patients in the first decade, 4 in the second, 7 in the third, 9 in the fourth, 9 in the fifth, 10 in the sixth, 5 in the seventh, and 3 in the 8th decade. Females outnumbered males in a ratio of 3:1. In the AFIP OTR from 1976 through 1985, the ages ranged from 5 through 73 years, with an average age at onset of 44 years. There were 11 females to 9 males. In Miller's series (68) of 55 patients, the middle ear was listed as the most common site of occurrence with the rare involvement of the tympanic membrane and external auditory canal. In the AFIP OTR, 10 patients were listed with the middle ear cleft area as the anatomical site of occurrence; 5 had external canal lesions, and 3 had lesions involving the pinna. One patient had an inner auditory canal hemangioma. Managham et al. (69) presented 10 patients with intratemporal histologically benign vascular neoplasms: 6 of these neoplasms originated in the internal auditory canal; 3, from the geniculate ganglion; and 1, from the petrous apex area. The clinical presentation of these patients was mainly one of facial nerve paralysis, facial twitching, tinnitus, and hearing loss. The histology supported either a capillary or a cavernous hemangioma or what was termed a vascular malformation. These tumefactions invaded the facial nerve. Complete surgical excision was the treatment of choice, which would usually require severance and repair of the involved facial nerve.

Clinical presentations of vascular tumors of the external canal (Fig. 21.38), eardrum, or middle ear cleft were accompanied by symptoms such as tinnitus or pulsing tinnitus, loss of

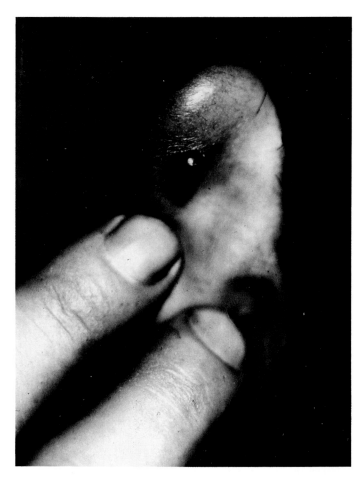

Figure 21.38. Clinical picture of primary small hemangioma occurring on the external auricle of a middle-aged adult.

hearing, and pain. Signs were a red eardrum membrane, a polypoid hemangiomatous mass in the external canal, bleeding from the ear, otorrhea, and involvement of cranial nerves. In any of the *systemic hemangiomastoses,* such as *Rendu-Osler-Weber disease and Sturge-Weber disease,* the external ear including the external auditory canal can be involved with the hemangiomatous lesions. Obiako (70) presented a 28-year-old man with a history of a steadily enlarging left auricle that probably dated back to trauma to the area following a soccer accident as a young boy. Although pain was not a problem, the enlarged appearance was cosmetically disturbing. Physically, the involved ear was warmer than the right and revealed on auscultation a continuous bruit with systolic accentuation. A left carotid angiography was done and confirmed the presence of an arteriovenous fistula. Surgical ligation of the vessels contained in the mass including the posterior occipital artery and vein led to an apparent cosmetic cure.

Histologically, the hemangioma is a benign noncircumscribed lesion consisting of proliferating blood vessels of various types (Fig. 21.39). Micromorphologic distinction between tissue malformations (hamartomas) and true tumors is especially difficult. The capillary hemangioma (juvenile hemangioma) is composed predominantly of small vascular channels, mostly of capillary size, lined by a single layer of benign endothelial cells (Fig. 21.40). The cavernous hemangioma is composed predominantly of cavernous vascular structures lined by a single layer of endothelial cells. The intervascular tissue is usually that of an acellular fibrous nature. The hemangiomatosis that accompanies

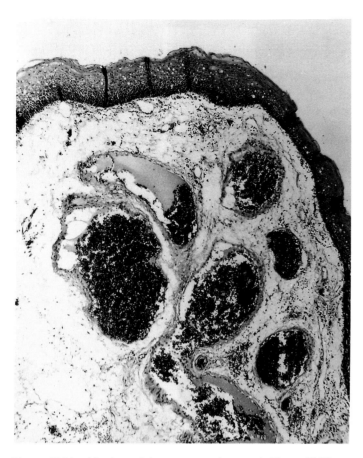

Figure 21.39. Histology of the same neoplasm as in Figure 21.38 supports a proliferation of benign vascular structures consistent with hemangioma. (Hematoxylin and eosin, ×63.)

the Rendu-Osler-Weber disease or Sturge-Weber disease is a regional or diffuse proliferation of capillaries or thin-walled vascular structures. The granuloma pyogenicum or the sclerosing hemangioma is usually a raised lesion of the skin or mucosal surface that has the microscopic appearance of a lobulated capillary hemangioma or richly vascular granulation tissue (Fig. 21.41). Secondary features such as surface ulceration, chronic inflammation, and fibrosis are common. The tendency to occur during adult life and occasionally during pregnancy helps to distinguish it from capillary hemangioma (2).

Therapy, particularly in the younger patients, has been somewhat conservative, with the idea that there is the potential for natural regression in many of these benign vascular lesions, essentially in the young (67). Previously recommended modes of therapy included the utilization of radiation, carbon dioxide, liquid nitrogen, tattooing, diathermy, electrocoagulation, and sclerotic agents. If there is reason to believe that there is no resolution of the tumor after reasonable observation or if there is significant airway obstruction, rapid hemangioma growth, hemorrhage, and ulceration or severe deformity, then surgery, with or without embolization, or embolization alone should prove a safe and effective method of treatment of these lesions (67). In the series of Miller (68) of hemangiomas of the ear and mastoid, the follow-up information in 22 of the patients reported revealed that at least 8 patents died as a result of the tumor and 14 patients recovered or were considered improved.

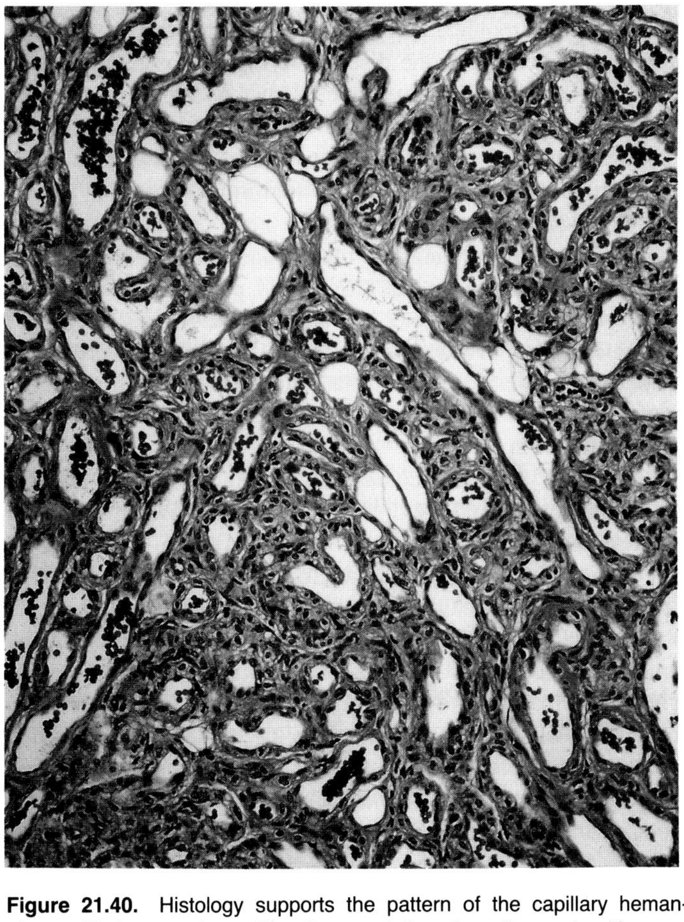

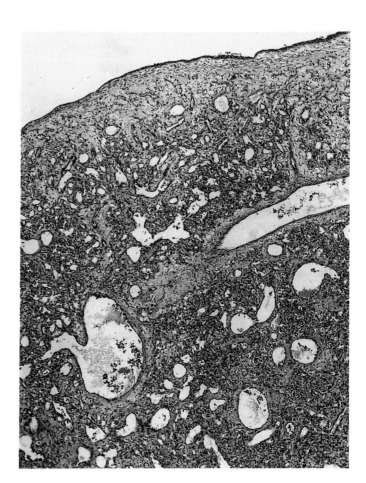

Figure 21.40. Histology supports the pattern of the capillary hemangioma with the vascular proliferation consisting of small vessels with prominent endothelial cells. (Hematoxylin and eosin, ×160.)

Figure 21.41. The histologic architecture of this so-called pyogenic granuloma looks like that of a hemangioma but with a pattern of large central vessels with surrounding feeder vessels. (Hematoxylin and eosin, ×63.)

men more than women in a ratio of 3:1 and has a predilection for people of Jewish and Mediterranean ancestry between 50 and 80 years of age (mean age at diagnosis of 63 years); 75% of these patients will have the initial lesions on the lower extremity and 22% will have them on the upper extremity and trunk. It is not uncommon that as the disease progresses, nodules appear on the head, neck, and mucosal membranes or internally as visceral lesions. In the classic Kaposi's sarcoma there appears to be a susceptibility in patients that have received immunosuppressive agents for renal transplants and those who have received steroid treatment. Lymphoma and other malignancies may also accompany the classical disease (79). The average survival time for patients with classical Kaposi's sarcoma is 8–13 years, with a small percentage of patients dying of complications of bowel involvement. There is a form of classical Kaposi's sarcoma occurring in Africa with a predominance for men that affects younger persons including children and adolescents and follows a more fulminating course.

The other manifestation of Kaposi's sarcoma is its occurrence in patients with the acquired immunodeficiency syndrome (AIDS). In this form the lesions present mainly on the upper body, including the arms, torso, head and neck, and the viscera. The lesion involves patients at an earlier age than the classical variety, from 22 to 52 years with a mean age at onset of 38 years. The prognosis, age of onset, and generalized systemic involvement are similar to the lymphadenopathy form of Kaposi's sarcoma seen in African children and young adults. Over a quarter of the patients with Kaposi's sarcoma associated with AIDS are dead within 2 years.

Gnepp et al. (79) were able to gather data from the medical literature on 74 patients and from the AFIP OTR on 9 patients who had classical Kaposi's sarcoma involving the head and neck. Seventy percent of the patients were 50 years of age or older, while 11 patients were under 16 years of age, with the majority of this latter group having African Kaposi's sarcoma. In this series of 83 patients there were 9 who had involvement of the external ear. As was noted, most of the patients developed head and neck lesions following discovery of Kaposi's sarcoma elsewhere, mainly the lower extremities, but some lesions of the

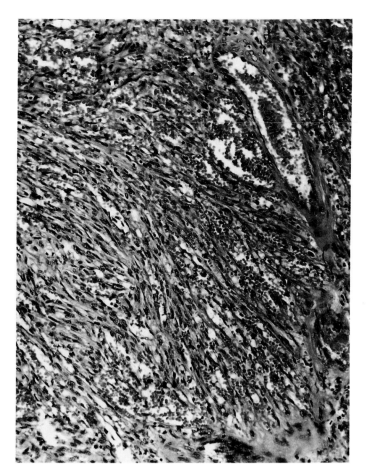

Figure 21.46. Histology of a Kaposi's sarcoma is demonstrated by the fibrosarcomatous micromorphology with the incorporated intracellular slit-like spaces filled with erythrocytes. (Hematoxylin and eosin, ×160.)

head and neck appeared simultaneously with lesions on the extremities. Abramson and Simons (80) recorded 8 of 12 patients with Kaposi's sarcoma of the ear who also had involvement of the extremities. Clinically, the Kaposi's sarcoma begins as one or several reddish-blue nodules or macules and may have associated edema of the involved part (Fig. 21.45). Ulceration may occur, and the lesions may also spontaneously regress. Pain is usually not a factor unless the lesion is on the weight-bearing body area, such as the sole of the foot. Histologically, in the typical lesion there is a moderately delineated nodule in the dermis and upper subcutaneous tissue. Under high magnification the characteristic vascular slit pattern is seen. This is the critical finding without which the diagnosis of Kaposi's sarcoma cannot be made (81). The vascular slit pattern is composed of interlacing sweeps of fusiform cells separated by slit-like spaces containing erythrocytes. The slits have no identifiable endothelial lining (Figs. 21.46 and 21.47). Mitoses are rare. The surface may be ulcerated with acute inflammatory cell infiltrates that suggest a granuloma pyogenicum. In older lesions there are fibrosis and deposition of hemosiderin pigment. In the differential diagnosis, the pyogenic granuloma, hemangioma, spindle cell squamous carcinoma, or other sarcomas may be difficult to differentiate histologically.

The Kaposi's sarcoma associated with AIDS may be the first manifestation of the disease in the patient. This was the case in 9 of the 13 patients studied by Patow et al. (82). The clinical behavior of this Kaposi's sarcoma commonly presents on the

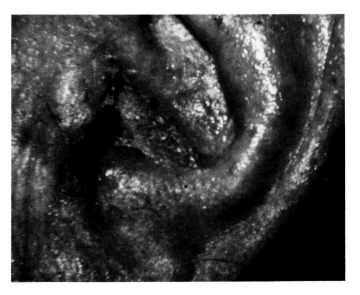

Figure 21.45. Elderly man with classical Kaposi's sarcoma on external auricle. A hemorrhagic papule occupies the antitragus.

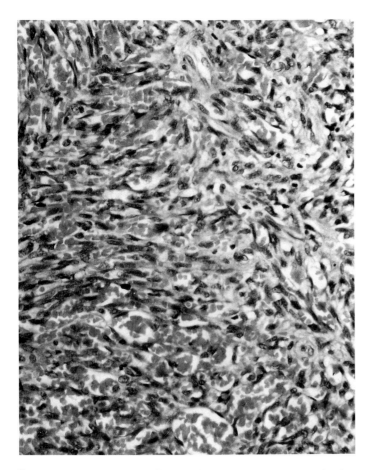

Figure 21.47. Higher magnification of a Kaposi's sarcoma emphasizes the vascular slits between the dysplastic fibrocytic cells (Hematoxylin and eosin, ×250.)

upper body including the arms, skin of the head and neck, and the oral or oropharyngeal mucous membranes (79). Multiple tumors, generalized lymphadenopathy, and visceral involvement are common.

The treatment of the classical Kaposi's sarcoma has been gratifying. Gnepp et al. (79) maintains that patients with Kaposi's sarcoma did not die because of it. Treatment has been simple excision or local radiation therapy. In the difficult cases with classical Kaposi's sarcoma involving the viscera, apparently chemotherapy (vinblastine) therapy has proven beneficial in half of these patients. Patients with the Kaposi's sarcoma associated with the AIDS, because of the visceral involvement and opportunistic infections, have an extremely poor prognosis. It is important to consider Kaposi's sarcoma in the differential diagnosis of any mucosal or skin tumor arising in the head and neck area.

CARTILAGINOUS NEOPLASMS

Cartilaginous neoplasms occur sporadically in the temporal bone area. Those cartilaginous neoplasms of the temporal bone that can be classified as benign are chondroma, osteochondroma (osteocartilaginous exostosis), chondromyxoid fibroma, and chondroblastoma. The last mentioned has also been described in a malignant form. The malignant cartilaginous neoplasms of the temporal bone are the chondrosarcoma and, possibly, the mesenchymal chondrosarcoma.

Chondroma

The AFIP OTR lists 10 patients with chondroma (enchondroma or osteochondroma) of the temporal bone area. Two had auricular tumors, 1 patient each had an external canal tumor and a middle ear tumor, and 6 patients had their chondromas occurring in the temporal bone only. The literature contains mention of 2 patients with chondromas or osteochondromas arising from the middle fossa surface of the petrous bone (83) and 1 patient with multiple osteochondromas arising from the skull surface, extremities, and bilateral external auditory canals (84). This latter patient was under 21 years of age, but those of Schater et al. (83) were 35–61 years of age. The sex ratio is even in some large series, while in others either males or females predominate. The clinical or gross appearance of these benign cartilage tumors is of a usually bony hard exophytic protuberance from a bone surface. The shape may resemble a cauliflower shoot with a surface that is lobulated or knobby and has a grayish-blue sheen (41). The microscopic picture of the chondroma or enchondroma or ecchondroma is characterized by the formation of mature cartilage (Figs. 21.48 and 21.49) but lacks the histologic characteristics of the chondrosarcoma (high cellularity, pleomorphism, and the presence of large cells with double nuclei or mitosis). The osteochondroma (osteocartilaginous exostosis) is a cartilage-capped bony projection on the external surface of a bone. The chondroma or the osteochondroma, if not causing symptoms, is not removed. Rarely do these lesions undergo malignant degeneration.

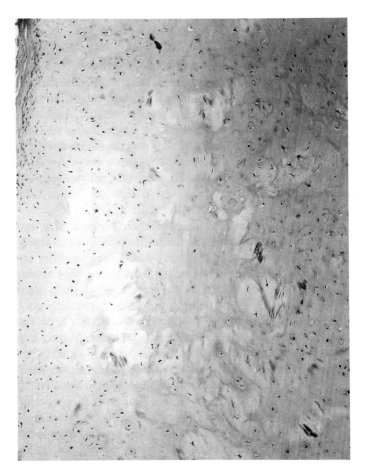

Figure 21.48. Histology of a chondroma will reflect the normal micromorphology of the parent tissue. (Hematoxylin and eosin, ×63.)

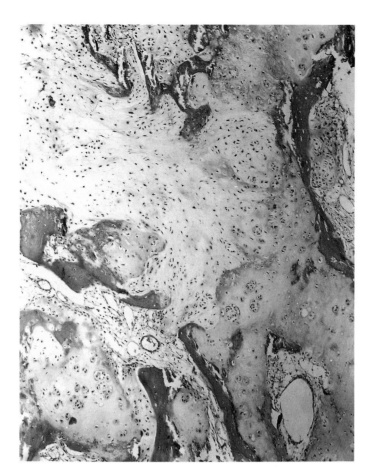

Figure 21.51. Low-grade chondrosarcoma will reflect the cartilaginous histology but with an increase in chondrocytes and pleomorphism, compared with the pattern of the chondroma. (Hematoxylin and eosin, ×63.)

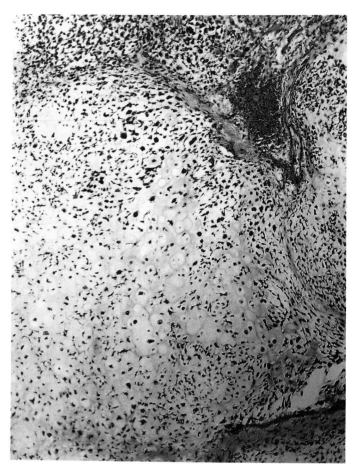

Figure 21.52. Higher-grade chondrosarcoma will usually contain such pleomorphism of the cellular element that the resemblance to cartilage is lost. (Hematoxylin and eosin, ×160.)

not practical because of the position of the tumor and the surrounding neural structures. The neoplasm is relatively radioinsensitive, and the dose of radiation that could be administered is limited by the possible damage to adjacent neural structures. The use of proton beam therapy for the chondrosarcoma has been encouraging.

Mesenchymal Chondrosarcoma

There were no patients in the AFIP OTR with mesenchymal chondrosarcoma, nor could an example be found in the literature. Since this particular malignant cartilaginous neoplasm does occur in the head and neck, it is included here.

Mesenchymal chondrosarcoma is a malignant tumor of bone, presenting elements of malignant cartilage and undifferentiated stroma (41). Huvos et al. (94) presented 35 patients with mesenchymal chondrosarcomas in bones or in soft tissue. In this study the histologies were separated into a small cell undifferentiated type and into one with a hemangiopericytomatoid growth pattern.

In this series (94), the ages ranged from 6 to 70 years for 20 males and from 13 to 64 years for 15 females. The average age at onset was 24.7 years. Thirty of the patients had skeletal tumors, and 3 of these were in the skull, although they were not mentioned as involving the temporal bone. In the AFIP OTR, no patient with mesenchymal chondrosarcoma of the temporal

bone was reported. Of the 35 patients in the series of Huvos et al. (94), pain was the most common complaint, with the recognition of a mass being the next most common symptom. The tumors averaged 12.5 cm, and on gross inspection they varied from gray to gray pink, and their consistency varied from firm to soft. They were usually relatively circumscribed masses separable from surrounding osseous or soft tissue. Varying amounts of necrosis and hemorrhages could be seen. Radiologically, the predominant pattern of bone destruction was permeative and osteolytic. During clinical evaluation of mesenchymal chondrosarcoma, both hematogenous and lymphatic metastases complicated the course either immediately or after a long delay. The histology was characterized by the presence of scattered areas of more or less differentiated cartilage (Figs. 21.53 and 21.54) together with a round small cell undifferentiated "mesenchymal" tissue or a tissue with a highly vascular spindle-cell pattern suggesting a hemangiopericytoma.

In the series of Huvos et al. (94), treatment of small cell undifferentiated histologically mesenchymal chondrosarcoma consisted of the local therapy of radiation, then radical surgery followed by the chemotherapy regimen that was recommended for Ewing's sarcoma. The more differentiated hemangiopericytomatoid tumors received preoperative chemotherapy, then definitive surgery, and then usually more of the same chemotherapy. This therapeutic regimen would be similar to that utilized in osteosarcoma of bone. The median survival rate of this series

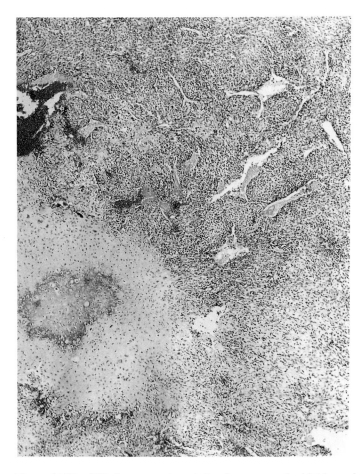

Figure 21.53. With the mesenchymal chondrosarcoma, the histology of malignant cartilage is difficult to identify. The main appearance is that of a malignant small cell infiltrate. (Hematoxylin and eosin, ×25.)

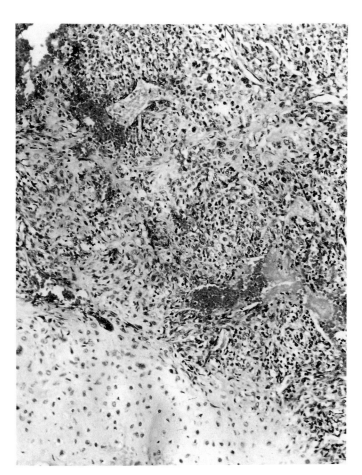

Figure 21.54. Higher-power magnification of the same view as in Figure 21.53, showing an area of malignant cartilage together with the undifferentiated malignant cell pattern. (Hematoxylin and eosin, ×160.)

of 32 patients followed was a 37.9-month average, with a 3-year survival rate of 50%, a 5-year survival rate of 42%, and a 10-year survival rate of 28%.

In 16 of the 35 patients, there were regional and distant lymph node metastases. Ten patients had pulmonary metastases, and 4 had osseous spread.

LIPOMATOUS NEOPLASMS

Lipomatous neoplasms (also known as lipoma, hibernoma, and liposarcoma) are probably one of the rarest mesenchymal tumors involving the temporal bone area. Lipomas are one of the most common tumors that occur in humans (95) but not in the ear. There are 3 patients with lipomas of the temporal bone area listed in the AFIP OTR, 2 with tumors involving the internal auditory canal and 1 with a tumor in the petrous portion of the bone. The literature lists 2 patients with lipomas of the internal auditory canal (95) (probably the same patients listed in the AFIP OTR), 4 patients with lipomas in the area of cerebellar pontine angle (95), and 5 patients with liposarcomas of the temporal bone area (96–98).

The lipoma is defined as a benign growth made up exclusively of mature adipose tissue cells showing no evidence of cellular atypia (Fig. 21.55). Some tumors will be encapsulated, but others may be infiltrating adjacent tissue with no demarcation or encapsulation. Some lipomas undergo a myxoid change

that should not be confused with a myxoid liposarcoma. *Hibernoma* is a benign, lobular, encapsulated tumor made up of granular or vacuolated, round acidophilic cells suggesting a brown fat. The shoulder or neck region of young adults may be involved. Liposarcoma is a malignant infiltrating neoplasm characterized by the presence of atypical lipoblasts in varying stages of differentiation, varying from well-differentiated to cellular or extremely pleomorphic types (2). The biologic behavior varies with the degree of differentiation.

Olsen et al. (95) described 2 patients, a 42- and a 59-year-old man, with lipoma of the internal auditory canal who clinically presented with the signs and symptoms of an acoustic neurilemoma of the anatomical area. Both patients underwent surgical removal with satisfactory results. The histology was that of mature adipose tissue intermixed with nerve bundles and ganglion cells. In the additional 4 patients with lipoma of the cerebellar pontine angle (95), 3 had probably incidental findings, and 1, a 26-year-old woman, underwent successful surgical removal of a cerebellar pontine angle lipoma. The case listed in the AFIP OTR was of a 35-year-old man who underwent successful surgical removal of a lipoma in the petrous portion of the temporal bone. Agarwal et al. (96) presented the case of a liposarcoma of the mastoid in a 4-year-old boy who required extensive surgery, but the child did not survive the operation. A review of the literature by Dahl et al. (98) for liposarcoma of the head and neck region revealed 56 patients. Three liposarcomas were designated as occurring in the temporal area, 1 was designated as occurring

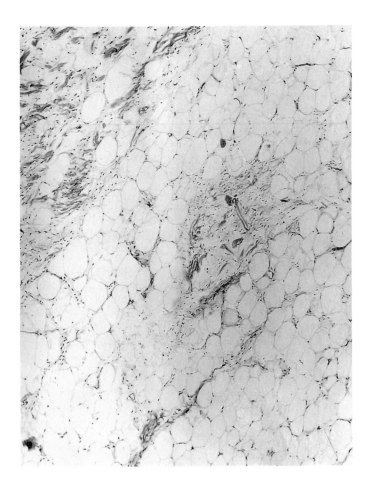

Figure 21.55. Histologic section of lipoma reflecting normal human fat micromorphology. (Hematoxylin and eosin, ×63.)

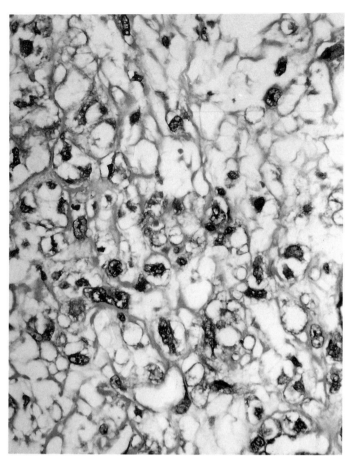

Figure 21.56. Poorly differentiated liposarcoma revealing anaplastic nuclei admixed with cells histologically supportive of fatty tissue (Hematoxylin and eosin, ×400.)

in the mastoid cavity (96), and 1 was designated as occurring in the postauricular neck. The liposarcoma is histologically divided into the predominantly well differentiated, myxoid, round cell, and the poorly differentiated or pleomorphic types (Fig. 21.56) and the mixed type. As mentioned above, there is a correlation of histopathology related to behavior of the liposarcoma.

Olsen et al. (95) have suggested that the origin of lipomatous tumors in the temporal bone area are possibly due to the displacement of presumptive embryonic mesenchymal cells, hyperplasia of normal fat cells within the pia, and lipomatous metaplasia of connective tissue or of pial cells. The lipoma in the petrous portion of the temporal bone brought to mind the possibility of origin of this lipoma from the fatty tissue normally found in among the fibers of the tensor tympanum muscle.

The number of cases of the lipomatous neoplasms of the temporal bone area are too few to be of statistical significance, but apparently these lipomas have been successfully treated surgically. The histories of the liposarcomas of the temporal bone have included the patient of Agarwal et al. (96) and the 4-year-old boy who died in the immediate postoperative period. A 22-year-old male patient of Saunders et al. (97) with a 1-cm primary liposarcoma of the right postauricular region of the neck died of metastases approximately 1 year following surgical treatment. Of the 2 patients of Enterline et al. (99) with liposarcoma of the temporal area, a 53-year-old woman and a 61-year-old man, the former had no recurrence 6 years following surgical removal, while the latter still had tumor present 11 years following multiple surgical removals.

References

1. Naufel PM. Primary sarcomas of the temporal bone. Arch Otolaryngol 1973;98:44–50.
2. Enzinger FM, Lattes R, Torloni H. Histological typing of soft tissue tumors. Int Histolog Classif Tumors 1969(3).
3. Feldman BA. Rhabdomyosarcoma of the head and neck. Laryngoscope 1982;92:424–440.
4. Prat J, Gray GF. Massive neuraxial spread of aural rhabdomyosarcoma. Arch Otolaryngol 1977;103:301–303.
5. Angervall L, Dahl I, Ekedahl C. Embryonal rhabdomyosarcoma in the external ear. Acta Otolaryngol 1972;73:513–520.
6. Friedman J. Pathology of the ear. Oxford: Blackwell Scientific Publications, 1974.
7. Willis R. Pathology of tumors. London: Butterworth and Co, 1953.
8. Russell DS, Rubenstein LJ. Pathology of tumors of the nervous system. 4th ed. Baltimore: Williams & Wilkins, 1977.
9. Smith MT, Armbrustmacher VW, Violett TW. Diffuse meningeal rhabdomyosarcoma. Cancer 1981;47:2081–2086.
10. Canalis RF, Gussen R. Temporal bone findings in rhabdomyosarcoma with predominantly petrous involvement. Arch Otolaryngol 1980;106:290–293.
11. Enzinger FR, Weiss SW. Soft tissue tumors. St Louis: CV Mosby, 1983.
12. Hyams VJ, Batsakis JG, Michaels L. Tumors of the upper respiratory tract and ear. In: Atlas of tumor pathology. 2nd series, Fascicle 25. Washington, DC: Armed Forces Institute of Pathology, 1988.
13. Enzinger FM, Shiraki M. Alveolar rhabdomyosarcoma. Cancer 1969;24:18–31.
14. Ragab AH, Heyn R, Tefft M, Hays DN, Newton WA, Beltangady M. Infants younger than 1 year of age with rhabdomyosarcoma. Cancer 1986;58:2606–2610.
15. Newman AN, Rice DH. Rhabdomyosarcoma of the head and neck. Laryngoscope 1984;94:234–239.

16. Goepfert H, Cangir A, Lindberg H, Ayala A. Rhabdomyosarcoma of the temporal bone. Is surgical resection necessary? Arch Otolaryngol 1979;105:310–313.

17. Sutlow WW, Lindberg RD, Gehan EA, Ragab AH, Raney RB Jr, Ruymann F, Soule EH. Three-year relapse-free survival rates in childhood rhabdomyosarcoma of the head and neck. Report from the Intergroup Rhabdomyosarcoma Study. Cancer 1982;49:2217–2221.

18. Shimade H, Newton WA, Soule EH, Beltangady MS, Maurer HM. Pathology of fatal rhabdomyosarcoma. Report from the Intergroup Rhabdomyosarcoma Study (IRS-I and IRS-II). Cancer 1987;59:459–465.

19. Raney RB Jr, Lawrence W Jr, Maurer HM, Lindberg RD, Newton WA, Ragab AH, Tefft M, Foulkes MA. Rhabdomyosarcoma of the ear in childhood. A report from the Intergroup Rhadomyosarcoma Study-I. Cancer 1983;51:2356–2361.

20. Soule EH, Newton W Jr, Moon TE, Tefft M (For the Intergroup Rhabdomyosarcoma Study Committee). Extraskeletal Ewing's sarcoma. Cancer 1978;42:259–264.

21. Hand R, O'Connor GB. Myxoma of the external auricle. Ann Otol Rhinol Laryngol 1938;47:1096–1100.

22. Stout AP. Myxoma, the tumor of primitive mesenchyme. Ann Surg 1948;127:706–719.

23. Becker W, Buckingham RA, Holinger PH, Kortin GW, Lederer FL. Atlas of otorhinolaryngology and bronchoesophagology. Philadelphia: WB Saunders, 1969.

24. Dahl I, Jarlstedt J. Nodular fasciitis in the head and neck. A clinicopathological study of 18 cases. Acta Otolaryngol 1980;90:152–159.

25. Bernstein KE, Lattes R. Nodular (pseudosarcomatous) fasciitis, a nonrecurrent lesion: clinicopathologic study of 134 cases. Cancer 1982;49;1668–1678.

26. Lever WF, Schaumberg-Lever G. Histopathology of the skin. 5th ed. Philadelphia: JB Lippincott, 1975.

27. Hutter RVP, Stewart FW, Foote FW Jr. Fasciitis. A report of 70 cases with follow-up proving the benignity of the lesion. Cancer 1962;15:992–1003.

28. Mackenzie DH. The fibromatoses. A clinicopathological concept. Br Med J 1972;4:277–281.

29. Neito CS, Forcelledo FF, Cortes JCC, Ablanedo AP, Fernandez de Leon R. Aggressive fibromatosis of the sphenoid. Arch Otolaryngol 1986;112:326–328.

30. Conley J, Healey WV, Stout AP. Fibromatosis of the head and neck. Am J Surg 1966;112:609–614.

31. Morioka WT, Health VC, Cantrell RW. Juvenile fibromatosis. Ann Otol Rhinol Laryngol 1979;88:324–326.

32. Wold LE, Weiland LH. Tumefactive fibro-inflammatory lesions of the head and neck. Am J Surg Pathol 1983;7:477–482.

33. Krishna B, Kacker AK. Dermatofibroma of the external auditory canal. Arch Otolaryngol 1968;87:246–248.

34. Barnes L, Coleman JA, Johnson JT. Dermatofibrosarcoma protuberans of the head and neck. Arch Otolaryngol 1984;110:398–404.

35. Swain RE, Sessions DG, Ogura JH. Fibrosarcoma of the head and the neck. Ann Otol Rhinol Laryngol 1974;83:439–444.

36. Lattes R. Tumors of the soft tissues. In: Atlas of tumor pathology. 2nd series, Fascicle 1. Washington, DC: Armed Forces Institute of Pathology, 1982.

37. Fretzin DF, Helwig EB. Atypical fibroxanthoma of the skin. A clinicopathologic study of 140 cases. Cancer 1963;31:1541–1552.

38. Blitzer A, Lawson W, Biller HF. Malignant fibrous histiocytoma of the head and neck. Laryngoscope 1977;87:1479–1499.

39. Cheng LH. Keloid of the ear lobe. Laryngoscope 1972;82:673–681.

40. Bartolomeo JR. The petrified auricle: comments on ossification, calcification and exostoses of the external ear. Laryngoscope 1985;95:566–575.

41. Spjut HJ, Dorfman HD, Fechner RE, Ackerman LV. Tumors of bone and cartilage. In: Atlas of tumor pathology. 2nd series, Fascicle 5. Washington, DC: Armed Forces Institute of Pathology, 1971.

42. Caron AS, Hajdu SI, Strong EW. Osteogenic sarcoma of the facial and cranial bones. Am J Surg 1971;122:719–725.

43. Huvos AG, Sundaresan N, Bretsky SS, Butler A. Osteogenic sarcoma of the skull. A clinicopathologic study of 19 patients. Cancer 1985;56:1214–1221.

44. Schajowicz F, Ackerman LV, Sissons HA, Sobin LH, Torloni H. Histological typing of bone tumours. Int Histolog Classif Tumors 1972(6).

45. Dorfman HD, Weiss SW. Borderline osteoblastic tumors: problems in the differential diagnosis of aggressive osteoblastoma and low grade osteosarcoma. Semin Diagn Pathol 1984;1:215.

46. Wells WE, Fechner RE. Tumors and tumorlike lesions of the craniofacial bones and cervical vertebrae. In: Gnepp DR, ed. Pathology of the head. New York: Churchill Livingstone, 1988.

47. Pindborg JJ, Kramer IR, Torloni H. Histological typing of odontogenic tumours, jaw cysts, and allied lesions. Int Histolog Classif Tumors 1971(5).

48. Stecker RH. Ossifying fibroma of the middle ear. Arch Otolaryngol 1871;94:80–82.

49. Kridel RWH, Miller RH, Greenberg SD. Ossifying fibroma: diagnostic clarification. Otolaryngol Head Neck Surg 1983;91:568–573.

50. Fu Y-S, Perzin KH. Non-epithelial tumors of the nasal cavity, paranasal sinuses, and nasopharynx: a clinicopathologic study. II. Osseous and fibro-osseous lesions, including osteoma, fibrous dysplasia, ossifying fibroma, osteoblastoma, giant cell tumor and osteosarcoma. Cancer 1974;33:1289–1305.

51. Lund VJ. Ossifying fibroma. A case report. J Laryngol Otol 1982;96:1141–1147.

52. Smith AG, Zavaleta A. Osteoma, ossifying fibroma and fibrous dysplasia of facial and cranial bones. Arch Pathol 1952;54:507–524.

53. Dahlin DC. Giant cell tumor (osteoclastoma). In: Bone tumors. 2nd ed. Springfield, Illinois: Charles C Thomas, 1967.

54. Goldenberg RR, Campbell CJ, Bonfiglio M. Giant-cell tumor of bone. An analysis of two hundred and eighteen cases. J Bone Joint Surg 1970;52A:619–664.

55. Hirschl S, Katz A. Giant cell reparative granuloma outside the jaw bone. Hum Pathol 1974;5:171–181.

56. Rhea JT, Weber AL. Giant-cell granuloma of the sinuses. Radiology 1983;147:135–137.

57. Jaffee HL. Giant-cell reparative granuloma, traumatic bone cyst, and fibrous (fibro-osseous) dysplasia of the jawbones. Oral Surg 1953;6:159–175.

58. Fechner RE, Fitz-Hugh GS, Pope TL Jr. Extraordinary growth of giant cell reparative granuloma during pregnancy. Arch Otolaryngol 1984;110:110–116.

59. Saltzman EI, Jun MY. Aneurysmal bone cyst of the mandible: report of a case. J Surg Oncol 1981;17:385–394.

60. Arafat M, Ellis GL, Adrian JC. Ewing's sarcoma of the jaw. Oral Surg Oral Med Oral Pathol 1983;55:589–596.

61. Rappaport H. Tumors of the hematopoietic system. In: Atlas of tumor pathology. 3rd series, Fascicle 8. Washington, DC: Armed Forces Institute of Pathology, 1966.

62. Conley SF, Staszak C, Clamon GH, Maves MD. Non-Hodgkin's lymphoma of the head and neck: the University of Iowa experience. Laryngoscope 1987;97:291–300.

63. Kruger GRF, Medina JR, Klein HO, Konrads A, Zach J, Rister M, Jnik G, Evers KG, Hirano T, Kitamura H, Bedoya VA. A new working formulation of non-Hodgkin's lymphomas. A retrospective study of the new NCI classification proposal in comparison to the Rappaport and Kiel classifications. Cancer 1983;52:833–840.

64. Paparella MM, ElFiky FM. Ear involvement in malignant lymphoma. Ann Otol Rhinol Laryngol 1972;81:352–363.

65. Takehara T, Sando I, Bluestone CD, Myers EN. Lymphoma invading the anterior Eustachian tube. Temporal bone histopathology of functional tubal obstruction. Ann Otol Rhinol Laryngol 1986;95:101–105.

66. Wolfe D. Wherry Memorial Lecture. The vascular pathology of the temporal bone. Trans Am Acad Ophthalmol Otolaryngol 1949;37–64.

67. Persky MS. Congenital vascular lesions of the head and neck. Laryngoscope 1986;96:1002–1015.

68. Miller MV. Hemangioma of the ear and mastoid process. Report of two cases. Arch Otolaryngol 1949;49:535–545.

69. Managham CA, Carberry JN, Brackmann DE. Management of intratemporal vascular tumors. Laryngoscope 1981;91:867–876.

70. Obiako MN. Arteriovenous fistula of the auricle. Ear Nose Throat J 1988;67:604–607.

71. Barnes L. Surgical pathology of the head and neck. New York: Marcel Dekker, 1985.

72. Farr HW, Carandang CM, Huvos AG. Malignant vascular tumors of the head and neck. Am J Surg 1970;120:501–503.

73. Hodgkinson DJ, Soule EH, Woods JE. Cutaneous angiosarcoma of the head and neck. Cancer 1979;44:1106–1113.

74. Panje WR, Moran WJ, Bostwick DG, Kitt VV. Angiosarcoma of the head and neck: review of 11 cases. Laryngoscope 1986;96:1381–1384.

75. Cochran JH, Fee WE Jr. Angiosarcoma of the head and neck. Otolaryngol Head Neck Surg 1979;87:409–416.

76. Cole LE. Haemangioendothelioma of the head and neck. J Laryngol Otol 1982;96:545–558.

77. Maddox JC, Evans HL. Angiosarcoma of skin and soft tissue: a study of forty-four cases. Cancer 1981;48:1907–1921.

78. Graham WJ, Bogardus CR. Angiosarcoma treated with radiation therapy alone. Cancer 1981;48:912–914.

79. Gnepp DR, Chandler W, Hyams VJ. Primary Kaposi's sarcoma of the head and neck. Ann Intern Med 1984;100:107–114.

80. Abramson AL, Simons RL. Kaposi's sarcoma of the head and neck. Arch Otolarygol 1970;92:505–507.

81. Wood JH. Vascular tumors of the skin. Int Acad Pathol Monogr 1971(1):578–596.

82. Patow CA, Steis R, Longo DL, Reichert CM, Findlay PA, Potter D, Masur H, Lane C, Fauci AS, Macher AM. Kaposi's sarcoma of the head and neck in the acquired immune deficiency syndrome. Otolaryngol Head Neck Surg 1984;92:255–260.

83. Schater IB, Wortz G, Noyer AM. The clinical and radiological diagnosis of cartilaginous tumors of the base of the skull. Can J Otolaryngol 1975;4:364–377.

84. Jones HM. Cartilaginous tumours of the head and neck. J Laryngol Otol 1973;87:135–151.

85. Harner SG, Cody DTR, Dahlin DC. Benign chondroblastoma of the temporal bone. Otolaryngol Head Neck Surg 1979;87:229–236.

86. Kingsley TC, Markel SF. Extraskeletal chondroblastoma. A report of the first recorded cases. Cancer 1971;27:203–206.

87. Dahlin DC. Chondromyxoid fibroma with emphasis on its morphological relationship to benign chondroblastoma. Cancer 1956;9:195–203.

88. Coltrera MD, Googe PB, Harrist TJ, Hyams VJ, Schiller AL, Goodman ML. Chondrosarcoma of the temporal bone. Diagnosis and treatment of 13 cases and review of the literature. Cancer 1986;58:2689–2696.

89. Sanerkin NG. The diagnosis and grading of chondrosarcoma of bone. A combined cytologic and histologic approach. Cancer 1980;45:582–594.

90. Salisbury JR, Isaacson PG. Demonstration of cytokeratins and an epithelial membrane antigen in chordomas and human fetal notochord. Am J Surg Pathol 1985;9:791–797.

91. Miettinen M, Lehio V, Dahl D, Virtanen I. Differential diagnosis of chordoma, chondroid and ependymal tumors as aided by anti-intermediate filament antibodies. Am J Pathol 1983;112:160–169.

92. Valderrama E, Lipper S, Kahm LB, Marc J. Chondroid chordoma: electron microscopic study of two cases. Am J Surg Pathol 1983;7:625–632.

93. Povysil C, Matenovsy Z. A comparative study of chondrosarcoma, chondroid sarcoma, chordoma and chordoma periphericum. Pathol Res Pract 1985;179:546–559.

94. Huvos AG, Rosen G, Dabska M, Marcove RC. Mesenchymal chondrosarcoma. A clinicopathologic analysis of 35 patients with emphasis on treatment. Cancer 1983;51:1230–1237.

95. Olsen JE, Glasscock ME III, Britton BH. Lipomas of the internal auditory canal. Arch Otolaryngol 1978;104:431–436.

96. Agarwal PN, Hishra SD, Pratap VK. Primary liposarcoma of the mastoid. J Laryngol Otol 1975;89:1079–1082.

97. Saunders JR, Jaques DA, Casterline PF, Percarpia B, Goodloe S Jr. Liposarcoma of the head and neck. A review of the literature and addition of four cases. Cancer 1979;43:162–168.

98. Dahl EC, Hammond HL, Sequira E. Liposarcomas of the head and neck. J Oral Maxillofac Surg 1982;40:674–677.

99. Enterline HT, Culberson JD, Rochlin DB, Brady LW. Liposarcoma: a clinical and pathological study of 53 cases. Cancer 1960;13:932.

22/ Osteomas and Exostoses

In contrast to earlier opinions that regarded external auditory canal (EAC) osteomas and exostoses as synonymous (1, 2), more recent observations indicate that these lesions are clinically and histologically different (3–5).

OSTEOMAS

Definition

Osteomas represent a localized, hamartomatous proliferation of a usually very dense, although otherwise-normal intramembranous bone (6).

Localization, Age, and Sex Distribution

Because of their intramembranous, periosteal origin, osteomas arise from bones that develop by intramembranous ossification, and most of them are attached to the skull and facial bones. They are frequently found in the paranasal sinuses where, in decreasing frequency, they involve the frontal, ethmoidal, maxillary, and sphenoid sinuses. They occur on the mandible, anterior maxilla, and outer and inner tables of the calvaria. Their development on the internal surface of the mandible results in the formation of the bosselated mandibular torus, and their location on the undersurface of the hard palate results in the appearance of the nodular palatine torus.

Osteomas also arise from the outer surface of the temporal bone, within the EAC, in rare instances within the mastoid (Fig. 22.23), and from the outer table of the squamous portion of the temporal bone in close proximity to a suture line (Figs. 22.1–22.5). Their size may vary from that of a cherry stone to that of a walnut, and they are slow growing. They manifest themselves as a hemispherical or, rarely, a spherical ivory-hard protrusion with a smooth surface. Except for the noticeable postauricular or supra-auricular deformity, they are initially asymptomatic but may eventually become painful (Figs. 22.4, 22.6, and 22.18).

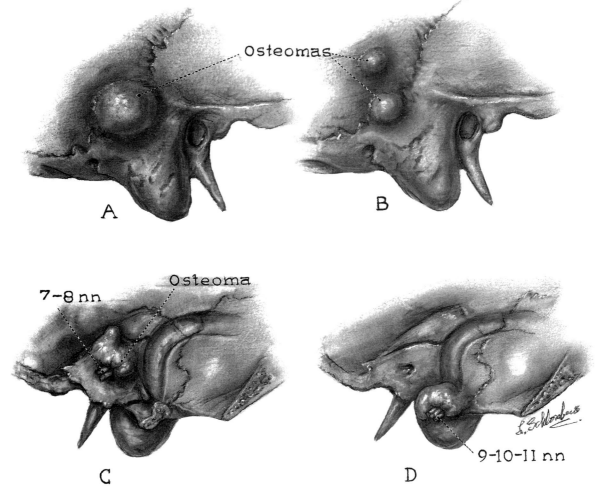

Figure 22.1. Illustration of preferential locations of osteomas on outer surface of temporal bone near suture lines (**A** and **B**) and on inner aspects of petrous pyramid in vicinity of porus acusticus and jugular foramen (**C** and **D**)

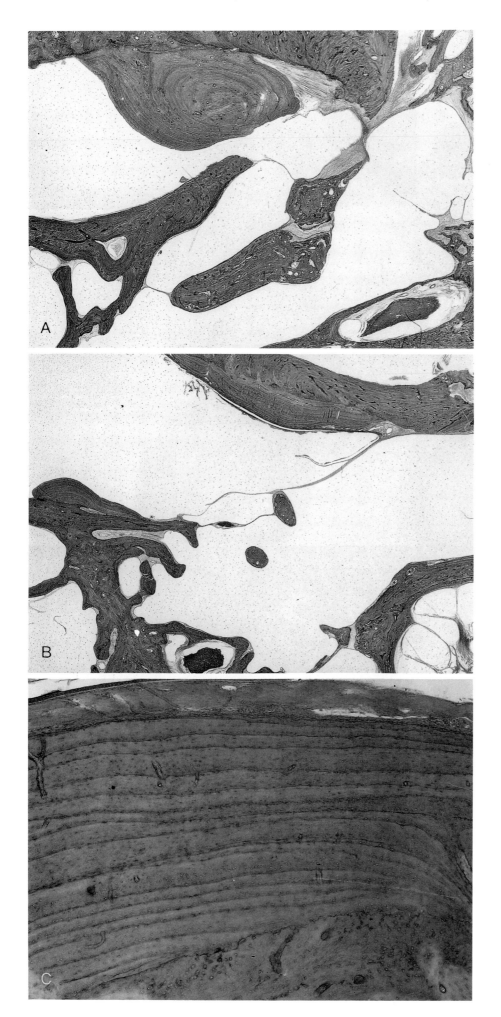

Figure 22.9. **A.** Horizontal section through left temporal bone of an adult male at level of incudomalleolar articulation. An almost spherical exostosis arises from the anterosuperior canal wall near the annulus. (Hematoxylin and eosin, ×10.)

Figure 22.9. **B.** Horizontal section at level of oval window. Two facing broad-based compact exostoses arise from the anterior and posterior canal wall near the annulus. (×8.)

Figure 22.9. **C.** The exostoses consist of subperiosteal lamellar bone with no marrow spaces. (×65.)

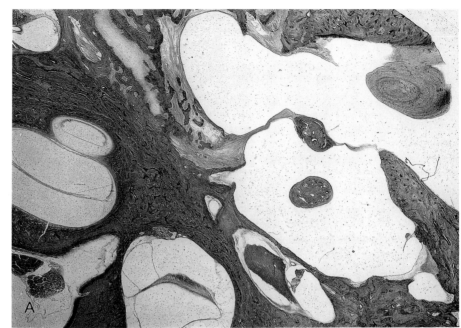

Figure 22.10.   A. Horizontal section through right temporal bone of the same patient as in Figure 22.9 at level of superior oval window margin. A pedunculated spherical exostosis arises from the anterosuperior canal wall near the annulus. (Hematoxylin and eosin, ×10.)

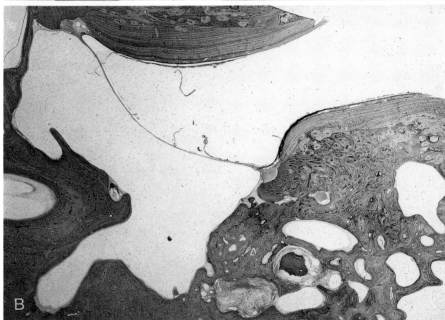

Figure 22.10.   B. Horizontal section at level just above round window niche. Two opposite broad-based compact exostoses arise from the anterior and posterior canal wall at the annulus. (×7.)

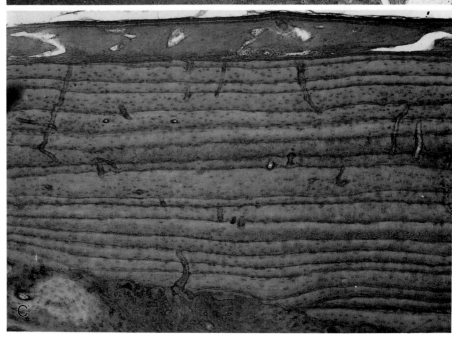

Figure 22.10.   C. The exostoses are made up of subperiosteal, lamellar bone without marrow spaces. (×65.)

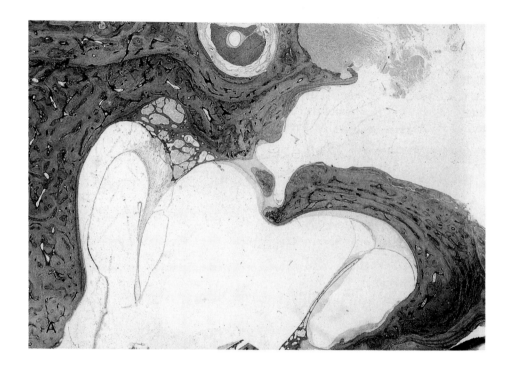

Figure 22.12.   A. Vertical section through right petrous pyramid at level of anterior margin of vestibular fenestra in an adult male. (Hematoxylin and eosin, ×16.)

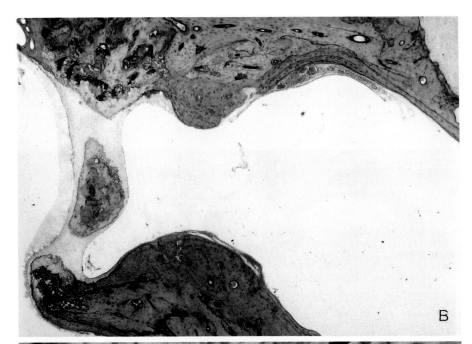

Figure 22.12.   B. The superior and inferior window margins display a hemispherical hyperostosis of subperiosteal bone that someday could impinge on the anterior crus of the stapes as it continues to grow. (Hematoxylin and eosin, ×55.)

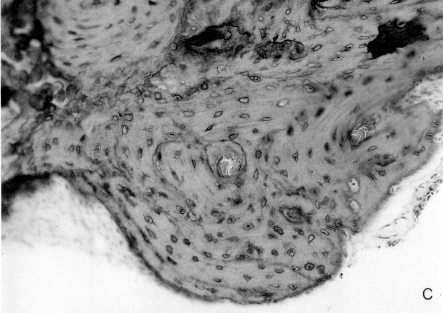

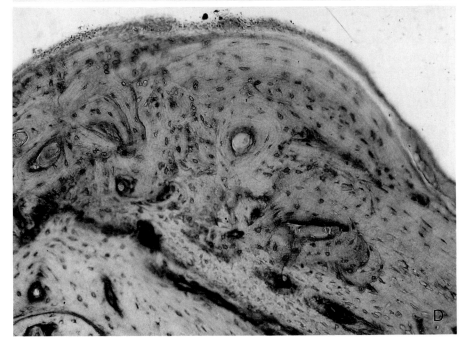

Figure 22.12.   C and **D.** The superior hyperostosis **(C)** consists predominantly of lamellar bone gradually blending into parallel lamellar bone of the periosteal layer of the promontory. The inferior hyperostosis **(D)** reveals an identical structure. These lesions are similar in appearance to those found in very circumscribed "healed or inactive" otosclerotic processes. However, there is no evidence of otosclerosis in this patient. (×250 and ×160, respectively.)

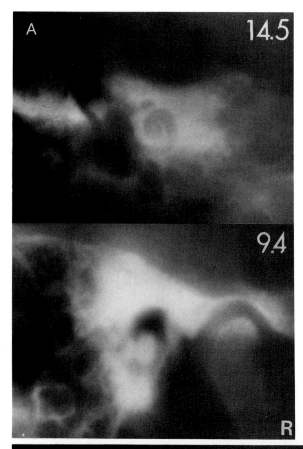

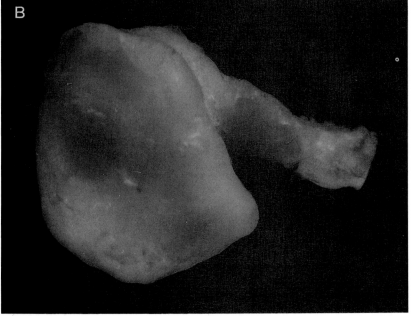

Figure 22.15. **A.** Multidirectional AP and lateral polytomograms of right temporal bone of a 23-year-old man with pedunculated, spherical osteoma in EAC. The osteoma had occluded most of the canal lumen.

Figure 22.15. **B.** The osteoma was removed with a small segment of the posterior inferior canal wall from which it had originated.

Case Reports

Case 1. *Pedunculated osteoma of right EAC with origin from the lateral, postero inferior meatal wall at 8 o'clock.*

The patient was a 23-year-old man with a history of recurrent right external otitis after swimming, who 3 months prior to admission developed otalgia, loss of hearing in the right ear, and a transient episode of dizziness. He presented to the referring otologist with a large osteoma in the right outer ear canal, a diffuse external otitis, and a maximal conductive hearing loss. As the external ear infection subsided, hearing returned to normal. On admission, a cherry stone-sized, spherical, pedunculated osteoma was found in the right EAC. It had originated from the lateral, posteroinferior osseous meatal wall and had obliterated about 90% of the canal lumen (Fig. 22.15A). The left outer ear canal was normal. The osteoma was removed in conjunction with a circumscribed portion of the bony canal wall from which it had arisen (Fig. 22.15B). A considerable amount of keratinous debris and cerumen had accumulated between the medial end of the osteoma and the tympanic membrane. Histologic examination revealed that the osteoma consisted of compact lamellar bone (Fig. 22.16A–C).

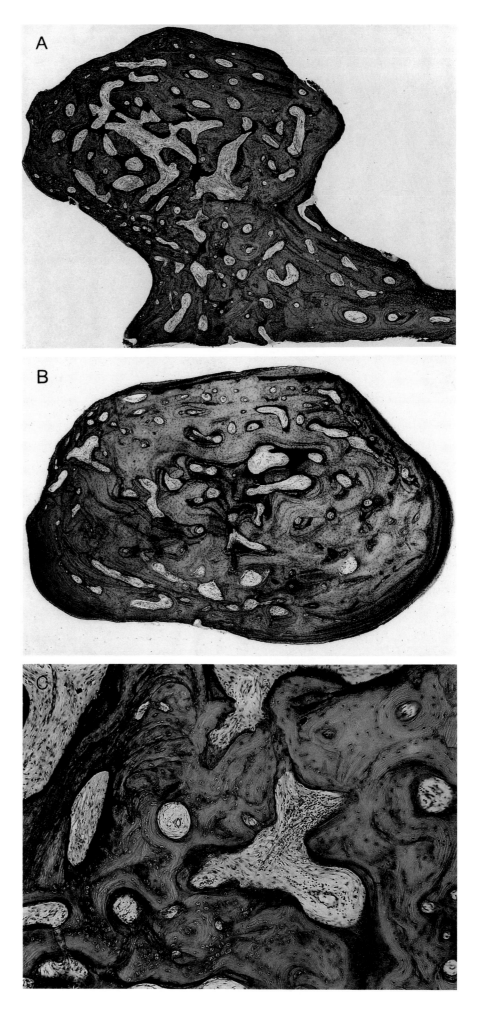

Figure 22.16.   A–C. The osteoma consists of compact lamellar bone with numerous Haversian systems. (Hematoxylin and eosin, ×20, ×20, and ×100, respectively.)

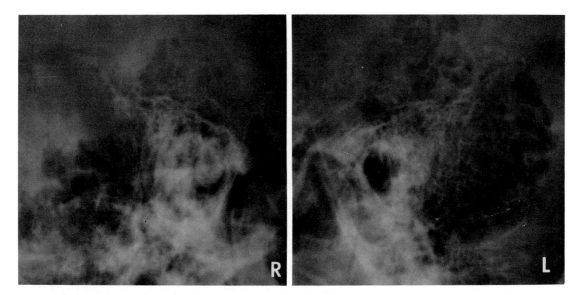

Figure 22.17. Lateral (Schüller) projection of temporal bones of a 27-year-old man with broad-based osteoma almost completely obliterating the right external canal.

Case 2. *Extensive, recurrent, broad-based, predominantly compact osteoma of right EAC with attachment along entire length of posterosuperior canal wall, near-total obstruction of meatus, and impingement on tympanic membrane. Chronic external otitis and secondary external cholesteatoma of right ear. History of extensive swimming and recurrent external otitis for years. Severe conductive hearing loss of right ear.*

A 27-year-old man with recurrent external otitis was seen. Both he and his brother and sister were on swimming teams and had suffered from recurrent external otitis. His father had what appeared to be an external cholesteatoma. The patient swam daily and had suffered from chronic recurrent right external otitis and intermittent obstruction of the right ear canal for years. Elsewhere, he had had a bone growth removed from his right ear canal for partial obstruction. During the past 12 months, he had developed a progressive loss of hearing and tinnitus in the right ear.

On *admission*, the patient presented with a large, single, elongated bone growth in the right EAC that almost totally occluded the lumen of the canal. There was a chronic external otitis and an external cholesteatoma. Audiometric studies revealed a maximal conductive hearing loss in the right ear.

The lateral projections and multidirectional anteroposterior (AP) and lateral polytomograms of the right temporal bones showed a large 20 × 9 × 9-mm osteoma originating from the posterosuperior canal wall along its entire length and impinging on the tympanic membrane (Figs. 22.17 and 22.18*A* and *B*).

At *operation*, the ivory-hard osteoma was attached to the posterosuperior canal wall. It was impinging medially on the tympanic membrane, displacing it somewhat into the middle ear cavity. The osteoma consisted primarily of compact bone (Fig. 22.19). Postoperatively, hearing returned to normal.

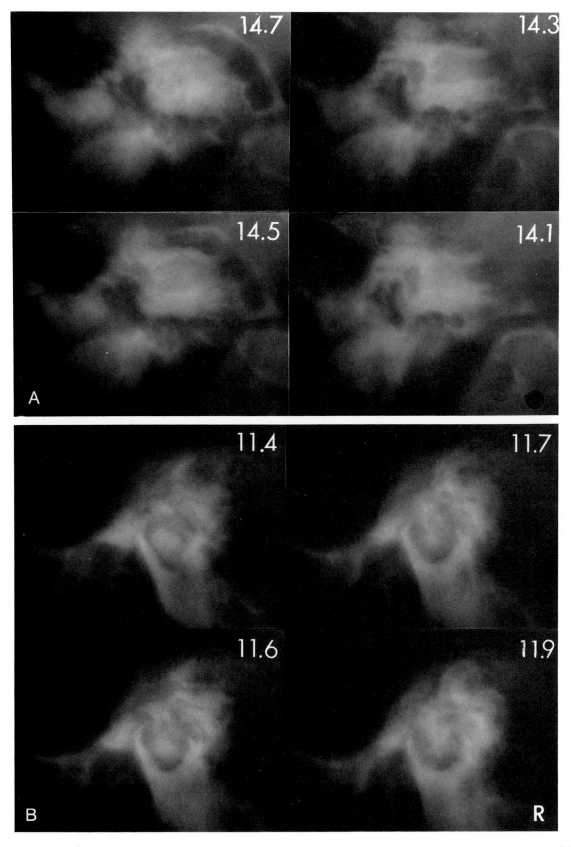

Figure 22.18. Multidirectional polytomograms of the right temporal bone in the AP **(A)** and lateral **(B)** projections show the origin of the osteoma along the roof of the canal and the medial displacement of the lower tympanic membrane.

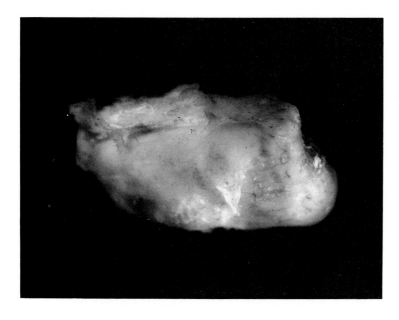

Figure 22.19. The osteoma measured 20 × 9 × 7 mm and consisted of compact lamellar bone.

Case 3. *Extensive, recurrent, broad-based osteoma of left EAC, measuring 20 × 5 × 5 mm, with origin from anteroinferior meatal wall. Extension through central pars tensa perforation into middle ear cavity, which was filled with adherent granulation tissue and firmly embedded the ossicular chain. Chronic hyperplastic tympanomastoiditis and external otitis. Maximal conductive hearing loss of left ear.*

The patient was a 38-year-old white man who at age 13 had noticed the onset of a progressive hearing loss in the left ear that by age 33 had developed into a maximum conductive loss and who was found to have an obliterating bone growth in that ear. The tumor was subsequently removed elsewhere, but hearing was not improved. During the ensuing 5 years, the growth recurred, the EAC gradually closed, the patient developed repeated episodes of external otitis, requiring the removal of a polyp from the meatus on one occasion, and had intermittent malodorous otorrhea and left-sided headaches and facial pains.

On *admission,* the left EAC was almost totally obliterated by an irregularly hard bone growth that had arisen from the anteroinferior meatal wall. Its surface was irregular and covered by inflamed meatal skin that showed some localized ulcerations. The residual canal lumen was filled with malodorous exudate and epithelial debris. The audiogram revealed a maximal 60-dB, flat conductive hearing loss with normal bone conduction in the left ear.

Radiologic examination demonstrated a spherical bone density occupying the left EAC and generalized haziness throughout a slightly underdeveloped left mastoid air cell system (Fig. 22.20*A*). AP and lateral multidirectional polytomograms showed the smoothly rounded bone density filling almost the entire EAC and extending halfway into the middle ear cavity (Fig. 22.20*B* and *C*).

At *operation,* the osteoma was found to extend through a large central pars tensa perforation into the middle ear, which was filled with firmly adherent granulation tissue that had solidly embedded what appeared to be an intact ossicular chain. Postoperatively, hearing in that ear had returned to near normal. Histologically, the tumor proved to be an osteoma (Fig. 22.20*D*). The osteoma consisted primarily of cancellous bone.

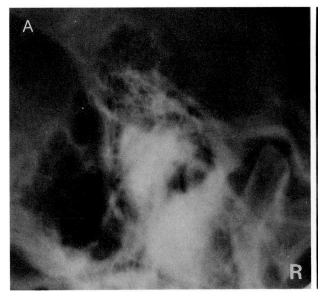
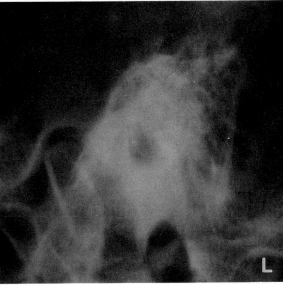
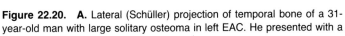

Figure 22.20. **A.** Lateral (Schüller) projection of temporal bone of a 31-year-old man with large solitary osteoma in left EAC. He presented with a history of increasing discomfort and a maximal conductive hearing loss in that ear.

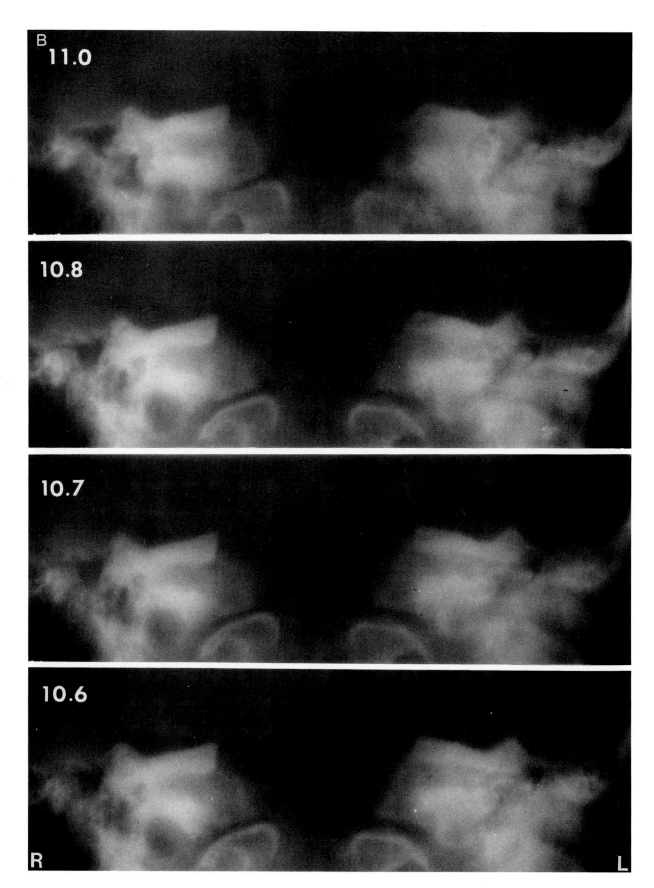

Figure 22.20. **B** and **C.** Multidirectional polytomograms of the left temporal bone of the same patient as in Figure 22.20*A* in the AP **(B)** and lateral **(C)** projections display the size and configuration of the osteoma. It had originated from the roof of the external meatus and caused a considerable medial displacement of the tympanic membrane.

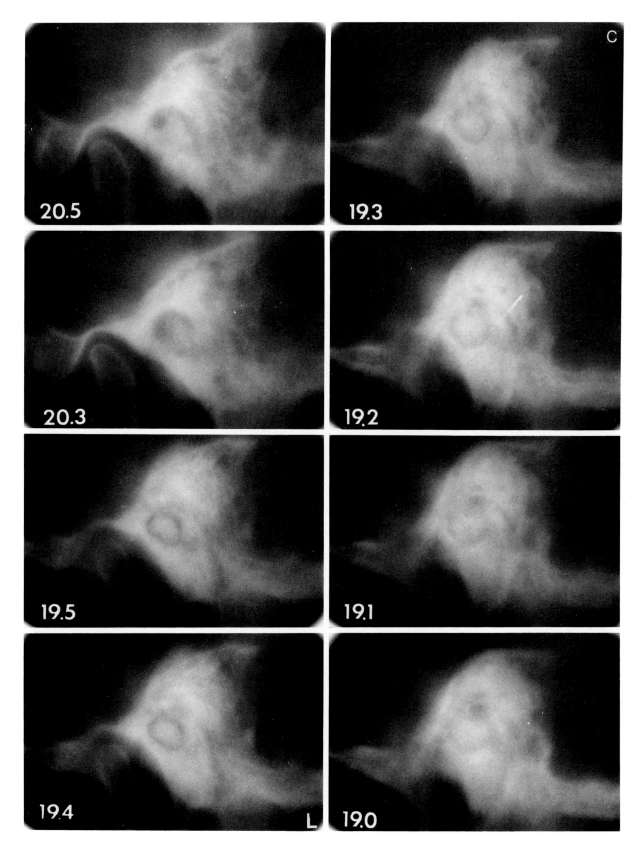

Figure 22.20.   C.

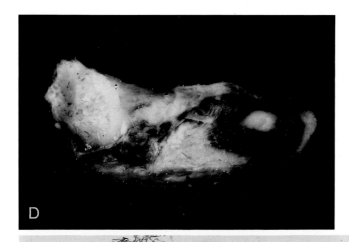

Figure 22.20. **D.** The osteoma of the same patient as in Figure 22.20*A* measured 29 mm in length and 10 mm in greatest diameter and consisted of compact lamellar bone.

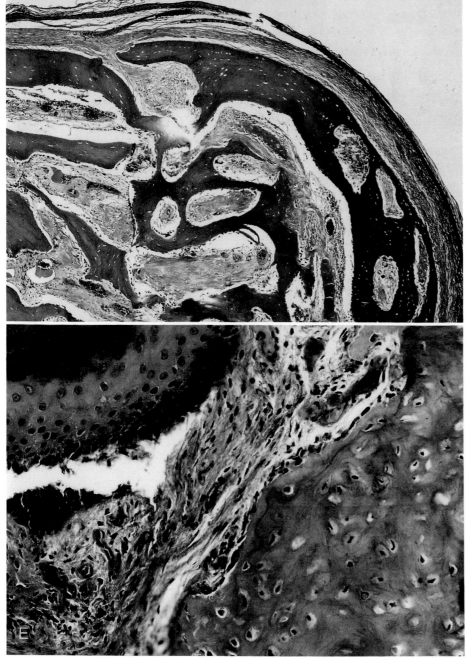

Figure 22.20. **E.** Histologically, the osteoma is made up of compact lamellar bone. (Hematoxylin and eosin, ×50.)

Case 4. *Hemispherical osteoma with origin from left mastoid cortex near the asterion.*

A 16-year-old girl who had noticed a hard, initially painless, gradually increasing swelling of the bone in the left postauricular area, which in recent months had grown more rapidly and had become tender, was seen.

Examination of the left postauricular area disclosed a firm hemispherical swelling measuring 2 × 1 × 1 cm in the area of the junction of the mastoid-occipitoparietal sutures (asterion), which had the characteristics of an osteoma.

On *radiologic examination,* a conventional radiograph of the left temporal bone confirmed the clinical diagnosis (Fig. 22.21*A* and *B*).

At *operation,* projections of abnormally sclerotic bone extended from the undersurface of the cortical osteoma medially into the lateral and medial cortex of the petrous pyramid and toward the sinodural angle (Fig. 22.21*B*). Histologic examination revealed an osteoma (Fig. 22.21*C*).

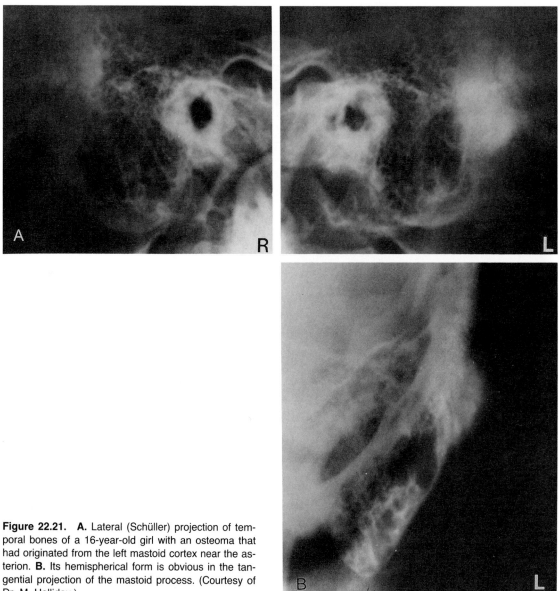

Figure 22.21. **A.** Lateral (Schüller) projection of temporal bones of a 16-year-old girl with an osteoma that had originated from the left mastoid cortex near the asterion. **B.** Its hemispherical form is obvious in the tangential projection of the mastoid process. (Courtesy of Dr. M. Holliday.)

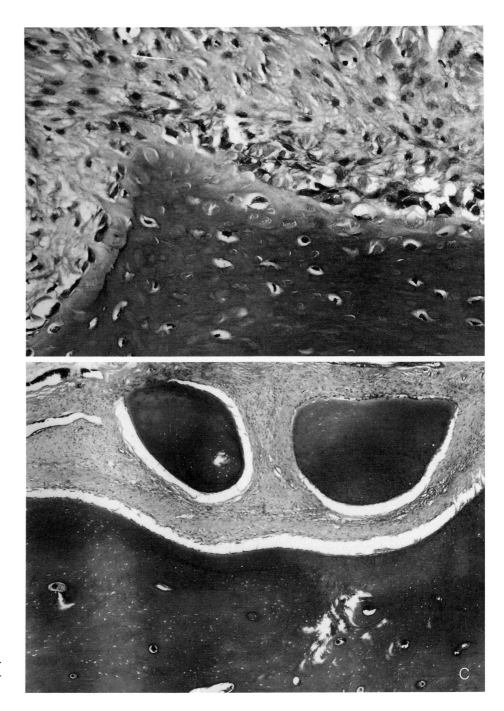

Figure 22.21. C. Microscopically, the osteoma is made up of compact lamellar subperiosteal bone. (Hematoxylin and eosin, ×280.)

Case 5. *Large, diffuse, broad-based exostosis arising from antero-inferior wall of left EAC, with subtotal occlusion of lumen of EAC. External cholesteatoma extending through anteriosuperior pars tensa perforation into middle ear and down into Eustachian tubal orifice. Chronic tympanomastoiditis with obliteration of middle ear cavity by granulation tissue and encasement of ossicular chain. Maximal conductive hearing loss of left ear; bilateral benign positional nystagmus.*

A 75-year-old white man who 5 years ago, when examined for an external otitis, was found to have a stenosis of left external auditory canal was seen. He had had recurrent external ear infections with occlusion, requiring repeated antibiotic treatments, and had noticed progressive loss of hearing in the left ear.

Otologic examination revealed an almost complete obstruction of the left EAC by a broad-based exostosis arising from the anterior canal wall with a cholesteatoma behind it. The left ear disclosed a maximal conductive hearing loss with normal discrimination. There was a bilateral benign paroxysmal positional nystagmus.

On *radiologic examination,* serial axial computed tomography (CT) scans of the temporal bones revealed a diffuse, dense, hemispherical bone growth arising from the left anterior canal wall close to the annulus. It obstructed the canal lumen significantly (Fig. 22.22).

At *operation,* after removal of the bone growth, the cholesteatoma was found to extend through an anterosuperior pars tensa perforation into the middle ear and Eustachian tube. The middle ear was filled with fibrous granulation tissue that solidly encased the ossicular chain. Postoperatively, hearing was much improved.

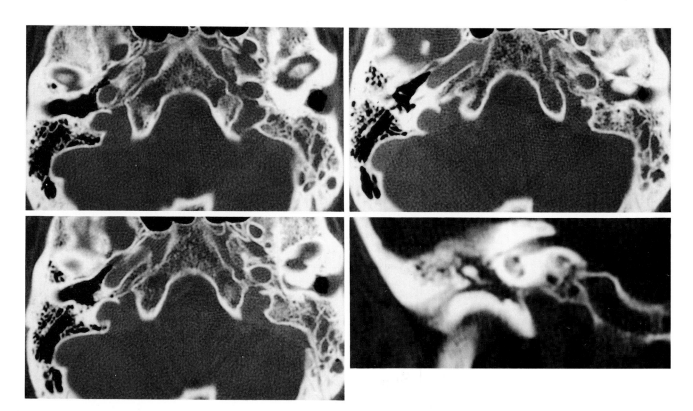

Figure 22.22. Axial CT scans of temporal bones of a 75-year-old white man with diffuse exostosis arising from anterior wall of left EAC. The exostosis had almost totally occluded the canal lumen and was associated with an external cholesteatoma that had extended through the anterior tympanic membrane into the Eustachian tube. (Courtesy of Dr. D. Mattox.)

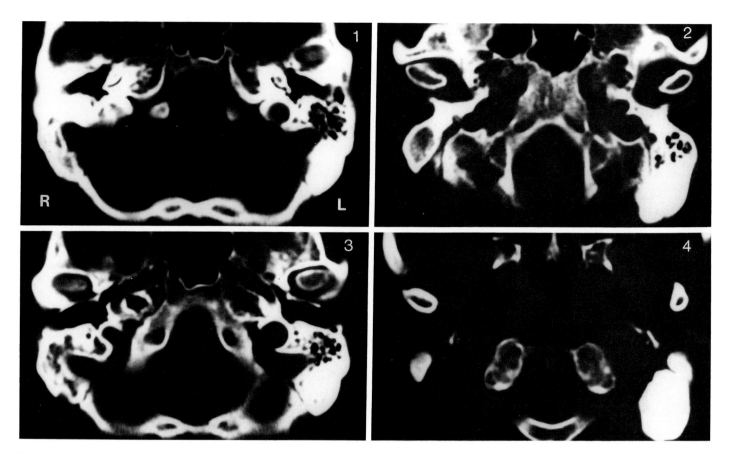

Figure 22.23. Axial CT scans of temporal bones of a 34-year-old woman with an 8-year history of a painless gradual increase in size of her left mastoid process that had suddenly become tender during the past 2 weeks prior to admission. The left mastoid process reveals a uniform sclerotic compact osteoma measuring about 2½ × 2 × 2 cm that involves the lateral and medial cortex as well as the air cells of the lower half of the mastoid bone. It has markedly enlarged the mastoid tip and extends downward below it for about 1½ cm. The remaining mastoid air cells are unremarkable. The osteoma was successfully removed, and histologic examination confirmed the diagnosis.

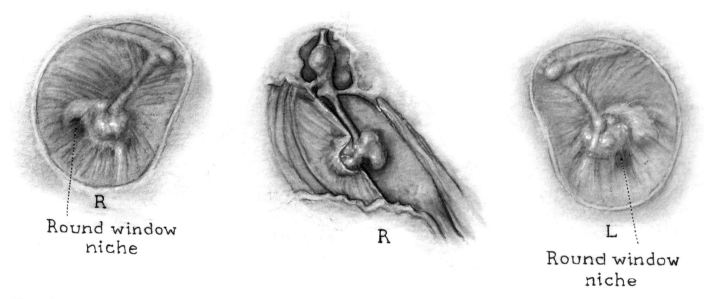

Figure 22.24. Drawing of bilateral symmetrical compact osteomas arising from superior and anterior margin of round window niche in a 41-year-old man who was being evaluated for a left-sided progressive conductive hearing loss. The osteomas elevated the central portion of the tympanic membrane about 1½ mm, and the one on the left was impinging on the undersurface of the umbo of the handle of the malleus. The audiogram showed a 30-dB conductive hearing loss on the left.

References

1. Virchow R. Über Exostosen des Meatus auditorius externus. Klin Wochenschr 1893;30:635.
2. Friedman I. Pathology of the ear. Oxford: Blackwell Scientific Publications, 1974.
3. Graham M. Osteomas and exostoses of the external auditory canal. Ann Otol Rhinol Laryngol 1979;88:566–72.
4. Sheehy JL. Diffuse exostoses and osteomata of the external auditory canal. Otolargyngol Head Neck Surg 1982; 90:337–342.
5. Hyams VJ, Batsakis JG, Michaels L. Tumors of the upper respiratory tract and ear. In: Atlas of tumor pathology. 2nd series, Fascicle 25. Washington, DC: Armed Forces Institute of Pathology, 1971:2306–6006.
6. Aegerter E, Kirkpatrick JJA. Orthopedic diseases. Physiology, pathology, radiology. 3rd ed. Philadelphia: WB Saunders, 1958.
7. Spjut HJ, Dorfman HD, Feckmer RE, Ackerman LV. Tumors of bone and cartilage. In: Atlas of tumor pathology. 2nd series, Fascicle 5. Washington, DC: Armed Forces Institute of Pathology, 1971.
8. Van Gilse PHG. Des observations ultérieurs sur la genèse des exostoses du conduit externe par l'irritation d'eaud froid. Acta Otolaryngol (Stockh) 1938;26:343.
9. Harrison DF. The relationship of osteomata of the external auditory meatus to swimming. Ann R Coll Surg Engl 1962;31:187.
10. Kessel CS. Exostosenstammbaum. Z Hals-Nasen-Ohrenheilkd 1924;8:266.
11. Ruttlin E. Über Exostosen und Hyperostosen des Gehörganges. Acta Otolaryngol (Stockh) 1933;18:281.
12. Nager GT. Paget's disease of the temporal bone. Ann Otol Rhinol Laryngol Suppl 22 1975;84(4):1–33.

SECTION IV

Tumors of the Nerve Sheath, Meninges, Brain, and Other Space-Occupying Lesions of the Temporal Bone

23/ Acoustic Schwannomas

UNILATERAL ACOUSTIC SCHWANNOMAS

Morphology of Cranial Nerve VIII

The morphologic structure of cranial nerves III–XII as they emerge from the central nervous system resembles initially that of a fiber bundle within the brain with abundant neuroglial supporting elements: oligodendrocytes, astrocytes, and microglia (1). This proximal neuroglial portion of the cranial nerve root ends, however, with the penetration of the nerve through the pia. On penetrating the pia, the neuroglia is abandoned, and the nerve root acquires its reticulin and Schwann cell components. From that point on, Schwann cells sheath the axons to their terminations.

The distance from the cerebral axis to the level at which the nerve penetrates the pia mater varies considerably among the different cranial nerves. In cranial nerve VIII the neuroglial portion may measure up to 10 mm (2).

In cranial nerve VIII the location of the neuroglial-neurolemmal junction is in most instances within the porus acusticus (Figs. 23.1 and 23.2). Occasionally, it is located more distally, closer to the fundus of the internal acoustic meatus. At times, it may be located more proximally, medial to the porus acusticus, and therefore outside the temporal bone. This neuroglial-neurolemmal connection displays a somewhat irregular, sickle-shaped, centrally concave configuration (Figs. 23.1 and 23.2). Islands of glial tissue are often found beyond the neuroglial-neurolemmal union in the distal portion of the nerve as far peripherally as Scarpa's ganglion (Fig. 23.2) (2).

Incidence, Age, and Sex Distribution

Eighth nerve tumors represent the third largest group of intracranial tumors following gliomas and meningiomas (3). They account for 7–10% of all intracranial neoplasms (4–8). They embody the overwhelming majority of intracranial schwannomas and represent about 75–85% of all space-occupying lesions in the cerebellopontine angle (3).

Eighth nerve tumors are most frequently found in the middle decades of life. Their age peak is between 35 and 45 years. Only exceptionally do they occur during childhood. In later decades of life, they are occasionally detected incidentally during a postmortem examination or a review of serially sectioned temporal bones (Figs. 23.3–23.5) (9). These tumors are about twice as common in females as in males (8).

Case Reports

Cases 1–3 are examples of asymptomatic eighth nerve tumors. They illustrate the site of origin of these lesions and their relation to adjacent structures.

Case 1. *Early asymptomatic schwannoma arising from inferior division of left vestibular nerve near Scarpa's ganglion (Fig. 23.3).*

This 30-year-old man had essentially normal hearing bilaterally as tested with pure tones and speech. He made a definite statement that he had had no tinnitus, imbalance, or vertigo. He had no spontaneous nystagmus or past pointing. Special vestibular tests had to be postponed because of his severe cardiac condition, which caused his death 1 month after the otologic examination.

Microscopic examination of the left temporal bone reveals a schwannoma originating from the inferior division of the vestibular nerve, measuring about 2.5 mm in diameter. This vestibular schwannoma is so small that it had not exerted pressure on the adjacent nerves or eroded the bony wall of the internal auditory canal (9).

Case 2. *Asymptomatic schwannoma of right eighth cranial nerve with location between cochlear and inferior divisions of vestibular nerve near Scarpa's ganglion (Fig. 23.4).*

This 78-year-old man had had an audiogram 3½ months prior to death, which revealed a gradual bilateral sensorineural high-tone loss compatible with his age. It was difficult to obtain a reliable history because of his senile dementia. He had no spontaneous nystagmus, and caloric responses were normal bilaterally.

Microscopic examination of the right temporal bone reveals a schwannoma measuring less than 1 mm in diameter. It was located between the cochlear and the inferior division of the vestibular nerve (9).

Case 3. *Asymptomatic schwannoma arising from saccular branch of inferior division of left vestibular nerve at macula of saccule (Fig. 23.5).*

This 45-year-old woman had no history of hearing loss, imbalance, or vertigo. She died from a metastasizing carcinoma of the cystic duct of the gallbladder before her cochlear and vestibular function could be evaluated.

Microscopic examination of the temporal bones reveals small, symmetrical, inactive nonankylosing otosclerotic lesions anterior to the oval window and large symmetrical active otosclerotic lesions at the round window with secondary new bone formation in the adjacent lower basal turn of the cochlea. In addition, it reveals an asymptomatic schwannoma arising from the left saccular nerve at the macula of the saccule.

Historical Findings

The first description of an acoustic neurinoma was by Sandifort (10) in 1777. Wishart (11) reported the first patient with bilateral eighth nerve tumors associated with neurofibromatosis in 1822. Virchow (12) (1864–1865) was much interested in these tumors. Sternberg (13) (1900) and, above all, Henschen (14) (1915) and Cushing (15) (1917) wrote the classical monographs. Numerous important contributions appeared thereafter in the literature on the clinical, pathologic, and surgical aspects of these neoplasms. Toynbee (16) first reported a small primarily intracanalicular tumor in 1853. Similar observations were made

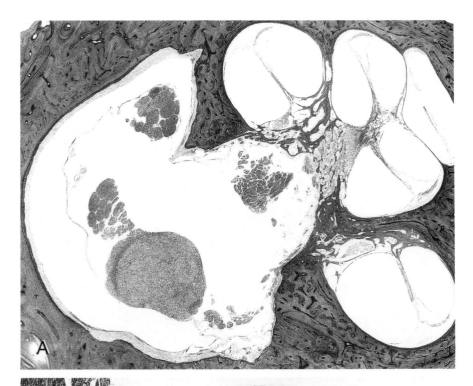

Figure 23.3. **A.** Vertical midmodiolar section through left petrous pyramid, demonstrating the location and size of the asymptomatic schwannoma and its relation to adjacent structures. (Hematoxylin and eosin, ×12.)

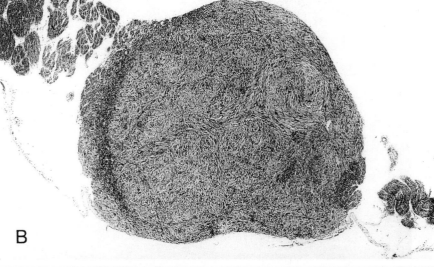

Figure 23.3. **B.** The tumor originates from the inferior division of the vestibular nerve near Scarpa's ganglion. It has assumed an eccentric position with regard to its parent nerve and ganglion, which are spread out in a crescent-shaped band over its left circumference. (×50.)

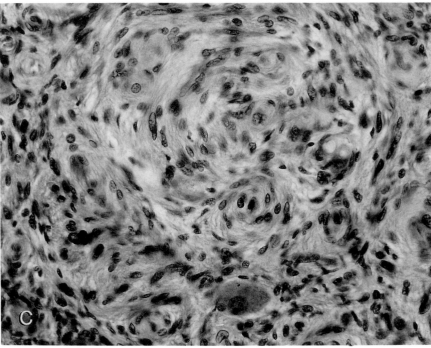

Figure 23.3. **C.** The cellular architecture of the schwannoma discloses cell patterns in streams, loops, and whorls. (×400.)

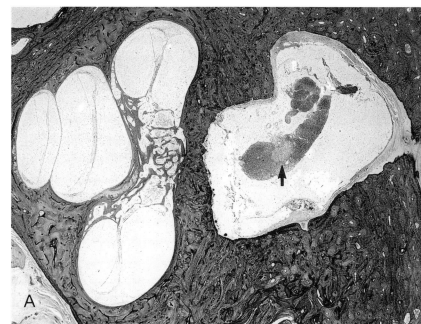

Figure 23.4. A. Vertical paramodiolar section through right petrous pyramid to show the location and size of the small asymptomatic schwannoma *(arrow)* and its relation to adjacent nerves within the internal auditory canal. (Hematoxylin and eosin, ×12.)

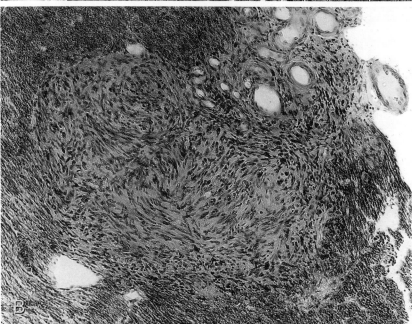

Figure 23.4. B. The schwannoma is embedded between the cochlear nerve in the left upper corner and the inferior division of the vestibular nerve in the right lower corner. The tumor is attached to both nerves without having invaded either of them. Its exact origin remains unclear. (×120.)

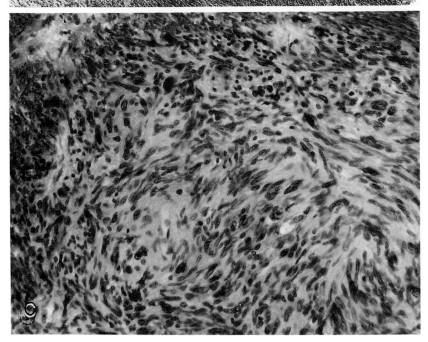

Figure 23.4. C. The cellular architecture of the schwannoma discloses the fibrillary structure of the type "A" tissue (Antoni). Several large atypical hyperchromatic nuclei are scattered throughout the tumor field and recognized in the left upper corner. (×300.)

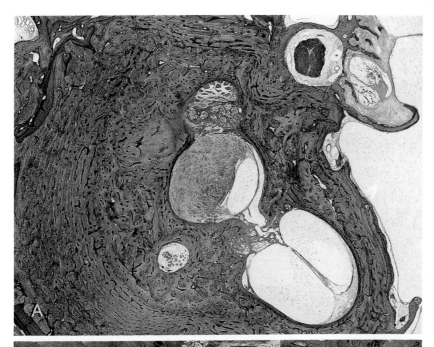

Figure 23.5. A. Vertical section through left petrous pyramid anterior to oval window, demonstrating the site and extent of the asymptomatic schwannoma. (Hematoxylin and eosin, ×12.)

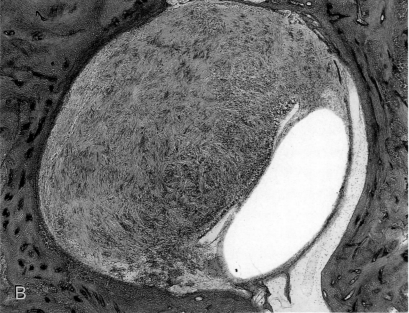

Figure 23.5. B. The schwannoma arises from the saccular nerve just after the nerve has entered the anterior vestibule. It occupies the spherical recess of the vestibule and invades the macula of the saccule. (×50.)

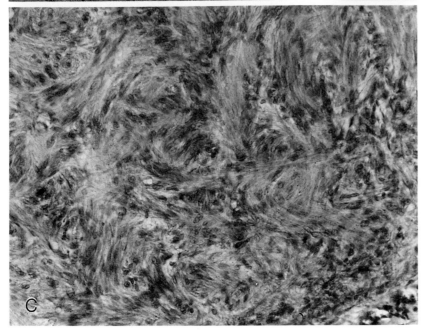

Figure 23.5. C. The tumor cells are arranged in fascicles, loops, and whorls, and there is palisading of the cell nuclei. (×300.)

thereafter by Habermann (17) (1891), Alexander (18) (1907), Henschen (2) (1910), Hardy and Crowe (9) (1936), Fowler (19) (1936), and others.

Origin and Local Behavior

Eighth nerve tumors arise in the distal neurolemmal portion of the nerve. The majority originate in the vestibular division of the nerve. Most neuropathologists today agree that the principal cell of origin of these tumors is the Schwann cell. Some investigators accept, with a certain reservation, the alternative possibility; i.e., that the perineural cells that are morphologically identical with Schwann cells, except for their lack of a direct relationship to the axon from which they are separated by the endoneurium, could be the cells of origin for these lesions (20). Harkin and Reed (21) consider the perineural cells to be a form of Schwann cells. They believe that schwannomas may arise from either or both cell types. Since the tumor represents a neoplasia of the Schwann cells, it should correctly be referred to as a schwannoma.

The tumor generally arises within the nerve trunk, gradually grows out of it, and, as it increases in size, assumes a peripheral position (Fig. 23.3). The nerve fibers, therefore, are not evenly distributed over the tumor surface but rather frequently course over a limited area, usually flattened out to a thin ribbon and incorporated in the tumor capsule (Fig. 23.6).

In most instances, the tumor arises inside the internal acoustic meatus (Figs. 23.3 and 23.4) and, following the direction of least resistance, grows out of it into the cerebellopontine angle, where it may reach a considerable size. The tumor therefore consists of two portions: a stalk, which represents the canalicular portion, and a larger extratemporal portion in the cerebellopontine angle (Figs. 23.6 and 23.12). Tumors without a stalk are exceptional (Fig. 23.7). They arise from the extratem-

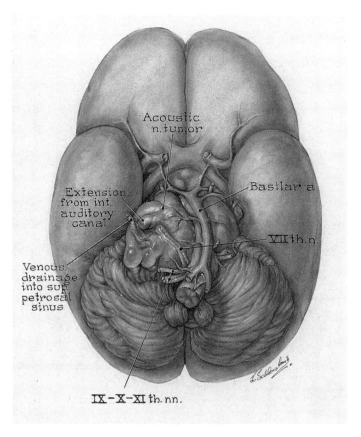

Figure 23.6. Illustration of indentation and deformation of pons and medulla and displacement and distortion of cerebellum, cranial nerves, and basilar and vertebral arteries by large right-sided acoustic schwannoma. The right seventh and eighth cranial nerves, flattened out to look like a ribbon, course over the anterior inferior surface of the tumor. Three arachnoid cysts are attached to the caudal pole of the tumor. The schwannoma derives its arterial supply from the basilar and vertebral arteries (anterior inferior cerebellar artery, etc.). The venous flow returns through the petrosal vein into the superior petrosal sinus.

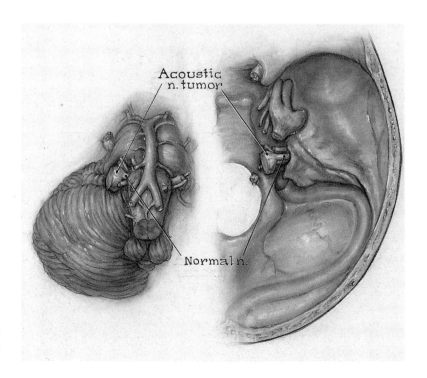

Figure 23.7. Illustration of rare instance of "medially" located neurinoma of right vestibular nerve. Although situated outside the temporal bone, the position of the tumor is still distal to the neuroglial-neurolemmal junction, which in this situation is medial to the porus of the internal acoustic meatus.

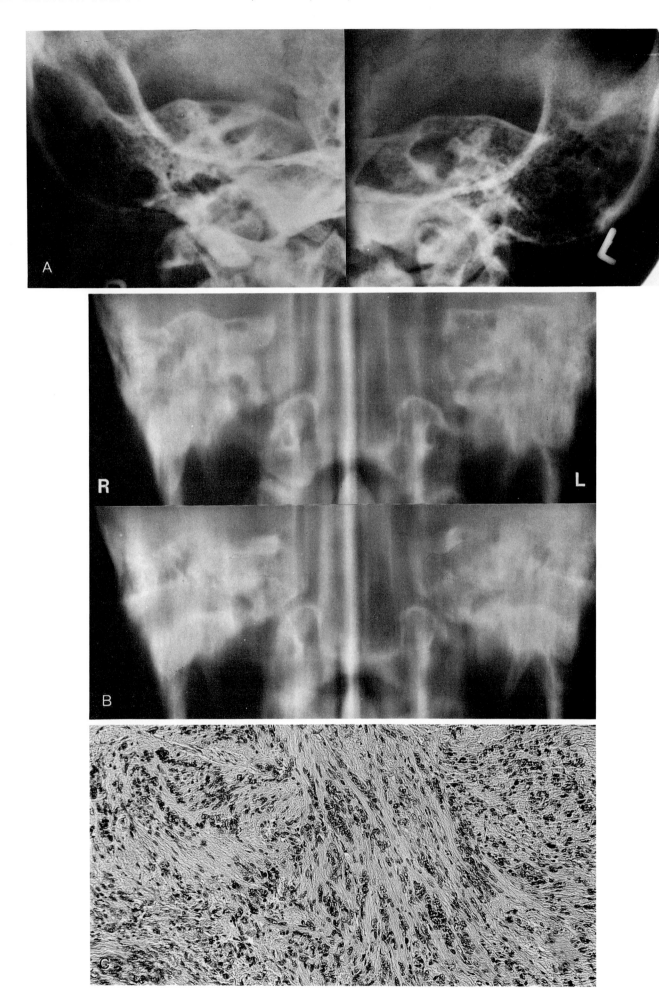

poral segment of the eighth nerve. Although located outside the temporal bone, they still arise distal to the neuroglial-neurolemmal junction.

Once a tumor fully occupies the internal auditory meatus, it begins to erode the walls of the canal and to enlarge its lumen (see Figs. 23.11, 23.16, and 23.18). The resulting enlargement may be regular, funnel-shaped, or quite irregular and may include a large portion of the petrous pyramid. In a rare situation the tumor can develop entirely inside the temporal bone, without presenting in the cerebellopontine angle (Fig. 23.8). In such instances a vast portion of the petrous pyramid can become hollowed out (22, 23). on the other hand, if the tumor arises from the extratemporal segment of the eighth nerve, it may develop primarily in the cerebellopontine angle, and the configuration of the internal meatus may remain unaffected or only minimally altered (Fig. 23.7).

The extratemporal portion of the tumor may produce considerable deformation of the brain stem and the cerebellum (Fig. 23.6). The axial distortion of the ipsilateral cerebellar hemisphere may lead to the formation of a superior and inferior cerebellar pressure cone. Large tumors may present a sizeable supratentorial extension and may occasionally project inferiorly as far as the foramen magnum (Fig. 23.16). The adjacent cranial nerves and vessels are stretched over the surface of the tumor. The compression and distortion of the fourth ventricle may eventually produce an increase in intracranial pressure and result in an internal hydrocephalus.

Eighth nerve tumors, as a rule, are slow-growing lesions. Certain degenerative mechanisms, such as edema, cyst formation, and hemorrhages into the tumor tissue, may indicate a more rapid rate of growth. On the other hand, certain acoustic schwannomas actually cease to grow or even decrease in size. Of Olivecrona's 83 partially removed tumors, for instance, 50% remained asymptomatic (24). Furthermore, the advanced age of 78 years of one of our three asymptomatic patients with schwannomas (Case 2, Fig. 23.4) might indicate that certain small tumors may remain inactive for a long period or even never develop into a symptomatic space-occupying lesion.

Macroscopic Appearance

Eighth nerve tumors are, generally, well-demarcated encapsulated neoplasms, initially with a pale color and a firm consistency. Smaller tumors tend to be spheroidal, display a smoother surface and a lighter color, are semitranslucent or opaque, and are elastic (Fig. 23.12). Larger tumors exhibit an irregular nodular and lobulated surface (Fig. 23.6). Their color and consistency vary with the amount of regressive changes. These changes are frequent and include fatty and hyalin degeneration, old and recent hemorrhages, ectatic vascular formations, edema, and cyst formations. Such regressive changes often lend these tumors a multicolored appearance. The texture can accordingly be either firm and rubbery or soft and brittle; it can also be partially or mainly cystic. The eighth nerve tumor derives its arterial supply from branches of the basilar and vertebral arteries, mainly from the former. The entire venous flow generally returns through the petrosal vein that drains into the superior petrosal sinus. One or several arachnoidal cysts are frequently found around the caudal pole of larger tumors (Fig. 23.6).

Figure 23.8.   A. Longitudinal (Stenvers) projection of petrous pyramids of a 37-year-old man in whom the development of a left acoustic schwannoma had been entirely inside the petrous bone at the time of this radiograph. The neurosurgeon, during the suboccipital craniectomy, found the left porus acusticus unaltered and free of tumor tissue. **B.** Linear antero-posterior (AP) tomograms of petrous pyramids. The intrinsic destruction of the left internal acoustic meatus and the erosion and invasion of the petrous pyramid are well visualized. **C.** The intrapetrosal tumor has the characteristics of a schwannoma. (Hematoxylin and eosin, ×300.)

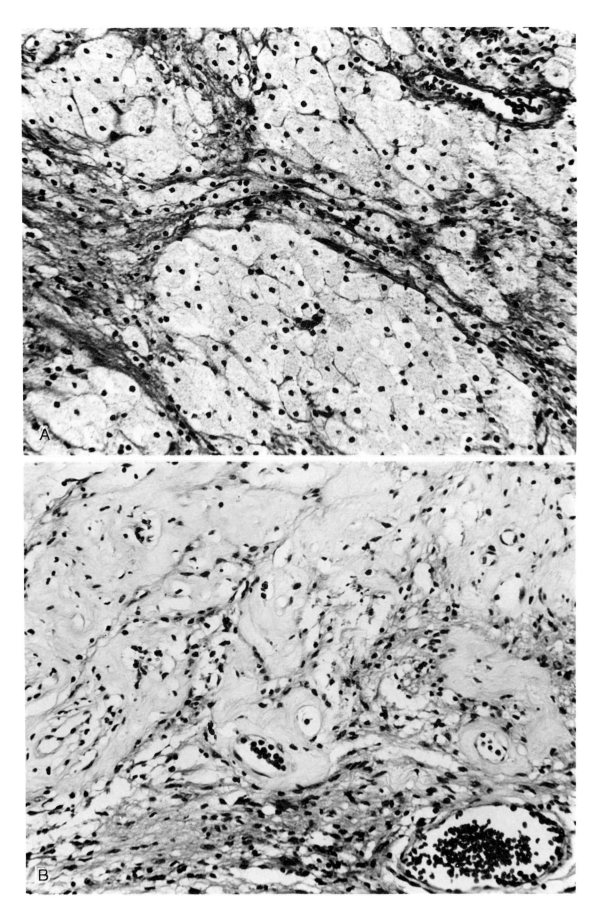

Figure 23.10. **A.** Fatty degeneration in reticular tissue. Increasing accumulation of lipids results in a honeycombed appearance of tumor cells in which the pyknotic nuclei are frequently eccentrically located. **B.** Hyaline degeneration in reticular tissue. It is characterized by great reduction of cell content and the transformation of tumor tissue into hyaline masses. (Hematoxylin and eosin, ×300 for both.)

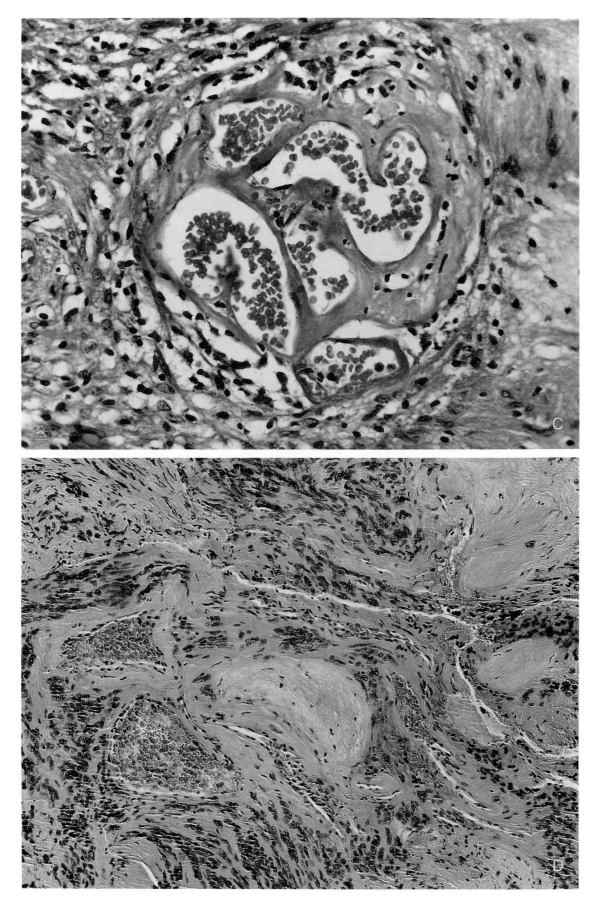

Figure 23.10. C. Sinusoidal dilatation of blood vessels in acoustic schwannoma. The wall of the vessel lacks the usual layered structure and consists of a single endothelium. **D.** Blood vessels in acoustic schwannoma whose walls have undergone regressive changes with hyaline thickening. This process often results in spontaneous thrombosis or complete obliteration of the vascular lumen. (×400 and ×200, respectively.)

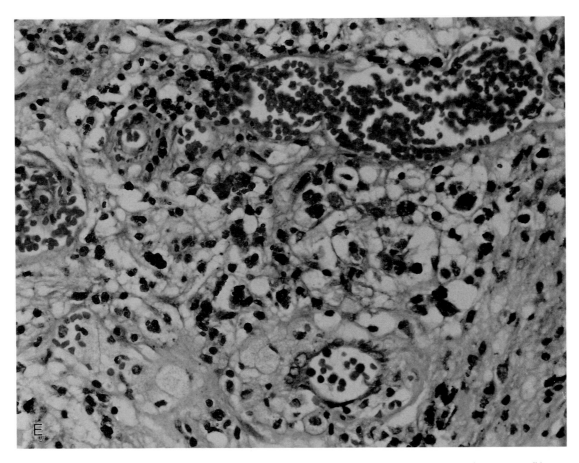

Figure 23.10. **E.** Numerous macrophages containing varying amounts of hemosiderin. They are residues of old hemorrhages and common morpho-logic features in a large acoustic schwannoma. (Hematoxylin and eosin stain, ×450.)

Case Reports

In Cases 4–6, computed tomography scanning (CT) and magnetic resonance imaging (MRI) illustrate the radiologic and histologic aspects of acoustic schwannomas.

Case 4. *Schwannoma of vestibular division of left eighth cranial nerve. Compression and distortion of brain stem and cerebellum.*

A 25-year-old man with a 5-month history of tightness over the left side of his face, numbness of the left side of his tongue, and a sensation as if his mouth was drawn to the left was seen. He subsequently developed some difficulties with control of balance. His gait deviated to the left, and he bumped into objects on his left side. He began to experience deep-seated occipital headaches and intermittent slurring of speech.

On admission to another hospital, *physical examination* had revealed some difficulties with jaw movements on the left, weakness and absence of deep tendon reflexes involving the left arm, and left cerebellar ataxia, but there was no loss of hearing, no tinnitus, and no spontaneous nystagmus or facial weakness on the left. A CT scan of the head had demonstrated an enhancing mass in the left cerebellopontine angle, measuring about 2 × 2 cm, extending into an enlarged left internal auditory canal (Fig. 23.14). The fourth ventricle was indented on the left and displaced to the right, and there was a slight internal hydrocephalus. As the initial exploration of the left cerebellopontine angle at that hospital was unsuccessful and inconclusive, the patient was transferred to our institution.

Reexploration of the left cerebellopontine angle revealed a large cystic schwannoma that could only be subtotally removed. Three months later the remaining intracanalicular portion of the tumor was removed through a translabyrinthine approach. The histologic diagnosis was of schwannoma (Fig. 23.15).

Case 5. *Large left acoustic schwannoma with supratentorial herniation and extension into foramen magnum. Impingement on fifth cranial nerve, anterior, lateral, and posterior compression of brain stem, and indentation of left cerebellar hemisphere.*

A 20-year-old man was seen who had a 1-year history of progressive loss of hearing and tinnitus in the left ear, unsteadiness, numbness over the entire left side of the face, double vision on left lateral gaze, loss of dexterity in the left hand, slurred speech, difficulties on swallowing, and occipital headaches.

On admission, *neurologic examination* revealed: involvement of left cranial nerves V–X; left cerebellar ataxia and a wide-based gait with a tendency to fall to the left; and bilateral papilledema without motor or sensory impairment. The audiologic evaluation disclosed a severe distorting sensorineural loss on the left with no ability to interpret speech and every evidence of a retrocochlear lesion.

The CT scan demonstrated a large contrast-enhancing lesion in the left cerebellopontine angle with extension above the tentorium, to the petrous apex, and into the foramen magnum (Fig. 23.16). The cerebral angiogram identified a branch of the left middle meningeal artery and a large meningohypophyseal vessel from the left internal carotid artery as the major feeding vessels of the tumor (Fig. 23.16D).

At *operation,* the tumor, which histologically proved to be a schwannoma (Fig. 23.17), was totally removed in two stages.

Case 6. *Schwannoma measuring 3.5 × 2 × 1.5 cm of left eighth cranial nerve with impingement on brain stem and left cerebellar hemisphere and compression of fourth ventricle. History of sudden loss of hearing in left ear, tinnitus, and negative CT scan 7 years prior to admission.*

A 52-year-old man who 7 years prior to admission had experienced a sudden loss of hearing with tinnitus in the left ear was seen. A CT scan at the time was reported to show no evidence of a space-occupying lesion in the left cerebellopontine angle and internal auditory canal. Six years later, he suffered a head injury as a result of a motor vehicle accident that left him with increased tinnitus in that ear, disequilibrium when walking up stairs, and intermittent lightheadedness. The MRI ordered by the otolaryngologist disclosed a large, enhancing tumor in the left cerebellopontine angle that extended into the left internal auditory canal (Fig. 23.18A). The tumor was removed through a left suboccipital craniectomy and proved to be a schwannoma (Fig. 23.18B).

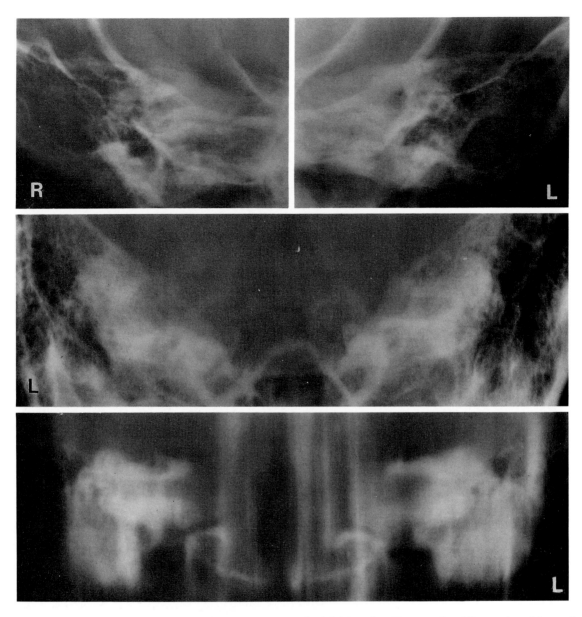

Figure 23.11. Stenvers occipital (Towne) and AP multidirectional tomographic views of petrous pyramid of a 23-year-old woman with left-sided acoustic schwannoma. The medially wider, funnel-shaped enlargement of the left internal auditory canal and the erosion of the posterior canal wall are well recognized.

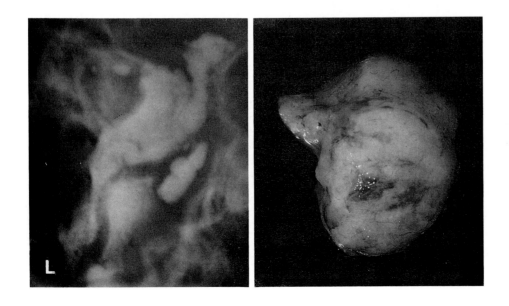

Figure 23.12. On the *left,* the contrast cisternogram displays a filling defect produced by the extratemporal portion of the tumor. On the *right,* there is a photograph of the tumor whose greatest vertical diameter measured 1.6 cm. The cone-like tumor projection, pointing to the left, represents the intracanalicular tumor portion.

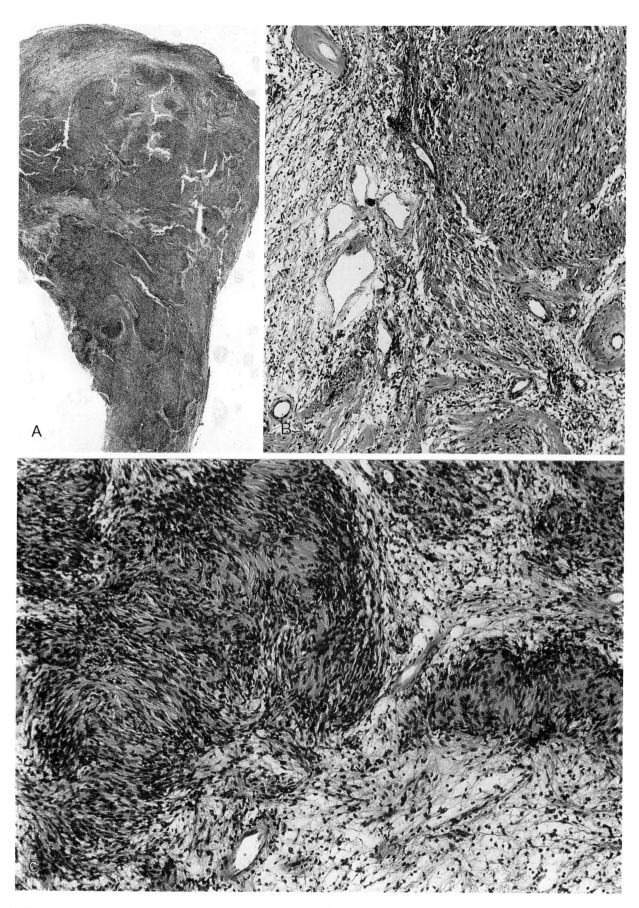

Figure 23.13.   A. Low-power photomicrograph of vertical cross-section through entire acoustic schwannoma in the same 23-year-old woman as in Figure 23.12. *Darker areas* represent the type A tissue of Antoni; *lighter areas* represent the type B tissue of Antoni. **B.** The type B tissue on the left displays examples of microcystic degeneration and hyalin thickening of the vessel walls. On the right is the type A tissue (Antoni). **C.** Type A and type B tissue (Antoni) are shown side by side with a tendency toward nuclear palisading in the type A tissue on the left. (Hematoxylin and eosin, ×7, ×125, and ×175, respectively.)

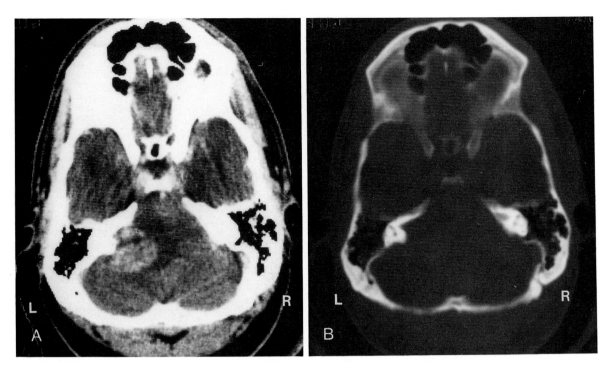

Figure 23.14. Enhanced axial CT scan **(A)** of a 25-year-old man with a left-sided acoustic schwannoma that caused considerable enlargement of the internal auditory canal **(B)**.

BILATERAL ACOUSTIC SCHWANNOMAS

Bilateral acoustic schwannomas or eighth nerve tumors account for about 5–6% of all acoustic tumors. Some 20 families have been reported in which two or more members have been afflicted (26). In 4 of the 20 families, bilateral eighth nerve tumors were the chief manifestation. No other associated tumors of the central nervous system were mentioned, but no complete postmortem examinations had been performed. Most other families revealed more extensive neoplastic involvement, with schwannomas found in other cranial and spinal nerves; meningiomas and additional tumors were, in most instances, an expression and the presenting symptom of what was formerly regarded as the central form of neurofibromatosis. In only about 2–4% of patients were they a manifestation of what once was regarded as the peripheral form of neurofibromatosis (27). About 2% of these patients had a unilateral eighth nerve tumor (28). Therefore, patients with bilateral eighth nerve tumors may have had what was formerly known as either the central or the peripheral form of the disorder.

In the statement of a recent National Institutes of Health Consensus Development Conference in neurofibromatosis, the forms formerly known as peripheral and central neurofibromatosis were reclassified as neurofibromatosis-1 (NF1) and neurofibromatosis-2 (NF2), respectively (29). Both are genetically transmitted in an autosomal dominant manner. Each offspring of a parent afflicted with NF1 and NF2 has a 50% chance of inheriting the disease.

NF1 is the more frequent form with a prevalence of 30–40/100,000 people. It affects approximately 80,000 people in the United States and occurs in 1 of every 2500–3300 live births (30, 31). The gene for NF1 is located near the centrosome of the long arm of chromosome 7 (31–33). Genetically, it has a penetrance of 95% with a widely variable expression. The diagnostic criteria for NF1 classification include findings of any two of the following in an individual: (*a*) six or more café au lait macules over 5 mm in diameter in prepubertal patients and over 15 mm in greatest diameter in postpubertal patients; (*b*) two or more neurofibromas of any type or one plexiform neurofibroma; (*c*) freckling in the axillary, inguinal, or perimammary regions; (*d*) optic glioma; (*e*) two or more Lisck nodules (hamartomas of the iris); (*f*) a distinctive osseous lesion such as a sphenoid dysplasia or thinning of long bone cortex, with or without pseudarthrosis; or (*g*) a first-degree relative with NF1 (34).

NF2, the less common form, has a prevalence of about 1/100,000 people. A few thousand people are affected in the United States. Genetically, it has a high penetrance but a low mutation rate. The gene for NF2 classification is found in any person who has (*a*) bilateral eighth nerve tumors as confirmed by appropriate imaging techniques (MRI) or (*b*) a first-degree relative with NF2 and either a unilateral eighth nerve mass or two of the following: neurofibroma, meningioma, glioma, schwannoma, or juvenile posterior subcapsular lenticular opacity (34, 35). Fifty percent of patients with NF2 have no family history of the disease. Although in some instances the disease may have been present in the parent of an affected offspring or as a "forme fruste" and hence escaped clinical detection, there is good evidence that many of these occurrences represent spontaneous mutations transmitted in an autosomal dominant fashion.

The principal similarities between NF1 and NF2 are their genetic mode of autosomal dominant transmission and their propensity to produce tumors derived from neural crest elements. They are, however, distinctly different entities with entirely different clinical manifestations. As a result of the remarkable variation of their clinical symptoms, differentiation between NF1 and NF2 may become difficult. Variant forms of the disease also exist, and a combination of the two forms has been documented (36, 37).

NF1 is often associated with a glioma of the optic nerve but usually spares all other cranial nerves. NF2, in contrast, can

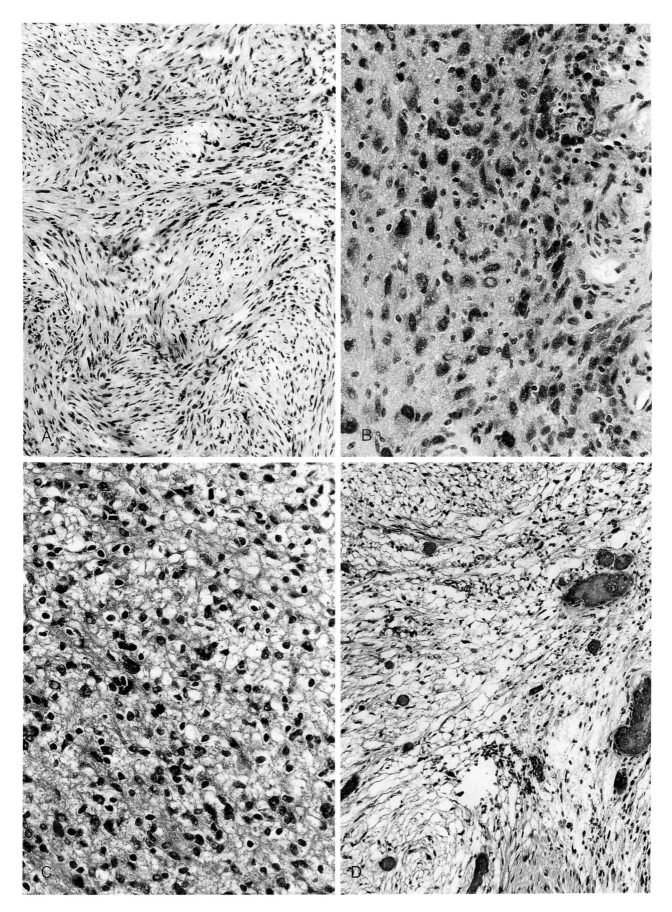

Figure 23.15. The schwannoma displays areas of the type A tissue **(A)**, with focal regions of numerous mononucleated and multinucleated giant cells with large, atypical, hyperchromatic nuclei **(B),** and of the type B tissue **(C)** that includes zones of greater vascularity **(D).** (Hematoxylin and eosin, ×145, ×335, ×260, and ×190, respectively.)

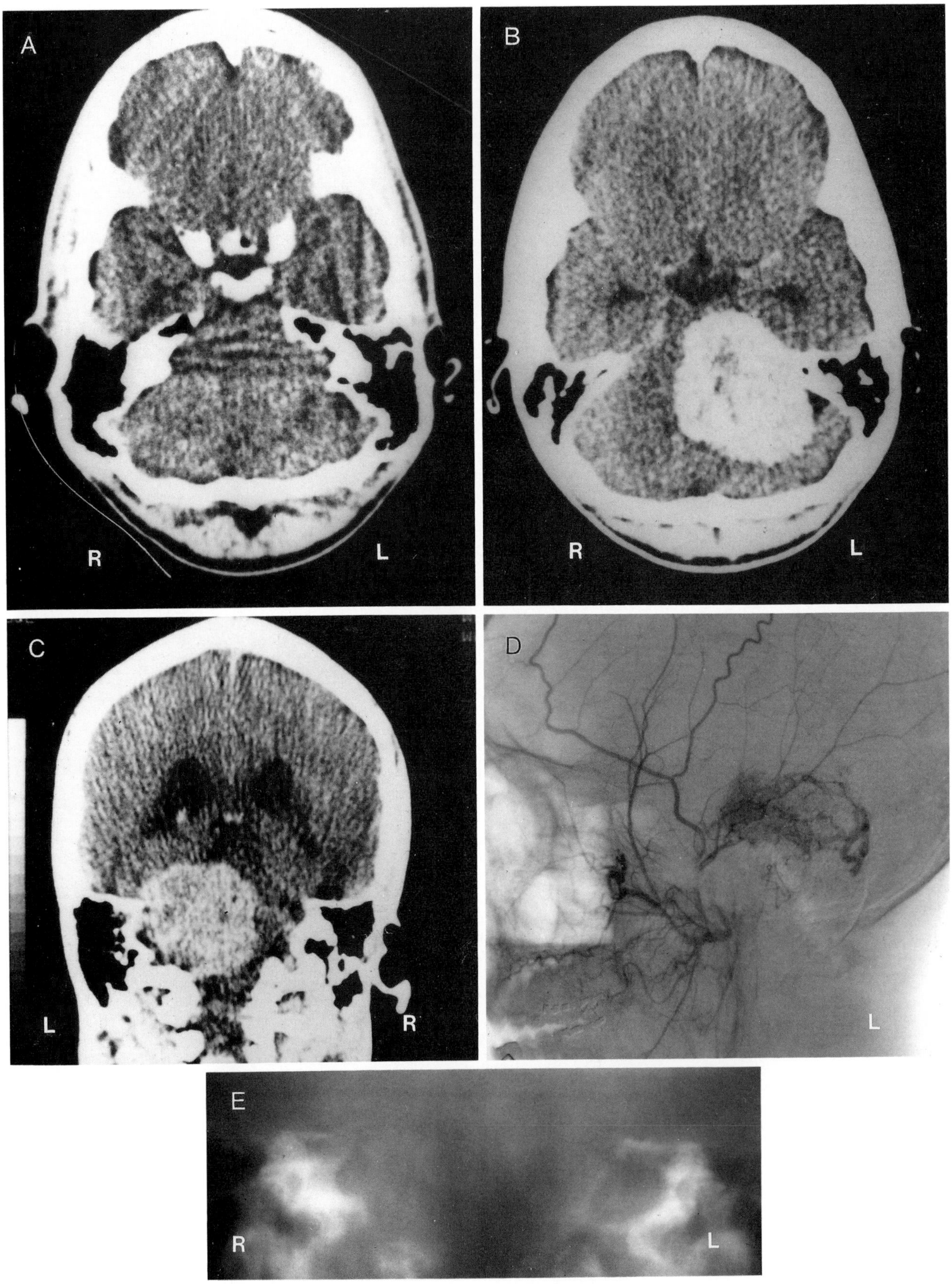

Figure 23.16. **A–C.** Enhanced axial and coronal CT scans of a 20-year-old man with a large left acoustic schwannoma. **D.** The unusually vascular capsular area of the schwannoma receives its main blood supply from a large meningohypophyseal vessel of the left internal carotid artery and from a branch of the left middle meningeal artery. **E.** The multidirectional AP tomogram of the petrous pyramids demonstrates the enormous enlargement of the left internal auditory canal.

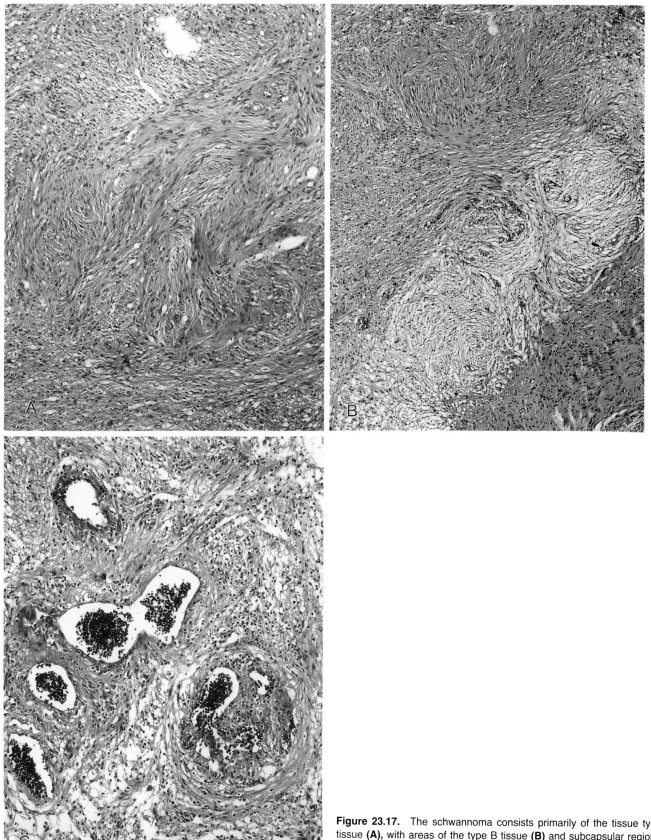

Figure 23.17. The schwannoma consists primarily of the tissue type A tissue **(A)**, with areas of the type B tissue **(B)** and subcapsular regions of enormous vascularity **(C).** (Hematoxylin and eosin, ×120, ×35, and ×130, respectively.)

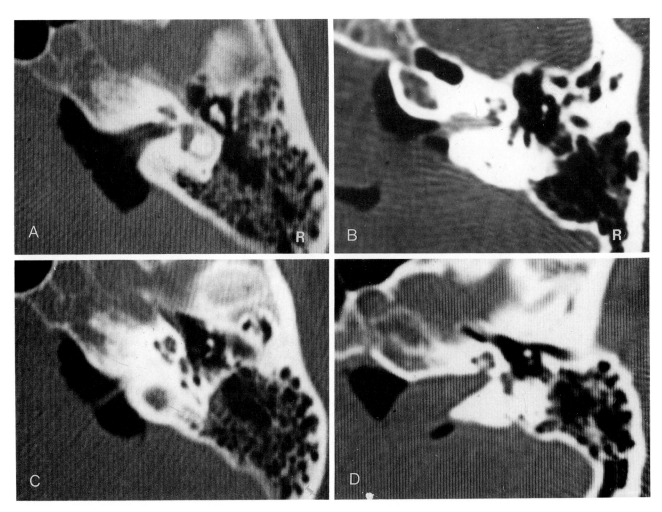

Figure 23.19. **A** and **C.** Axial CT scans of right temporal bone with air contrast cisternogram of lateral recess and internal auditory canal in an adult woman with essentially normal findings. The seventh and eighth nerves are well recognized within the internal meatus. **B** and **D.** Axial CT scans of right temporal bone with air contrast cisternogram of small intracanalicular acoustic tumor in a 41-year-old man **(B)** and of a medium-sized eighth nerve tumor in a 37-year-old man **(D).** (Courtesy of Drs. R. Gayler and J. Zinreich.)

involve any of the cranial nerves, most commonly the acoustic nerve. More than 90% of patients have bilateral eighth nerve tumors. NF2 is associated with intracranial meningiomas, gliomas, and tumors involving the spinal cord. NF1 generally presents at birth, while NF2 usually manifests itself in late adolescence or early adulthood. NF2 patients may have café au lait spots and cutaneous neurofibromas, but they are fewer and less severe than in NF1 patients (38).

Bilateral eighth nerve tumors differ in several ways from the unilateral eighth nerve tumor. The onset of clinical symptoms is much earlier, generally occurring around age 20. The tumors may reach a remarkable size and cause severe distortion of the brain stem. The changes involving the internal acoustic meatus and inner ear capsule are more extensive. The internal meatus may be markedly enlarged. Its walls can be irregularly eroded. The roof of the canal may become destroyed, allowing the tumor to grow extradurally into the middle cranial fossa (Figs. 23.24, 23.27, 23.32, 23.40, and 23.45). The tumor has a tendency to invade adjacent marrow spaces and pneumatic cells (Figs. 23.28 and 23.46). It may invade the cochlear modiolus and extend into the basal turn of the cochlea (Figs. 23.40 and 23.45). In some instances, all branches and end organs of the vestibular nerve, selected bundles of the cochlear nerve, the facial nerve, and almost every other cranial and peripheral nerve within the

temporal bone are affected by a proliferation of Schwann cells, which may be localized, diffuse, or both (Figs. 23.26, 23.31, 23.39, and 23.44). These lesions obviously display a multicentric growth pattern. In other instances, the schwannomas are more limited and involve only the cranial nerves within the internal auditory canal (Fig. 23.49). The association of schwannomas in the internal auditory canal and neural compartment of the jugular foramen with a meningioma is a common observation (Figs. 23.26, 23.27, 23.31, 23.33, 23.39, 23.41, 23.49, and 23.51). In some instances, the microscopic structure of an acoustic schwannoma displays a conspicuously whorled pattern strongly resembling that of certain meningiomas (Figs. 23.40 and 23.45). On the other hand, a meningioma may, in some areas, exhibit certain features that bear such a close resemblance to a schwannoma that the two become almost indistinguishable, particularly when they are so closely associated in the internal auditory canal. The simultaneous development of schwannomas and meningiomas in NF2 and the overlapping of their histologic appearance constitute a fairly characteristic feature of this condition (39) and become more readily understandable, considering the fact that the parent cell of each tumor shares a common ancestor in the neural crest (40).

The otolaryngologist should realize that an acoustic schwannoma in a young individual or a family history of eighth

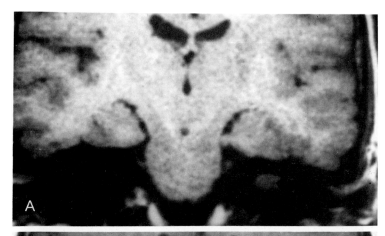

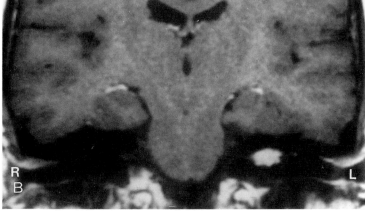

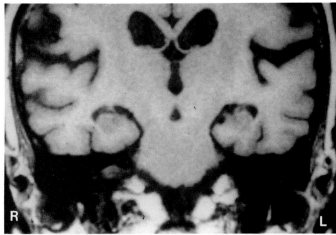

Figure 23.20. *(top left* and *bottom left)* Coronal MRI scans of a woman's brain with T1-weighted pulse sequences without **(A)** and with **(B)** gadolinium enhancement. They show a small enhancing tumor in the left internal auditory canal that histologically proved to be a schwannoma. (Courtesy of Dr. J. Zinreich.)

Figure 23.21. *(top right)* Coronal MRI scan of a man's brain, nonenhanced with T1-weighted pulse sequences. It shows a right intracanalicular tumor that on microscopic examination proved to be an acoustic schwannoma. (Courtesy of Dr. J. Zinreich.)

nerve tumors strongly suggests bilateral disease. Also, a patient with bilateral disease should be carefully observed for other central nervous system tumors, and relatives should be examined for manifestations of the same condition. Similarly, the presence of multiple meningiomas should arouse the suspicion of NF2 and the association with bilateral eighth nerve tumors. As a rule, acoustic schwannomas, neuroblastomas, retinoblastomas, and paragangliomas are generally sporadic and nonfamilial when they present unilaterally, but they are frequently genetically determined and transmitted as an autosomal Mendelian dominant when they present bilaterally (26).

Case Reports

Cases 7–9 are examples of bilateral eighth nerve tumors associated with NF2. In Case 9, these tumors may well have been asymptomatic, since they were only detected during the examination of the temporal bones, which at that time were routinely studied in patients who succumbed to a brain tumor. Cases 7–9 illustrate the differences between bilateral and unilateral eighth nerve tumors in their regional behavior and relation to adjacent structures. The otolaryngologist has to be familiar with this condition, since the initial symptoms and disabilities of the disease are prone to bring the patient to a member of this specialty first. He or she must be aware that bilateral eighth nerve tumors represent one of the most important features of the kaleidoscopic disorder known as NF2.

Case 7. *Neurofibromatosis-2 (NF2) (possibly combined with NF1). Large en plaque meningioma, predominantly fibrous with origin from falx. Several small meningotheliomatous and fibrous meningiomas coating the falx, right cerebellar hemisphere, and both Gasserian ganglia. Multiple schwannomas involving the right second, left third, and the seventh to eleventh cranial nerves bilaterally. Polar spongioblastomas involving the cerebellum. Distor-*

tion of brain stem and internal hydrocephalus secondary to large right eighth nerve tumor. Intracranial aneurysmal dilatation of right internal carotid artery. Numerous schwannomas involving the dorsal and ventral spinal roots, ganglia, and peripheral nerves. Schwannomas and neurofibromas involving the larynx, axilla, intestines, and paravertebral and sacral plexuses (Figs. 24.25, 24.26, and 24.31).

The patient was a 22-year-old man whose *neurologic examination* at age 17 revealed: (*a*) chorioretinitis of the right eye with secondary optic nerve atrophy and bilateral congenital cataracts: (*b*) bilateral oculomotor nerve palsy; (*c*) palsy of the left abducent nerve; (*d*) bilateral, peripheral facial nerve paresis; (*e*) bilateral absence of caloric responses; (*f*) bilateral sensorineural hypacusis; (*g*) bilateral complete vocal cord palsy; (*h*) paresis of the left spinal accessory nerve; (*i*) bilateral paresis of the hypoglossal nerve; (*j*) extensive, symmetrical wasting and weakness of distal portions of all limbs; (*k*) impairment of the sense of touch, tactile discrimination, temperature, vibration, and position, more pronounced in the distal portion of all four extremities; (*l*) absence of deep tendon reflexes; (*m*) early trophic changes and vasomotor instability of the skin; (*n*) adenoma sebaceum involving the central portion of the face; and (*o*) a few café au lait spots and two soft tissue masses over the trunk.

Radiologic examination showed enlargement of both internal auditory canals, especially of the lateral portion on the right (Figs. 23.24 and 23.25).

A subcutaneous nodule was removed from the left pectoral region and interpreted by the pathologist as a neurofibroma.

After age 17, the patient was no longer able to stand, walk, or write and had to be hospitalized permanently. At age 22, he underwent multiple dental extractions under general anesthesia, and the following day developed dysphagia and dyspnea. A chest film revealed infiltrations throughout the right lower lobe. Death occurred 24 hours later from cardiac arrest secondary to atelectasis and widespread pneumonitis.

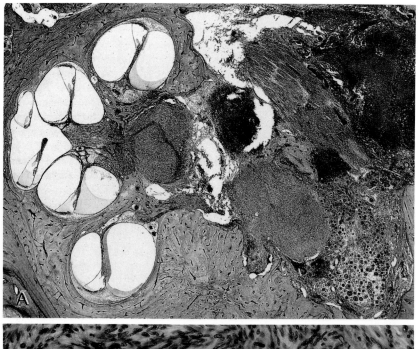

Figure 23.41. A. Vertical midmodiolar section through right petrous pyramid, illustrating the sizeable remaining schwannomas involving the cochlear, vestibular, and facial nerves and their association with an extensive meningioma within the internal acoustic meatus. (Hematoxylin and eosin, ×12.)

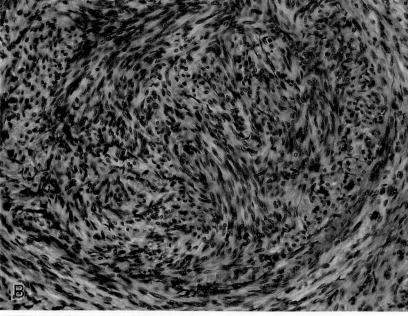

Figure 23.41. B. The cochlear schwannoma displays the fibrillary structure of the type A tissue (Antoni), with the tumor cells arranged in streams and loops. (×225.)

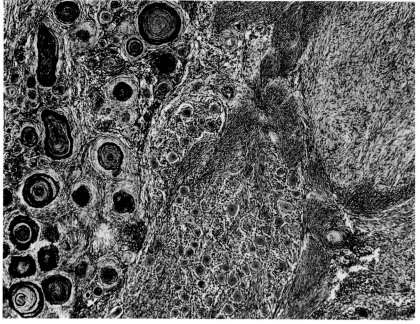

Figure 23.41. C. This section demonstrates the association of a psammomatous meningioma on the left with the superior ganglion of the glossopharyngeal and vagus nerves in the middle and the schwannomas involving the vagus and spinal accessory nerves on the right, inside the neural compartment of the jugular foramen. (×75.)

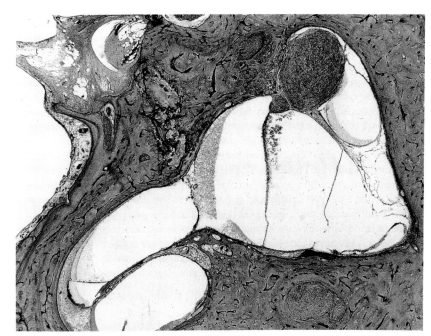

Figure 23.42. Vertical section through right petrous pyramid just anterior to oval window. The large schwannoma arising from the utricular nerve and invading the macula utriculi is continuous anteriorly with a schwannoma of the saccule (not shown here). (Hematoxylin and eosin, ×16.)

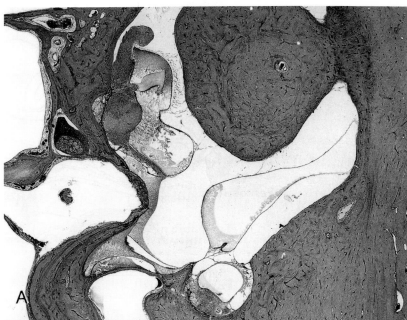

Figure 23.43. **A.** Vertical section through right petrous pyramid at approximate level of ampullae of all three semicircular canals. The schwannomas arising from branches to the superior and lateral ampullae form a conglomerate. A smaller schwannoma involves the posterior ampulla. (Hematoxylin and eosin, ×10.)

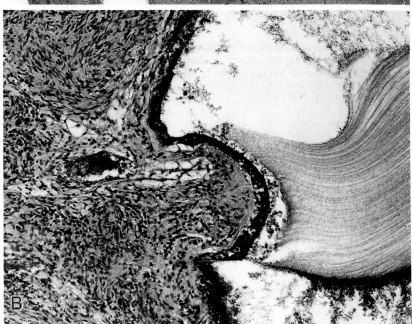

Figure 23.43. **B.** The schwannoma involving the crista of the superior ampulla displays the fibrillary type of tumor structure. (×160.)

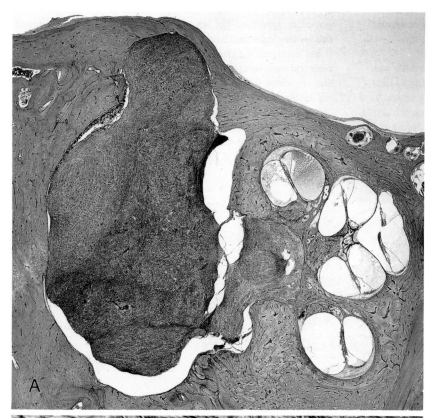

Figure 23.45.   A. Vertical midmodiolar section through left petrous pyramid, demonstrating the conglomerate of schwannomas involving the cochlear, vestibular, and facial nerves and the erosion and invasion of the floor and roof of the internal auditory canal. The cochlear schwannoma extends through the spiral foraminous tract into the basal turn of the cochlea. (Hematoxylin and eosin, ×8.)

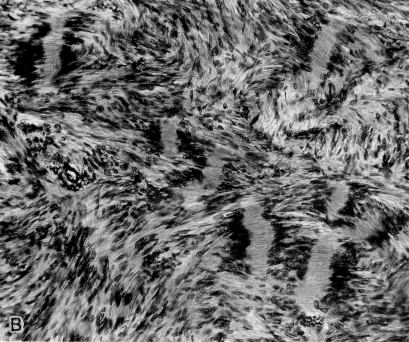

Figure 23.45.   B. The cochlear schwannoma reveals the tumor cells arranged in fascicles and loops and the palisading of cell nuclei. (×200.)

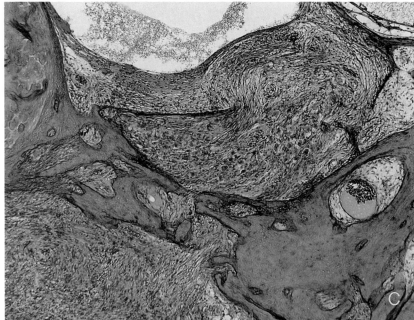

Figure 23.45. C. The cochlear schwannoma in the upper basal turn exhibits a cellular arrangement in streams and loops. (×90.)

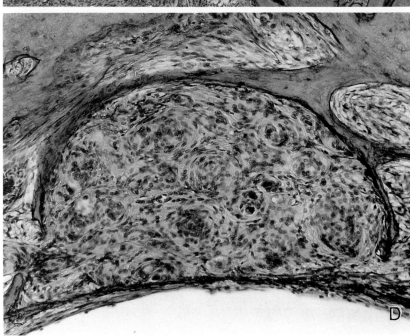

Figure 23.45. D. The cochlear schwannoma in the lower basal turn displays a cellular arrangement in concentric whorls and cell clusters. (×200.)

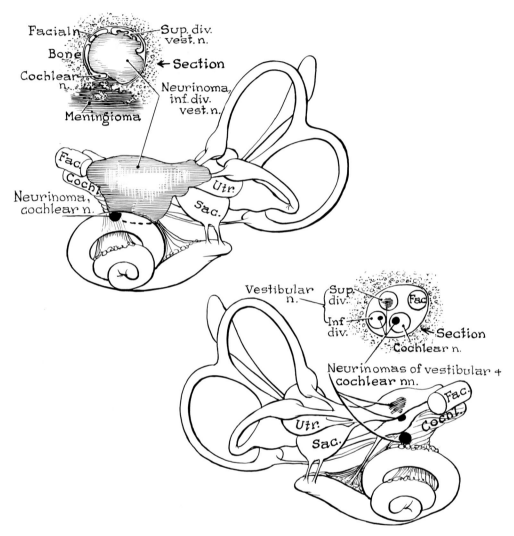

Figure 23.49. Schematic representations of the localization, extent, and relation of probably asymptomatic bilateral cochlear and vestibular schwannomas and their association with a meningioma in the left internal auditory canal of the 54-year-old man with the central form of neurofibromatosis (NF2).

Differential Diagnosis

Eighth nerve tumors must be differentiated from other lesions, above all from meningiomas that account for about 13–18% of all cerebellopontine angle tumors (41, 42). Meningiomas may arise from the porus acusticus, along the lateral and petrosal sinuses, from Meckel's cave, and occasionally within the internal acoustic meatus and jugular foramen (28). Less frequent nearby sites of origin include: (a) the tentorium, (b) the clivus, (c) the cerebellar convexity, and (d) the foramen magnum. Radiographically, meningiomas may reveal a combination of bony erosion and sclerosis, whereas eighth nerve tumors rarely show sclerosis.

The cerebellopontine angle is the most important predilective site for epidermoids, which account for about 6–7% of tumors in that area (3, 41, 42). They arise not only in that location but also on the outer aspect and within the temporal bone (43). The erosion of the internal acoustic meatus by an epidermoid with origin in the petrous apex or in the cerebellopontine angle characteristically begins outside the canal, and its location is usually medial to the one caused by an acoustic neurinoma. Furthermore, the sharply defined destruction of the petrous apex in epidermoids is not typical for schwannomas of the eighth cranial nerve.

Next in frequency are the gliomas, which account for about 5–6% of tumors in the cerebellopontine angle (3, 41). They may originate in the pons, cerebellar flocculus, or lateral recess. The types of gliomas found in that area are, in decreasing frequency, astrocytomas, medulloblastomas, ependymomas, and glioblastomas. They may involve the petrous pyramid via the jugular foramen and the internal acoustic meatus, or they may invade it directly and, in a rare instance, even destroy it (44).

Other tumors less frequently found in the cerebellopontine angle include schwannomas of the other cranial nerves (III, V–VII, IX–XI) (43), glomus tumors, hemangiomas, papillomas, teratomas, oteomas, lipomas, meningeal sarcomas, and metastatic tumors (carcinomas, sarcomas, hypernephromas, melanomas (45, 46). In addition, a number of other space-occupying lesions have to be considered: granulomas (tuberculous luetic, sarcoid, and other granulomas and the fungus lesions), cholesterol granulomas, arachnoid cysts, parasites, arteriovenous malformations, and abscesses.

Clinical Diagnosis

The neurologic manifestations produced by acoustic schwannomas can be divided into localized symptoms, symptoms involving adjacent structures, and symptoms of increased intracranial pressure. The localized symptoms, impairment of cochlear and vestibular function, are the predominant manifestations. Unilateral loss of hearing is present in 95% of patients, and in 75% it is the initial symptom. In most instances it is progressive in nature, but in up to 10% it may be of sudden onset. Five percent of the patients may have normal hearing. Impairment of discrimination often precedes the pure-tone loss. The detection may be incidental during a telephone conversation. Tinnitus is present in 70% of patients but is observed as an initial symptom in only 10–20%. Seventy percent of patients have some form of disequilibrium; only 5%, however, present with this symptom. Most patients describe it as a mild unsteadiness, often following change of position, but a few complain of rotary vertigo. Fullness, discomfort, and even pain in the affected ear are mentioned by 10–15% of patients and may reflect pressure on the sensory fibers of the seventh cranial nerve. Disturbance of facial sensation, noticed by 30% of or fewer patients, facial twitching or facial weakness, and loss of taste, described by 10% of patients, are manifestations of pressure by the tumor on the trigeminal and facial nerves.

Cochlear function studies identify the unilateral or asymmetrical sensorineural loss in most instances as retrocochlear in nature. The higher frequencies are generally involved first, and discrimination is frequently affected. Recruitment is usually absent, and there may be evidence of an abnormal threshold shift. However, about 10% of patient with acoustic schwannomas have a positive recruitment phenomenon, and 25% have good discrimination. At present, a very accurate and noninvasive test for identification of a tumor, regardless of its size, is the brain stem auditory evoked response (BAER). Ninety-five percent to 98% of patients with a tumor display an abnormal BAER. Therefore, a normal BAER almost always rules out the presence of a space-occupying lesion. The only limitation of the BAER is that the patient must have enough hearing in the affected ear. As the average pure-tone hearing loss approaches 70 dB, the results lose their validity (34).

Vestibular function studies reveal a diminished or absent response to caloric stimulation of the affected labyrinth in about 90% of patients. Thus about 10% of patients, primarily with small tumors, may have normal caloric responses.

In the past, air contrast cisternography and CT with the use of an intravenous contrast for enhancement of the tumor were the methods of choice for demonstrating acoustic neurinomas above a certain size (Figs. 23.11, 23.12, 23.14, 23.16, and 23.19C and D). More recently, MRI with gadolinium enhancement has become the best diagnostic method for the identification of these lesions (Figs. 23.18 and 23.20–23.23).

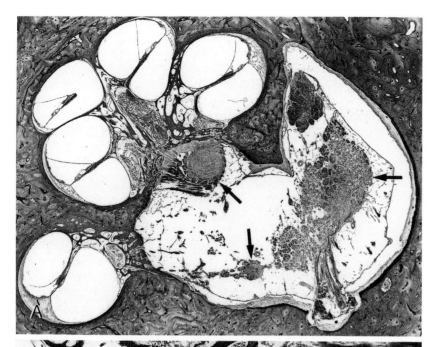

Figure 23.50. **A.** Vertical midmodiolar section through right petrous pyramid, to show the three schwannomas in the internal auditory canal. One originates from the cochlear nerve, one originates from the superior division of the vestibular nerve, and one originates from the inferior division of the vestibular nerve *(arrows)*. (Hematoxylin and eosin, ×12.)

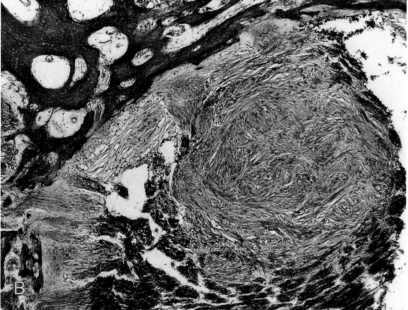

Figure 23.50. **B.** The cochlear schwannoma measures 1 mm in diameter. It arises at the spiral foraminous tract from fibers supplying the upper basal turn. (×85.)

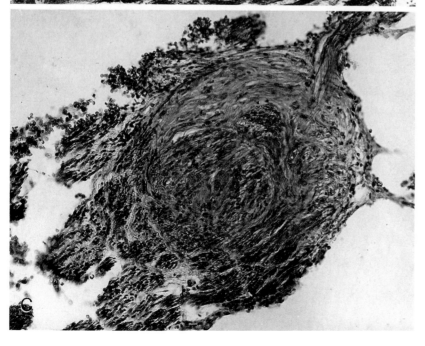

Figure 23.50. **C.** This schwannoma measures 0.3 mm in diameter. It originates from the inferior division of the vestibular nerve distal to the inferior portion of Scarpa's ganglion. (×200.)

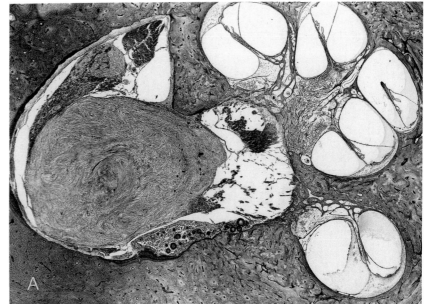

Figure 23.51. **A.** Vertical midmodiolar section through left petrous pyramid, to demonstrate a large schwannoma arising from the inferior division and a much smaller schwannoma arising from the superior division of the vestibular nerve. The schwannomas are associated with a meningioma along the floor of the internal auditory meatus, which has invaded adjacent perilabyrinthine marrow spaces. (Hematoxylin and eosin, ×13.)

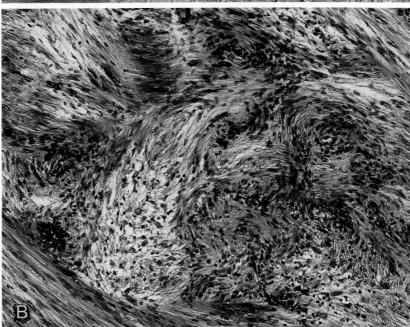

Figure 23.51. **B.** In the large vestibular schwannoma the dense fibrillary structure of the type A tissue and the loosely reticular, less cellular structure of the type B tissue are seen side by side. In the type A tissue (Antoni) the cells form long and wavy streams, whorls, and palisades. (×200.)

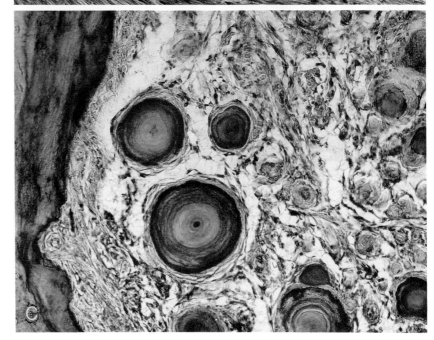

Figure 23.51. **C.** The meningioma is of the endotheliomatous variety and contains multiple psammoma bodies. (×200.)

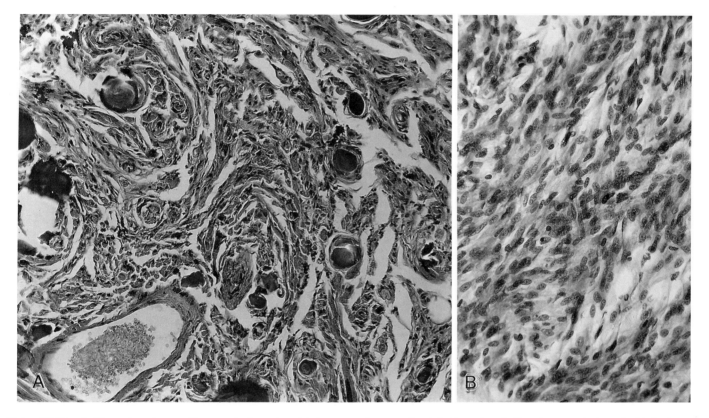

Figure 23.52. **A.** Biopsy from large solitary meningioma (en globe) covering the floor of the left middle cranial fossa. It is a very vascular meningotheliomatous meningioma with numerous psammoma bodies. **B.** Biopsy from nearby globoid meningotheliomatous meningioma that is far less vascular with very few calcifications, resembling the fibrous variety of meningiomas. (Hematoxylin and eosin, ×200 and ×300, respectively).

References

1. Tarlov IM. Structure of nerve root; differentiation of sensory from motor roots; observation on identification of function on roots of mixed cranial nerves. Arch Neurol 1937;37:1338–1355.

2. Henschen F. Über Gesehwülste der hinteren Schädelgrube, insbesondere des Kleinhirnbrücuenwinkels. Dissertation, University of Jena, 1910.

3. Gonzales-Revilla A. Neurinomas of the cerebellopontine recess; clinical study of 160 cases including operative mortality and end results. Bull Johns Hopkins Hosp 1947;80:254–296.

4. Walsh FMR. Intracranial tumors: a critical review. Q J Med 1931;24:587–640.

5. Cushing H. Intracranial tumors. Springfield, Illinois: Charles C Thomas, 1935.

6. Marburg O. Die Tumoren im Bereiche des Cochlear-Vestibularsystems und Kleinhirns. In: Handbuch der Neurologie des Ohres. Wien: 1926;3:1–166.

7. Olivecrona H. Acoustic tumors. J Neurol 1940;3:141–146.

8. Zülch KJ. Brain tumors: their biology and pathology. 3rd ed. Berlin: 1986.

9. Hardy M, Crowe SJ. Early asymptomatic acoustic tumors: report of six cases. Arch Surg 1936;32:292–301.

10. Sandifort E. De duro quodam corpusculo nervo auditorio adherente. In: Observationes anatomico-pathogicae. Leiden: Chap. 9, 1777:116–120.

11. Wishart J. Cases of tumors in the skull, dura mater and brain. Edinburg Med Surg J 1822;18:393–397.

12. Virchov R. Die krankhaften Geschwülste. Berlin: 1864–1865;2:116, 151, 295.

13. Sternberg C. Beitrag zur Kenntnis der sogenanten Geschwülste des Nervus acusticus. Z Heilk Abt Path Anat 1900;21:163–186.

14. Henschen F. Zur Histologie und Pathogenese der Kleinhirnbrückenwinkel Tumoren. Arch Psychiatr Nervenkr 1915;56:21–122.

15. Cushing H. Tumors of the nervus acusticus and the syndrome of the cerebello-pontine angle. New York: Hafner, 1963.

16. Toynbee J. Neuroma of the auditory nerve. Trans Pathol Soc Lond 1853;4:259–260.

17. Habermann JE. Über Nervenatrophie im inneren Ohr Z Heilk 1891;12:357–394.

18. Alexander G. Zur Kenntnis der Akustikustumoren. Z Klin Med 1907;12:447–456.

19. Fowler EP. Acousticus tumors within the internal auditory meatus. Laryngoscope 1936;46:616–627.

20. Rubinstein LJ. Tumors of the central nervous system. In: Atlas of tumor pathology. 2nd series, Fascicle 6. Washington, DC: Armed Forces Institute of Pathology, 1982.

21. Harkin JC, Reed RJ. Tumors of the peripheral nervous system. In: Atlas of tumor pathology. 2nd series, Fascicle 3. Washington, DC: Armed Forces Institute of Pathology, 1982.

22. Adelstein LJ. Tumor of the acoustic nerve within the petrous bone; operative removal. Arch Neurol 1944;51:268–270.

23. Nager GT. Acoustic neurinomas. Pathology and differential diagnosis. Arch Otolaryngol 1969;89:252–279.

24. Olivecrona H. Analysis of results of complete and partial removal of acoustic neurinomas. J Neurol Neurosurg Psychiatry 1950;13:271–272.

25. Antoni NRE. Über Rückenmarkstumoren und Neurofibrome. Wiesbaden: JF Bergmann, 1920.

26. Young DF, Eldridge R, Nager GT, Deland FH, McNew J. Hereditary bilateral acoustic neuroma (central neurofibromatosis). Birth Defects 1971 VII(4):73–86.

27. Holt GR. ENT manifestations of von Recklinghausen's disease. Laryngoscope 1978;88:1617–1632.

28. Rubenstein AF. Neurofibromatosis. A review of the clinical problems. Ann N Y Acad Sci 1986;426:1–13.

29. National Institutes of Health Conference Statement. Neurofibromatosis. Arch Neurol 1988;45:575–578.

30. Crowe FW, Schull WJ, Neel JV. A clinical, pathological and genetic study of multiple neurofibromatosis. Springfield, Illinois: Charles C Thomas, 1956.

31. Glasscock ME III, Heart MJ, Vrobec JT. Management of bilateral acoustic neuroma. Otolaryngol Clin North Am 1992;25(2):449–458.

32. Barker D, Wright E, Ngugen L, et al. Gene for von Recklinghausen neurofibromatosis is in the pericentromeric region of chromosome 17. Science 1987;236:1100–2102.

33. Seizinger BR, Roulean GA, Ozelius LJ, et al. Genetic linkage of von Recklinghausen neurofibromatosis to the nerve growth factor receptor gene. Cell 1987;49:589–594.

34. Baldwin RL, LeMaster K. Neurofibromatosis-2 and bilateral acoustic neuromas: distinction from neurofibromatosis-1 (von Recklinghausen's disease). Ann J Otol 1989;10(6):439–442.

35. Roulean GA, Wertelecki W, Haines JL, et al. Genetic linkage of bilateral acoustic neurofibromatosis to a DNA marker on chromosome 22. Nature 1987;329:246–248.

36. Sadeh M, Markinovitz G, Goldhammer Y. Occurrence of both neurofibromatosis-1 and -2 in the same individual with a rapidly progressive course. Neurology 1989;39:282–283.

37. Michaels VV, Whismont JP, Garriti JA. Neurofibromatosis type I with bilateral acoustic neuromas. Neurofibromatosis 1989;2:213–217.

38. Riccardi VM. Is NF-1 always distinct from NF-2? Neurofibromatosis 1989;2:193–194.

39. Russell DS, Rubinstein LJ. Pathology of tumors of the nervous system. 5th ed. Baltimore: Williams & Wilkins, 1989.

40. Nager GT. Meningiomas involving the temporal bone. Clinical and pathological aspects. Springfield, Illinois: Charles C Thomas, 1964.

41. Thomalske G, Kienow-Rieg I, Mohr G. Critical observations concerning the diagnosis and clinical features in and 100 cases of tumors in the cerebellopontine region. Adv Neurosurg 1973;7:252–259.

42. Fromm H, Huf H, Schafer M. Operations and results in 102 tumors of the cerebello-pontine angle. Adv Neurosurg 1973;7:260–261.

43. Nager GT. Epidermoids involving the temporal bone (congenital cholesteatomas). In: English GM, ed. Otolaryngology. New York: Harper & Row, 1981;43:1–18.

44. Nager GT. Gliomas involving the temporal bone. Clinical and pathological aspects. Laryngoscope 1967;77:454–488.

45. Nager GT. Neurinomas of the trigeminal nerve. Am J Otolaryngol 1984;5:301–333.

46. McShane D. Acoustic neuroma. Case presentation and diagnostic review. Proceedings of the Irish ORL Society 24th Annual Meeting, September 1983. Irish J Med Sci 1983;39–47.

the presence of large, hyperchromatic, occasionally multinucleated giant cells (Fig. 24.17*B* and *C* (Case 4)) with no important adverse effect (22). Mitotic figures are detected rarely, indicating the slow growth of schwannomas.

The ganglion cells tend to be distributed to localized areas on the surfaces of the tumors (5, 31, 32), a phenomenon also observed in acoustic schwannomas (28, 33). Because of the rostral location of these ganglion cells in reference to the bulk of the tumor, it was believed that the site of origin of the neoplasms was proximal to the ganglion, a common finding in spinal schwannomas. That tumors may occasionally also arise from nerve fibers distal to the ganglion has been clearly documented (Fig. 24.4*D*) (11, 23, 25). In several instances, tumors were found to have arisen in the maxillary or mandibular nerve (Figs. 24.7*F* and 24.11 (Case 2)). The most frequent site of origin, however, remains the area in which the sensory root joins the ganglion. Trigeminal schwannomas thus share a centripetal predilection with the spinal, posterior root tumors.

RADIOGRAPHIC MANIFESTATIONS

The radiographic methods used in the past for identification of trigeminal schwannomas included: *(a)* conventional views of the skull and petrous pyramids; *(b)* axial and coronal complex motion tomograms of the petrous pyramids and middle cranial fossa; *(c)* cerebral angiography; and, sometimes, *(d)* selective contrast encephalography combined with tomography. More recently, computed tomography (CT) and magnetic resonance imaging with contrast enhancement have become the diagnostic procedures of choice (10, 12, 17, 19, 30, 34–41).

In tumors located predominantly in the middle cranial fossa, the most frequent observation is a sharply defined bone defect involving the medial half of the floor of the middle cranial fossa (Fig. 24.10*A* (Case 2)). The defect may involve and even totally include the basal foramina. Equally frequent features are enlargement of the trigeminal impression and erosion, excavation, and finally destruction of the superior, lateral, and medial portions of the petrous apex (Fig. 24.12*A* and *B* (Case 3)). Erosion of the petrous tip often, but not always, reflects tumor extension from the middle cranial fossa into the posterior cranial fossa or from the posterior cranial fossa to the middle cranial fossa. Anterior extension of the schwannoma is reflected by erosion of the medial portion of the sphenoid wing, by enlargement or destruction of the superior orbital fissure, by distortion and destruction of the inferior margin of the optic canal, by erosion of the anterior clinoid process, and by amputation of the orbital apex. Inferior extension of the tumor may result in invasion of the pterygopalatine fossa, anterior displacement of the posterior wall of the maxillary sinus, invasion of that sinus, and destruction of the pterygoid process (Figs. 24.6 (Case 1) and 24.12*C* (Case 3)). Tumor extension in a medial direction may destroy the adjacent floor and dorsum of the sella and the posterior clinoid process. It may produce a medial displacement and erosion of the lateral wall of the sphenoid sinus (Figs. 24.16, *cut 11* (Case 4), and 24.18 *(cut 22)* (Case 5)) and invasion of the adjacent and opposite sinuses. Erosion of the adjoining clivus is clear evidence that the schwannoma is extending into the posterior cranial fossa. Regardless of the extent of erosion or destruction of the petrous

apex, the configuration of the internal auditory canal remains unchanged. This is a determining factor in the differentiation between trigeminal and acoustic schwannomas.

Once a schwannoma of the middle cranial fossa has reached a certain size, it often produces structural changes of the orbital apex. Enlargement of the superior orbital fissure and erosion of the inferior margin of the optic canal are generally considered characteristic bony alterations (17).

Similar to the experience with acoustic schwannomas, earlier reports of trigeminal schwannomas concerned very large neoplasms with extensive bone erosion (24, 25). As the number of reports of smaller tumors increased, the incidence of detectable bone erosion diminished (38, 42).

With larger tumors, carotid and vertebral angiography may show rather characteristic distortion of the vascular architecture. The typical features of schwannomas located in the middle cranial fossa are the anterior, medial, and inferior displacement of the ganglionic and intracavernous segments of the internal carotid artery, stretching of the siphon and the supraclinoid segment of that vessel, and curved elevation of the middle cerebral artery (Fig. 24.13 (Case 3)) (17, 36). Enlarged cavernous carotid branches related to the tumor were observed in the majority of patients. The characteristic features of schwannomas located in or extending into the posterior cranial fossa on vertebral angiography are posterior and contralateral displacement of the basilar artery, dorsocranial displacement of the posterior cerebral artery and superior cerebellar artery, and downward deflection of the anteroinferior cerebellar artery (36). An hourglass-shaped schwannoma may appear to be encircled above by the posterior cerebral artery and below by the superior cerebellar artery (18, 25). Not every schwannoma, however, produces such typical angiographic features (43).

A characteristic feature on venograms is the laterobasal displacement of the petrosal vein. Large tumors may produce a severe compression of that vein and slowing of the circulation in the posterior cranial fossa (36).

Naidich et al. (37) examined 47 extra-axial posterior fossa lesions, including three trigeminal schwannomas, using CT. All trigeminal schwannomas were located closer to the tip than were the acoustic schwannomas. They were clearly demarcated, appeared to extend through the tentorial incisura, and were confluent with the anteroposterior aspect of the petrous pyramid. Two were slightly denser than the surrounding normal brain tissue without contrast medium and, after contrast infusion, showed homogeneous increase in density. The third tumor was cystic, with a clearly demarcated zone of decreased density. All tumors produced changes involving the fourth ventricle and basal cisterns similar to those observed with acoustic schwannomas.

Many schwannomas in the head and neck area are quite vascular on account of their content of large vascular channels and sinusoidal dilatation of smaller blood vessels (Figs. 24.9 (Case 1), 24.13 (Case 3), and 24.19*A* (Case 5)) (28, 33). Of 32 schwannomas, 22 (68%) showed abnormal tumor vascularity (35). The angiographic observations included: *(a)* simultaneous occurrence of vascular and avascular areas in close proximity, *(b)* puddling of contrast medium, *(c)* less specific vascular patterns, and *(d)* the presence of capsular vessels. The trigeminal schwannoma derives its blood supply from branches of the internal carotid and middle meningeal arteries that normally supply the fifth cranial nerve and the Gasserian ganglion.

CLINICAL SYMPTOMS AND SIGNS

The insidious onset, the often atypical sequence of clinical manifestations, and the protracted course account for the frequently observed delays in recognizing trigeminal schwannomas. The initial symptoms are usually an expression of trigeminal nerve dysfunction, primarily irritation and changes in facial sensation. They are observed in about two-thirds of these patients (23). Numbness and paresthesia may gradually spread from one division to all three divisions of the nerve and are more common than pain in the early stage of the illness (11). Pain may be present, although it is not a constant feature. It can be intermittent or continuous and may be manifested as a burning or crawling sensation or an aching, or it can mimic tic douloureux. At times it is localized behind the eye or in the ear. Some investigators believe that tumors originating in the ganglion tend to produce constant pain, while schwannomas arising from the posterior sensory root rarely cause pain (8, 9, 14, 24). Quite often the patient is unable to chew food on the corresponding side of the mouth or does so with difficulty. Recurrent episodes of neuralgia are relatively infrequent, occurring in 50% or less of patients. Neurologic examination may disclose hypesthesia or hypalgesia in one division or all divisions of the nerve and decreased or absent corneal sensation. In addition, weakness or atrophy of the masticatory muscles may be present. The degrees of trigeminal dysfunction, as well as the relations between impairment of sensation and motor function, may vary considerably. Involvement of trigeminal nerve function as an initial clinical manifestation is observed in about 40% of patients. As a schwannoma originating at the ganglion extends into the cavernous sinus, grows through the superior orbital fissure into the orbit, or invades the optic canal, about half of the patients experience optic symptoms. These symptoms, in order of decreasing frequency, are: *(a)* paralysis of the abducent, trochlear, and oculomotor nerves; *(b)* ipsilateral exophthalmos; and *(c)* loss of vision. Occasionally, diplopia due to paralysis of one of the three oculomotor nerves, especially the sixth nerve, may be the first presenting symptom (14, 44). Involvement of the oculomotor nerves has been observed in about 50% of patients. The abducent nerve is involved most frequently. Ipsilateral exophthalmos, also a frequent finding, may occasionally be the first presenting sign. In such instances the superior orbital fissure generally appears to be enlarged and distorted. Ipsilateral impairment of vision reflects compression of the optic nerve, frequently associated with erosion of the inferolateral border of the optic canal. Bilateral loss of vision results from intracranial hypertension and papilledema and is usually a late symptom (45). Trophic disturbances with neuroparalytic keratitis have been observed in about 30% of patients. Two-thirds or more of the patients show evidence of erosion of the petrous apex and of the floor of the middle cranial fossa. In about half of the patients, symptoms and signs indicate involvement of the posterior cranial fossa, reflecting a schwannoma either originating in the posterior sensory root or arising at the ganglion with an hourglass configuration. Signs of posterior fossa involvement, including *(a)* tinnitus and impairment of hearing and *(b)* cerebellar ataxia, may occasionally be the initial clinical manifestations. Ataxia is thought to be the result of pressure on the cerebellar peduncles rather than on the cerebellar hemispheres (11). Occasionally, the seventh nerve may be involved in the form of a palsy or facial spasm, and at times, symptoms of ninth, tenth, and eleventh cranial nerve involvement may also be observed. Signs of increased intracranial pressure, headaches, and papilledema have been observed in about 40% of patients but are, as expected, late manifestations.

ASSOCIATION OF TRIGEMINAL SCHWANNOMAS WITH THE CENTRAL FORM OF NEUROFIBROMATOSIS

Von Recklinghausen's neurofibromatosis is a relatively common, dominant, widespread phakomatosis found predominantly in females. It is characterized by the presence of multiple nerve sheath tumors (neurofibromas, schwannomas, and malignant neurogenic tumors), by changes in the skin (café au lait patches, elephantiasis), by changes in bone and joints (scoliosis, pseudarthrosis), by changes in the central nervous system (meningiomas, schwannomas, central gliomas), and by a series of so-called central changes including rachischisis, syringomyelia, heterotopia of nerve cells, displacement of cortical layers, fibrinomyelinic plaques, excessive atypical glia, small angiomatous malformations, and connective tissue inclusions. The disease may also be associated with neoplasms arising from the neural crest, such as peripheral neuroblastomas, adrenal ganglioneuromas, and pheochromocytomas (46). The condition used to be conveniently divided into four categories, each with characteristic clinical and pathologic features: a central form (NF2), a peripheral form (NF1), a visceral form, and a forme fruste (46). Although these forms may incorporate some degree of overlap, patients with the central form (NF2) generally display few or none of the peripheral signs; conversely, patients with the peripheral form (NF1) rarely exhibit the central manifestations of the disease (22). All forms may be represented in the members of a family (22). The forme fruste, in which health is not impaired and the lesions are limited, often escapes clinical detection.

It is the central form (NF2) of neurofibromatosis that is of primary interest to the otologist because of its frequent association with mutiple and, almost invariably, bilateral cranial nerve tumors (schwannomas), multiple meningiomas, gliomas, and hamartomas (22, 33, 47–49). The eighth nerves are affected most frequently, but it is not uncommon for other cranial nerves, especially the trigeminal nerve and the Gasserian ganglion, to be involved either in association with the eighth nerves or independently (50, 51). In a rare instance, schwannomas of the Gasserian ganglion and of the eighth cranial nerve can develop ipsilaterally side by side. In such a situation, radiographs of the pyramid may disclose erosion of the petrous apex and enlargement of the internal acoustic meatus (52). The motor roots are, in general, implicated less often than the sensory roots. In many patients, bilateral eighth nerve tumors are the principal or only manifestation of the disease (53). Otologists should be aware that a benign or malignant trigeminal schwannoma or a neurofibroma may be a manifestation of a central form (NF2) or forme fruste of neurofibromatosis.

MALIGNANT SCHWANNOMAS OF THE TRIGEMINAL NERVE

In rare instances, schwannomas of the trigeminal nerve may display the characteristic features of malignant tumors. Cueno

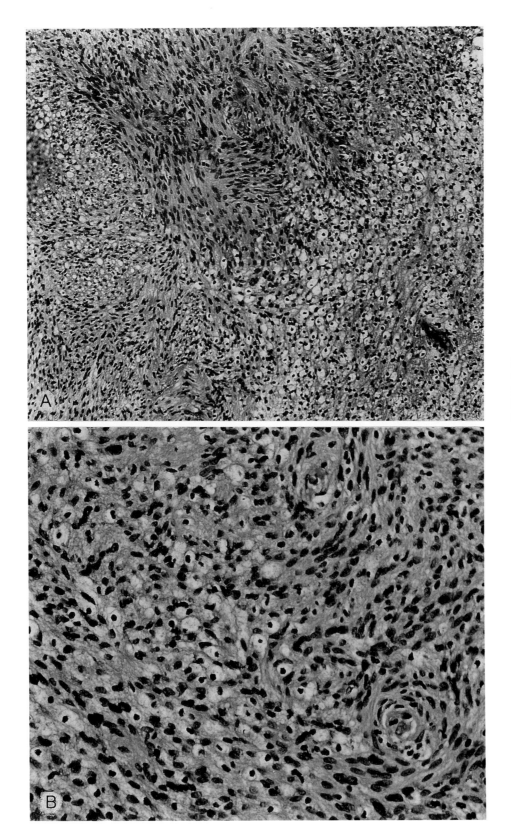

Figure 24.8. **A.** Schwannoma of left maxillary nerve, with Antoni type A tissue with prominent palisades of nuclei in left upper half and Antoni type B tissue in right lower half of field. (Hematoxylin and eosin, ×200.)

Figure 24.8. **B.** Antoni type A tissue with compactly arranged spindle cells with oval nuclei forming interlacing fascicles. (×350.)

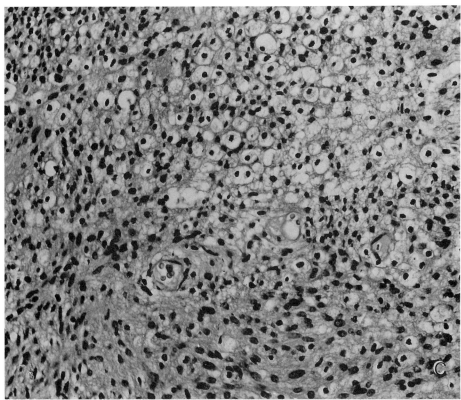

Figure 24.8.   C. Area of transition from Antoni type A to type B tissue with occasional lipid-filled foam cells. (×350.)

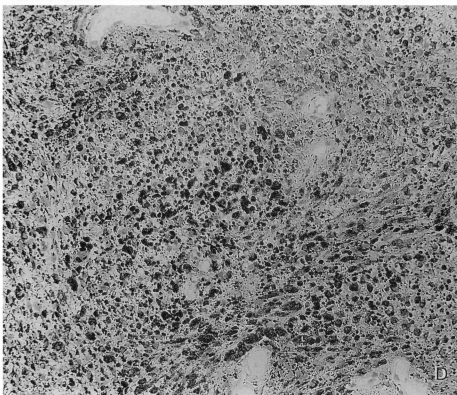

Figure 24.8.   D. Area of earlier hemorrhage with hemosiderin-laden macrophages. (×350.)

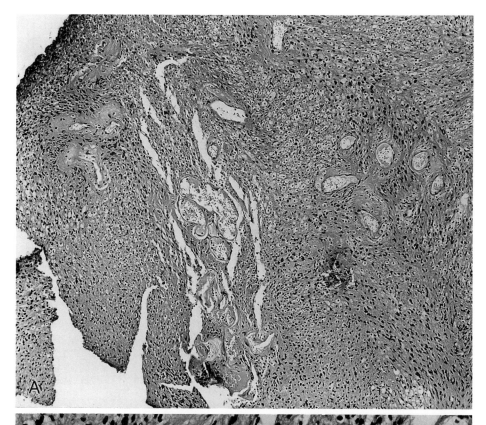

Figure 24.9. A. Low-power view, for orientation, from another field of the same tumor shown in Figure 24.8, revealing some vascular changes. (Hematoxylin and eosin, ×100.)

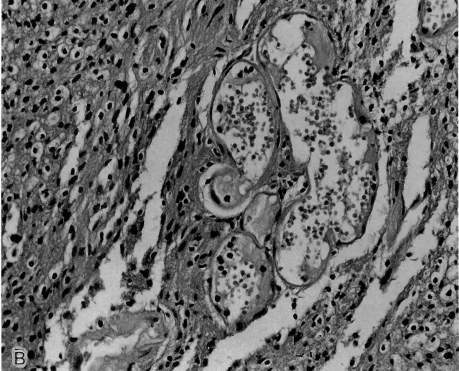

Figure 24.9. B. Focal sinusoidal dilatation. (×350.)

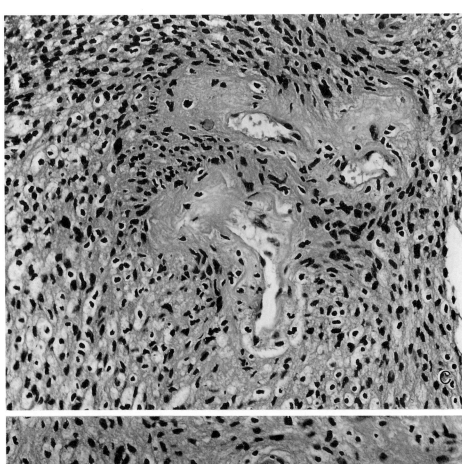

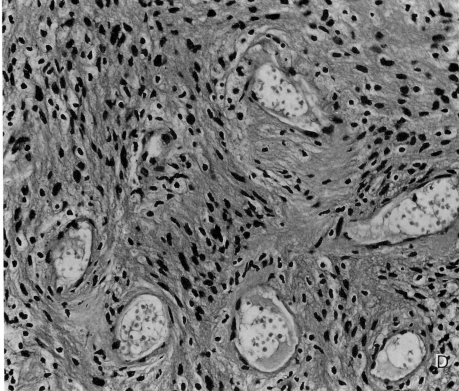

Figure 24.9. C and **D.** The walls of these vessels consist of a single layer of endothelium that has undergone regressive changes with irregular hyaline thickening. (×350.)

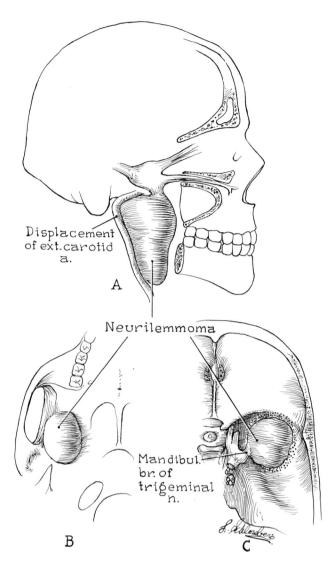

Displacement of ext.carotid a.

A

Neurilemmoma

Mandibul. br. of trigeminal n.

B

C

Figure 24.11. Large schwannoma originating in mandibular division of right trigeminal nerve. It eroded the floor of the middle cranial fossa and occupies the pterygomaxillary and retromandibular fossa.

Case 3. *Hourglass-shaped intracranial and extracranial schwannoma originating at left Gasserian ganglion.*

A 25-year-old man had had three transient episodes involving a sensation of fullness and decreased hearing in the left ear during the preceding 3 years. Each episode resolved within 8–10 days. Six months prior to admission, he had experienced the same symptoms, as well as a persistent high-pitched tinnitus in the left ear. A left aspiration myringotomy and placement of a tympanostomy tube resulted in partial relief. The patient also recalled several brief episodes of decreased sensation over the left side of the lower jaw and left side of the neck. On admission, the patient complained of a moderate sensation of fullness, pressure, slight loss of hearing, continuous high-pitched tinnitus, and an occasional deep-seated lancinating pain in the left ear.

Otologic examination revealed an inflamed, bulging left tympanic membrane without landmarks and a purulent exudate draining through a tympanostomy tube. The audiogram showed a mild pure conductive hearing loss in the left ear with a speech reception threshold of 15 dB and a discrimination score of 100%. Vestibular function studies disclosed reduced caloric response on the left. On nasopharyngoscopy, an extrinsic submucosal mass was seen protruding into the left fossa of Rosenmüller, compressing, rotating, and displacing the Eustachian tubal orifice almost to the midline and obliterating its lumen. There was no decrease of sensation to touch, pain, or temperature over the left side of the face, tongue, palate, or buccal

mucosa. The corneal reflexes were normal. There was no weakness or atrophy of the temporalis or masseter muscles on the left, and the extraocular movements were full, without diplopia or nystagmus. There was obvious weakness on the left side of the palate, with marked deviation of the uvula to the right. Pharyngeal sensation and reflexes and the mobility of the left vocal cord were normal.

Neurologic examination was normal except for paresis of the left ninth and tenth cranial nerves.

Radiologic examination of the left temporal bone revealed generalized haziness throughout a well-developed cellular system (Fig. 24.12). The petrous apex was eroded, with a thin bony shelf above and below that extended posteriorly to the anterior margin of the porus acusticus. The base of the skull contained a large defect in the left middle cranial fossa. It extended anteriorly to the sphenoid wing and included the foramina ovale and rotundum. The left pterygoid plate was destroyed. On tomograms of the base of the skull, the destruction of the floor of the middle fossa corresponded to a smoothly rounded hole about 4 cm in diameter that extended from the petrous to the sphenoid ridge and from the midline to the lateral margin of the middle fossa. The lateral and medial plates of the pterygoid process were completely destroyed. On anteroposterior polytomograms of the left petrous pyramid, the destruction of the petrous apex appeared as an anteromedial concave excavation. The transfemoral cerebral angiogram revealed: *(a)* medial displacement of the intracavernous segment of the left internal carotid artery; *(b)* a space-occupying lesion in the left middle fossa, elevating the main middle cerebral artery and its trifurcation without producing identifiable displacement of the midline structures or elevation of the major portion of the Sylvian fissure; and *(c)* no vascular staining or abnormally increased vascular supply (Fig. 24.13). On the echoencephalogram the midline structures exhibited a 3-mm lateral shift to the right. CT was not available to us at that time (1974). The differential diagnosis included: a long-standing, possibly congenital, expanding process such as an epidermoid or teratomatous cyst; a tumor arising in the bone (chondroma, chondrosarcoma) or in the nasopharynx; a meningeal or an arachnoid cyst; and a metastasis, a meningioma, or a schwannoma of the trigeminal nerve. A schwannoma of the left fifth cranial nerve was thought to be the most likely possibility.

A left temporal craniotomy was performed, and a left trigeminal schwannoma was subtotally removed. Extradural exploration of the left temporal fossa disclosed a spheric, encapsulated, rather firm, grayish-white tumor with a smooth surface located above the foramen ovale. The anteroposterior diameter was about 4 cm, and the mediolateral diameter was about 3 cm; the tumor elevated the temporal lobe about 2 cm. It extended anteriorly as far as the anterior pole of the middle fossa, posteriorly to the tentorium, abutted medially against the cavernous sinus and extended about 2 cm through a large defect in the floor of the middle fossa into the retromaxillary fossa (Fig. 24.14). Incision of the avascular capsule exposed a grayish-yellow tumor with a soft, granular consistency. It had the gross appearance of a schwannoma, a diagnosis that was subsequently confirmed with frozen and permanent sections (Fig. 24.15). Ninety-five percent of the neoplasm could be removed, leaving some tumor nodules adherent to the lateral wall of the cavernous sinus and the lining of the retromaxillary fossa. The maxillary and mandibular division of the fifth nerve were visualized and appeared to be intact. The remaining space in the retromaxillary fossa and the defect in the floor of the middle fossa were filled with sheets of absorbable gelatin sponge. The postoperative course was uneventful.

Four years later, a CT scan of the head showed no evidence of recurrent intracranial tumor. The neurologic deficit was limited to a small area of hypesthesia in the distribution of the maxillary nerve and to persistent paresis of the left ninth and tenth cranial nerves. The narrowing of the left fossa of Rosenmüller and the compression of the orifice of the left Eustachian tube had not changed. Testing of the left ear revealed a speech reception threshold of 15 dB and a discrimination score of 100%.

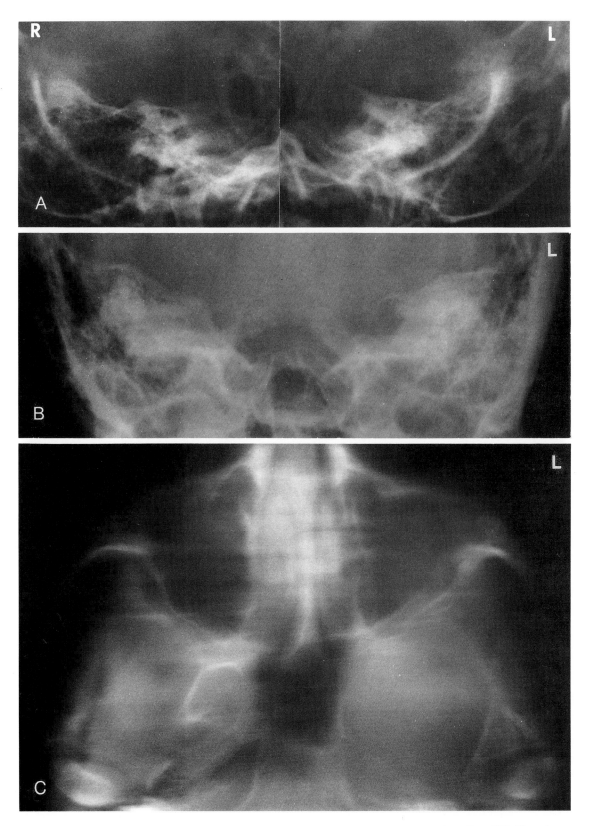

Figure 24.12.   The generalized haziness throughout the air cell system of the left temporal bone reflects the serous otitis media resulting from extrinsic compression of the Eustachian tube **(A).** The destruction of the left petrous apex appears as an excavation extending posteriorly to the anterior rim of the porus acusticus **(A** and **B).** The schwannoma extending through a large defect in the floor of the left middle cranial fossa completely destroyed the left pterygoid process **(C).**

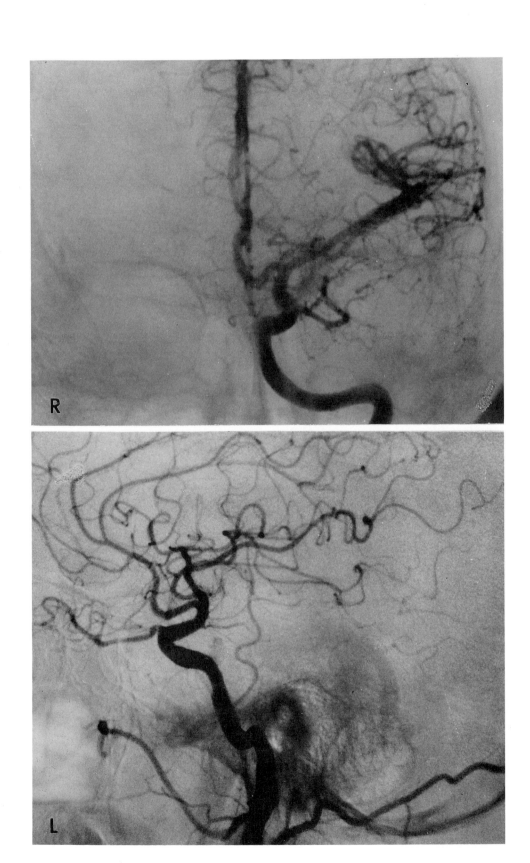

Figure 24.13. Carotid angiograms revealing medial displacement of intracavernous segment of left internal carotid artery and elevation of left middle cerebral artery.

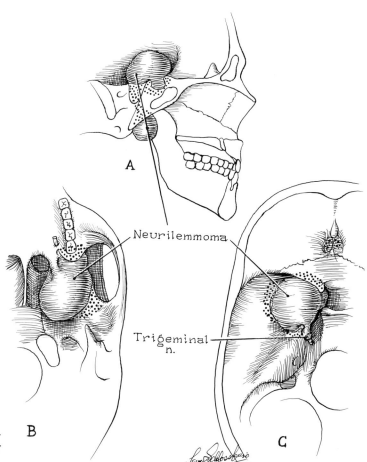

Figure 24.14. Dumbbell-shaped schwannoma originating at left Gasserian ganglion, with a larger intracranial portion in the middle and a smaller extracranial portion in the pterygomaxillary fossa.

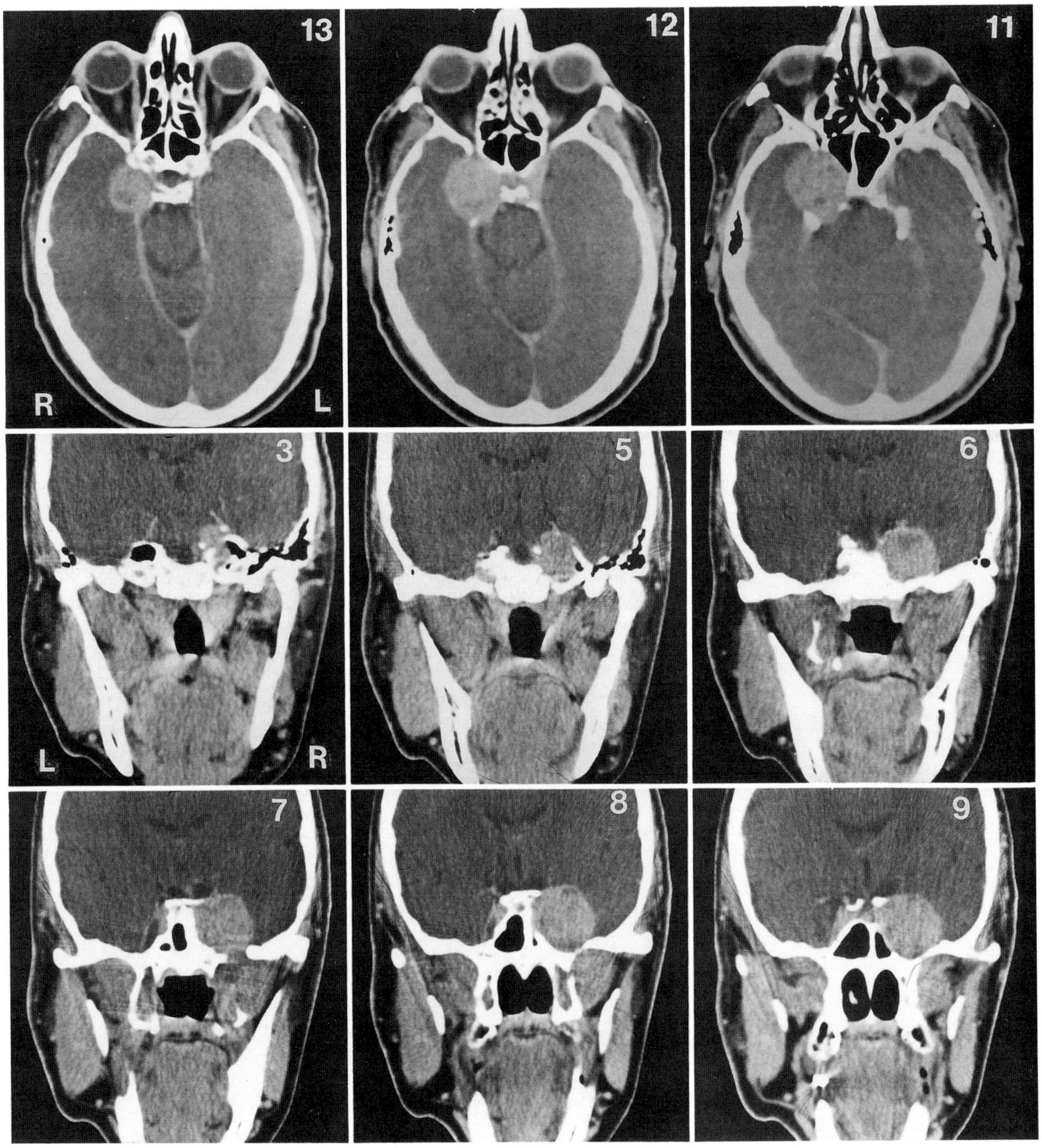

Figure 24.16. CT scans of the head in axial and coronal planes disclose the schwannoma in the right middle cranial fossa, eroding the lateral aspect of the sella, the lateral wall of the sphenoid sinus, and the floor of the middle cranial fossa around the right foramen ovale. (Courtesy of Dr. E. Walker.)

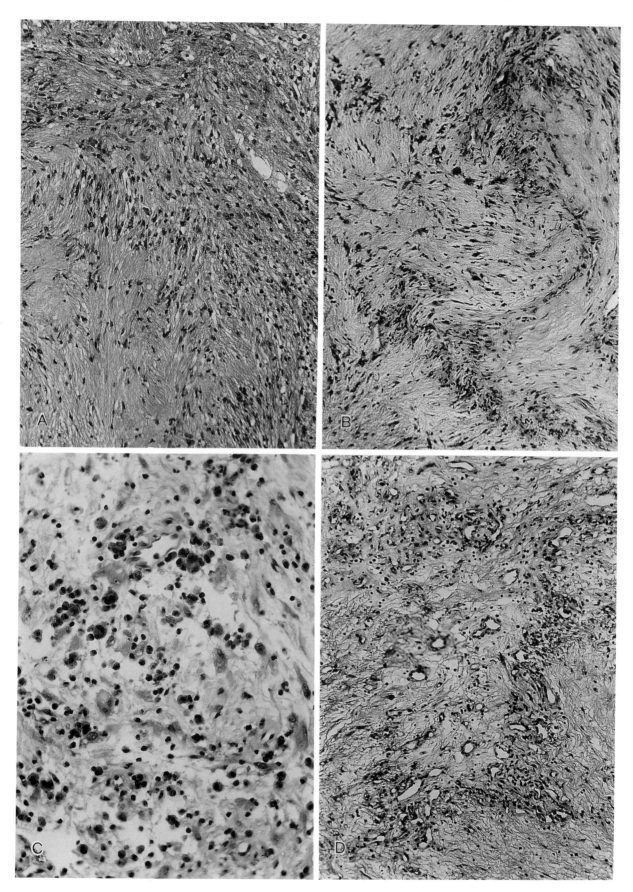

Figure 24.17.   A. Antoni type A tissue with increasing hyalinization of connective tissue (lower left of field). **B.** Antoni type A tissue with large, plump, atypical hyperchromatic nuclei irregularly distributed throughout field. **C.** Area containing numerous hemosiderin-laden macrophages, lymphocytes, and mast cells. **D.** Area of Antoni type B tissue with numerous vascular convolutions. (Hematoxylin and eosin, ×160, ×140, ×300, and ×150.)

Case 5. *Schwannoma arising from left Gasserian ganglion.*

A 45-year-old woman experienced intermittent diplopia, especially when tired, for which she had been examined by an ophthalmologist 3 years prior to admission. The diplopia resulting from a left lateral abduction paresis eventually became continuous and was no longer correctable with prisms. Three years later she began to notice paresthesia over the left side of the face, and a CT scan of the head showed a left parasellar tumor.

Neurologic examination on admission revealed a left sixth nerve palsy and decreased sensation in the maxillary division of the left fifth cranial nerve. There was no weakness of the ipsilateral masticatory muscles. The remaining cranial nerves on that side and cerebellar function were normal. A repeat head scan disclosed a markedly and homogeneously enhancing mass over the medial floor of the left middle cranial fossa, extending posteriorly from about the level of the foramen rotundum across an eroded petrous apex slightly into the posterior cranial fossa. It measured about 3.5×2 cm and was pressing medially on the left cavernous sinus (Fig. 24.18).

At *operation,* a left temporal craniotomy was performed. A somewhat nodular subdural mass covered the floor of the middle cranial fossa in the parasellar region. The mass extended from the medial portion of the greater sphenoid wing into the anterior portion of the cerebellar fossa. After internal decompression, the tumor and its capsule were totally removed with an ultrasonic suction device. The Gasserian ganglion and the posterior root of the trigeminal nerve were identified and appeared normal. Histologic examination showed the tumor to be a schwannoma (Fig. 24.19). A 6-month postoperative examination revealed, except for a persistent left sixth nerve palsy and hypesthesia in the maxillary division of the left fifth nerve, no neurologic deficit. A repeat head scan showed no residual tumor tissue. The patient's diplopia was subsequently corrected by recession of the left medial rectus and resection of the right lateral rectus muscle.

Clinically, trigeminal schwannomas display considerable variation, depending on the site of origin, the location of the predominant tumor portion, and the local behavior of the tumor. A schwannoma arising in the middle fossa is often associated with dysfunction of sensation in the distribution of that cranial nerve. Signs of irritation (paresthesia and neuralgia), generally constant and lasting for several hours or days but occasionally paroxysmal, or signs of loss of the ability to recognize light tactile, thermal, and painful sensations in the face are the presenting symptoms in more than half of the patients (14, 16). On the other hand, it is not uncommon for a trigeminal schwannoma to lack fifth nerve symptoms completely (8, 13, 14, 42). The suggestion was made earlier that schwannomas arising from the ganglion are frequently accompanied by pain, whereas those arising from the sensory root are not (8, 14). Since that time, however, a number of tumors originating solely in the dorsal root that did produce facial pain have been reported (69, 70). Weakness and atrophy of the masticatory muscles, occasionally with deviation of the jaw toward the side of the lesion, are common observations (8, 11, 13, 14, 25). One-fourth of trigeminal schwannomas initially produce posterior fossa symptoms. Involvement of the cerebellum, cerebral peduncle, and the lower cranial nerves and nystagmus are the most common signs.

At times it may be difficult to differentiate between a trigeminal and an acoustic schwannoma. In acoustic tumors, however, impairment of cochlear and vestibular function and enlargement of the internal acoustic meatus are the salient features, and involvement of the fifth nerve function is much less common. In contrast, in trigeminal tumors of the posterior fossa, impairment of fifth nerve function is more marked than cochlear and vestibular dysfunction. Also, trigeminal tumors frequently erode the superior aspect of the petrous apex, whereas the internal auditory canal remains unaltered. Nevertheless, in a rare situation, a posterior fossa trigeminal schwannoma may lack evidence of fifth nerve involvement.

As a middle fossa schwannoma extends to the optic canal, superior orbital fissure, or cavernous sinus, atrophy of the optic nerve, exophthalmos, or isolated sixth, fourth, or third nerve palsy may become the initial symptom. Similarly, if the tumor extends to the lacerated foramen and produces extrinsic compression of the Eustachian tube, a serous middle ear effusion may be the initial manifestation.

Emphasis is obviously on early recognition of trigeminal schwannomas in patients with facial pain and numbness at the stage when the tumor may still be relatively small and when total removal with little or no morbidity is possible. The hitherto classic radiologic features associated with large schwannomas—erosion of the floor of the middle fossa, of the orbita and petrous apex, and of the sella and clivus and displacement of the internal carotid artery and its branches and of the anterior horn of the ventricle—have lost significance. Instead, high-resolution CT head scans in axial and coronal planes, aided by air contrast cisternography and magnetic resonance imaging now enable the recognition of a trigeminal schwannoma before it has caused significant structural changes or bone erosion (38).

The neurotologist is expected to be well acquainted with the behavior and manifestation of tumors that arise in the vicinity of the temporal bone. The differential diagnosis of eighth nerve tumors, for example, includes not only meningiomas, epidermoids, and gliomas but also a relatively large group of infrequent space-occupying lesions in the cerebellopontine angle (33). One of these lesions is the trigeminal schwannoma. As this tumor invades the sensory portion of the nerve, it may produce typical and atypical pain sensations or loss of sensation in the cutaneous, mucosal, and dural distribution of the nerve, and loss of corneal and sternutatory reflexes. Otalgia, for instance, may represent neuralgia of the third division of the fifth nerve. Involvement of the motor fibers may cause paralysis and atrophy of the masticatory muscles with deviation of the jaw. With growth of the tumor into the posterior cranial fossa, symptoms and signs of involvement of the lower cranial nerves, cerebellum, and medulla develop. Expansion within the middle cranial fossa may lead to involvement of the ocular motor nerves (VI, IV, and III), the optic nerve, and the orbit. Pressure on the adjacent bone will give rise to the characteristic erosions at the base of the skull. Extracranial extension or extracranial origin of the tumor may result in invasion of the retromaxillary and retromandibular fossae, infiltration of the nasopharynx with extrinsic compression and distortion of the Eustachian tubal orifice, and the presentation of a submucosal mass in the nasopharynx and oropharynx. The tumor may also extend into the sphenoid (71) and maxillary sinuses. A schwannoma originating within the inferior alveolar canal may appear as an endoral submucosal mass over the buccal or lingual aspect of the mandible.

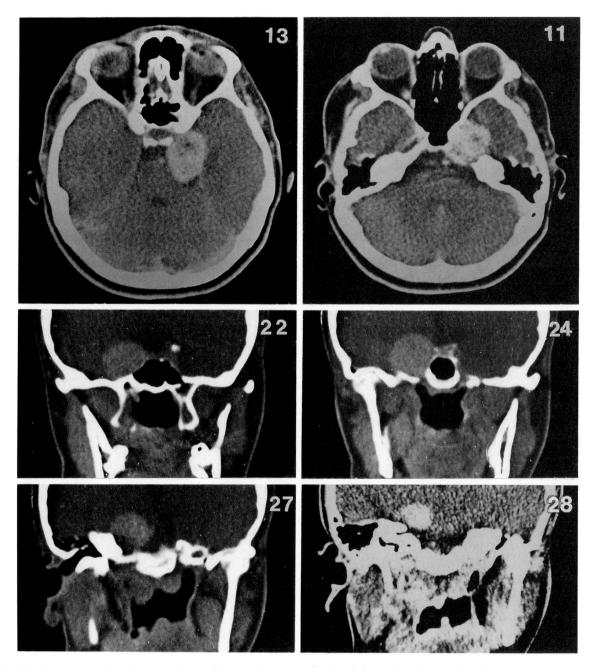

Figure 24.18.   Head scans in axial and coronal planes disclose a homogeneously enhancing schwannoma originating at the left Gasserian ganglion. The major portion of the schwannoma is in the middle cranial fossa. It extends in an hourglass configuration across the eroded left petrous apex *(cut 11)* into the posterior cranial fossa to the level of the internal auditory canal *(cut 28)*. (Courtesy of Dr. Donlin Long.)

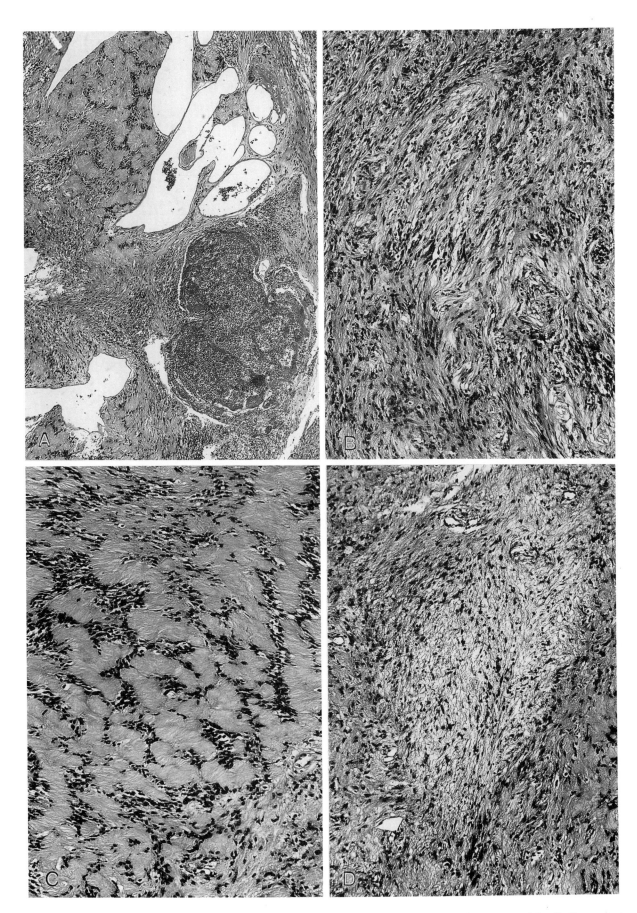

Figure 24.19.   A. The vessel in the lower right of the field contains a recently formed thrombus. Above it is a conglomerate of cysts, to the left of which is an area of marked palisading of cell nuclei. **B.** Antoni type A tissue. **C.** Orderly grouping of cells, creating an organoid pattern. The nu-clei are arranged in palisades separated by fibrillary cytoplasmic processes. **D.** Antoni type B tissue in center, surrounded by type A tissue. (Hematoxylin and eosin, ×60, ×150, ×150, and ×125.)

References

1. Dixon J. Tumor of Gasserian ganglion. Med Clin Trans Lond 1846;29:131.

2. Marchand F. Beitrag zur Kenntnis der Geschwülste des Ganglion Gasseri. In: Festschrift für G.E. v. Rindfleisch. Leipzig: 1907:265–290.

3. Sacks E. Tumors of the Gasserian ganglion. Ann Surg 1917;66:152–159.

4. Smith RW. A treatise on the pathological diagnosis and treatment of neuroma [Thesis]. Dublin: Royal College of Surgeons, 1849.

5. Altmann F. Zur Kenntnis der primären Geschwülste des Trigeminus und des Ganglion Gasseri. Beitr Pathol Anat Allg Pathol 1928;80:261–403.

6. Novotny K, Uiberall H. Zur Kenntnis der Neurinome des Trigeminus. Z Gesamte Neurol Psychiatrie 1934;150:75–99.

7. Gaal A. Zur Röntgendiagnose des Neurinoma trigemini. Rontgenpraxis 1935;7:546–550.

8. Krayenbühl H. Primary tumors of the root of the fifth cranial nerve: their distinction from tumors of the Gasserian ganglion. Brain 1936;59:337–352.

9. Krayenbühl H. Das Neurinom des Nervus trigeminus. Schweiz Akad Med Wissensch 1959;15:89–106.

10. Lindgren E. Das Röntgenbild bei Tumoren des Ganglion Gasseri. Acta Clin Scand 1941;85:181–194.

11. Jefferson G. Trigeminal neurinomas with some remarks on malignant invasion of the gasserian ganglion. Proc Congr Neurol Surg 1955;1:11–54.

12. Loew F, Tönnis W. Klinik und Behandlung der Neurinome des Nervus trigeminus. Zentralbl Neurochir 1954; Hl/2:32–41.

13. Olive I, Svien HJ. Neurofibromas of the fifth cranial nerve. J Neurosurg 1957;14:484–505.

14. Schisano G, Olivercrona H. Neurinomas of the Gasserian ganglion and trigeminal root. J Neurosurg 1960;17:306–322.

15. Dieckmann H. Zur Klinik und Diagnostik der trigeminus Neurinome. Nervenarzt 1959;30:357–362.

16. Morniroli G. Das trigeminus Neurinom. Schweiz Arch Neurol Neurochir Psychiatrie 1970;107:47–86.

17. Mello LR, Tanzer A. Some aspects of trigeminal neurionomas. Neuroradiology 1972;4:215–221.

18. de Benedittis G, Bernasconi V, Ettore G. Tumors of the fifth cranial nerve. Acta Neurochir 1977;38:37–64.

19. Glasauer FE, Tandon PN. Trigeminal neurinomas in adolescents. J Neurol Neurosurg Psychiatry 1969;32:562–568.

20. Amirchanjan SE, Lebedev AN. Röntgendiagnostik der trigeminus Neurinome. Radiol Diagn 1979;20:78–85.

21. Tarlov IM. Structure of the nerve root: I. Nature of the junction between the central and the peripheral nervous system. Arch Neurol 1937;37:555–583.

22. Rubinstein LJL. Tumors of the central nervous system. In: Atlas of tumor pathology. 2nd series, Fascicle 6. Washington, DC: Armed Forces Institute of Pathology, 1972.

23. Cohen J. Tumors involving the Gasserian ganglion. J Nerv Ment Dis 1933;78:492–499.

24. Montaut J. Les neurinomes du Trijumeau [Thèse]. University of Nancy, 1962; cited in Ref 25.

25. Paillas JE, Grisoli F, Farnarier P. Neurinomes du trijumeau: a propos de 8 cas. Neurochirurgie 1973;20:41–54.

26. Zülch KJ. Brain tumors: their biology and pathology. 2nd American ed. New York: Springer Verlag, 1957.

27. Cushing H, Eisenhardt L. Meningiomas: their classification, regional behavior, life history and surgical end results. Springfield, Illinois: Charles C Thomas, 1938.

28. Henschen F. Tumoren der Hirneven III–XII. In: Handbuch der speziellen pathologischen Anatomie und Histologie. Berlin: Springer Verlag, 1955:13(3).

29. Bormal J, Pellegrin J. Volumineux neurinome du trijumeau gauche en sablier occupant les fosses moyenne et posterieure, guérison operatoire. Neurochirurgie 1957;32:112–122.

30. Noyek AM, Kassell EE, Wortzman G, et al. Clinically directed CT in occult-disease of the skull base involving foramen ovale. Laryngoscope 1982;92:1021–1027.

31. Hellsten ML. Ein Fall von Ganglion Gasseri Tumor. Nervenheilkunde 1914;53:290–305.

31. Gjertz E, Hellerstrom S. Tumeur du Ganglion de Gasser. Acta Med Scand 1925;63:7–23.

33. Nager GT. Acoustic neurionomas: pathology and differential diagnosis. Arch Otolaryngol 1969;89:68–95.

34. Palacios E, MacGee EE. The radiographic diagnosis of trigeminal neurinomas. J. Neurosurg 1972;36:153–156.

35. Moscow NP, Newton TA. Angiographic features of hypervascular neurinomas of the head and neck. Radiology 1975;114:635–640.

36. Wullenweber R, Traupe H, Scharz G. Angiographic demonstration of a trigeminal neurinoma. Neuroradiology 1976;10:225–229.

37. Naidich TP, et al. Computed tomography in the diagnosis of extra-axial posterior fossa masses. Radiology 1976;120:333–339.

38. Leventhal R, Bentson JR. Detection of small trigeminal neurinomas. J Neurosurg 1976;45:568–575.

39. Goldberg R, Byrd S, Winter J, et al. Varied appearance of trigeminal neuromas on CT. Am J Radiol 1980;134:57–60.

40. Delenge D, Heon M. The internal carotid artery. In: Newton TH, Potts DG, eds. Radiology of the skull and brain. St. Louis: CV Mosby, Book 2, Chap 2, 1974;2:1221–1224.

41. Takahashi M. The anterior inferior cerebellar artery. In: Newton TH, Potts DG, eds. Radiology of the skull and brain. St Louis: CV Mosby, Book 2, Chap 70, 1974;2:1806.

42. Knudson V, Kolze V. Neurinoma of the gasserian ganglion and the trigeminal root: report of four cases. Acta Neurochir 1972; 26:159–164.

43. Westberg G. Angiographic changes in neurinoma of the trigeminal nerve. Acta Radiol (Diagn) 1963;1:513–520.

44. Yamashita J, Asato R, Handa H, et al. Abducens nerve palsy as initial symptom of trigeminal neurinoma. J Neurol Neurosurg Psychiatry 1977;40:1190–1197.

45. Gordy PD. Neurinoma of the Gasserian ganglion: report of a case and review of the literature. J Neurosurg 1965;22:90–94.

46. Harkin JC, Reed RJ. Tumors of the peripheral nervous system. In: Atlas of tumor pathology. 2nd series, Fascicle 3. Washington, DC: Armed Forces Institute of Pathology, 1969.

47. Nager GT. Meningiomas involving the temporal bone: clinical and pathological aspects. Springfield, Illinois: Charles C Thomas, 1964.

48. Nager GT. Association of bilateral eighth nerve tumors with meningiomas in von Recklinghausen's disease. Laryngoscope 1964;74:1120–1264.

49. Nager GT, Heroy J. Hoeplinger M. Meningiomas invading the temporal bone with extension to the neck. Am J Otolaryngol 1983;4:297–324.

50. Alexander WS. Central neurofibromatosis: report of a case presenting as trigeminal neuralgia. N Z Med J 1947;46:264–272.

51. Arena S, Hilal EY. Neurilemmomas of the infratemporal space. Arch Otolaryngol 1976;102:180–184.

52. Vaquero J, Cabezudo JM, Leunda G, et al. Simultaneous posterior and middle cranial fossa neurinomas. Acta Neurochir 1981;55:321–327.

53. Gardner WJ, Turner O. Bilateral acoustic neurofibromas: further clinical and pathological data on hereditary deafness and Recklinghausen's disease. Arch Neurol 1940;44:76–99.

54. Cueno HM, Rand CW. Tumors of the Gasserian ganglion: tumor of the left Gasserian ganglion associated with enlargement of the mandibular nerve. J Neurosurg 1952;9:423–431.

55. Hedeman LS, Levinsky BS, Lockridge GK, et al. Primary malignant schwannoma of the Gasserian ganglion. J Neurosurg 1978;48:279–283.

56. Karmody CS. Malignant schwannoma of the trigeminal nerve. Otolaryngol Head Neck Surg 1979;87:594–598.

57. Eversole LR. Central benign and malignant neural neoplasms of the jaws: a review. J Oral Surg 1969;27:716–721.

58. David DJ, Speculand B, Vernon-Roberts B, et al. Malignant schwannoma of the inferior dental nerve. Br J Plast Surg 1978;31:323–333.

59. Katz AD, Passy V, Kaplan L. Neurogenous neoplasms of major nerves of the face and neck. Arch Surg 1971;103:51–56.

60. Grinberg FG, Levy NS. Malignant neurilemmoma of the supraorbital nerve. Am J Ophthalmol 1974; 78:489–492.

61. Liwnicz BH. Bilateral trigeminal neurofibrosarcoma. J Neurosurg 1979;50:253–256.

62. Laxorthes G, Espagno J, Arbus L. Tumeurs du trijumeau. Encycl Med Chir Systeme Nerv 1966;10:9, 1736A.

63. Nager GT. Epidermoids involving the temporal bone. In: English GM, ed. Otolaryngology. Philadelphia: Harper & Row, Chap 43, 1981;1:1–18.

64. Maspes PE. Tumori del ganglio di Gaser: due casi di emangioma. Minerva Neurochir 1957;1:1–4.

65. Papo I, Salvolini, V, Vecchi A. Tumeur vasculaire du cavum de Meckel. Neurochirurgie 1972;4:271–381.

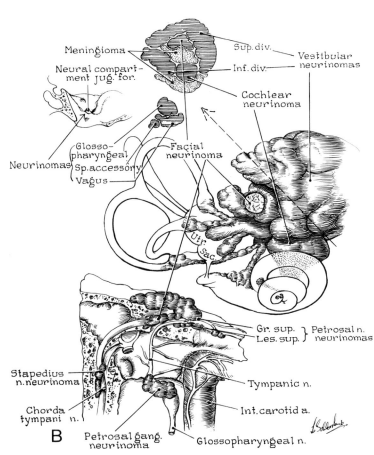

Figure 25.5. Illustrations to show the gross relations, sites, and extent of schwannomas involving the right and left seventh to eleventh cranial nerves and their branches in a 22-year-old man with the central form of von Recklinghausen's neurofibromatosis (NF2).

RADIOLOGIC MANIFESTATIONS

Intratemporal schwannomas are best visualized radiographically in axial and coronal computed tomography scans (CT) and by magnetic resonance imaging (MRI) (Figs. 25.10 and 25.11). Pneumatization, as a rule, is normal. The initially smooth enlargement of the descending portion of the Fallopian canal, the subsequent erosion of the perifacial cells, and the destruction of the posteroinferior bony canal wall and posterior floor of the hypotympanum are the salient features (6). Malignant transformation and recurrences of facial schwannomas after total resection are rare (13).

A progressive facial paresis, especially when preceded or accompanied by hemifacial spasms, must arouse suspicion of a facial schwannoma, although an epidermoid or cholesterol granuloma can present identical features. As an acoustic tumor can occasionally manifest itself with a sudden loss of hearing, so a facial tumor can present as a sudden paresis or paralysis. On the other hand, at least 50% of facial schwannomas show no evidence of facial nerve dysfunction (29–34).

High-resolution CT and MRI with gadolinium contrast enhancement are the diagnostic procedures of choice in identifying the lesion, determining its local behavior, and selecting the surgical approach. After resection of the tumor, the continuity of the nerve is restored either by rerouting of the nerve or by interposition of a cable graft generally procured from the greater auricular nerve.

Case Report

Case 1. *Solitary neurofibroma involving distal one-third of tympanic segment and entire mastoid segment of left facial nerve.*

An 8-year-old girl with a 2-year history of slowly progressive left-sided facial paresis with initial involvment of the lower nerve branches was seen. No history of ear disease or impairment of hearing and equilibrium was given.

Neuro-otologic examination revealed a left lower facial paresis involving the buccal, orbicularis oris, and lower orbicularis oculi muscles, but normal frontalis muscle function and impairment of taste over the left anterior portion of the tongue. Cochlear function studies disclosed a normal audiogram, acoustic reflexes, and acoustic brain stem responses. There was no nystagmus, and gait and the Romberg test were normal. The other cranial nerves and the rest of the neurologic examination including motor, sensory, and cerebellar testing were essentially normal. There were no café au lait spots or a family history of von Recklinghausen's disease.

On *radiologic examination,* serial axial and coronal CT scans of the temporal bones showed a longitudinal enlargement of the distal tympanic and entire mastoid segment of the left Fallopian canal measuring about 5 mm in diameter (Fig. 25.6).

At *operation,* the left facial nerve was exposed in its tympanic and mastoid portions following an intact canal mastoidectomy with a facial recess exposure. An oblong tumor was found that occupied the distal one-third of the tympanic portion and the entire mastoid portion of the facial nerve. The original nerve could not be identified within the tumor and separated from it. The nerve was resected from the midtympanic segment to the stylomastoid foramen and reconstructed with a graft. Histologically, the tumor proved to be a neurofibroma (Fig. 25.7).

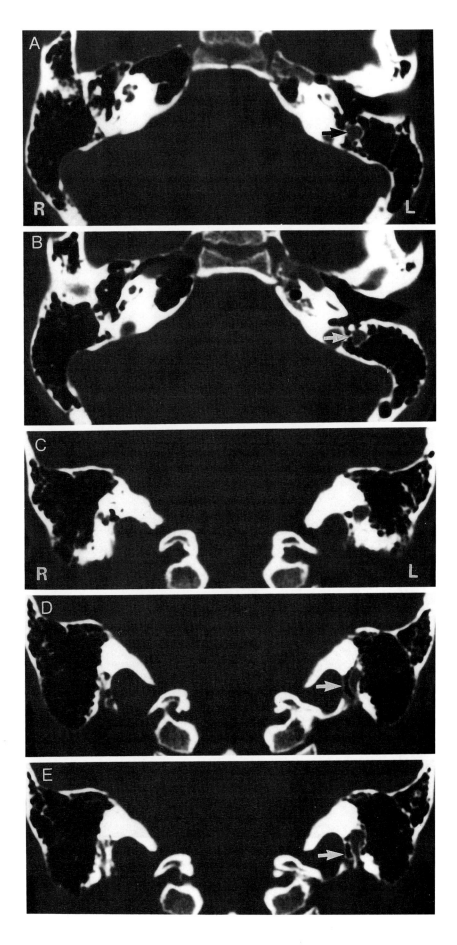

Figure 25.6. Serial axial **(A** and **B)** and coronal **(C–E)** CT scans of both temporal bones. The neurofibroma that originated in the mastoid segment of the left facial nerve has created an even, spindle-shaped enlargement of the Fallopian canal to about 4 times its normal diameter *(arrows).* (Courtesy of Dr. D. Mattox.)

26/ Glossopharyngeal, Vagus, Spinal Accessory, and Hypoglossal Schwannomas

Solitary intracranial schwannomas may originate in any cranial nerve, except for the olfactory and optic nerves, and in any location where the parent nerve possesses a Schwann cell sheath. The sensory nerves tend to be selectively affected. Most of these schwannomas arise in the acoustic nerve, with most, but not all, developing in the superior and the inferior division of the vestibular nerve. They account for about 96% of all intracranial schwannomas and for about 7–10% of all intracranial neoplasms. Trigeminal schwannomas are less frequent. They represent about 2–3% of all intracranial schwannomas and about 0.2% of all intracranial tumors. About 200 cases have so far been reported. Schwannomas of the facial nerve are even less frequent; some 100–150 cases are recorded in the literature. Solitary schwannomas originating in the remaining cranial nerves (III, IV, VI, and IX–XII), in the absence of von Recklinghausen's neurofibromatosis-2 (NF2), are even more exceptional. Up to now about 60 instances of sporadic schwannomas involving the jugular foramen, arising presumably from the glossopharyngeal, vagus, or accessory nerves, have been published (1). These lesions assume a dumbbell configuration with an intracranial component and, often, a much larger extracranial component. They characteristically produce an even or "benign" enlargement of the jugular foramen. Similarly, a hypoglossal schwannoma is recognized by the widening of the hypoglossal canal. A schwannoma arising in the extracranial segment of these nerves is generally accompanied by corresponding clinical manifestations. A glossopharyngeal tumor may be associated with dysgeusia, and a vagal tumor may be associated with paralysis of the soft palate and vocal cord, hoarseness, and dysphagia. A spinal accessory tumor is accompanied by a shoulder drop, and a hypoglossal tumor is accompanied by ipsilateral fasciculation and atrophy of the tongue. The majority of schwannomas in the neck arise in the sympathetic trunk and manifest themselves with a Horner's syndrome.

Solitary glossopharyngeal schwannomas are exceptionally rare. A recent review of 35 cerebellopontine angle tumors observed during a period of 16 months included 26 acoustic neurinomas, 6 meningiomas, and 2 epidermoids, with only 1 glossopharyngeal schwannoma (2). Their early manifestations are rather discrete. As they originate in the neural compartment of the jugular foramen and extend into the posterior cranial fossa, their symptoms and signs are very similar to the ones of acoustic schwannomas (3).

Solitary vagus schwannomas are also uncommon. In a recent survey of 36 vagal tumors, paragangliomas accounted for 50%; schwannomas, for 31%; neurofibromas, for 14%; and neurofibrosarcomas, for 5% (4). The majority were localized in the upper cervical or parapharyngeal region. Most were detected incidentally. Some extended to the skull base and into the posterior cranial fossa. Another location for these tumors was the thoracic region, where most (16 of 19) were identified as schwannomas, and 3 of 19 were identified as neurofibromas. Over 50% were located in the left upper mediastinum (6).

In neurofibromatosis-2 (NF2), formerly known as the central form of neurofibromatosis, any of the cranial nerves may become involved in solitary or multiple schwannomas and neurofibromas, unilaterally and bilaterally. Bilateral acoustic schwannomas are a pathognomonic feature and occasionally the sole manifestation. Although schwannomas and neurofibromas in all likelihood share a common cell of origin, their recognition is clinically important; it is especially important to recognize whether a neurofibroma represents a solitary lesion or a manifestation of NF2. The location of the tumor, its association with other lesions involving the central nervous system, and the family history, in addition to or in the absence of the microscopic examination, provide valuable information. In a rare instance a tumor may display features of a schwannoma and a neurofibroma. For such a lesion the term "solitary benign nerve sheath tumor" may be most appropriate (7).

For the neuro-otologist, schwannomas of the jugular foramen are of particular interest, since they represent one of the, although exceedingly rare, lesions in the cerebellopontine angle.

Case Reports

Cases 1–3 illustrate the clinical, radiologic, and pathologic aspects of these types of schwannomas.

Case 1. *Large schwannoma originating from right ninth and tenth cranial nerves. Marked enlargement of right jugular foramen. Extension into right lower cerebellopontine angle with compression and displacement of brain stem. Paresis of right cranial nerves VII–X. History of three suboccipital craniectomies for removal of initial, residual, and recurrent tumor. Postoperative right transtemporal exploration of right jugular foramen with complete removal of residual schwannoma.*

A 29-year-old man who at age 19 presented with a several month history of right suboccipital headaches, repeated episodes of blurred vision, disequilibrium, and bilateral papilledema was seen.

Neurologic examination on admission revealed a paresis of the right cranial nerves VII, IX, and X. There was evidence of retrocochlear involvement of the right cochlear nerve, reflected by normal hearing for pure tones but impairment of discrimination and absence of the stapedial reflex. There was diminished response to caloric stimulation of the right labyrinth, right cerebellar ataxia, and bilateral papilledema. The computed tomography (CT) scan showed an enlargement of the right jugular foramen, associated with a large enhancing tumor occupying the lower portion of the right cerebellopontine angle. It extended laterally into the jugular foramen and medially into the foramen magnum and across the midline (Figs. 26.1 and 26.2). The patient underwent initially a two-stage suboccipital craniectomy with subtotal removal of schwannoma of the right ninth and tenth cranial nerves. This was followed 4 years later by a

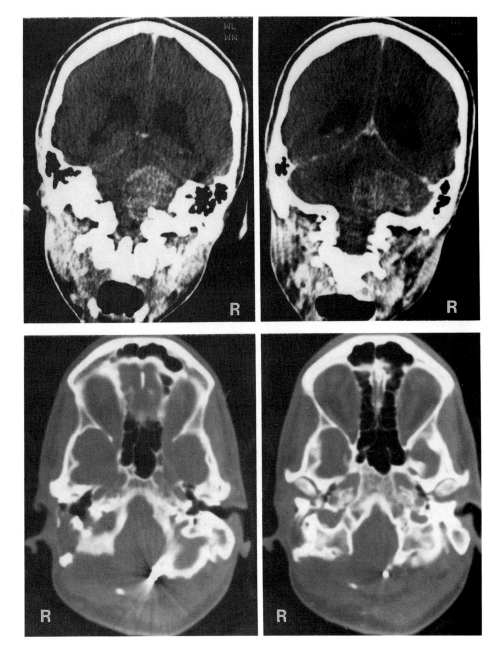

Figure 26.1. Cranial contrast CT scans show an enhancing mass in the right cerebellopontine angle, compressing the anterior medial portion of the cerebellar hemisphere. The mass displaces the fourth ventricle to the opposite side and is associated with a moderate hydrocephalus.

Figure 26.2. Axial noncontrast CT scans of the skull, taken 5 years after three right suboccipital craniotomies and a right transtemporal exploration of the jugular foramen, demonstrate marked enlargement of the jugular foramen.

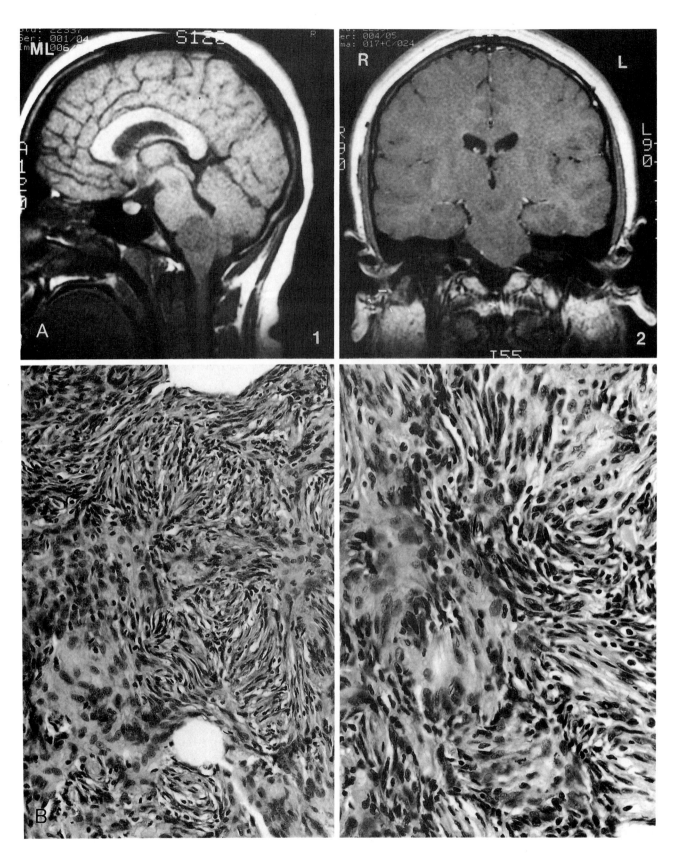

Figure 26.8. **A.** Sagittal *(1)* and coronal *(2)* enhanced MRI of the same patient as in Figure 26.7. The schwannoma in the right cerebellopontine angle, while distorting and displacing the brain stem, does not extend into or widen the right internal auditory canal *(2)*. **B.** The tumor shows the characteristics of a schwannoma consisting predominantly of the type A tissue of Antoni. (Hematoxylin and eosin, ×180 and ×400, respectively.)

References

1. Ho KL. Schwannoma of the trochlear nerve. J Neurosurg 1981;55:132.
2. Kelly DL Jr, Britten BH, Branch CLJ. Cooperative neuro-otologic management of acoustic neuromas and other cerebellopontine angle tumors. South Med J 1988;81:557–61.
3. Anderson T, Ulsoe C, Overgaard J, Ringsted J. Intracranial glossopharyngeal schwannoma, a tumor imitating an acoustic schwannoma. J Laryngol Otol 1986;100:831–835.
4. Green JD, Olsen KD, DeSanto LW, Scheithauer BW. Neoplasms of the vagus nerve. Laryngoscope 1988;98:648–654.
5. Shirakusa T, Tsutsui M, Montonaga R, Takota S, et al. Intrathoracic tumors arising from the vagus nerve. Review of resected tumors in Japan. Scand J Thorac Cardiovasc Surg 1989;23:173–175.
6. Besznyak I, Toth L, Szende B. Intrathoracic vagus nerve tumors: a report of two cases and review of the literature. J Thorac Cardiovasc Surg 1985;83:462–465.
7. Harkin JC, Reed RJ. Tumors of the peripheral nervous system. In: Atlas of tumor pathology. 2nd series, Fascicle 3. Washington, DC: Armed Forces Institutes of Pathology, 1968.

27 Meningiomas

GENERAL INFORMATION

Definition and Origin

Meningiomas are hamartomatous, not truly neoplastic, tumors that arise from cell elements forming the meninges and their derivatives in the meningeal spaces. They may originate from dural fibroblasts and pial cells, although the majority develop from the arachnoid cells that constitute the core of the arachnoid villi (1). Arachnoid villi are finger-like projections of arachnoid mesothelium that protrude through the walls into the lumen of the dural veins and sinuses. The lumen is continuous with the subarachnoid space and contains a spongy network of arachnoid cells. The arachnoid villi, in all likelihood, provide the main pathway for the drainage of the cerebrospinal fluid into the venous circulation. Arachnoid villi may also protrude through the dura lining the base of the skull and the inner table of the calvaria, where they cause localized bone resorption recognized as foveolae granulares.

Location and Incidence

The preferential sites of meningiomas correspond closely to the locations where arachnoid villi are most frequently found, namely, along the major venous sinuses and their contributory veins, at the foramina of exit of the cranial nerves, and at the exits of the spinal nerve routes from their meningeal sleeves. In addition to arachnoid villi, meningiomas may arise from arachnoid cells anywhere along the arachnoid membrane. Within the cerebral hemispheres, meningiomas may originate from stroma cells within the spaces surrounding the perforating blood vessels. The intraventricular meningiomas arise from meningeal cells in the intracerebral infoldings of the leptomeninges that form the vela interposita and the stroma of the choroid plexus (Fig. 27.1) (1).

Meningiomas account for about 16.6–18% of all primary intracranial tumors (1, 2). The majority are found in the cerebral chamber; only 8–9% are situated in the cerebellar chamber. In the posterior fossa, the cerebellopontine angle is the most common location, and the posterior surface of the petrous pyramid is the most frequent site of dural attachment (3, 4). Two-thirds of the posterior fossa meningiomas arise at the porus acusticus or medial to it, near the superior petrosal sinus. Of all intracranial meningiomas, about 6–7% arise from the posterior or anterior surface of the petrous bone (3).

Meningiomas can also originate within the temporal bone. The four locations within the petrous pyramid in which they originate are: (a) the internal acoustic meatus, (b) the jugular foramen, (c) the region of the geniculate ganglion, and (d) the sulcus of the greater and lesser superficial petrosal nerves (Fig. 27.2) (3, 4). In all these locations, arachnoid cells and granulations are regularly found. Thus, the temporal bone may become involved by meningiomas arising not only in adjacent structures and on the outer surface of the petrous bone but also within the petrous pyramid.

Age and Sex Distribution

Meningiomas occur at any age, although most are diagnosed in patients between 20 and 60 years old, with a peak incidence occurring between 45 and 55 years of age. Intracranial meningiomas affect women more frequently than men, by a ratio of about 2:1. Small, asymptomatic meningiomas are a frequent incidental observation during postmortem examination of elderly persons; they show no particular sex preference (Case 2, Fig. 27.9) (1).

Macroscopic Appearance

Macroscopically, meningiomas have a fairly characteristic appearance. The majority are well circumscribed, globular ("en-globe" of Cushing (5)), ovoid or lobulated, usually with a smooth surface, varying in size and shape, and clearly demarcated from the brain. On cut surface they appear gray or pink, with a fairly homogeneous dense tissue, an indistinct lobular pattern, and a very firm consistency (Cases 1, 3–5, and 8; Figs. 27.12, 27.22, 27.23, and 27.37). A well-recognized variant of this usual gross appearance is the more diffuse, flat type ("en-plaque" of Cushing) (5)). These lesions are not greatly raised above the level of the convexity of the brain or the dura of the base of the skull (Cases 6–8; Figs. 27.23, 27.25, 27.26, 27.32, 27.37, 27.40, and 27.41). Cranial nerves and blood vessels at the base can be surrounded by the tumor's carpet-like outgrowth. These tumors are notably prone to invade the underlying bone. Involvement of the bone, however, is by no means limited to the en plaque meningioma. In fact, most lesions reported to have caused extensive destruction of the temporal bone have been of the en globe variety (3). The simultaneous occurrence of a globular and flat meningioma may also be observed (Case 8, Fig. 27.37). Meningiomas that come in contact with the skull may produce local overgrowth of bone, either of the calvaria or of the base (Figs. 27.11A and B, 27.25, 27.26, 27.28, and 27.35A). Such new bone formation may be minimal or so extensive that the contours of the head may be altered. The hyperostosis is due to the extensive new bone formation that frequently is but may not necessarily be associated with invasion of the marrow spaces by the meningioma cells.

Microscopic Appearance

The microscopic appearance of meningiomas varies greatly. On the basis of their morphologic patterns, meningiomas may be divided into the following subgroups: (a) meningotheliomatous

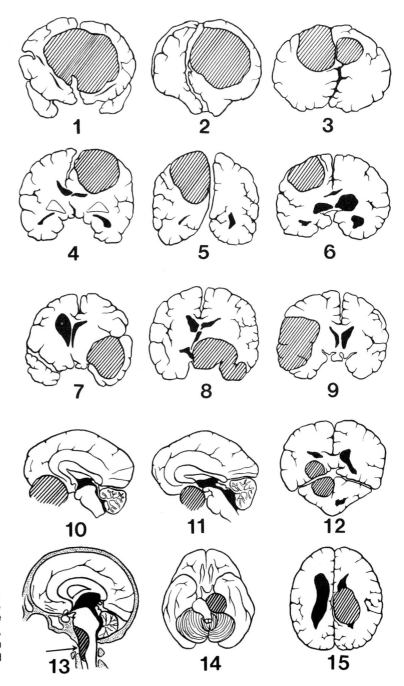

Figure 27.1. Preferential locations of intracranial meningiomas: *1,* falx, bilateral; *2,* falx, unilateral; *3,* anterior third of the sagittal sinus, bilateral; *4,* middle third of the sagittal sinus; *5,* posterior third of the sagittal sinus; *6,* convexity; *7,* sphenoid, "en-globe"; *8,* sphenoid, "en-plaque"; *9,* Sylvian fissure; *10,* olfactory groove; *11,* tuberculum sellae; *12,* tentorium; *13,* clivus (craniospinal); *14,* petrous pyramid (cerebellopontine angle); and *15,* lateral ventricle.

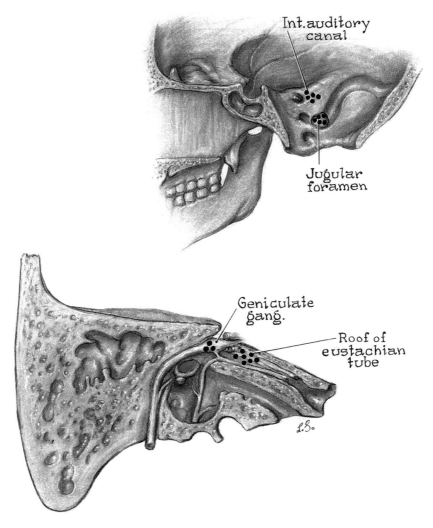

Figure 27.2. Schematic representation of four sites of origin for meningiomas within temporal bone. These areas are: (*a*) within the internal acoustic meatus, (*b*) within the jugular foramen, (*c*) the region of the geniculate ganglion, and (*d*) the sulcus of the greater and lesser superficial petrosal nerves.

(endotheliomatous), *(b)* fibrous (fibroblastic), *(c)* transitional, *(d)* psammomatous, *(e)* angiomatous, *(f)* papillary, and *(g)* "anaplastic" (malignant dedifferentiated) meningiomas (1, 2). The fundamental cell of origin for all subgroups is the meningothelial arachnoid cell. The morphologic variation of the subgroups simply reflects the adaptive potential of the normal arachnoid cell. As a result, different areas within the same tumor may frequently exhibit two or more of the subgroups as well as the transitional forms (1). The various subgroups have no prognostic significance. All of them have the propensity to invade the temporal bone, but the meningotheliomatous subgroup accounts for most of these tumors.

In the meningotheliomatous meningioma, the cell masses are arranged into islands, strands, nests, and other cell complexes, divided by only a small amount of connective tissue (Figs. 27.3B, 27.8B–D, 27.9B, 27.11C–D, 27.14C, 27.19, and 27.40). The similarity to the clusters of normal arachnoidal endothelium is their significant characteristic. The tumor cells frequently form a syncytium (Fig. 27.6B). They have an ill-defined cell membrane and delicate round or oval nuclei with a thin nuclear membrane, with a pale nucleoplasm, and often with one or two small conspicuous nucleoli. The cell nests often display a typical whorl formation in which the cells are wrapped around one another closely, suggesting the appearance of a transversely cut onion or of rings in which psammoma bodies develop (Figs. 27.8B, 27.14C, and 27.40B). Some areas of meningotheliomatous meningiomas frequently fade inconspicuously into the next histologic subgroup (1).

The fibrous meningioma consists of long spindle-shaped cells arranged in streams and whorls. These interlacing bundles and loop-shaped formations of tumor cells are arranged around capillaries. Their distinctive features are the rich development of reticular and stout collagen fibers between the individual cells. Psammoma bodies do occur but are more often shaped like spears or clubs.

The transitional meningioma represents an intermediate form between the meningotheliomatous or syncytial and the fibrous or fibroblastic subgroups. Their salient feature is their cellular arrangement in the form of concentric whorls. The tumor cells are elongated and crescent-shaped, occasionally surrounding a capillary blood vessel. Hyalin degeneration and secondary calcification of degenerating tumor cells in the center of the whorls result in the formation of psammoma bodies. The tumors in which these psammoma bodies are especially numerous and predominate are sometimes recognized as a separate histologic subgroup and referred to as psammomatous meningiomas or psammomas.

The angiomatous meningioma is the least common of the subgroups. It is characterized by the large number of blood vessels and by its highly cellular content. The blood vessels may be dilated or, more frequently, compressed or partially occluded by the rather plump endothelial cells. The tumor cells have an ill-defined cytoplasm with densely packed distinct ovoid nuclei. The characteristic feature is the abundance of reticular fibers forming the vessel walls and branching between the adjacent stroma cells (1).

The papillary meningioma is a tumor in which the papillary cell pattern prevails.

The "anaplastic" or malignant meningioma is extremely rare. Its growth is accelerated, and the destruction of adjacent structures is more extensive than that from nonmalignant meningioma. The tumor is more cellular and vascular, the architecture is disorganized, and mitotic figures may be observed. It represents a transition to the fibrosarcoma and may eventually metastasize in distant organs (1).

Very rarely, regressive processes, i.e., fatty, mucoid, or cystic degeneration and the formation of cartilaginous or bony tissue, may be found in a meningioma (Fig. 27.11C). A well-known feature of the intracranial meningioma is that it frequently invades the dural venous sinuses but so rarely results in dissemination.

MENINGIOMAS INVOLVING THE TEMPORAL BONE

The temporal bone may become involved by meningiomas arising in its vicinity, on its outer surface, or within the petrous pyramid (3, 4). Meningiomas in the vicinity of the temporal bone may originate from the sphenoid ridge, the parasellar region, the tentorium, the clivus, the convexity of the cerebellum, and the cerebellopontine angle. Meningiomas on the outer surface of the temporal bone may arise from the floor of the middle cranial fossa and the Gasserian envelopes or from the posterior aspect of the pyramid along the transverse, lateral, superior, and inferior petrosal sinuses and at the porus of the internal acoustic meatus. The petrous pyramid may also be involved by meningiomas originating within its own confines in the four locations mentioned earlier (3).

Development of meningiomas involving the temporal bones shows a clear predilection for the middle and later decades of life. Women are more frequently affected than men, by a ratio of about 2:1.

Extension of the Meningioma within the Temporal Bone

Extension of the meningioma within the temporal bone does not occur randomly and precipitously; rather, it is a slow process that follows a regular pattern. A meningioma with origin in the dura of the floor of the middle cranial fossa, invading the tegmen, gradually protrudes with finger-like projections into neighboring spaces. Invasion of adjacent marrow spaces occurs along preformed spaces, hiatus, and vascular channels. The vascular channels are the nutrient vessels of the bone, the central blood vessels of the Haversian system, and the perforating canals of Volkmann. Gradually, more marrow spaces are invaded until occasionally the tumor has spread throughout the temporal bone (Figs. 27.14, 27.17, and 27.38–27.40).

Within invasion begins resorption of bone (Figs. 27.4, 27.5, 27.7, and 27.20). Initially, a loose connective tissue is found in a marrow space between the ingrowing tumor and the bone. As the tumor expands, the meningioma cells come in direct apposition to the osseous tissue with their long axes arranged parallel to the surface of the bone. The adjacent osseous tissue is gradually being resorbed in the form of irregular shallow pits. The marrow space thus enlarges, and the bony wall or the partition that may separate it from an adjacent marrow space becomes thinner and may gradually disappear. This mechanism of resorption whereby bone appears to "melt away" under the influence of expanding tumor tissue is prevailing. Areas of typical lacunar erosion with osteoclastic giant cells in Howship's lacunae are a significant exception.

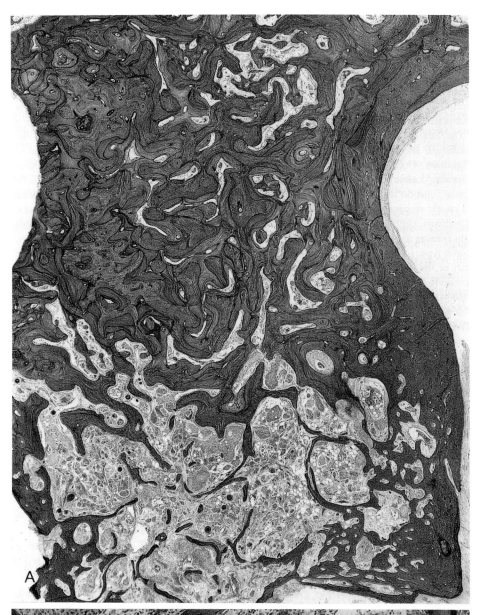

Figure 27.3. A. Vertical section through anterior portion of right petrous pyramid, showing widespread infiltration of marrow spaces in apical and infralabyrinthine areas by meningioma. (Hematoxylin and eosin, ×10.)

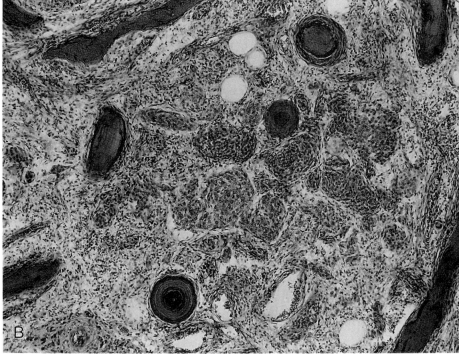

Figure 27.3. B. The meningioma is of the meningotheliomatous subgroup. Islands of solid masses of tumor cells are surrounded by numerous blood vessels and psammoma bodies. (×10.)

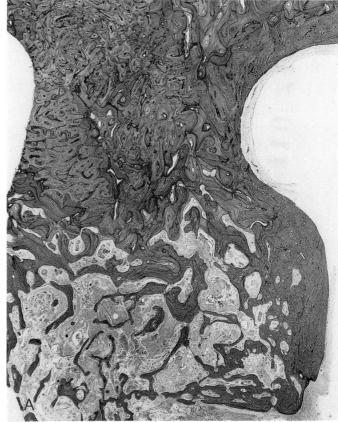

Figure 27.4. **A.** Vertical section through anterior portion of right petrous pyramid, illustrating resorption of bony partition between adjacent marrow spaces. **B.** The invasion of bone occurs along the nutrient vessels of the bone. **C.** The meningioma cells appear to act as osteoclasts without noticeably changing their morphologic appearance. The adjacent osseous tissue is gradually being resorbed in the form of irregular shallow pits. (Hematoxylin and eosin, ×10, ×100, and ×400, respectively.)

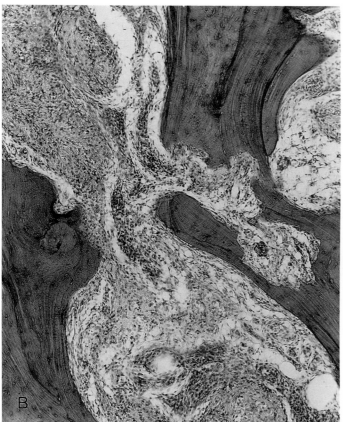

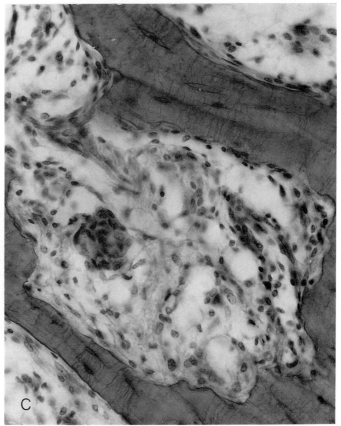

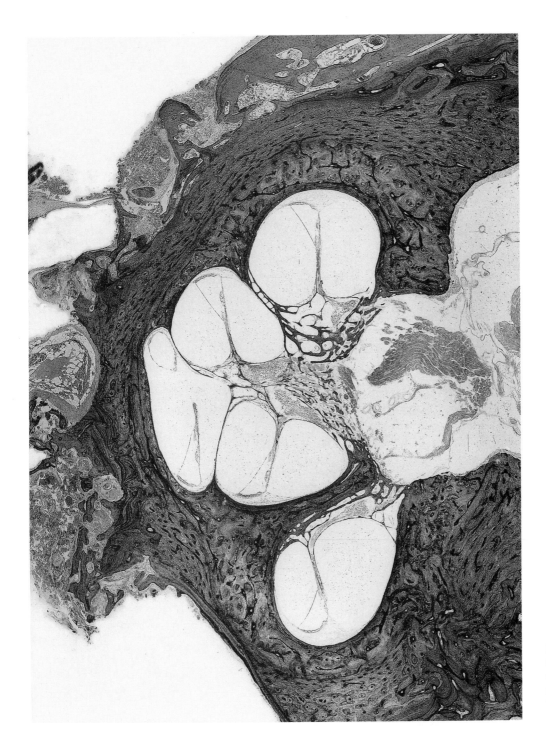

Figure 27.5. Vertical midmodiolar section of right cochlea. The erosion of the cochlear capsule occurs from adjacent marrow spaces, along the Haversian and the perforating canals of Volkmann. (Hematoxylin and eosin, ×10.)

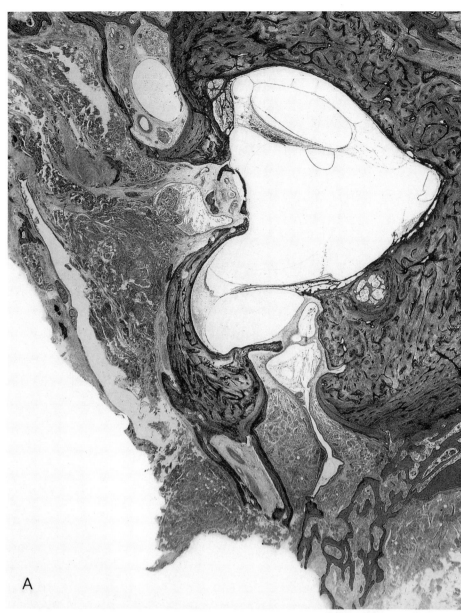

Figure 27.6. A. Vertical section through right petrous pyramid at level of oval and round windows. Expansion of the meningioma within the tympanic cavity is predominantly along the submucosal plane. Despite the massive tumor infiltration of the mucoperiosteum, the overlying mucosa often remains intact, as seen in the niche to the round window. (Hematoxylin and eosin, ×10.)

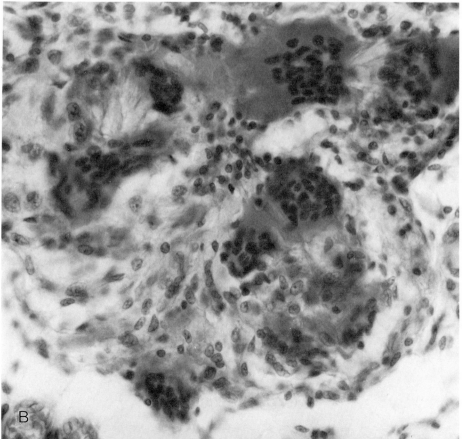

Figure 27.6. B. In some syncytial tumor cell complexes, shown here in a peripheral marrow space, the cell nuclei tend to congregate and cluster in one area. These formations resembling "multinucleated giant cells" are the precursors of psammoma bodies. (×400.)

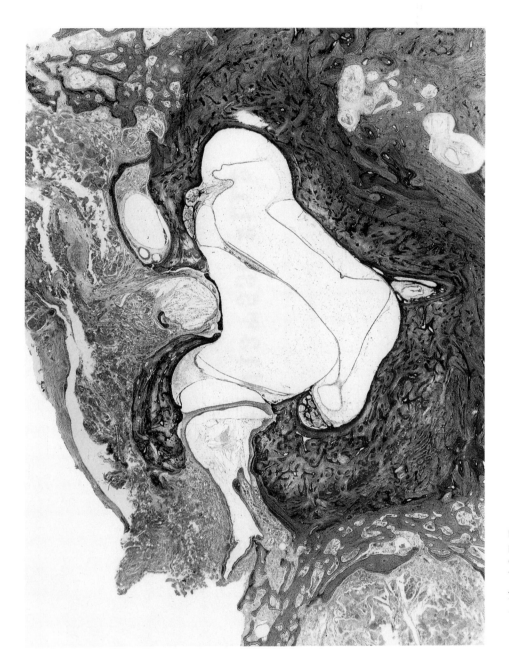

Figure 27.7. Vertical section through right petrous pyramid at level of oval and round windows. Although the meningioma has invaded the marrow spaces of the petrous pyramid, the jugular fossa, the hypotympanum, and the entire middle ear, there is no invasion of either the round window membrane or the stapedial footplate or the annular ligament. (Hematoxylin and eosin, ×10.)

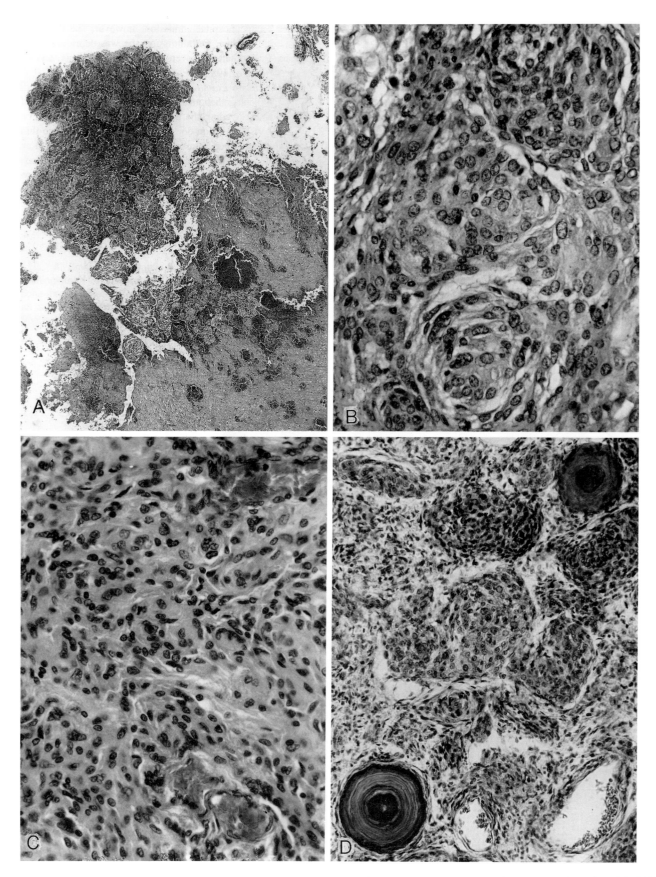

Figure 27.8. **A.** Section of meningotheliomatous meningioma that originated from the right sphenoid ridge, compressed the right frontal and temporal lobes, and extensively invaded the underlying bones of the cranial base, including the right and left temporal bones. **B.** The architecture reveals a somewhat lobulated arrangement of solid tumor cell masses with ill-defined cell membranes and delicate oval and round nuclei. **C.** Numerous blood vessels are encountered throughout the tumor. **D.** A section of the meningioma within the right temporal bone displays the identical cytoarchitecture. (Hematoxylin and eosin, ×20, ×400, ×400, and ×200, respectively.)

Case 3. *En globe, dumbbell-shaped meningotheliomatous meningioma with possible origin from right transverse sinus at transition to sigmoid sinus. Infiltration of dura over right transverse sinus and right middle cranial fossa. Invasion of adjacent tentorium with supratentorial extension of tumor. Invasion of mastoid, petrous, and squamous portions of right temporal bone. Right suboccipital craniectomy with removal of infratentorial tumor portion. Uneventful postoperative course. Patient alive 15 years later.*

A 54-year-old woman was seen who during the 12 months prior to admission developed, in succession, progressive loss of hearing and tinnitus in the right ear, occipital headaches, unsteadiness of gait, clumsiness of her right hand movements, and progressive nausea and vomiting.

Otologic examination revealed bilaterally normal tympanic membranes, a severe sensorineural hearing loss and absence of caloric responses in the right ear, paresis of the right fifth and, possibly, seventh cranial nerves, and no abnormalities in the nasopharyngeal and parapharyngeal spaces.

Neurologic examination showed, in addition to the cranial nerve involvement mentioned above, a staggering gait.

Radiographic examination of the right temporal bone exhibited hyperostosis and sclerosis of the petrous pyramid with ill-defined contours of the internal auditory canal and areas of radiolucencies in the adjacent bone (Fig. 27.11*A* and *B*).

At *operation,* a globoid meningioma was found to invade the petrous pyramid and mastoid process (Fig. 27.11*C*). Since only the infratentorial portion of the tumor was removed, the patient received 25 radiation treatments postoperatively to the tumor site and 15 years later was still doing quite well.

Case 4. *Large globoid meningotheliomatous meningioma occupying the right cerebellopontine angle with attachment just below the porus acusticus and extension into the right internal acoustic meatus, jugular foramen, and hypotympanum (Fig. 27.12). Extension along cochlear nerve into modiolus, canal of Rosenthal, and scala tympani and along vestibular nerve to maculae of utricle and sac-*

cule and to crista of superior semicircular canal (Fig. 27.13). Invasion of facial nerve and perilabyrinthine marrow spaces. Severe compression and distortion of right cerebellar hemisphere and brain stem. Death 24 hours following right suboccipital craniectomy.

A 44-year-old woman was seen who during the 3 years prior to admission had developed, in succession, right frontal and facial pains, right occipital and mastoid headaches, progressive loss of hearing and tinnitus in the right ear, unsteadiness of gait, right facial paresthesias, right hemiparesis, vertigo, and rapid loss of vision in both eyes, resulting in total blindness.

Otologic examination revealed a slightly scarred but otherwise normal right tympanic membrane, a sensorineural hypacusis, and total absence of caloric responses in the right ear.

Neurologic examination revealed bilateral papilledema with optic nerve atrophy and amaurosis, involvement of the right fifth, seventh, and eighth cranial nerves, and right cerebellar ataxia.

At *operation,* a right suboccipital craniectomy was performed, and a large globoid meningotheliomatous meningioma was removed from the right cerebellopontine angle (Fig. 27.12). It was attached to the posterior surface of the petrous bone, below the porus acusticus. The patient died the following day.

Microscopic examination of the right temporal bone confirms the expected tumor extension into the right internal auditory canal and jugular foramen (Figs. 27.15*A*, 27.16*A*, and 27.17) and an obliteration of the lateral sinus by thrombosis. From the internal auditory canal the meningioma extends into the adjacent perilabyrinthine marrow spaces and pneumatic cells (Figs. 27.14, 27.17, and 27.21). It extends into the cochlear modiolus (Fig. 27.14*A* and *B*), the canal of Rosenthal (Figs. 27.15 and 27.16), and, in some areas, the habenulae perforata (Fig. 27.16*A* and *B*) and invades the scala tympani (Figs. 27.15A and *C* and 27.16*A*). It follows the vestibular nerve and its subdivisions to the respective end organs (Figs. 27.13, 27.18, and 27.20) and infiltrates the facial nerve (Fig. 27.16). From the jugular foramen it extends into the hypotympanic cells and protrudes into the middle ear (Fig. 27.17). The meningioma is of the meningotheliomatous variety (Fig. 27.19).

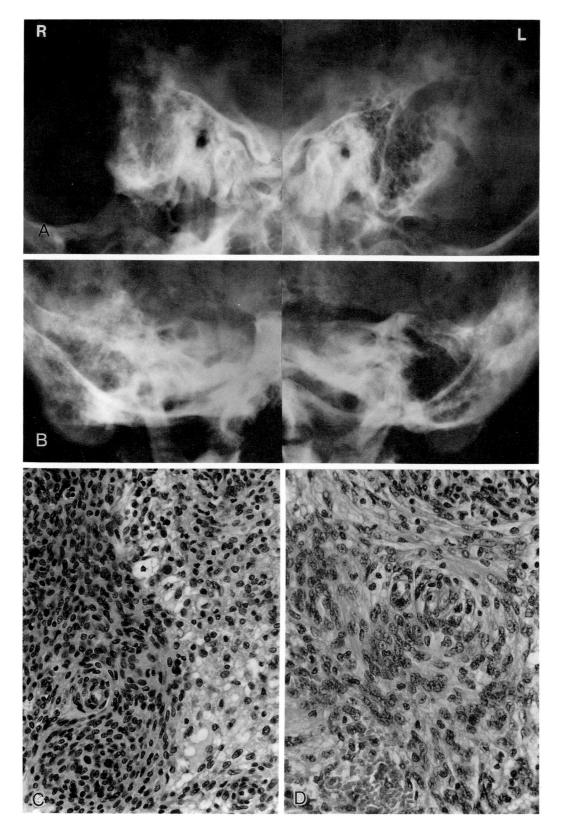

Figure 27.11. **A.** Lateral (Schüller) projection of temporal bones. The large bony defect on the right represents the earlier suboccipital craniectomy. The right mastoid process displays a peculiar pattern of spotty hyperostosis and dermineralization side by side, characteristic of meningiomatous invasion. **B.** Longitudinal (Stenvers) projection of petrous pyramids. The right petrous pyramid discloses the same moth-eaten pattern. The conspicuous irregularity of the superior border of the pyramid is caused by marked hyperostosis posterior to, and, by extensive osseous destruction, anterior to the arcuate eminence. **C.** Biopsy from tumor tissue in right mastoid process, disclosing a meningotheliomatous meningioma with areas of mucoid and hydropic degeneration. (Hematoxylin and eosin, ×400.) **D.** Section from meningotheliomatous meningioma originating at upper end of right sigmoid sinus. Its architecture is identical with the tumor encountered in the adjacent right mastoid process. (Hematoxylin and eosin, ×400.)

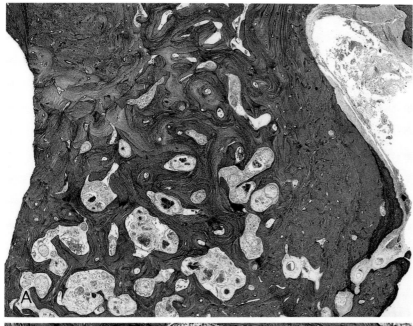

Figure 27.14. A. Vertical section through right petrous pyramid at level of anterior wall of internal acoustic meatus. The meningioma extends along the jugular foramen and has invaded the perilabyrinthine marrow spaces. (Hematoxylin and eosin, ×8.)

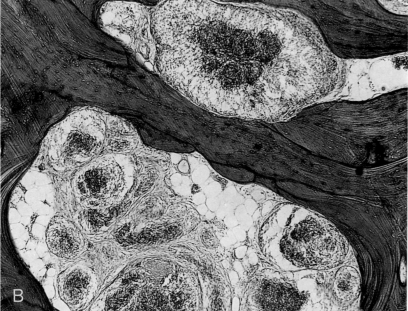

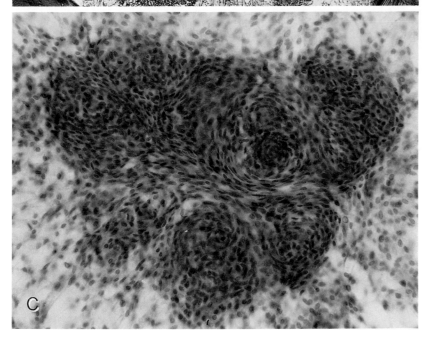

Figure 27.14. B. Two adjacent infralabyrinthine marrow spaces with tumor invasions. (×75.)

Figure 27.14. C. The meningioma cells display a tendency toward whorl formations. (×325.)

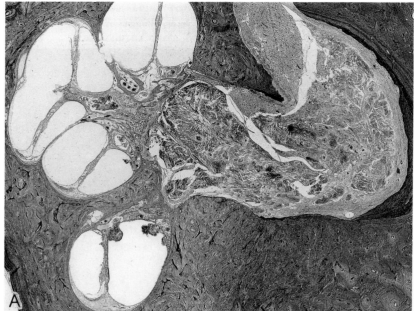

Figure 27.15.   A. Vertical midmodiolar section through right petrous pyramid. The meningioma has invaded the internal auditory canal. It follows the cochlear nerve fibers through the spiral foraminous tract and extends into the modiolus and canal of Rosenthal. (Hematoxylin and eosin, ×14.)

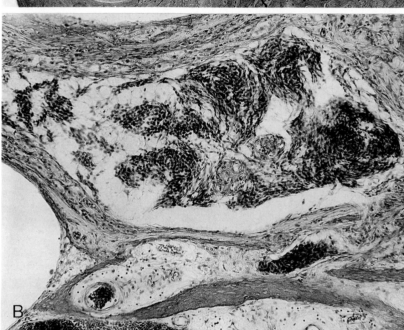

Figure 27.15.   B. Apical region of cochlear modiolus, revealing massive tumor infiltration. (×150.)

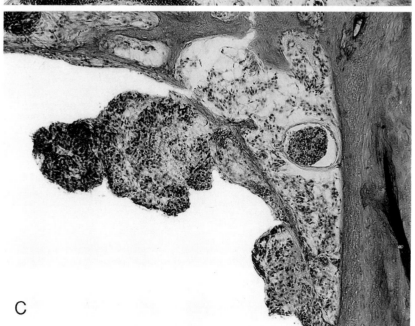

Figure 27.15.   C. From Rosenthal's canal the tumor is seen invading the scala tympani of the lower basal turn of the cochlea. (×150.)

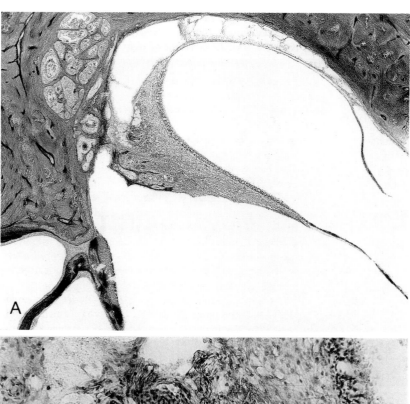

Figure 27.18. A. Vertical section through right petrous pyramid near center of oval window. The meningioma follows the utricular nerve to its end organ. (Hematoxylin and eosin, ×32.)

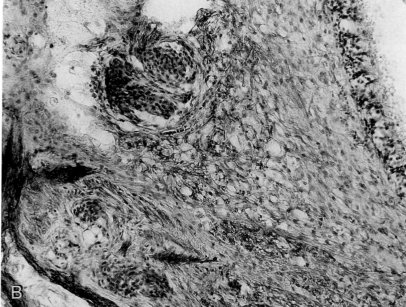

Figure 27.18. B. The macula of the utricle reveals extensive tumor infiltration. (×200.)

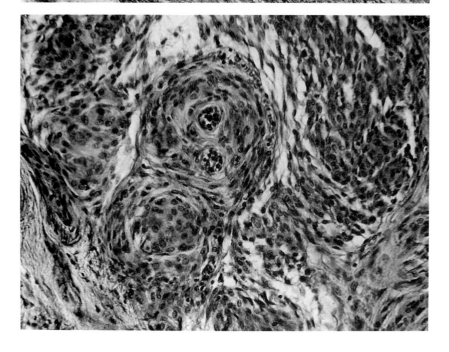

Figure 27.19. Higher magnification of the same tumor in the right internal auditory canal as seen in Figure 27.15A shows the tumor cells arranged in solid masses and whorls. (Hematoxylin and eosin, ×200.)

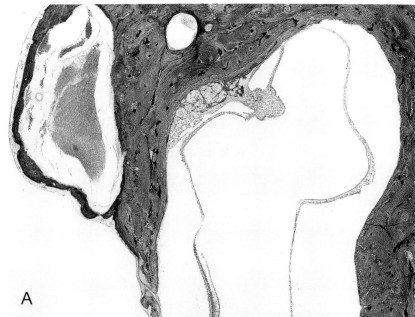

Figure 27.20. A. Vertical section through right petrous pyramid near posterior end of stapes footplate. The meningioma follows the vestibular branch of the superior ampulla to its end organ. (Hematoxylin and eosin, ×25.)

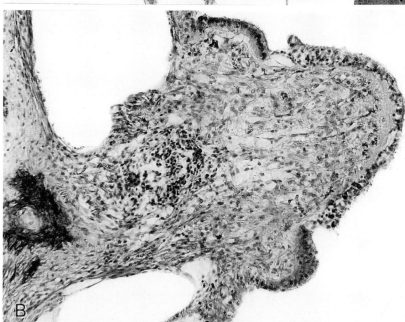

Figure 27.20. B. The crista of the superior semicircular canal displays islands and strands of tumor cell infiltration. (×200.)

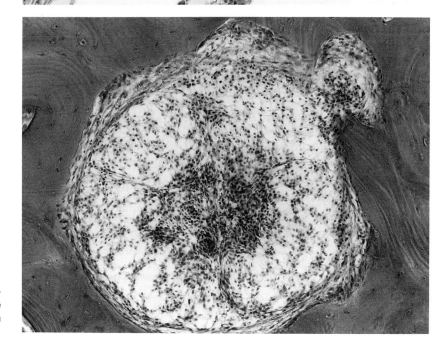

Figure 27.21. Resorption of bone by meningioma in infralabyrinthine marrow space. The adjacent osseous tissue is gradually being resorbed by the action of tumor cells (from Fig. 27.15A). (Hematoxylin and eosin, ×150.)

Clinical Aspects of Meningiomas Involving the Temporal Bone

CLINICAL SYMPTOMS

The predominant symptoms of meningiomas involving the temporal bone, in order of decreasing frequency, are: *(a)* progressive loss of hearing, *(b)* headaches, *(c)* vertigo, *(d)* tinnitus, *(e)* otorrhea, *(f)* otalgia, and *(g)* facial weakness and/or loss of taste. Less frequently noted are: *(h)* progressive loss of vision and double vision, *(i)* dysphagia, dysphonia, and dysarthria, *(j)* nausea and vomiting, *(k)* facial pains and paresthesias, *(l)* exophthalmos, *(m)* hemiparesis or paraparesis of the lower extremities, and *(n)* a periauricular swelling or mass in the neck (3).

OTOLARYNGOLOGIC MANIFESTATIONS

Once the tumor has gained access to the middle ear, symptoms of chronic tympanomastoiditis or of "acute otitis media" develop, and tumor tissue appears in the form of "polyps" and "granulation tissue" or is manifested by "hyperemia" and infiltration of the tympanic membrane or the middle ear mucoperiosteum. Middle ear structures such as the facial and chorda tympani nerves become involved, and sound conduction is affected (Fig. 27.16).

NEUROLOGIC MANIFESTATIONS

Neurologic symptoms are generally less uniform. The most frequently affected cranial nerves are the seventh and eighth, followed by the fifth, ninth, tenth, and eleventh. About 30% of patients have ipsilateral involvement of the cerebellum, and about 25% have brain stem involvement (3).

EXTRATEMPORAL EXTENSION

Once a meningioma gains access to the temporal bone, it extends farther in about 43% of patients (3). Invasion of the pericranium can proceed in several directions. The most common avenue is through the jugular and lacerate foramina into the nasopharyngeal, retromaxillary, retromandibular, and cervical spaces (Figs. 27.25–27.29, 27.32, 27.33, and 27.37). In the nasopharynx, the tumor generally presents as a downward-growing submucosal mass behind the lateral and posterior pharyngeal wall (Figs. 27.26, 27.27, and 27.33). At times, the meningioma may infiltrate the soft palate and the ipsilateral tonsil and extend into the piriform sinus (Figs. 27.27 and 27.33). Other routes are through the squamous portion of the temporal bone into the temporal fossa, through the root of the zygoma into the preauricular region, through the cortex into the postauricular area, or through the mastoid tip into the upper portion of the sternocleidomastoid muscle. Forward extension can involve the sphenoid bone and sphenoid sinus and the pterygopalatine fossa. Invasion of the orbit generally occurs through the optic foramen and supraorbital fissure. The origin of meningiomans extending outside the temporal bone does not differ from that of tumors remaining within its boundaries. Some arise within the temporal bone (geniculate ganglion, hypotympanic cavity, or jugular foramen), whereas others originate from the posterior or anterior aspect or from the apex of the petrous pyramid.

Meningiomas Involving the Temporal Bone with Extension to the Neck (6)

A meningioma in the parapharyngeal area can represent one of the following lesions:

1. An extracranial extension of a meningioma with an intracranial origin.
2. An extracranial extension of a meningioma arising in the jugular foramen, outside the cranial cavity but within the cranial base.
3. An ectopic, primary extracranial meningioma arising from an arachnoid cell cluster within the trunk or on the outer surface of a cranial nerve without any connection to either a neural foramen or the endocranium.
4. An extracranial metastasis to a cervical lymph node from a primary intracranial meningioma.

EXTRACRANIAL EXTENSION WITH AN INTRACRANIAL ORIGIN

Extracranial extensions of a primarily intracranial meningioma are by no means rare. Of 371 patients with an intracranial meningioma observed over a 30-year period, 71 (20%) had an extracranial extension of the tumor (7). In 30 patients, the tumor extended into the orbit; in 25, it extended through the external table of the calvaria into the overlying soft tissue; in 11, it extended into the nasal cavity and paranasal sinuses; and in 5, it extended into the parapharyngeal, parotid, or cervical region (7).

Intracranial meningiomas extend extracranially along well recognized avenues: *(a)* via the neural foramina in the base of the skull (Figs. 27.25–27.28, 27.30–27.31*(b)*, and 27.37), assuming an hourglass or dumbbell tumor configuration; *(b)* along preformed pathways and spaces such as the sutures in the calvaria and the pneumatic cells in the temporal bone; and *(c)* through the Haversian canals in the bony structures of the skull.

Case Reports

Cases 7–9 illustrate the pertinent clinical and pathologic aspects of meningiomas involving the temporal bone, extending to the nasopharynx and retromandibular space, and manifesting as neoplasms in the pharynx and neck.

Case 7. *En plaque meningioma arising from left sphenoid ridge with extension into anterior cranial fossa and across middle cranial fossa into posterior cranial fossa. Hyperostosis and sclerosis of underlying base of skull. Invasion of left temporal bone with extracranial extension through lacerated and jugular foramina into left retromandibular area. Involvement of left cranial nerves VII and IX–XII. Possibility of bilateral vestibular schwannomas. Syringomyelia of lower thoracic cord. Isolated cutaneous neurofibromas. Two café au lait spots. Neurofibromatosis-2 (Figs. 27.25 and 27.26).*

A 20-year-old college girl with a family history of neurofibromatosis (NF1) was seen. At age 16 she had had a thoracic laminectomy for syringomyelia and, following 7 years of "recurrent otitis media" affecting her left ear, underwent a radial mastoidectomy and was diagnosed as having a glomus tumor. She subsequently developed a firm nontender mass in the left anterior cervical triangle that protruded medially into the left oropharynx and responded temporarily to radiation therapy. During the next 3 years the patient developed otalgia, tinnitus, and left-sided facial twitching, vertigo, bifrontal headaches, and blurred vision.

Otologic examination showed a 4 × 3 × 3-cm mass in the left carotid triangle, extending medially into the pharynx and protruding under an intact mucous membrane superiorly to the base of the skull and inferiorly to the piriform sinus (Figs. 27.25–27.27). The left radical mastoid cavity contained a red vascular tumor tissue covered by a hyperemic squamous epithelium (Fig. 27.25). Cochlear function studies revealed a maximal conductive hearing loss on the left, and vestibular function studies showed no responses to caloric stimulation of either labyrinth.

Radiographic examination revealed marked sclerosis of the left base of the skull, areas of radiolucency and increased density in the left temporal bone, enlargement of both internal auditory canals with irregular erosions of the left canal wall, and a soft tissue density in the left jugular and lacerated foramina (Fig. 27.28).

At *operation,* exploration of the left neck disclosed a 4 × 3 × 3-cm fusiform tumorous enlargement involving the left cranial nerves IX–XII and the cervical sympathetic system (Fig. 27.29). The superior pole of the tumor extended to the lacerated and jugular foramina. Exploration of the left mastoid cavity revealed the remaining mastoid and perilabyrinthine cells and marrow spaces invaded by a dense vascular tumor tissue that could be traced through large bony defects in the tegmen to the original tumor in the left middle cranial fossa (Fig. 27.30). Biopsies from the tumors in the neck and temporal bone showed a meningotheliomatous meningioma with psammoma bodies (Fig. 27.31). Death occurred 5 years later from progressive intracranial extension of the large tumor.

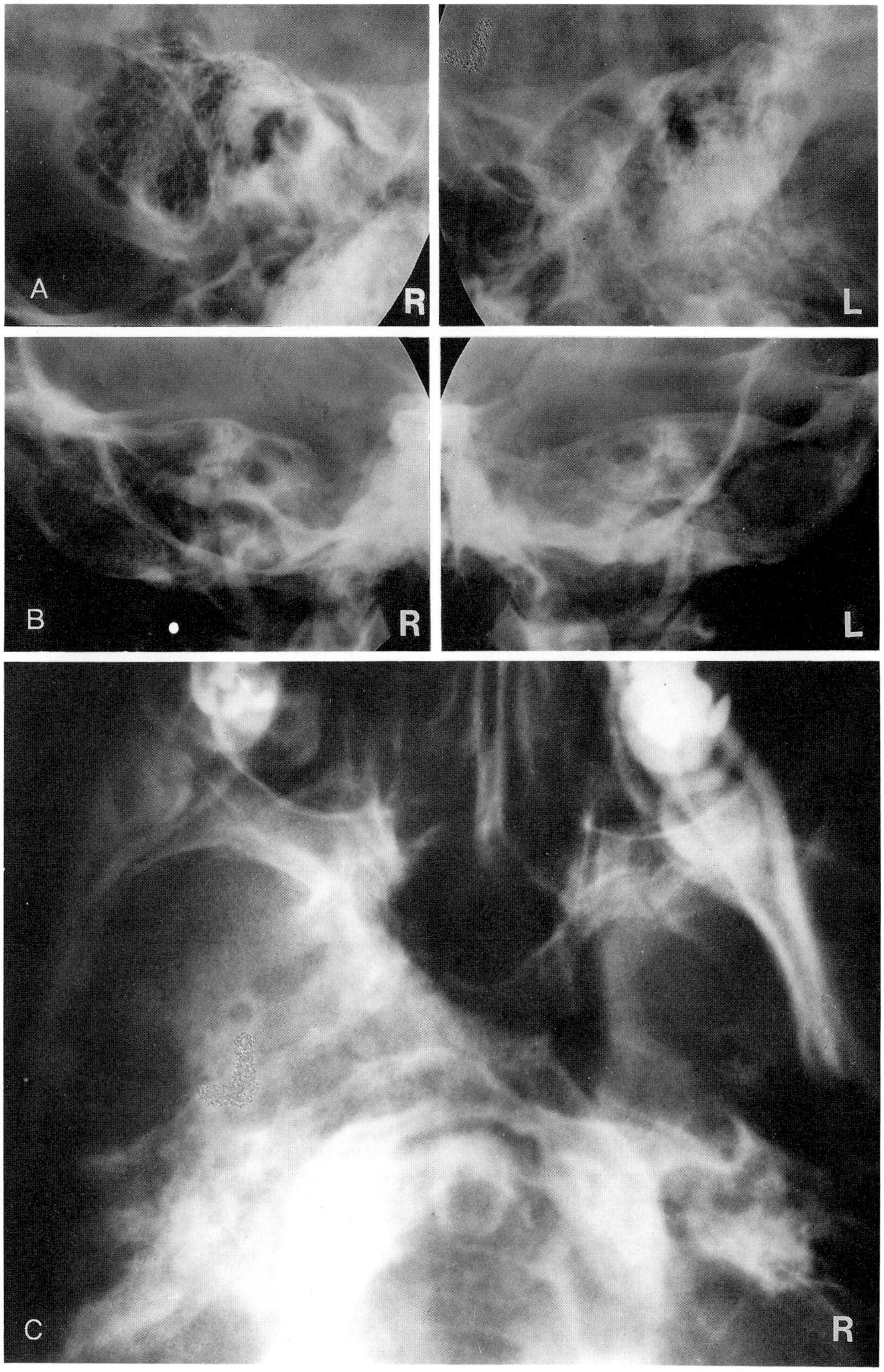

Figure 27.28. A. The left mastoid reveals an operative defect. Areas of increased density and radiolucency can be seen in the region of the sinodural angle and mastoid tip. **B.** Both internal auditory canals are enlarged. The enlargement on the left is caused by a meningioma and is characterized by irregular erosion of the canal wall. The widening of the right is produced by a vestibular schwannoma and is distinguished by regular contours of the canal wall. **C.** The sclerosis and hyperostosis involve the left sphenoid ridge, floor of the left middle cranial fossa, and left petrous pyramid.

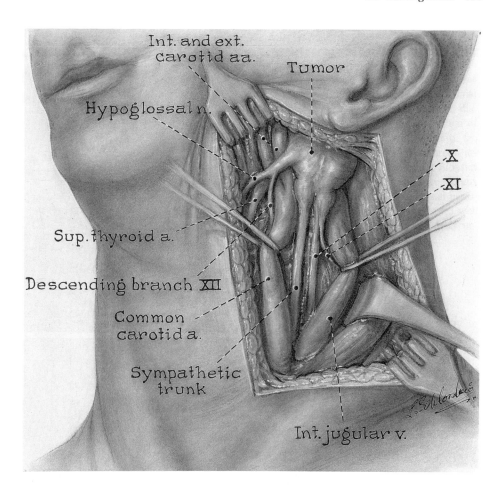

Figure 27.29. Fusiform enlargements involve left cranial nerves IX–XII and the left cervical sympathetic system. The tumor mass continues cephalad into the left lacerated and jugular foramina.

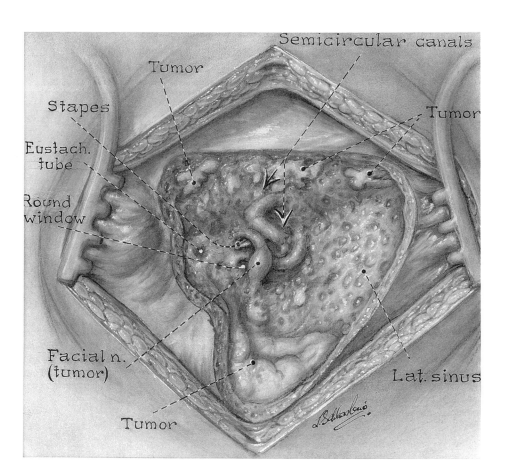

Figure 27.30. Massive invasion of entire left temporal bone by vascular tumor through extensive bone destruction in tegmental region. Notice the spindle-shaped tumor involving the upper mastoid segment of the facial nerve.

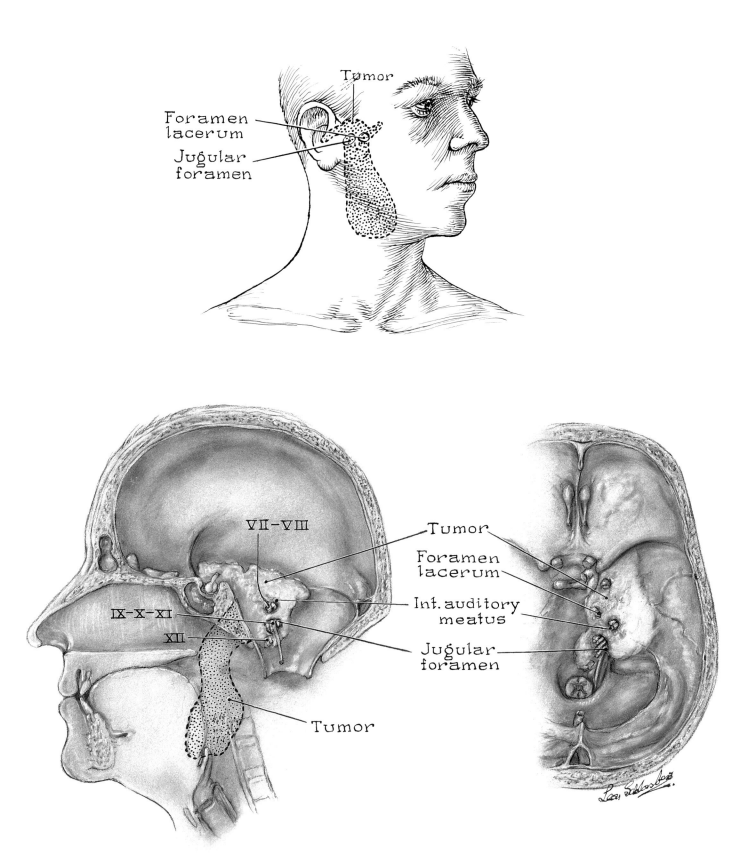

Figure 27.32. Illustration of origin of en plaque meningioma and its extension through lacerated and jugular foramina into the right side of the neck as visualized from radiographic, endoscopic, and surgical exposures.

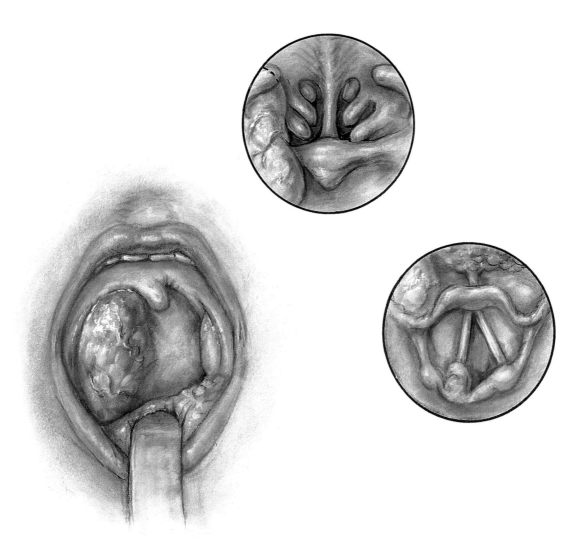

Figure 27.33. The submucosal tumor protrudes from the base of the skull lateral and anterior to the right tubal orifice and extends downward along the lateral and posterior pharyngeal wall into the right vallecula. Paralysis of the right vocal cord resulted from tumor involvement of the vagus nerve.

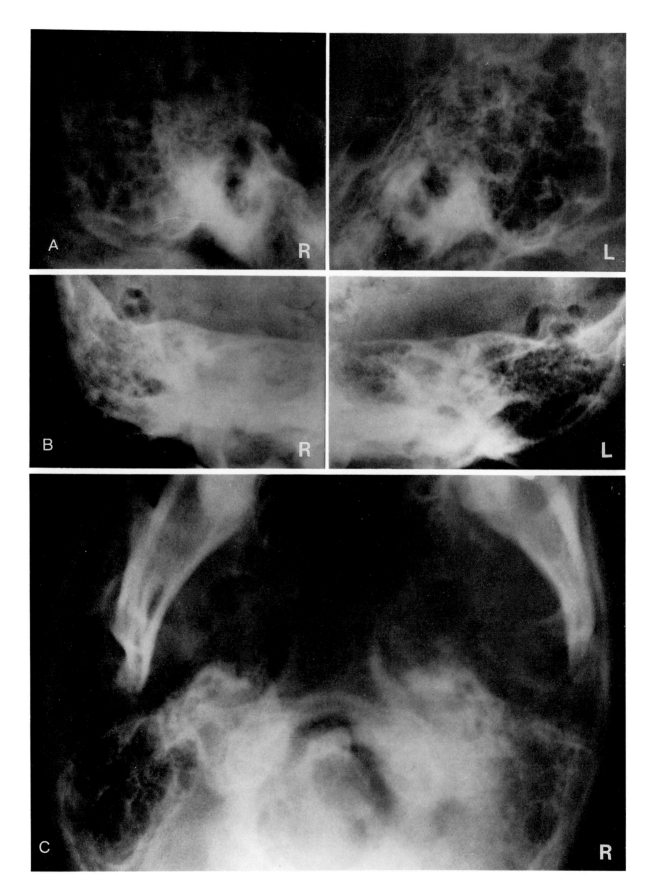

Figure 27.34. A. The right mastoid process shows generalized sclerosis and diffuse haziness throughout a well-developed cellular system. **B.** Irregular areas of radiolucency and increased density are evidence of mas-sive tumor invasion of the right temporal bone. **C.** The sclerosis of the right petrous pyramid and the widening of the right foramen ovale are recognizable.

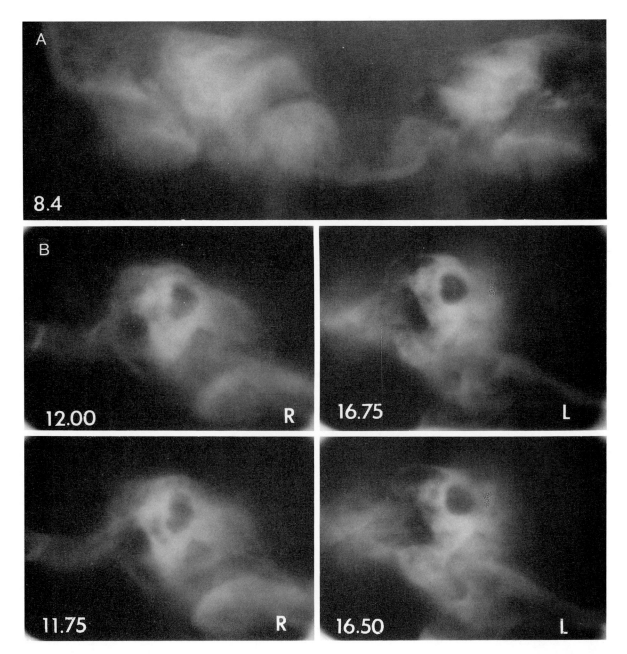

Figure 27.35. **A.** Anteroposterior polytomogram of petrous pyramids. The sclerosis and hyperostosis of right otic capsule and occipital condyle and the enlargement of the lateral portion of the right internal auditory canal are clearly visible. **B.** Lateral tomograms of petrous pyramids. The right internal auditory canal is enlarged, and its lumen displays a uniform increase in density.

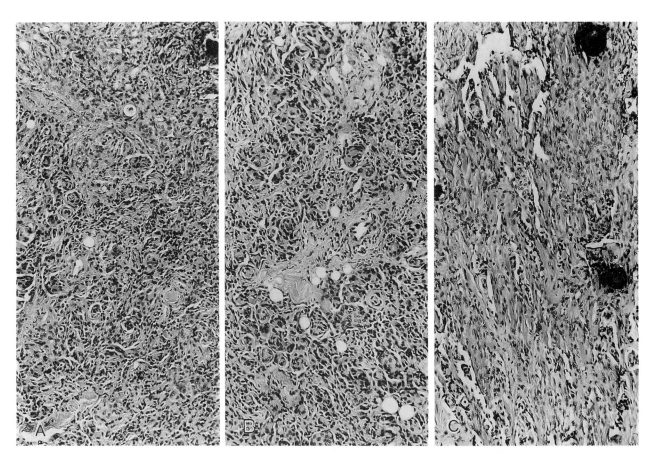

Figure 27.36. Biopsy specimens that identify the neoplasm as an extracranial extension of a meningotheliomatous meningioma from the nasopharynx **(A)**, oropharynx **(B)**, and right neck tumor **(C)**. (Hematoxylin and eosin, ×120, ×137, and ×120, respectively.)

Case 9. *En globe meningotheliomatous meningioma arising from the posterior aspect of the left petrous pyramid growing as an en plaque meningioma across the floor of the middle cranial fossa, invading the underlying left temporal bone, and extending through the lacerated and jugular foramina into the left retromandibular space and parotid gland. Compression of left cerebellar hemisphere, distortion and displacement of brain stem, and occlusive internal hydrocephalus. Pressure atrophy of left cranial nerves V and VII–XII. Death from exsanguination following erosion of bracheocephalic artery by tracheostomy tube (Fig. 27.37).*

A 7-year-old boy who after age 4 had developed signs of left "tympanomastoiditis," otalgia, and facial nerve palsy was seen. He was subsequently found to have palsies involving cranial nerves V and VII–XII. After a left facial nerve decompression, he developed headaches, vomiting, staggering, left-sided hemiparesis, and loss of bladder and bowel control.

Otologic examination revealed, in addition, a mass in the left carotid triangle.

Radiologic examination revealed a destruction of the left petrous pyramid, the floor of the left middle and posterior cranial fossae, and the left border of the foramen magnum.

Surgical exploration of the left neck showed a firm encapsulated tumor adherent to the skull base at the jugular foramen, compressing the major vessels and caudal group of cranial nerves (Fig. 27.37). The tumor, which had also invaded the parotid gland, proved to be a meningotheliomatous meningioma (Fig. 27.40*B*). The patient died, 5 weeks after tracheostomy, from a massive arterial hemorrhage through the tracheostoma.

Microscopic examination of the left temporal bone shows widespread invasion of the petrous pyramid and mastoid process by an extrinsic meningioma through the lateral, medial, and inferior aspects and through the internal acoustic meatus and jugular foramen. From the internal acoustic meatus the meningioma widely invades the floor and underlying bone (Figs. 27.38*A* and 27.39, *top*). Strands and clusters of tumor cells can be followed along remaining bundles of the cochlear nerve into the cochlear modiolus and Rosenthal's canal of the basal turn of the cochlea (Fig. 27.39, *top* and *bottom*). The meningioma invades the vestibular labyrinth in a similar manner. Invasion of the internal acoustic meatus resulted in compression and destruction of the seventh and eighth cranial nerves. In the mastoid segment of the facial nerve, the greater portion of the bony canal had been either removed during the nerve decompression or destroyed by tumor, to the extent that the facial nerve has become firmly embedded in tumor tissue (Fig. 27.40*A*). In the petrous apex, the meningioma extends into the bony canal of the carotid artery, causing a partial extrinsic compression of the vascular lumen. In the jugular foramen, cranial nerves IX–XII are embedded in tumor, and the neoplasm has invaded and obliterated the jugular bulb and extended through the hypotympanum into the tympanic cavity. From the hypotympanum it extends beneath the annulus fibrosus into the external auditory canal. The tumor occupies the entire middle ear space, obliterates the oval and round windows, and superficially erodes the cochlear and vestibular capsule (Figs. 27.38*B* and 27.39, *top*). Histologically, the meningioma is of the meningotheliomatous subgroup (Fig. 27.40*B*).

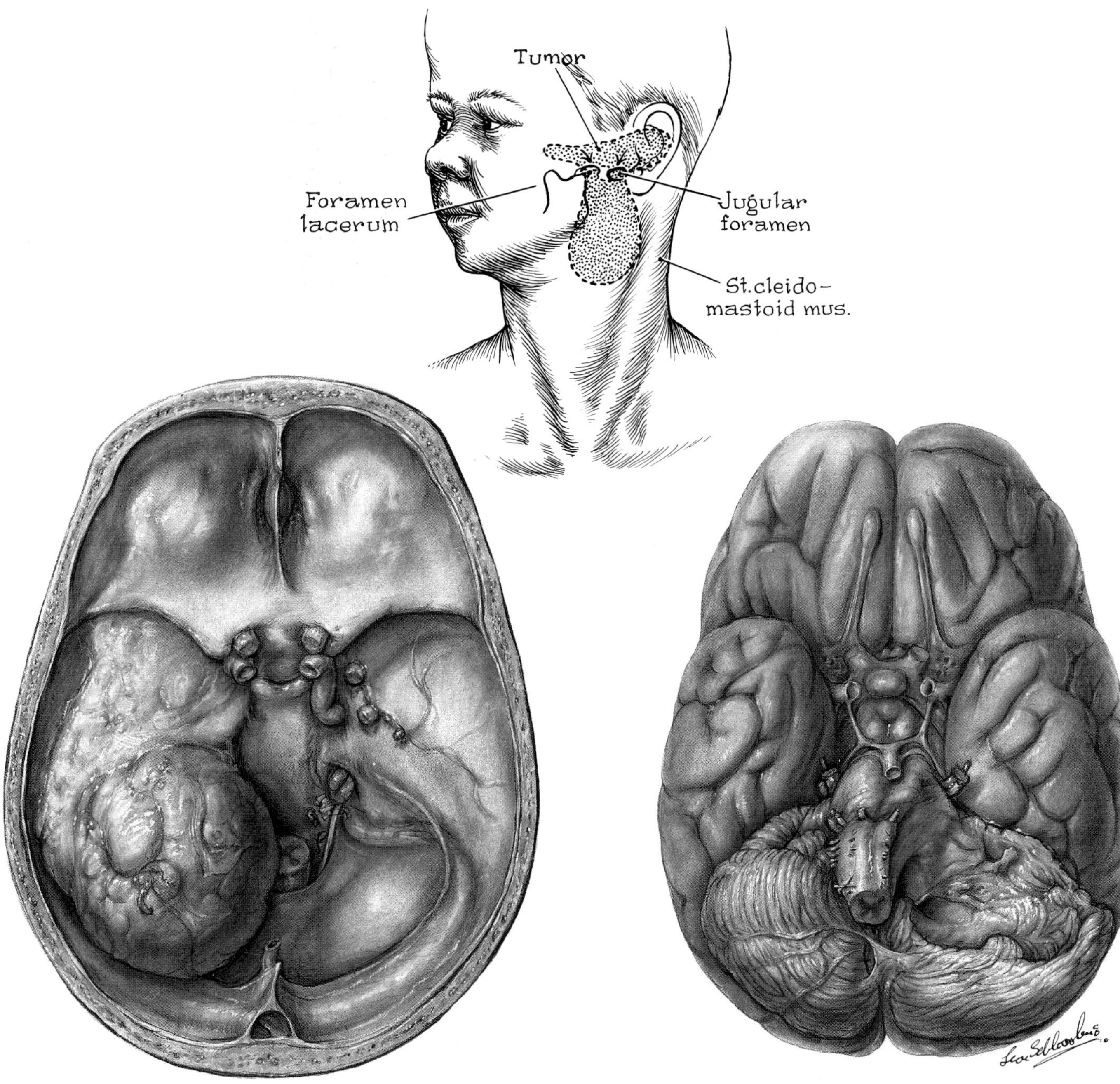

Figure 27.37. Illustration of meningotheliomatous meningioma as visualized at autopsy. Arising as an en globe meningioma from the posterior aspect of the left petrous pyramid, it compresses the left cerebellar hemisphere and distorts and displaces the brain stem to the opposite side. It grows as an en plaque meningioma across the floor of the left middle cranial fossa, invades the underlying temporal bone, and extends through the lacerated and jugular foramina into the left retromandibular space.

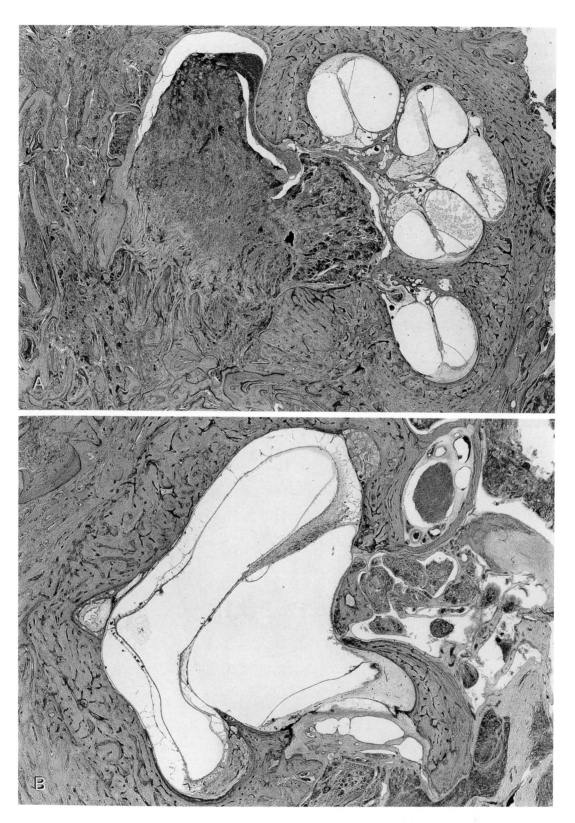

Figure 27.38.   A. Vertical midmodiolar section through left temporal bone. The meningioma invades the petrous pryamid from the posterior cranial fossa, extends into the auditory canal, and infiltrates the adjacent bone. **B.** Vertical section at level of oval and round windows. The meningioma occupies the entire middle ear cavity but does not invade the labyrinth or cochlea. (Hematoxylin and eosin, ×12.5 and ×16, respectively.)

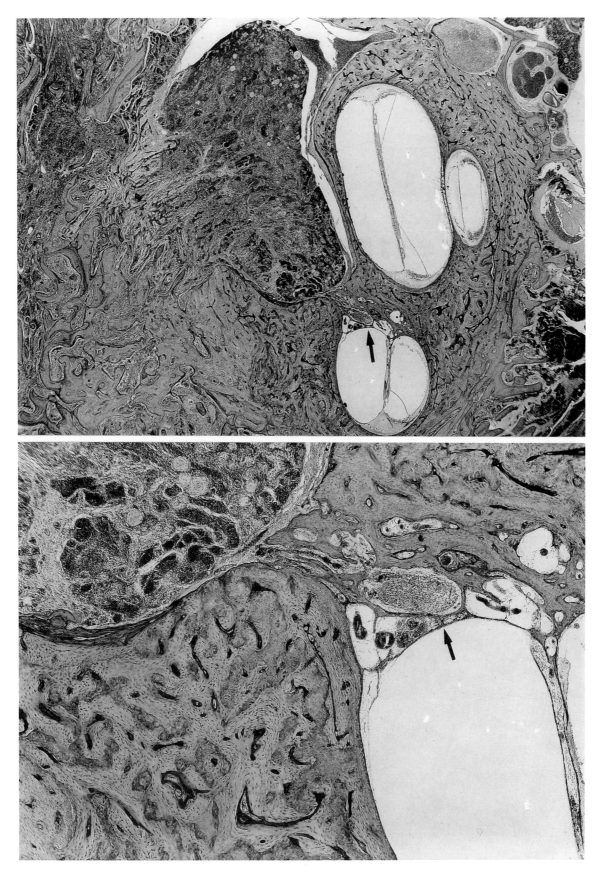

Figure 27.39. Vertical paramodiolar section through left temporal bone. The massive tumor invasion of the internal acoustic meatus resulted in compression and destruction of the seventh and eighth cranial nerves. Clusters of tumor cells follow remaining cochlear nerve fibers into Rosenthal's canal of the lower basal turn of the cochlea *(arrows)*. (Hematoxylin and eosin, *top*, ×13; *bottom*, ×50.)

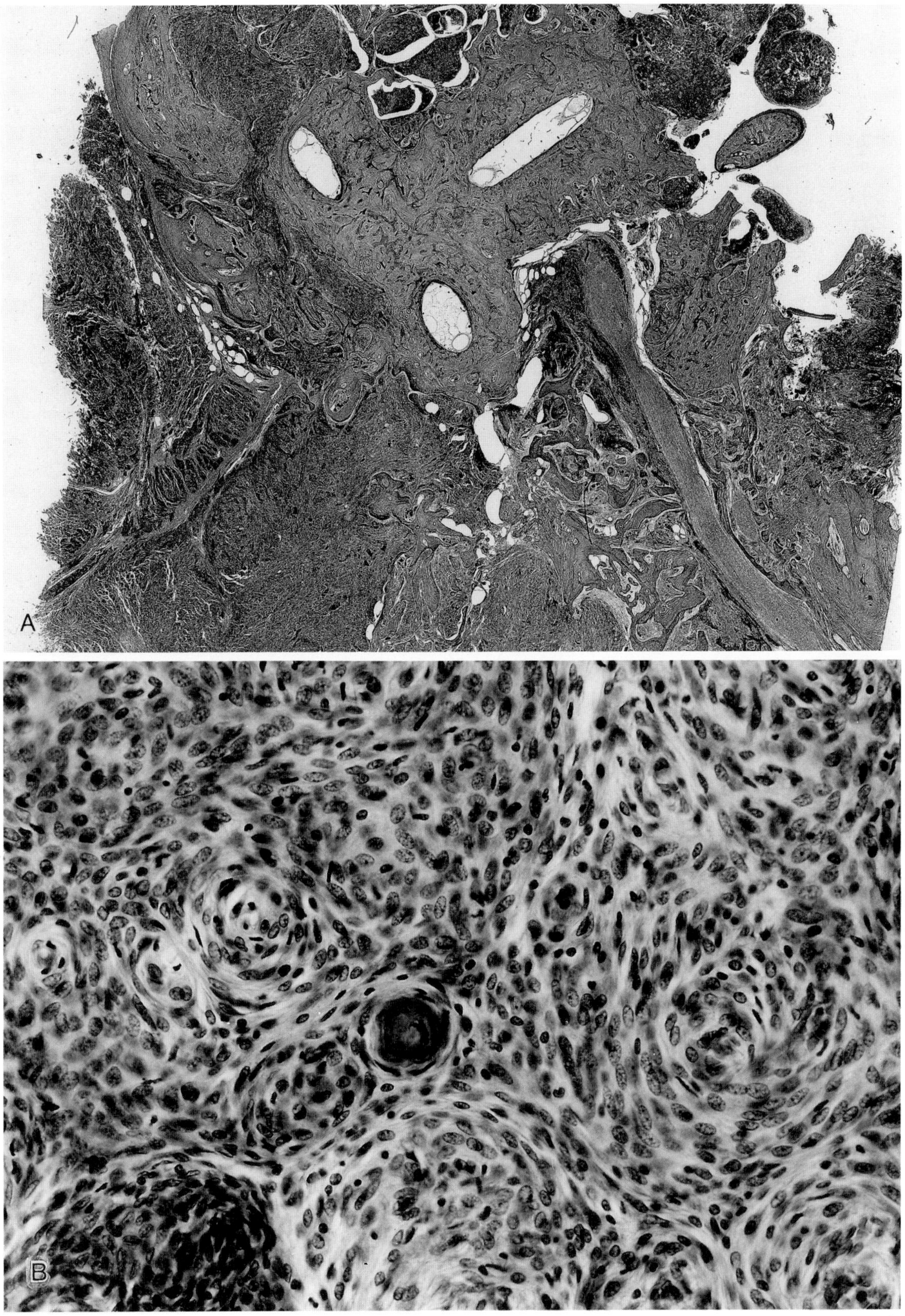

Figure 27.40. **A.** Vertical section through left pyramid at level of mastoid segment of facial nerve. The previous decompression widely exposed the facial nerve to the surrounding tumor masses. **B.** The meningioma in the left temporal bone is of the meningotheliomatous variety. (Hematoxylin and eosin, ×7 and ×400, respectively.)

EXTRACRANIAL EXTENSION FROM THE NEURAL COMPARTMENT OF THE JUGULAR FORAMEN

The jugular foramen is one of the four predilective sites of meningiomas that originate within the temporal bone (3). These tumors, as they increase in size, follow the direction of least resistance and extend extracranially to the parapharyngeal space and neck without entering the posterior cranial fossa (7–9).

The extracranial parapharyngeal location of these meningiomas, their firm attachment to the base of the skull in the area of the jugular foramen, and the absence of any tumor tissue in the cranial cavity strongly suggest that these neoplasms originate outside the cranial cavity but within the skull base in one of their predilective sites, namely, in the jugular foramen.

ECTOPIC, PRIMARILY EXTRACRANIAL MENINGIOMAS WITH NO CONNECTION TO EITHER A CRANIAL NERVE FORAMEN OR THE ENDOCRANIUM

Ectopic, primarily extracranial meningiomas are exceedingly rare. About 50 examples have been reported (7). The majority of these patients, however, did not have the benefit of the most sophisticated radiographic diagnostic studies to rule out the possibility of another origin. The predilective locations of these tumors included: (a) the orbit and the optic nerve; (b) the nasal cavity, the paranasal sinuses, and the nasopharynx; (c) the external surface of the calvaria with the overlying scalp and the skin and subcutis of the back; (d) the neck; and (e) the brachial plexus (3, 4, 8–16).

EXTRACRANIAL METASTASES FROM AN INTRACRANIAL MENINGIOMA TO A PARAPHARYNGEAL (CERVICAL) LYMPH NODE

Whereas direct extensions from a meningioma into adjacent soft tissues, salivary glands, muscles, nerves, blood vessels, and bone are fairly common, dissemination through the cerebrospinal fluid pathway and through the bloodstream to the periphery remains a rare occurrence. Among reported cases, the histologic appearance of both the primary tumor and its metastasis was remarkably benign. In a few instances the morphologic features were somewhat atypical, and they included occasional mitotic figures. Although no histologic type of primary tumor is exempt from a malignant transformation, the angiomatous meningioma has a greater predisposition and, therefore, a somewhat more guarded prognosis (1). Verified metastases from intracranial meningiomas have been reported in the cervical, supraclavicular, and mediastinal lymph nodes, the thymus, the lungs, and the liver (1, 2, 5, 17–26). Therefore, a meningioma in the neck area can be an extracranial metastasis, although this is exceedingly rare.

Regional Behavior of Intracranial Meningiomas with Extracranial Extension

Although meningiomas are generally considered to be locally limited neoplasms, this is not always the case. The examples discussed above illustrate that the presence of an extracranial extension places these tumors in a category of their own. They represent a more serious form of neoplasia, characterized by a tendency to more frequent local recurrence, to multicentric growth, to spread beyond the confinements of the skull, and to

frequent association with other neoplasms of the central nervous system, particularly schwannomas of other cranial nerves. These lesions are, therefore, often an expression of neurofibromatosis-2 (NF2) (6–17)

DIAGNOSTIC EVALUATION AND MANAGEMENT

CT and MRI are essential for the identification and delineation of meningiomas. They provide the necessary information concerning the extent of the endocranial and extracranial tumor growth, the degree of bone destruction and involvement, and the relation of the neoplasm to adjacent structures. The CT scans (Fig. 27.41) and magnetic resonance images (Fig. 27.42) of Case 10 and two other magnetic resonance images (Figs. 27.44 and 27.45) are good examples.

The aim of management of these lesions is total surgical excision. In instances in which complete extirpation is impossible or when the margins of resection are not entirely free of tumor, radiation therapy should be considered, since it may reduce the high recurrence rate.

Case Report

Case 10. *En plaque meningotheliomatous meningioma originating from right sphenoid wing. Massive infiltration and extensive reactive sclerosis and hyperostosis involving the right sphenoid wing, right temporal bone, right pterygoid plate, head of right condyloid process, and adjacent right base of skull. Bony occlusion of right external auditory meatus. Involvement of right Eustachian tube, middle ear, antrum, and mastoid process with complete obliteration of air spaces and air cells. Secondary subacute external otitis with external cholesteatoma. Chronic tympanomastoiditis and osteomyelitis. Involvement of right cranial nerves V and VII. Bilateral clinical otosclerosis.*

A 51-year-old woman with a history of bilateral progressive loss of hearing for about 23 years, requiring the use of a hearing aid for the past 19 years, was seen. She had had several exploratory tympanotomies on her right ear, elsewhere, for a stapes operation and removal of an unusually vascular "granulation tissue." Three years prior to admission, she developed intermittent purulent otorrhea, otalgia, a sensation of fullness and pressure in the right ear, and a constant pulsating tinnitus. She had also noticed some right-sided facial paresthesias and facial twitching. She has had a positive family history of otosclerosis and bony exostoses.

Otologic examination revealed a swelling and edema of the right periauricular area, especially over the root of the zygoma and in the postauricular region. The right external auditory canal revealed a marked concentric narrowing with a thread-like lumen filled with keratinous debris. After removal of this debris, clear pulsating fluid drained from the middle ear. Only a small central portion of an inflamed eardrum was visible. Cochlear function studies disclosed a bilateral conductive loss with a speech reception threshold of 60 dB. Discrimination was 100% bilaterally. There were no palpable masses in the right neck or retromandibular area, and there was no distortion in the right nasopharynx, oropharynx, and hypopharynx. The left eardrum was normal. There was a persistent twitching involving the right orbicularis oculi muscle.

At *radiologic examination,* the CT scans revealed an extensive sclerosis and hyperostosis involving the wing of the right sphenoid and right temporal bone, extending anteriorly to the foramen ovale and posteriorly into the mastoid (Fig. 27.41). The right external auditory canal was almost completely obliterated by proliferation of bone. The right middle ear cavity, attic, aditus and antrum, and the mastoid process were opacified by what appeared to be a soft

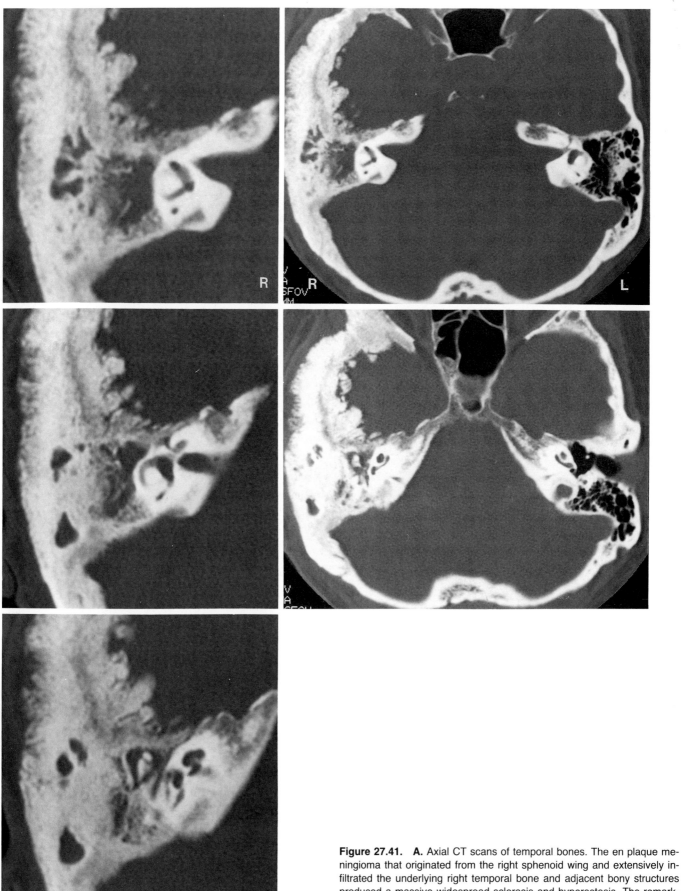

Figure 27.41.   A. Axial CT scans of temporal bones. The en plaque meningioma that originated from the right sphenoid wing and extensively infiltrated the underlying right temporal bone and adjacent bony structures produced a massive widespread sclerosis and hyperostosis. The remarkable bony spiculation of the hyperostotic bone is best visualized in the enlarged axial sections.

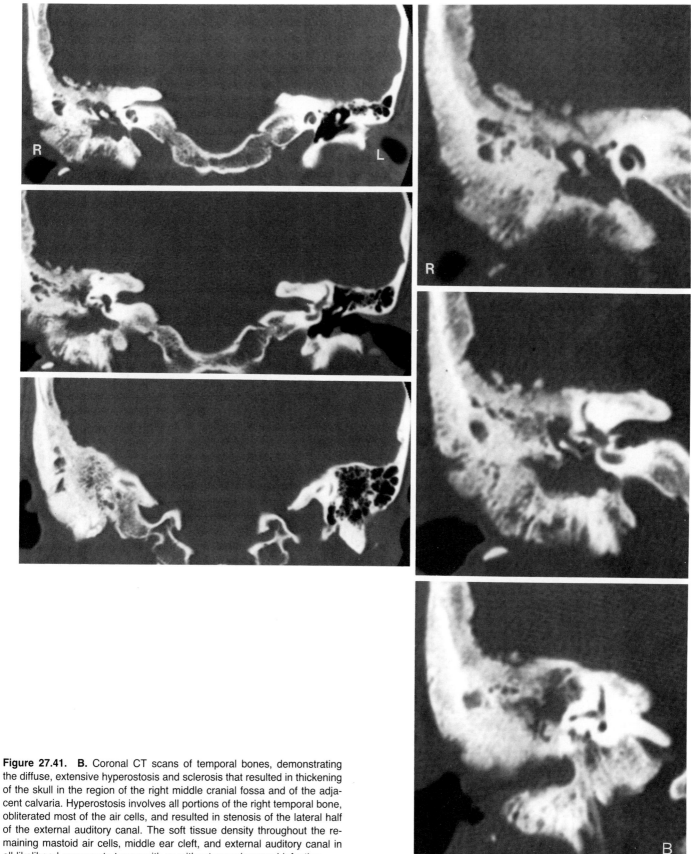

Figure 27.41. B. Coronal CT scans of temporal bones, demonstrating the diffuse, extensive hyperostosis and sclerosis that resulted in thickening of the skull in the region of the right middle cranial fossa and of the adjacent calvaria. Hyperostosis involves all portions of the right temporal bone, obliterated most of the air cells, and resulted in stenosis of the lateral half of the external auditory canal. The soft tissue density throughout the remaining mastoid air cells, middle ear cleft, and external auditory canal in all likelihood represents tumor with or without superimposed infection.

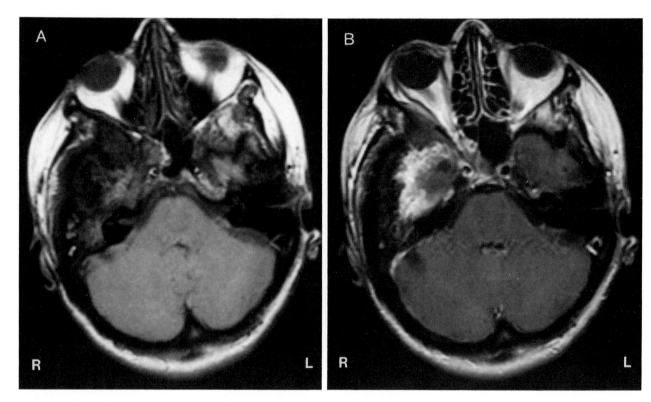

Figure 27.42. Axial magnetic resonance image of brain without **(A)** and with gadolinium **(B)** shows the tumor occupying the right middle cranial fossa, diffusely infiltrating the underlying temporal bone. It involves the petrous pyramid and mastoid process and extends forward through the lateral wall into the orbit, displacing the lateral rectus muscle slightly, into the right sphenoid sinus, and laterally to but not into the Sylvian fissure. There is diffuse enhancement of the tumor in the middle fossa and along the right dural margin **(B)**.

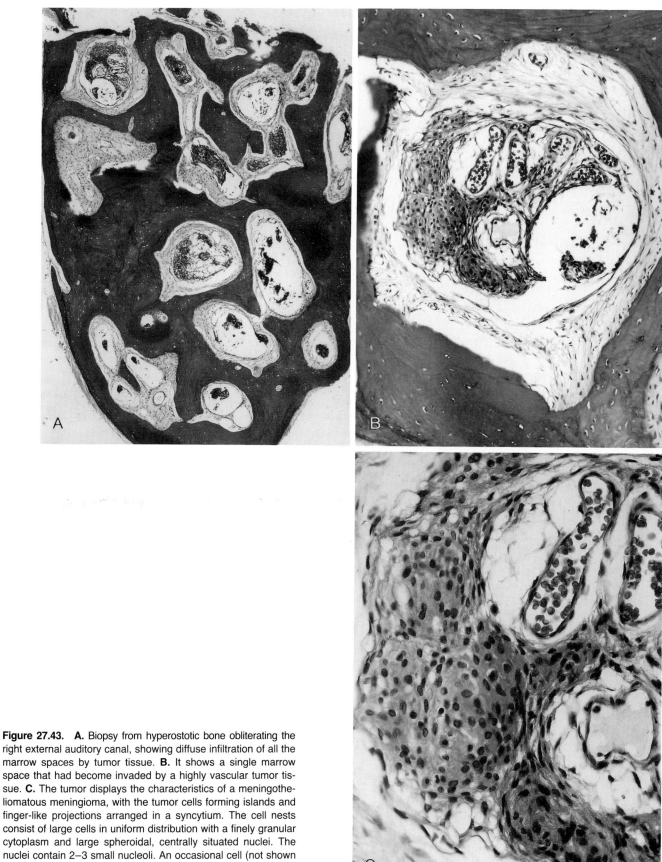

Figure 27.43.   A. Biopsy from hyperostotic bone obliterating the right external auditory canal, showing diffuse infiltration of all the marrow spaces by tumor tissue. **B.** It shows a single marrow space that had become invaded by a highly vascular tumor tissue. **C.** The tumor displays the characteristics of a meningotheliomatous meningioma, with the tumor cells forming islands and finger-like projections arranged in a syncytium. The cell nests consist of large cells in uniform distribution with a finely granular cytoplasm and large spheroidal, centrally situated nuclei. The nuclei contain 2–3 small nucleoli. An occasional cell (not shown here) displays a beginning concentric cellular arrangement. (Hematoxylin and eosin, ×90, ×140, and ×240, respectively.)

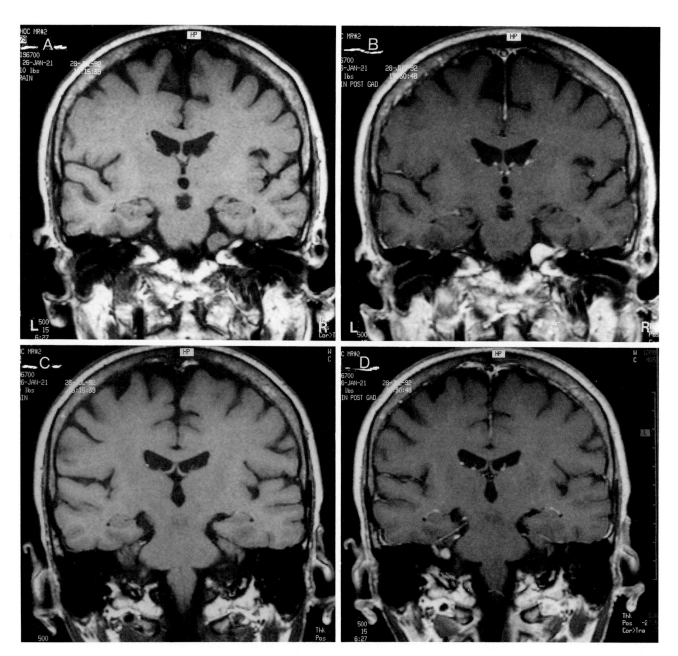

Figure 27.44. Coronal T2-weighted pregadolinium and postgadolinium magnetic resonance images of the brain of a 70-year-old woman with most likely bilateral meningiomas of the cerebellopontine angle. There is a 1.2 × 1.0 × 1.3-cm, slightly bright on T2, densely enhancing mass at the anterior margin of the left porus acusticus **(A** and **B).** A similar but smaller, 6 × 6 × 6-mm, slightly hyperintense on T2, densely enhancing mass is located at the posterior margin of the right porus acusticus **(C** and **D).** (Courtesy of Dr. M. Holliday.)

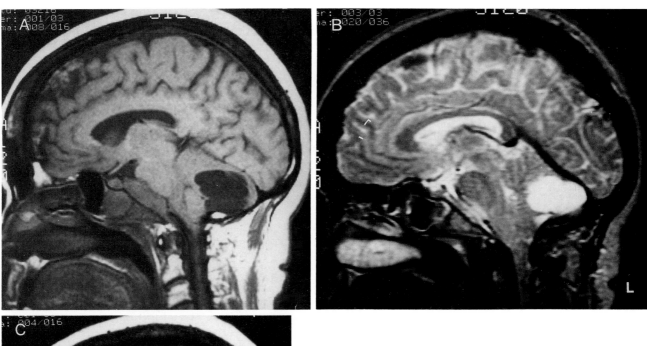

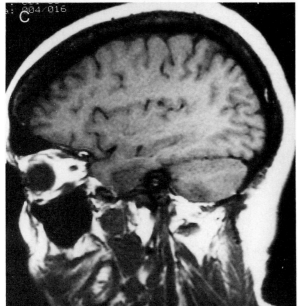

Figure 27.45. Sagittal and axial T1- and T2-weighted pregadolinium and postgadolinium magnetic resonance images of the brain of a 75-year-old woman with a meningioma arising from the clivus and an arachnoid cyst in the left cerebellar hemisphere. The meningioma is elevating the brain stem **(A)**; the arachnoid cyst displays increased signal intensely **(B)**; the tumor produced a marked indentation into the base of the overlying temporal lobe anterior to the left internal auditory canal **(C)**; the meningioma protrudes in a dumbbell fashion into the left middle and posterior cranial fossa, displacing the brain stem slightly toward the left, and is involving the left temporal bone **(D and E)**. It has partially destroyed the left petrous apex.

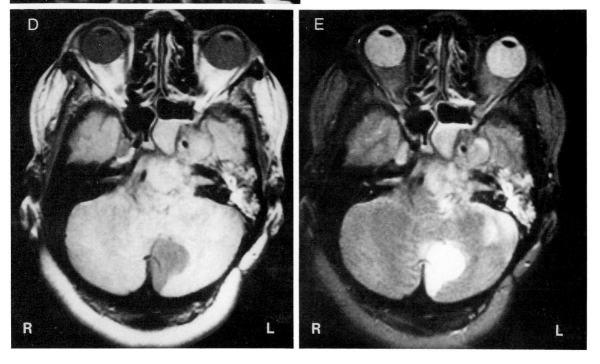

tissue mass occupying the air spaces and by reactive bone sclerosis. The right pterygoid plate and the condyloid process of the mandible exhibited the same sclerosis. Extensive bony overgrowth was also found in the condylar fossa surrounding the right temporomandibular articulation and in the adjacent left skull base, but the left temporal bone was not affected. A remarkable observation was the extensive bony spiculation of the hyperostotic bone in the skull base (Fig. 27.41). The T2-weighted magnetic resonance image showed an increased linear signal intensity in the right sphenoid and temporal bone, which is rather characteristic for a meningioma (Fig. 27.42).

At *operation,* the right external auditory canal was opened, and an external cholesteatoma was removed. The osseous canal was reconstructed, and a Silastic tubal stent to prevent future restenosis was inserted. The histologic examination confirmed the diagnosis of an en plaque meningioma of the meningotheliomatous variety (Fig. 27.43).

References

1. Rubinstein LJL. Tumors of the central nervous system. In: Atlas of tumor pathology. 2nd series, Fascicle 6. Washington, DC: Armed Forces Institute of Pathology, 1972.
2. Zülch KJ. Brain tumors: their biology and pathology. 3rd ed. Berlin: Springer Verlag, 1986.
3. Nager GT. Meningiomas involving the temporal bone: clinical and pathological aspects. Springfield, Illinois: Charles C Thomas, 1964.
4. Nager GT, Masica DN. Meningiomas of the cerebellopontine angle and their relation to the temporal bone. Laryngoscope 1970;80:863–895.
5. Nager GT. Meningiomas invading the temporal bone with extension to the neck. Am J Otolaryngol 1983;4:297–342.
6. Farr HW, Gray GF Jr, Vrana M, et al. Extracranial meningiomas. J Surg Oncol 1973;5:411–20.
7. Hoye SJ, Hoar CS, Murray JE. Extracranial meningioma presenting as a tumor of the neck. Am J Surg 1960;100:486–489.
8. Shuangshoti S, Netsky MG, Fitz-Hugh GS. Parapharyngeal meningioma with special reference to cell of origin. Ann Otol Laryngol Rhinol 1971;80:464–473.
9. Shaheen HB. Psammoma of the maxillary antrum. J Laryngol 1931;46:117.
10. Zachariae LA. A case of extracranial primary meningioma. Acta Pathol Microbiol Scand 1952;33:57–60.
11. Conley JJ, Jack GT, Trinidad SS. Surgical technique of removal of infratemporal meningioma. Laryngoscope 1956;66:540–549.
12. Pendergrass EP, Hope JW. An extracranial meningioma with no apparent intracranial source. Report of a case. Am J Roentgenol 1953;70:967–970.
13. Bain GO, Shnitka TK. Cutaneous meningioma (psammoma): report of a case. Arch Dermatol 1956;74:590–594.
14. Suzuki H, Gilbert EF, Zimmerman B. Primary extracranial meningioma. Arch Pathol 1967;84:202–206.
15. Hallgrimsson J, Bojoernsson A, Gudmundsson G. Meningioma of the neck: case report. J Neurosurg 1970;32:695–699.
16. Nager GT. Association of bilateral VIIIth nerve tumors with meningiomas in von Recklinghausen's disease. Laryngoscope 1964;74:1220–1261.
17. Craig WM, Geogela LH. Intraorbital meningioma: a clinicopathological study. Am J Ophthalmol 1949;32:1663–1680.
18. Russell DS, Rubinstein LG. Pathology of tumors of the nervous system. 5th ed. Baltimore: William & Wilkins, 1989.
19. Jurow HN. Psammomatous dural endothelioma (meningioma) with pulmonary metastasis. Arch Pathol 1941;32:222–226.
20. Opsahl R Jr. Meningioma with metastasis to cervical lymph nodes: case report. Acta Pathol Microbiol Scand 1965;64:294–298.
21. Robertson B. Case of meningioma with extracranial metastases. Acta Pathol Microbiol Scand 1970;48:335–340.
22. Shuangshoti S, Hongsaprabbas C, Netsky MG. Metastasizing meningioma. Cancer 1970;26:832–841.
23. Gibbs NM. Meningioma with extracranial metastasis. J Pathol Bacteriol 1958;76:285–288.
24. Kruse F. Meningeal tumors with extracranial metastasis. Neurology 1960;10:197–201.
25. Christensen E, Kiaer W, Winblad S. Meningeal tumors with extracranial metastases. Br J Cancer 1949;3:485–493.
26. Hamblet JB. Meningioma with metastases to liver. Arch Pathol 1944;37:216–218.

28/ Gliomas

The international classification of tumors of the central nervous system that are of neuroepithelial origin includes: astrocytic tumors, oligodendroglial, ependymal, and choroid plexus tumors, pineal cell tumors, neuronal tumors, and poorly differentiated and embryonal tumors (1). Each category contains several subgroups. Among these categories, there are a few tumors that are of interest to the neuro-otologist because they occasionally have to be considered in the differential diagnosis of cerebellopontine angle lesions and rarely may involve the temporal bone. The five tumors here reported include two glioblastomas, two astrocytomes, and a cerebellar medulloblastoma. All were diagnosed and classified by the pathologist. In all of them the autopsy of the brain was performed several decades ago. It is, therefore, conceivable that one or the other of these neoplasms might be classified differently today. Such a change, however, would in all likelihood involve only a shift in subgroup rather than one in category. The characteristic features of each of these three neoplasms are being mentioned briefly to facilitate the understanding of their biology and local behavior.

ASTROCYTOMAS

Astrocytomas display considerable variation in their gross appearance, morphology, stages of differentiation, and clinical behavior. According to their clinicopathologic features and biologic behavior, astrocytomas may be divided into the diffuse cerebral astrocytoma of adults, the solid and cystic cerebellar astrocytomas of children, the juvenile pilocystic astrocytoma of the third ventricle, hypothalamus, and chiasm of children and adolescents, the diffuse pontine astrocytoma of children, and the astrocytoma of the spinal cord (2).

Incidence, Age, and Sex Distribution

Astrocytomas constitute about 25–30% of all cerebral gliomas (2), which in turn account for about 45% of all intracranial tumors (1, 3). The various tumor locations often display a predilection for a certain age group. Thus, astrocytomas of the cerebral hemisphere are often found in the third and fourth decades of life, whereas lesions in the hypothalamic region, cerebellum, and pons are primarily observed in children and adolescents. Men are affected more often than women (2).

Clinical Symptoms

Astrocytoma of the cerebellum generally remains benign and only occasionally displays a tendency toward malignant degeneration. It produces symptoms and signs of a posterior fossa tumor. Astrocytoma of the pons often mimics a subacute brain stem encephalitis with involvement of cranial nerve nuclei and long tract signs (2).

Macroscopic Appearance

The astrocytoma of the cerebellum originates in either the lateral lobes or the vermis, frequently involving both. At times, it may be predominantly intraventricular. The tumors are usually well demarcated. Diffuse forms are rare and generally found in the older age groups.

The pontine astrocytoma of children typically presents as a gross, usually symmetrical, nodular enlargement of the pons and medulla. It may bulge into the fourth ventricle and extend, like a tongue, ventrally into the subarachnoid space (2).

GLIOBLASTOMA MULTIFORME

Glioblastoma multiforme exemplifies the most anaplastic form of a primary intracranial neoplasm in the adult. It is regarded as an extreme manifestation of anaplasia and dedifferentiation of a mature, predominantly astrocytic, glial tumor cell. In most instances, the glioblastoma probably arises by anaplasia from a preexisting small astrocytoma (2). It represents over 50% of all primary gliomas. Its highest incidence is in patients between ages 45 and 55. Males are affected more frequently than females, with the ratio being 3:2 (2).

Clinical Symptoms

Progressive rise of intracranial pressure and focal signs dependent on tumor localization, usually developing over a period of less than 6 months, characterize the rapid growth of the neoplasm.

Preferential Locations

Glioblastoma multiforme, which characteristically involves the white matter, may originate in any area of the central nervous system. The frontal lobes are most frequently involved, and many times, more than one lobe is affected. The deeper structures, especially the corpus callosum, are often affected. The "butterfly" pattern of a tumor presentation in coronal sections with tumor growth in either cerebral hemisphere, linked to the opposite side through the corpus callosum, is highly characteristic. The temporal lobe is next in frequency of involvement. The cerebellum, pons, and medulla are infrequent primary sites. Multiple foci are not infrequent and are observed in 2.5–5% of tumors (1, 2).

Macroscopic Appearance

The glioblastoma, when restricted to a single lobe, tends to be more or less spherical and appears relatively well circumscribed, with somewhat ill-defined margins. When several areas of the brain are involved, the outline becomes more irregular. One or more cysts are often found (1, 2).

Microscopic Appearance

The salient features of the glioblastoma multiforme, as its name suggests, are the high cellularity and either the relative uniformity or the extreme pleomorphism of the tumor cells with many intermediate stages. Anaplastic tumor cells of astrocytic lineage often tend to cluster around central areas of various stages of necrosis. This results in the classic formation of pseudopalisades that become a diagnostic feature in the identification of a glioblastoma multiforme (1–3).

The most typical vascular changes include: (a) the proliferation of the vascular endothelium; (b) the focal increase of thin-walled capillary blood vessels, producing a telangiectatic pattern; and (c) the increase of perivascular fibrous connective tissue, which creates a typical lacy pattern. A superficially located tumor tends to invade the adjacent meninges. There are two known instances in which a left parietal glioblastoma has invaded the adjacent sagittal sinus and its tributary veins (4). Likewise, direct extension to bone has been observed in the tegmental area of the temporal bone in a boy with a massive glioblastoma of the temporal lobe and in a girl with a temporal lobe glioblastoma that had eroded through the greater wing of the sphenoid and the sella turcica (1). There are also two instances of transdural extension of a glioblastoma of the temporal lobe with invasion and extensive destruction of the underlying temporal bone (5, 6).

MEDULLOBLASTOMA

Definition

The medulloblastoma is an embryonic tumor limited to the cerebellum and consisting of poorly differentiated cells whose origin has been attributed to two principal sources: the fetal external granular layer of the cerebellar cortex and the remnants of the primitive cells in the posterior and anterior medullary velum (2, 7–10). By the end of the first year of life, the cells that constitute the external granular layer have migrated inward to form the majority of neurons in the definitive internal granular cell layer; in addition, they differentiate and form the cortical neuroglia (1, 11, 12).

Incidence, Age, and Sex Distribution

Medulloblastomas represent the second most frequent brain tumor in children. Over 50% occur during the first decade of life, with a maximal incidence near the end of that period (1, 3, 10). About 30% develop between ages 15 and 35. The remaining few may be found in the fifth decade of life. Males are affected more frequently than females, with the ratio being about 4:3 (2). Familial occurrence has been reported (2, 13).

Locations

Most medulloblastomas, especially in children, are situated along the midline (2, 10), mostly adjacent to the cisterna magna and the cavity of the fourth ventricle. A minority are

located laterally in the cerebellar hemispheres, and these are mainly found in adults. In some instances, a medulloblastoma may develop in the region of the cerebellar tonsil or in the cerebellopontine angle (1, 2).

Macroscopic Appearance

The midline tumors in children are generally well demarcated. Tumors arising from the vermis may occupy the lumen of the fourth ventricle and infiltrate the floor. Tumors originating in the lateral hemisphere in adults are smooth or somewhat lobulated. They often appear on the surface of a hemisphere, frequently on its dorsal aspect. At times, a medulloblastoma may spread "en plaque" over the surface of the cerebellum, or it may infiltrate a hemisphere extensively in a diffuse manner (1).

Microscopic Appearance

The prominent features of the medulloblastoma are its extreme cellularity, the lack of a definite architectural pattern, the small, spheroidal, oval, or polar darkly stained cells with a scanty cytoplasm, and the round or oval hyperchromatic nuclei of various sizes. Mitotic figures are highly variable (1, 2).

Clinical Behavior

The cerebellar medulloblastoma is highly malignant. The laterally situated tumors in adults carry a more favorable prognosis over those located along the midline in children. The survival rate in adults varies from 6 months to 8 years. Infiltration of the subarachnoid space is frequent and develops early. Metastatic dissemination through the cerebrospinal fluid pathway is a common event. The spread may be diffuse or nodular. Intraventricular dissemination, more frequently nodular, is also common. Extraneural metastases have been documented, whereby a craniotomy has often paved the way. Remote metastases involve primarily the bone marrow and the regional cervical lymph nodes (2).

Case Reports

Case 1. *Giant cell glioblastoma of right temporofrontal region with extension to and beyond meninges and massive invasion and destruction of underlying temporal bone (Fig. 28.1). Protrusion of tumor through tympanic membrane into right external auditory canal. Secondary tympanomastoiditis. Several microscopic abscesses in right temporal and frontal lobes.*

A 41-year-old man was seen who 4 months prior to admission developed otalgia in the right postauricular region, increasing right occipital headaches, and unsteadiness with a tendency to fall. One month prior to admission, the patient noticed progressive loss of hearing and tinnitus in the right ear and right-sided facial twitching and purulent discharge from that ear. An otologic examination at that time disclosed a growth in the right external auditory canal. A biopsy was suggestive of a malignant tumor. The patient, however, did not return for another biopsy. Three days prior to admission, the patient developed a paralysis of the right face and difficulties with swallowing and speech. He was admitted to a regional Veterans' Administration hospital.

Neurologic examination revealed: (a) involvement of right cranial nerves V, VI, VII, and VIII, (b) unsteadiness of gait, (c) myosis of the right pupil, (d) motor weakness involving both upper extremi-

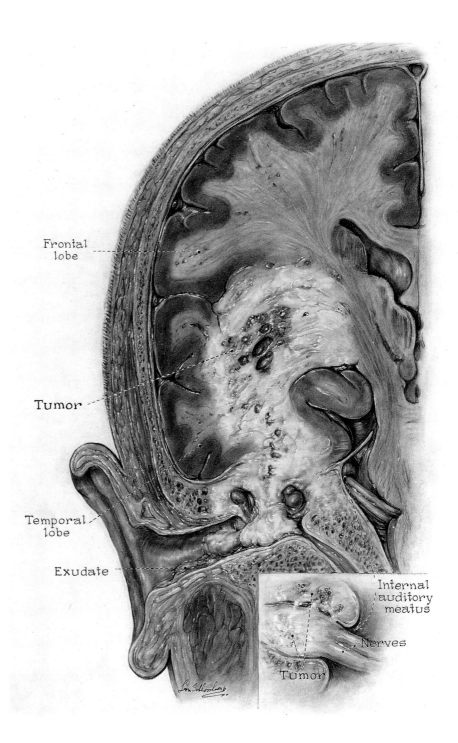

Figure 28.1.   Illustration of giant cell glioblastoma in right temporofrontal region and its extension to meninges, and massive invasion and obstruction of right temporal bone. The tumor protrudes from the middle ear through the tympanic membrane into the right external auditory canal.

ties, *(e)* slow cerebration and dysarthria, and *(f)* tenderness to percussion over the calvaria. Microscopic evaluation and chemical analysis of the cerebrospinal fluid and blood, except for an elevated sedimentation rate, were normal.

Otologic examination disclosed a reddish, soft tumor mass in the osseous portion of the right external auditory canal, tenderness of the right mastoid process, but no evidence of a postauricular infiltration or fluctuation. Cochlear function studies showed a profound mixed hearing loss in the right ear with a pure-tone average of 90 dB in the right ear and a mild sensorineural loss in the left ear. There was no spontaneous nystagmus.

Radiologic examination showed a large area of bone destruction involving the right middle ear, epitympanic recess, mastoid antrum, and petrous pyramid (Fig. 28.2).

The first biopsy was suggestive but not diagnostic of a malignant tumor. The second biopsy was diagnosed of anaplastic carcinoma (Fig. 28.3). The further course in the hospital was characterized by rapid deterioration of the patient's general condition, increasing intracranial pressure, and loss of consciousness. Death occurred in coma 26 days after admission. The postmortem examination revealed a softening in the anterior region on the right temporal lobe. The right temporal lobe was everywhere firmly attached to the dura lining the right middle cranial fossa and to the underlying right temporal bone. In the area where the temporal lobe was adherent to the base of the skull, the substance of the brain was friable and disclosed a grayish-green discoloration. Coronal cross-sections of the brain revealed the presence of tumor tissue in the inferior and anterior portions of the right temporal lobe, involving the subcortical and cortical regions of the brain and invading the overlying meninges (Fig. 28.1). Small hemorrhagic areas were present in the convolutions of the anterior portion of the temporal lobe, and a larger irregular hemorrhagic area was found in the subcortical region of the posterior portion of the right frontal lobe. The temporal horn of the right ventricle was slightly displaced; however, there was no evidence of a tumor extension to the ventricular wall.

Histologic examination of the right temporal and frontal lobes revealed extensive areas of necrosis and infiltration with polymorphonuclear leukocytes. Several abscesses of varying size were noted. Some of them were surrounded by foci of tumor cells. These tumor cells exhibited marked polymorphism with large, irregular, and bizarre cell forms, hyperchromatism, abundant mitotic figures, and many abnormal mitoses (Fig. 28.4). Tumor giant cells were found in several areas. The brain tumor, examined at an outside institution, had been erroneously interpreted as an undifferentiated carcinoma of the right middle ear with extension to the petrous pyramid, meninges, middle cranial fossa, and temporal and frontal lobes of the brain.

Microscopic examination of the right temporal bone reveals a massive invasion and extensive destruction by a neoplasm consisting predominantly of pleomorphic cells, some mixed with bizarre giant cells, separated into sheets and strands covered by a dense vascular connective tissue stroma (Fig. 28.5). The nuclei of the tumor cells are large and display great variation in form and chromatin content. The cytoplasm is abundant and has a coarse granular appearance. The cell boundaries are distinct. Mitoses are numerous, and atypical mitotic figures are frequent. In some areas, many bizarre hyperchromatic multinucleated giant cells are found (Fig. 28.5E). In certain regions the tumor cells are less pleomorphic, more uniform, and reminiscent of the spindle cell variety.

Two features of this tumor are remarkable: *(a)* the great amount of connective tissue formation and its diffuse distribution throughout the tumor; and *(b)* the marked proliferation of blood vessels of every caliber, from capillaries to large lacunar vessels, of predominantly venous type. Many of these vessels form numerous coils and loops. Some of these vessels are indigenous, but most are newly formed. Perivascular cell cuffs, i.e., tumor cells arranged in a multicellular layer around a blood vessel, are frequent (Fig. 28.5D). Smaller and larger areas of hemorrhages are seen throughout the tumor, and an occasional one is located around a rupture of the wall of such an ectatic newly formed vessel. Some vessels display proliferation of the intima and adventitia and some thrombotic occlusions; thus, necrosis of tumor tissue is frequently found, and the tumor cells are often arranged in pseudopalisades around such areas of necrosis (Fig. 28.5B, D, and E).

Invasion of the right petrous pyramid and mastoid process obviously occurred through the tegmen and the roof of the Eustachian tube where vast areas of bone have been destroyed and where tumor is continuous with the main portion of the neoplasm in the middle cranial fossa (Figs. 28.6–28.11). In the middle ear, the neoplasm completely destroyed the Fallopian canal and facial nerve and the semicanal of the tensor tympani muscle as well as the muscle itself (Figs. 28.5A and 28.8–28.11). Invasion of the canaliculus of the chorda tympani and of the petrotympanic fissure has caused the destruction of the chorda at several levels. The middle ear ossicles, although deeply embedded in the neoplasm, have remained intact (Figs. 28.9–28.11). Large tumor masses cover the oval and round window niches, but there is no invasion of the stapedial footplate, annular ligament, or round window membrane (Figs. 28.9 and 28.10). Wide areas of the tympanic membrane are infiltrated, and tumor tissue protrudes through the posterior half of the pars tensa into the external auditory canal (Figs. 28.10 and 28.11). The entire petrous apex and the overlying fifth and sixth cranial nerves are destroyed (Figs. 28.6). The destruction includes the entire osseous and part of the cartilaginous portion of the Eustachian tube as well as the entire bony canal of the carotid artery. Tumor cells surround the internal carotid artery and infiltrate the internal carotid and deep petrosal nerves (Fig. 28.6). Invasion of bone occurs along pneumatic cells, marrow spaces, preformed vascular and other channels, and, above all, by the destructive activity of the tumor cells (Figs. 28.5–28.10). In the otic capsule, infiltration of bone is limited to the periosteal and endochondral layers. Nowhere has the neoplasm advanced to the endosteal layer or actively invaded the perilymphatic or endolymphatic spaces. The internal auditory canal is completely occupied by tumor tissue (Figs. 28.5, 28.7, and 28.8), which extends along the labyrinthine segment of the Fallopian canal (Figs. 28.5 and 28.8) and through localized bone destruction in the roof into the epidural space along the roof of the internal meatus. As a result, the facial and vestibular nerves are completely destroyed, but the cochlear nerve shows only partial destruction. Tumor cells can be traced through the tractus spiralis foraminosus into the cochlear modiolus and through the superior and inferior vestibular areas along the subdivisions of the vestibular nerve. Extensive autolytic changes preclude evaluation of the cochlear and vestibular end organs, the stria vascularis, and the external sulcus cells. The vascular and neural compartments of the jugular foramen are free of tumor tissue.

Histologic examination of the left temporal bone reveals no evidence of tumor tissue anywhere. The bony structures and the membranous cochlea and vestibular labyrinth are intact.

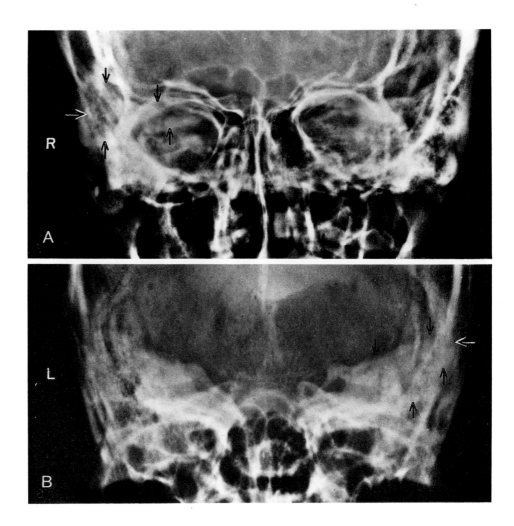

Figure 28.2. **A.** Transorbital projection (posteroanterior). **B.** Occipital projection (posteroanterior). *Arrows* point to the area of the right mastoid antrum and petrous pyramid where bone destruction and the tumor infiltration are obvious.

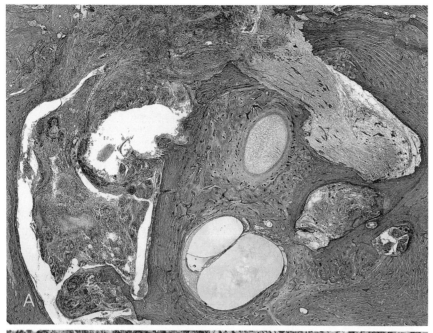

Figure 28.5. **A.** Vertical section through right temporal bone near posterior tangent of second turn of cochlea. The glioblastoma has invaded the tympanic cavity and the internal acoustic meatus through the tegmental region where it had caused extensive osseous destruction. (Hematoxylin and eosin, ×11.)

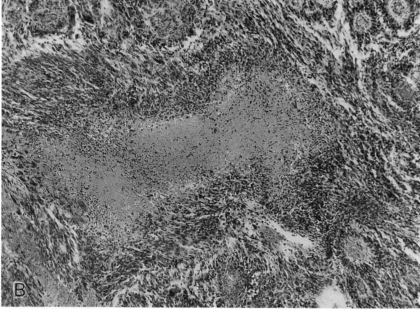

Figure 28.5. **B.** A higher magnification of the tumor in the middle ear shows a central region of necrosis surrounded by tumor cells arranged in pseudopalisades. (×100.)

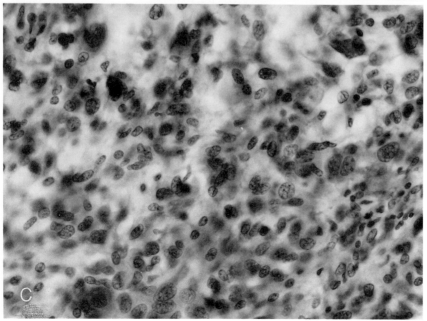

Figure 28.5. **C.** The nuclei of the tumor cells display great variation in size, form, and chromatin content. Mitoses are frequent and often atypical. (×450.)

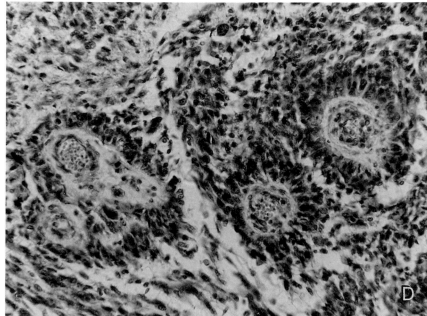

Figure 28.5. **D.** Numerous perivascular cell cuffs are found in this area. The perivascular arrangement of the tumor cells is probably due to the favorable nutrition in these locations. (×300.)

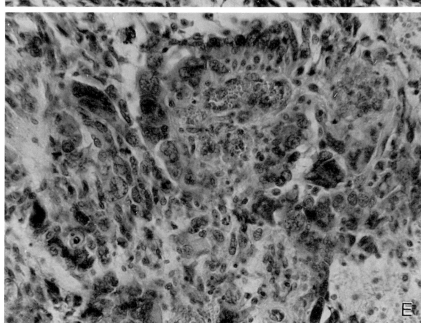

Figure 28.5. **E.** In this area the tumor cells are arranged in a crown-like pattern, radially, around a nutrient vessel; with their "vascular feet" some tumor cells are attached to the vessel wall. Note the numerous hyperchromatic, multinucleated giant cells. (×300.)

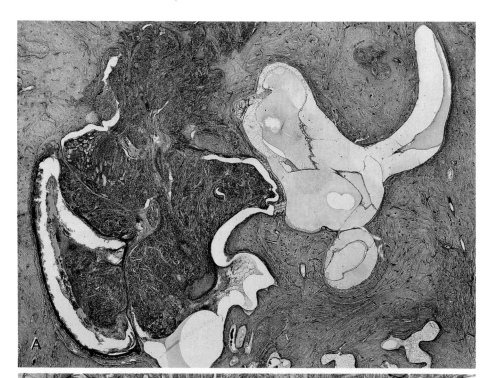

Figure 28.10.   A. Vertical section through right petrous pyramid near posterior end of oval window. The glioblastoma within the middle ear has invaded the tympanic membrane and the external auditory canal. (Hematoxylin and eosin, ×8.)

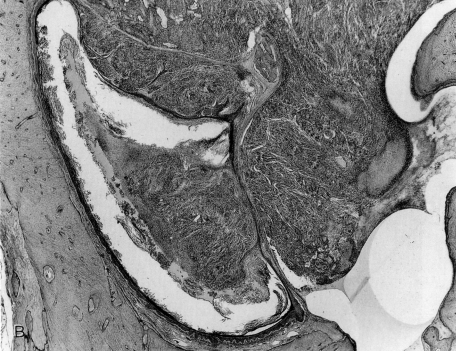

Figure 28.10.   B. In the upper portion of the tympanic membrane, a large tumor mass separates the epidermal from the fibrous layer of the pars tensa. (×18.)

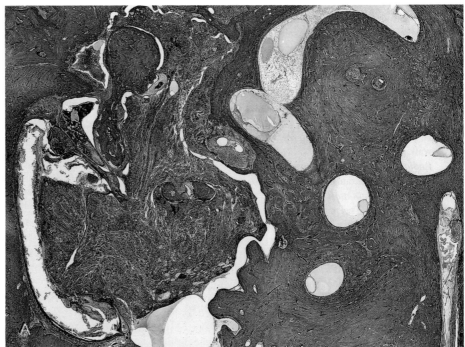

Figure 28.11.   A. Vertical section through right petrous pyramid at level of head of malleus and incudostapedial articulation. The glioblastoma extends from the middle ear through a perforation in the tympanic cavity into the outer ear canal. (Hematoxylin and eosin, ×8.)

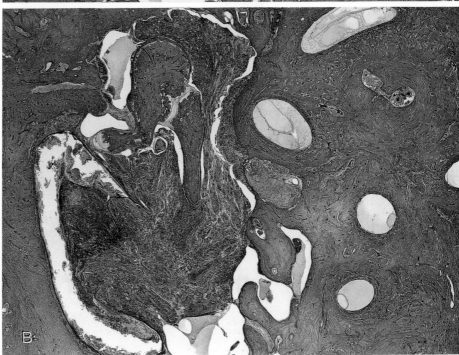

Figure 28.11.   B. Vertical section through right petrous pyramid at level of incudomalleolar articulation. The glioblastoma that invades the external auditory canal through a posterior pars tensa perforation has left the malleus and incus intact. (×8.)

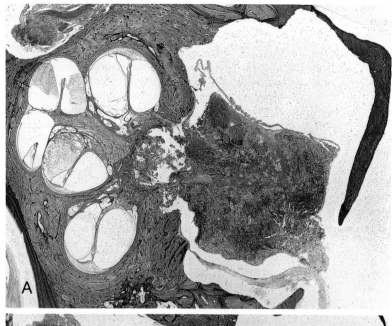

Figure 28.13.   A. Vertical midmodiolar section through right petrous pyramid. Long-standing increased intracranial pressure and erosion of bone by the glioblastoma resulted in marked irregular widening of the internal auditory canal and localized destruction of its roof. (Hematoxylin and eosin, ×11.)

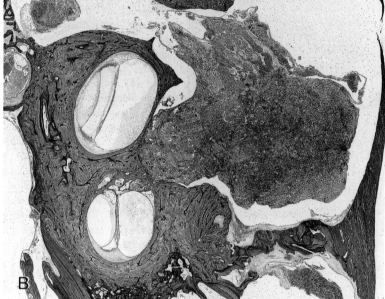

Figure 28.13.   B. Vertical section through right petrous pyramid at level of geniculate ganglion. The medulloblastoma extends to the geniculate ganglion along the labyrinthine segment of the Fallopian canal. The tumor has also invaded the jugular foramen. (×11.)

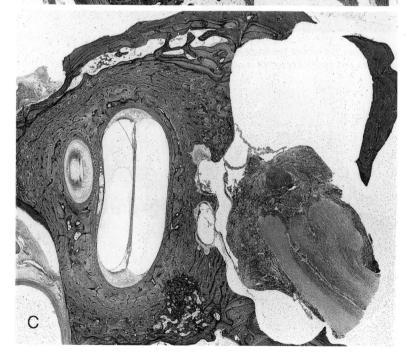

Figure 28.13.   C. Vertical paramodiolar section through right petrous pyramid. The medulloblastoma caused an irregular erosion of the walls of the internal auditory canal and a firm investment of the seventh and eighth cranial nerves. (×11.)

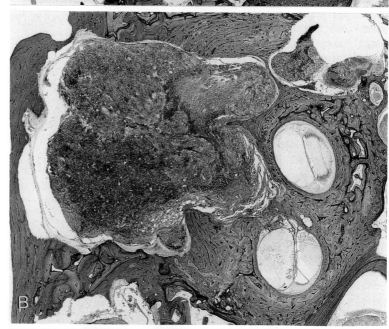

Figure 28.14. **A.** Vertical midmodiolar section through left petrous pyramid. The widening of the internal auditory canal and the partial erosion of its roof are very similar to the respective changes found on the opposite side. (Hematoxylin and eosin, ×11.)

Figure 28.14. **B.** The invasion of the geniculate ganglion by the medulloblastoma occurred along the Fallopian canal. The irregular enlargement of the neural compartment of the jugular foramen resulted from tumor invasion. (×11.)

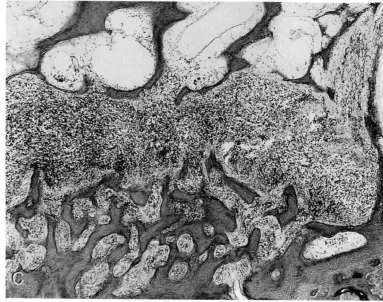

Figure 28.14. **C.** The medulloblastoma extends from the internal acoustic meatus to the cochlear modiolus along the cochlear nerve fibers. (×75.)

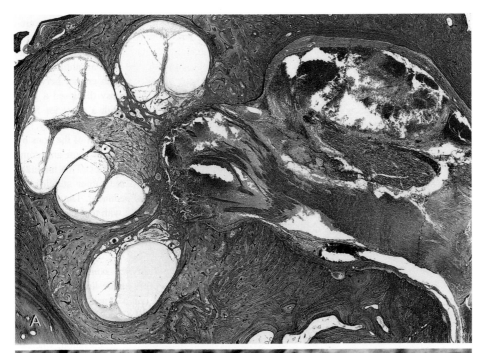

Figure 28.16. **A.** Vertical midmodiolar section through right petrous pyramid. The glioblastoma of the pons that had protruded into the right cerebellopontine angle and internal auditory canal produced a slight enlargement of the meatus and degeneration of the seventh and eighth cranial nerves. (Hematoxylin and eosin, ×14.)

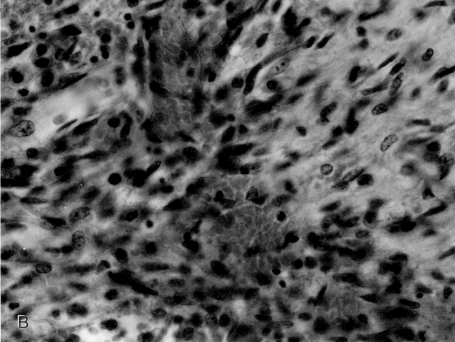

Figure 28.16. **B.** The tumor cells in this area are of the spindle cell variety. (×500.)

Case 4. *Astrocytoma of left temporal lobe with invasion of left lateral ventricle and diffuse metastases to meninges of cerebrum, cerebellum, brain stem, and cervical cord. Multiple cysts in pineal body (Fig. 28.17).*

A 33-year-old woman was seen who 2 months prior to admission had developed occipital headaches and projectile vomiting, 3 weeks later had developed weakness in her arms and legs, during the next 5 weeks had developed bilateral progressive loss of vision, and 1 week prior to admission had had difficulties on swallowing.

Neurologic examination revealed: *(a)* internal and subtotal external ophthalmoplegia, papilledema, and total loss of vision bilaterally; *(b)* generalized muscular weakness; *(c)* absence of deep tendon reflexes; *(d)* disorientation and slow cerebration; *(e)* nuchal rigidity; and *(f)* emaciation.

Otologic examination disclosed a history of recurrent otitis media in childhood, resulting in poor hearing in the right ear, with further

and progressive loss in that ear over the past 4–5 years. The left eardrum was normal, but the right was slightly retracted, thickened, and partially calcified. The pure tone audiogram by air conduction, performed in the usually noisy ward, disclosed a flat loss bilaterally with a pure tone average of 70 dB in the right ear and 50 dB in the left ear. No tuning fork tests were performed. Vestibular function studies disclosed no spontaneous nystagmus and a regular response to cold caloric stimulation of the left ear. Cold stimulation of the right ear induced no nystagmus to the left, on account of the patient's subtotal external ophthalmoplegia; there was a definite sensation of vertigo, however, when each ear was stimulated.

A ventricular estimation showed a block at the left foramen of Monro and in the Sylvian aqueduct. The patient's general condition rapidly deteriorated, and death occurred 8 days after admission.

Autopsy of the brain showed a 7×5×4-cm tumor in the left temporal lobe that extended from the anterior pole of the temporal lobe to within 1 cm from the posterior horn of the left lateral ventri-

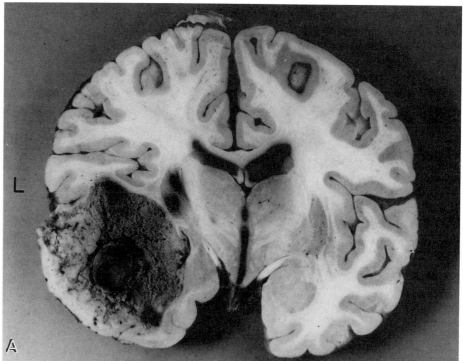

Figure 28.17. A. Coronal section through brain at midthalamus level, showing a large astrocytoma involving the left temporal lobe and a portion of the amygdala.

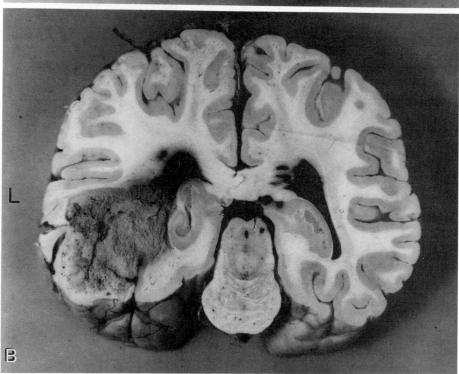

Figure 28.17. B. Coronal section of brain, showing the tumor involving the posterior temporal lobe and invading the left lateral ventricle.

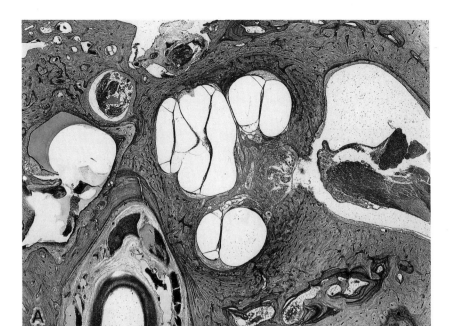

Figure 28.18.   A. Vertical paramodiolar section through right petrous pyramid. There is a metastasis in the subarachnoid space of the internal auditory canal. (Hematoxylin and eosin, ×10.)

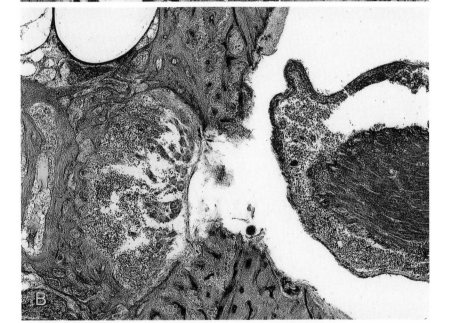

Figure 28.18.   B. The metastasis is from the astrocytoma in the left temporal lobe. It is located in the subarachnoid space and surrounds the right cochlear nerve. Note the presence of tumor cells within the cochlear modiolus. (×35.)

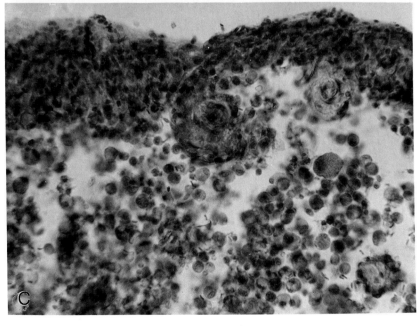

Figure 28.18.   C. Most tumor cells have a spherical cell body that varies considerably in size. Most tumor cells include vacuoles and 2 nuclei. (×300.)

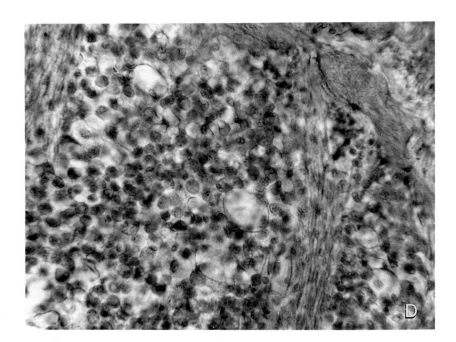

Figure 28.18.   D. The tumor is invading the cochlear modiolus through the tractus spiralis foraminosus along the perineural spaces. (×300.)

cle (Fig. 28.17). The tumor was sharply demarcated, its center was necrotic, and the tumor mass formed the wall of the posterior horn of the ventricle, where it became continuous with a blood clot that filled the ventricle. The meninges of the cerebellum showed areas of thickening suggesting tumor infiltration. The tumor proved to be an astrocytoma. Sections through the cerebrum, cerebellum, brain stem, and cervical cord disclosed extensive tumor infiltration of the meninges.

Microscopic examination of the temporal bones reveals almost identical observations. Metastases from the astrocytoma in the left temporal lobe are present in the subarachnoid space of both the internal acoustic meatus and the neural compartments of the jugular foramen (Figs. 28.18 and 28.19). The tumor formed a diffuse sheet attached to the arachnoid, which envelops portions of and infiltrates the seventh and eighth cranial nerves (Figs. 28.18*B* and *D* and 28.19*B* and *C*). Tumor cells can be followed through the tractus spiralis foraminosus into the cochlear mediolus (Fig. 28.18*B* and *D*) and

through the superior and inferior vestibular areas along the subdivision of the vestibular nerve. In the neural compartment of the jugular foramen, islands of tumor tissue surround the ninth, tenth, and eleventh cranial nerves. The tumor cells are closely packed, and the cell bodies have a spherical shape, varying considerably in size (Fig. 28.18*C* and *D*). Many include vacuoles. Their cytoplasm is coarsely granular. Their nuclei vary in size and chromatin content, and the majority display an eccentric position. Many cells contain 2 nuclei. Mitotic figures are fairly frequent, and a few multinucleated giant cells are seen. These metastases obviously reached the meninges along the cerebrospinal fluid pathway from the posterior horn of the left lateral ventricle, which was invaded by the tumor. Additional findings included a massive tympanosclerotic process completely obliterating the entire right middle ear, and an otosclerotic lesion involving the anterior inferior margin of the left oval window with some localized distortion of the vestibular fenestra but not causing an ankylosis of the stapes footplate.

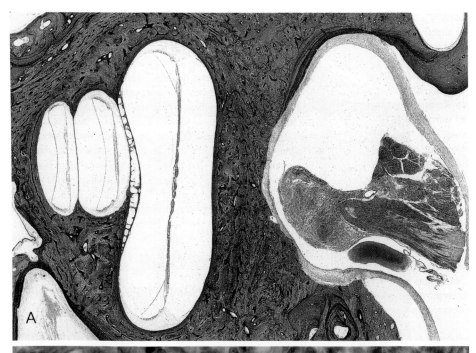

Figure 28.20.   A. Vertical paramodiolar section through right petrous pyramid, showing the location and extent of the metastasis in the internal acoustic canal. (Hematoxylin and eosin, ×15.)

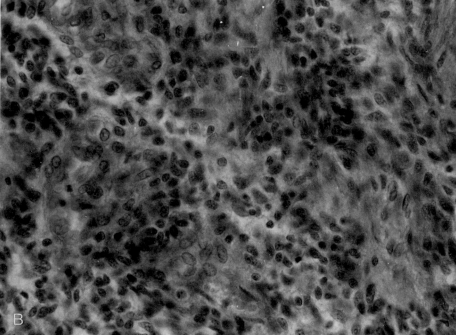

Figure 28.20.   B. The metastasis is from the astrocytoma in the tegmental region of the cerebellum. It is located in the subarachnoid space where it envelops the seventh and eighth cranial nerves. The morphology of the tumor is well recognized. (×500.)

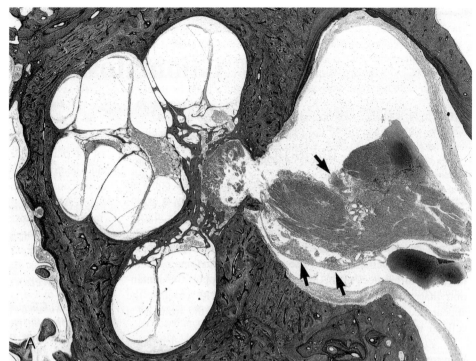

Figure 28.21.   A. Vertical midmodiolar section through right petrous pyramid. *Arrows* point to the sheets and islands of tumor cells in the internal auditory canal between the seventh and eighth cranial nerves. (Hematoxylin and eosin, ×14.)

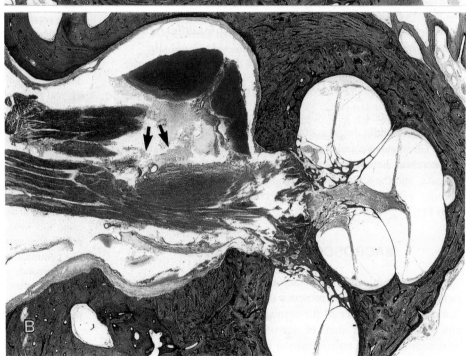

Figure 28.21.   B. Vertical midmodiolar section through left petrous pyramid. *Arrows* are the same as for Figure 28.21*A.* (×14.)

References

1. Russell DS, Rubinstein, LJ. Pathology of tumors of the nervous system. 5th ed. Baltimore: Williams & Wilkins, 1989.

2. Rubinstein LJ. Tumors of the central nervous system. In: Atlas of tumor pathology. 2nd series, Fascicle 6. Washington, DC: Armed Forces Institute of Pathology, 1972.

3. Zülch KJ. Brain tumors. Their biology and pathology. 3rd ed. Berlin: Springer-Verlag, 1986.

4. Rubinstein LJ. Development of extracranial metastases from a malignant astrocytoma in the absence of previous craniotomy. J Neurosurg 1967; 26:542–547.

5. Sanerkin NG. Transdural spread of glioblastoma multiforme. J Pathol Bacteriol 1962;84:228–233.

6. Nager GT. Gliomas involving the temporal bone. Clinical and pathological aspects. Laryngoscope 1967;77:454–488.

7. Stevenson L, Echlin F. Nature and origin of some tumors of the cerebellum-medulloblastoma. Arch Neurol Psychiatry 1934;31:93–109.

8. Kershman J. The medulloblast and the medulloblastoma: a study of human embryos. Arch Neurol Psychiatry 1938;40:937–967.

9. Raaf J, Kernohan JW. Relation of abnormal collections of cells in posterior medullary velum of cerebellum to origin of medulloblastoma. Arch Neurol Psychiatry 1944;52:163–169.

10. Ringertz N, Tola JH. Medulloblastoma. J Neuropathol Exp Neurol 1950; 9:354–372.

11. Fugita S. Quantitative analysis of cell proliferation and differentiation in the cortex of the postnatal mouse cerebellum. J Cell Biol 1967;32:277–288.

12. Kadin ME, Rubinstein LJ, Nelson JS. Neonatal cerebellar meduloblastoma originating from the fetal external granular layer. J Neuropathol Exp Neurol 1970;29:583–600.

13. Bickerstaff ER, Connolly RC, Woolf AL. Cerebellar medulloblastoma occurring in brothers. Acta Neuropathol 1967;8:104–107.

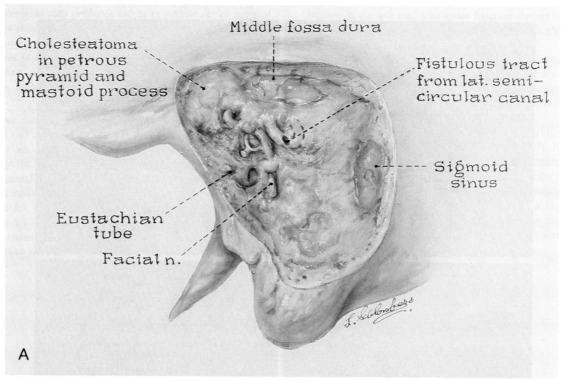

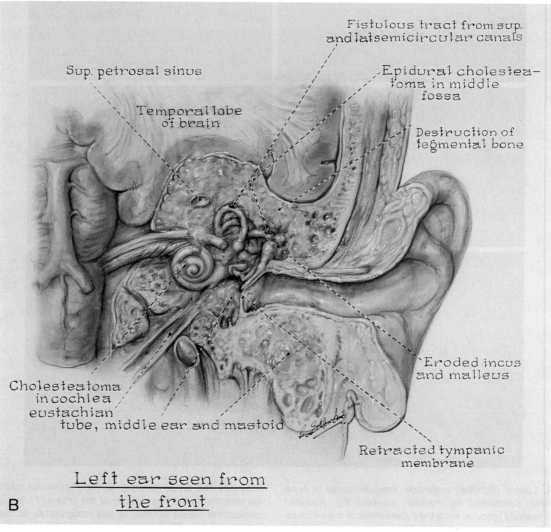

Figure 30.7. **A.** Illustration of epidermoid that had originated in the left mastoid process and had destroyed the major portion of the mastoid bone and posterior petrous pyramid. It had widely exposed the middle fossa dura and sigmoid sinus and had surrounded the facial nerve in each of its three intratemporal segments. **B.** Illustration of involvement of left temporal bone by epidermoid and of its extension through the anterior wall of the pyramid into the middle cranial fossa.

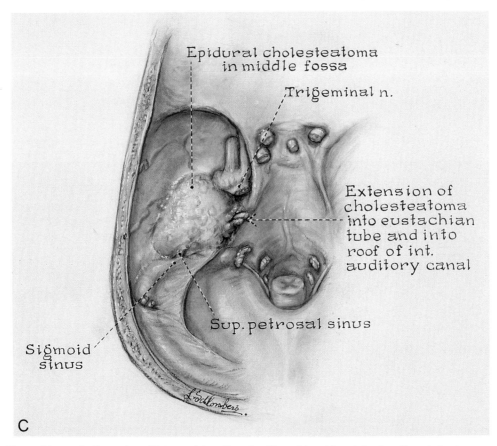

Figure 30.7.   C. Illustration of intracranial portion of epidermoid and its relation to adjacent structures.

Case 4. *Diploic epidermoid with origin in left occipital bone. Destruction of major portion of occipital squama, posterior half of petrous pyramid, mastoid process, and adjacent parietal bone. Extension posteriorly to external occipital protuberance and inferiorly to foramen magnum. Orange-sized lesion in left posterior cranial fossa, with compression and displacement of cerebellar hemisphere and exposure of descending portion of left Fallopian canal.*

For the past 10 years, the patient, a 60-year-old physician, had noticed some tenderness in the left postauricular area. For the past 2 months, he had had a persistent pulsatile tinnitus in his left ear, and more recently he had noticed some fullness in that ear and left-sided facial twitching. Throughout life he had suffered with diffuse headaches localized to the vertex, and he had become severely depressed. He attributed some difficulties to worsening of his Parkinson's disease, diagnosed 7 years previously. He reported no history of otalgia or otorrhea and had noticed no other cranial nerve involvement.

Otologic examination revealed intact tympanic membranes, normal cochlear function bilaterally, and evidence of some left-sided vestibular disturbance, not localizing centrally or peripherally. Facial twitching involving the left orbicularis oculi muscle was evident. A palpable marginal hyperostosis was noted along the border of the underlying osteolytic bony defect in the calvaria. Some firm, fibrous horizontal strands were palpable in the skin over the neck, extending between the mastoid tips, probably reflecting reactive connective tissue hyperplasia induced by the underlying irritating cyst.

Radiologic examination showed an extensive irregular radiolucent defect involving the greater part of the left occipital bone, adjacent parietal bone, posterior half of the petrous pyramid, and mastoid process (Fig. 30.8*A* and *B*). The defect extended posteriorly to the inion, inferiorly to the foramen magnum, and laterally to the area of the stylomastoid foramen. The margins were scalloped and sharply defined by a sclerotic rim, and islands of residual bone remained in the center (Fig. 30.8*C*). On CT scanning, a large, nonenhancing cyst was noted in the left posterior fossa, displacing the fourth ventricle anteriorly and to the right, and there was a moderate hydrocephalus (Fig. 30.9). The angiogram showed a massive avascular lesion, with displacement of the adjacent blood vessels and a complete extrinsic compression of the left lateral sinus.

At *operation*, an orange-sized diploic, extradural epidermoid that had eroded the posterior pyramid and exposed the vertical portion of the facial nerve was removed from the left posterior fossa (Fig. 30.10). The postoperative course was unremarkable except for transient right sixth cranial nerve paresis.

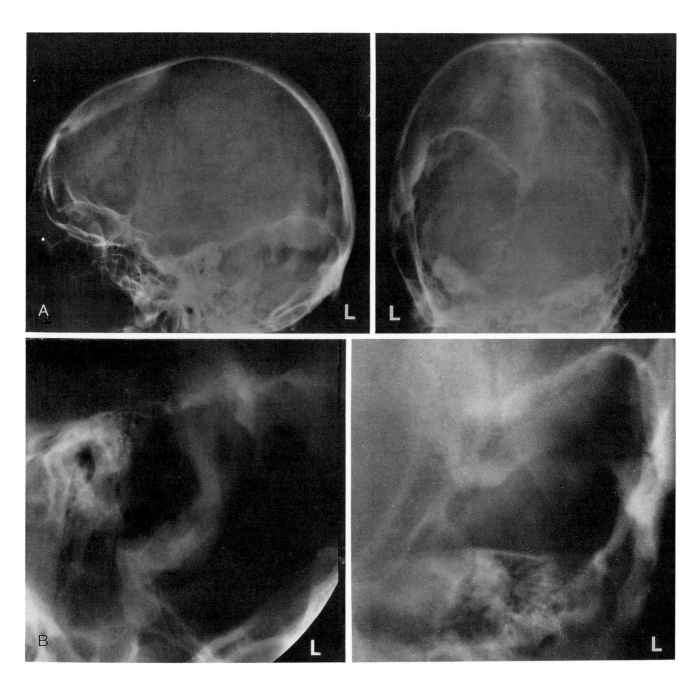

Figure 30.8. **A.** Left lateral and anteroposterior projections of skull. A large diploic epidermoid has destroyed almost the entire squamous portion of the left occipital bone and adjacent areas of the parietal and temporal bone. The bony defect is characterized by an irregularly scalloped, scle-rotic margin and a few remaining islands of bone tissue. **B.** In the lateral (Schüller) and longitudinal (Stenvers) projections the destruction involving the left posterior pyramid and mastoid process is clearly visible.

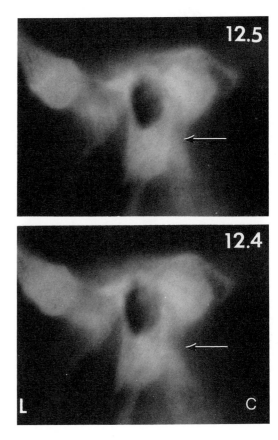

Figure 30.8.   C. The lateral multidirectional tomograms of the left temporal bone show the extension to and the involvement of the descending portion of the Fallopian canal *(arrows)* by the epidermoid.

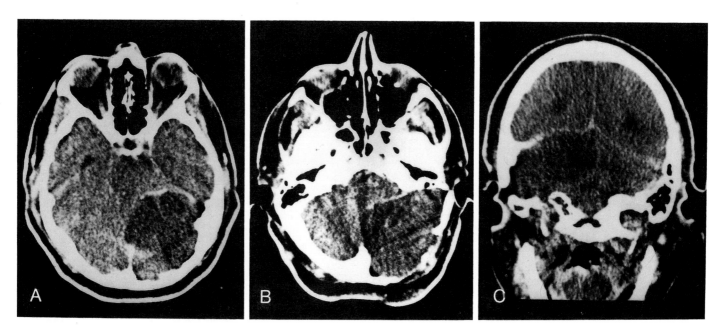

Figure 30.9.   A–C. CT scans display the overall dimensions and cystic nature of the epidermoid, bone destruction, and upward displacement of the left tentorium.

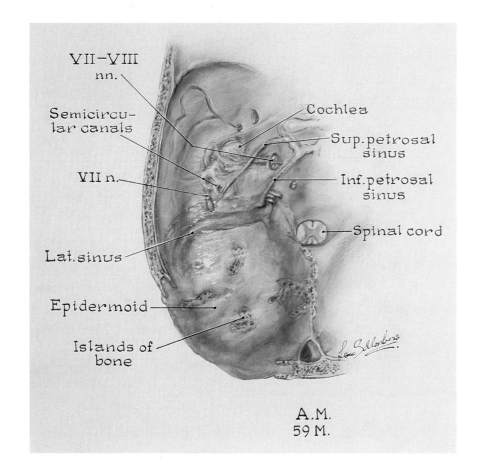

Figure 30.10. Illustration of magnitude of epidermoid occupying the left posterior cranial fossa, extent of bone destruction, and exposure of vertical segment of left facial nerve.

Case 5. *Epidermoid with origin in right mastoid process with widespread bone destruction. Extension to and partial erosion of posterior cortex of petrous pyramid, tegmen, mastoid cortex, posteroinferior bony wall of external auditory canal, and mastoid segment of Fallopian canal. Compression and obliteration of sigmoid sinus. No involvement of middle ear, attic, and antrum.*

A 52-year-old man was examined 7 months before, following an upper respiratory tract infection, had developed a scanty, somewhat malodorous discharge from his right ear. He had had no ear infections since childhood and had noticed no hearing loss, tinnitus, or disequilibrium. He had been aware of an occasional deep-seated pain in his right ear, however.

Otologic examination revealed a circular bony defect in the posteroinferior canal wall of the right external meatus (Fig. 30.13*B*), leading to a large cavity filled with slightly pulsating cholesteatomatous debris. The tympanic membrane appeared intact except for a slight redness of the epithelial lining. No fluid or hyperemia of the mucoperiosteum was found in the middle ear. Hearing was normal bilaterally except for a symmetrical 35-dB dip at 4000 cycles, compatible with a history of previous noise exposure.

Radiologic examination of the right temporal bone on plain films, coronal and lateral tomograms, and axial and coronal CT scans showed a very extensive irregular bony defect involving most of the mastoid process, with a sharply defined scalloped sclerotic margin (Fig. 30.11*A*). The defect included the posterior cortex of the petrous pyramid medially, the mastoid cortex laterally, and the tegmen superiorly, with extensive destruction of these structures (Fig. 30.12). The bone around the lower mastoid segment of the Fallopian canal was also involved (Fig. 30.11*C*). The mass occupying the bony defect appeared to have partially compressed the sigmoid sinus. It protruded slightly into the right posterior cranial fossa (Fig. 30.12). The middle ear and mastoid antrum, however, appeared not to be involved (Fig. 30.11*B* and *C*).

At *operation,* the epidermoid had eroded the mastoid cortex in three separate places. The destruction of the mastoid process had created a multiloculated defect filled with keratinous debris and cholesterol granulomas. The tumor surrounded and compressed the sigmoid sinus and extended into the occipital bone (Fig. 30.13*A*), under the external meatus, and, through its posteroinferior wall, into the canal. It had destroyed the lower vertical segment of the Fallopian canal, exposing the nerve (Figs. 30.11*C* and 30.13). The posterior fossa dura anterior and posterior to the lateral sinus was widely exposed. The exposure of the middle fossa dura was less extensive. Antrum, attic, and middle ear were free of disease.

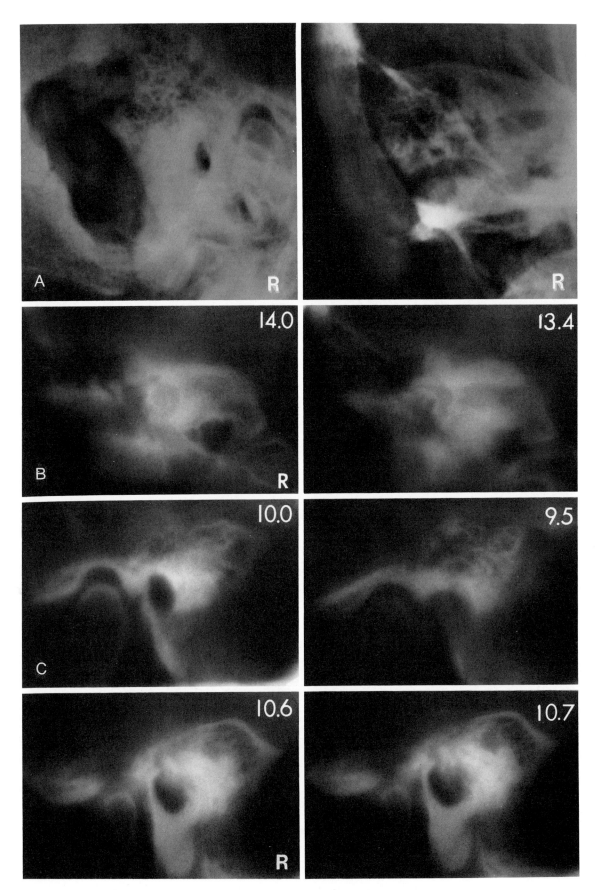

Figure 30.11. **A.** Lateral (Schüller) and longitudinal (Stenvers) projections of the right temporal bone show the massive destruction of the mastoid process and base of the petrous pyramid. The radiolytic defect displays characteristically scalloped and sclerotic margins. **B.** The anteroposterior polytomograms *(13.4* and *14.0)* prove that the right periantral cells, antrum, attic, and middle ear cavity have remained uninvolved. **C.** Lateral polytomograms of the right temporal bone *(9.5–10.7)* show epidermoid involvement of the descending portion of the facial nerve.

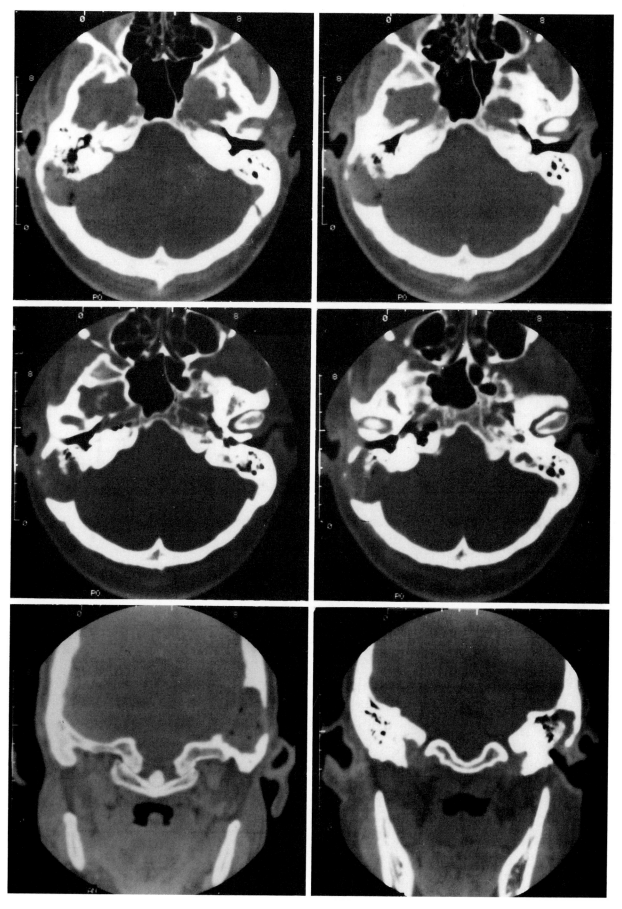

Figure 30.12.   Axial and modified coronal CT scans illustrate extensive destruction of the left mastoid cortex, mastoid process, posterior bony canal wall, and base and lateral aspect of left petrous pyramid.

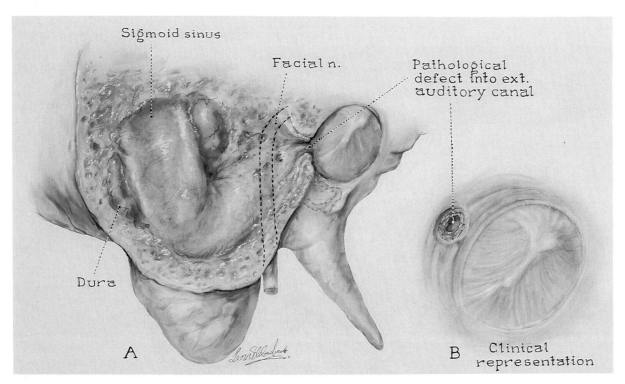

Figure 30.13. Illustration of epidermoid that originated in the right mastoid process and destroyed the major portion of the mastoid bone and posterior petrous pyramid. It extended into the adjacent occipital bone and external auditory canal through an erosion in its posterior canal wall. It widely exposed the middle and posterior fossa dura, the entire lateral sinus, and most of the descending portion of the facial nerve.

Case 6. *Epidermoid with origin in left cerebellopontine angle. Marked compression and invasion of left anterior cerebellar hemisphere. Distortion and displacement of pons, medulla, and basilar artery to opposite side. Extension into foramen magnum, left internal acoustic meatus, and, through the tentorium, into the undersurface of the left temporal and occipital lobe. Involvement of left fifth to eighth cranial nerves. Postoperative subtotal removal of large epidermoid from left anterior cerebellar hemisphere and cerebellopontine angle. Sudden death 12 days after operation from undetermined cause.*

A 42-year-old woman who for the past 25 to 30 years had noticed progressive loss of hearing and tinnitus in her left ear, unsteadiness, and staggering was seen. For 15–20 years she had had an internal strabismus involving her left eye and diplopia. For 15 years she had had ataxia involving her left arm and leg, and for 10 years she had noticed numbness involving the left side of her face and her left arm and leg. During the past 10 years she had developed left-sided facial spasms and progressive facial weakness, and during the past 2 years she had experienced difficulties with swallowing.

Neurologic examination on admission revealed: *(a)* a left internal strabismus, decreased vision in the left eye (20/70), and slight haziness of the left disc; *(b)* involvement of the left fifth to eighth cranial nerves; *(c)* a positive Romberg response with a tendency to fall to the left and ataxia in the left arm and leg; *(d)* weakness of the left arm and leg; and *(e)* a positive Babinski sign on the left.

Otologic examination disclosed: *(a)* normal tympanic membranes; *(b)* total loss of cochlear, vestibular, and facial nerve function on the left but no impairment on the right; and *(c)* a coarse, slow-beating spontaneous nystagmus of central (cerebellar) origin.

At *operation,* a large epidermoid was found in the left cerebellopontine angle and left cerebellar hemisphere. It had distorted, displaced, and surrounded the pons and medulla (Fig. 30.14*B*) and had extended into the foramen magnum, into the left internal acoustic meatus, and, through the tentorium, into the left temporal lobe (Fig. 30.14*A*). A subtotal removal was performed. Death occurred suddenly on the twelfth postoperative day from an undetermined cause.

Postmortem examination showed residual tumor tissue over the anterior surface of the markedly compressed left cerebellar hemisphere and adjacent meninges and over the undersurface of the left temporal lobe (Fig. 30.14*A*). The epidermoid had enlarged the left internal auditory canal and totally destroyed the seventh and eighth cranial nerves. In addition, a small endotheliomatous meningioma was found over the right Sylvian fissure, and an adenoma was found in the liver (Fig. 30.15*A–C*).

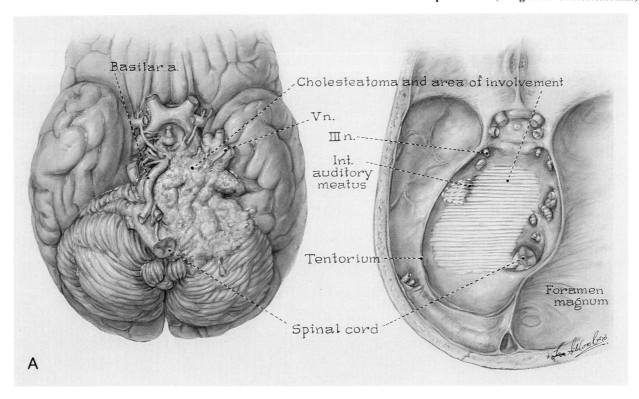

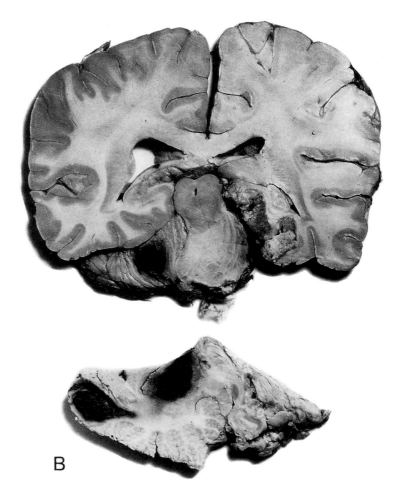

Figure 30.14. **A.** Illustration of epidermoid that originated in the left cerebellopontine angle, extended into the foramen magnum, and invaded the left internal auditory canal. **B.** Coronal section of brain with residual tumor in left cerebellopontine angle. The epidermoid is compressing and invading the anterior cerebellar hemisphere and the base of the temporal lobe. It distorts and displaces the pons and medulla to the opposite side.

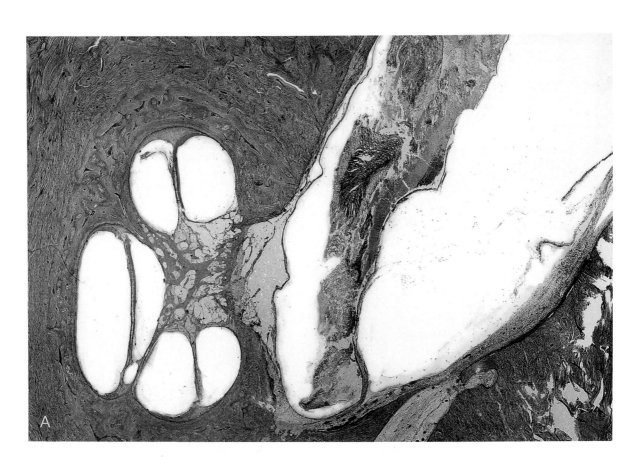

Figure 30.15.   A. Horizontal paramodiolar section of left petrous pyramid, showing extension of epidermoid into widened internal auditory canal. (Hematoxylin and eosin, ×12.)

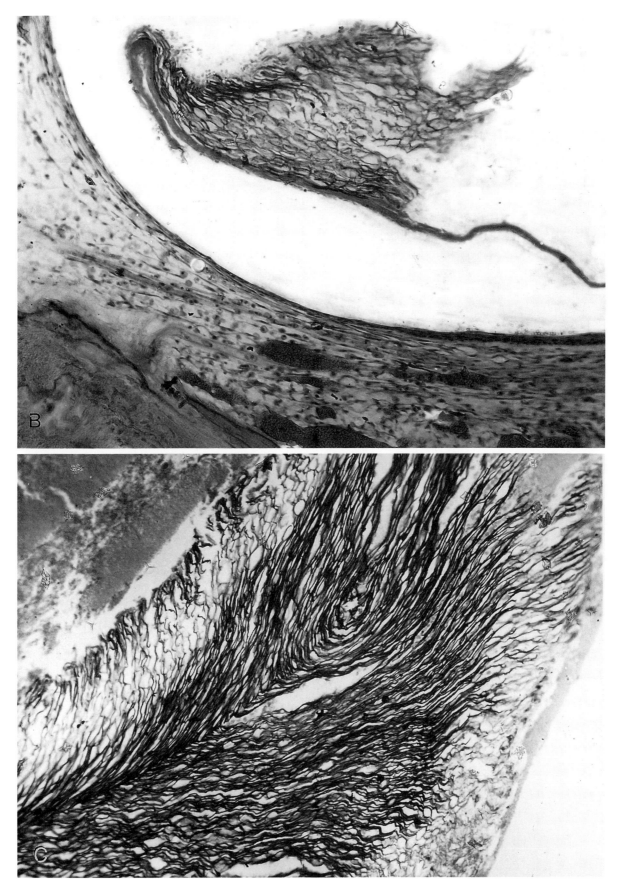

Figure 30.15.   B. The epidermoid occupies the subarachnoid space. Its thin capsule consists of the three layers of the epidermis. **C.** Continuous exfoliation of keratinous material from the epithelial lining, arranged in a lamellar onionskin-like fashion, forms the content of the cysts. (×150 for both *B* and *C*.)

Case 7. *Large epidermoid involving the anterior portion of the left petrous pyramid with possible origin near the geniculate ganglion. Massive destruction of superior petrous apex measuring about 2.5 cm in length. Perforation through superior cortex into left middle cranial fossa, elevating dura about 1 cm. Complete destruction of horizontal segment of bony canal of external carotid artery with wide exposure of artery. Extensive erosion of anterior and superior portions of cochlear basal turn, anterior and superior walls of internal auditory canal, medial wall of vestibule, tegmen tympani, and anterior wall of tympanic cavity. Extension of epidermoid into epitympanum with erosion of malleus and incus. Secondary perforative otitis media on left side. Involvement of left cranial nerves V, VII, and VIII.*

The patient was a 54-year-old white man with a 30-year history of gradual loss of hearing and tinnitus in his left ear, intermittent unsteadiness with a tendency to fall to the left for 1 year, and left otalgia and malodorous otorrhea for 1 week. Headaches subsided the moment the left ear began to drain.

Otologic examination revealed a chronically inflamed left tympanic membrane with a central anteroinferior pars tensa perforation, a reddish granular mass, and a straw-yellow exudate behind the mass. There was total loss of cochlear function on the left, a spontaneous paralytic nystagmus to the left, and absence of caloric responses on the left. There was a mild peripheral left facial weakness involving the ocular and buccal branches and hypesthesia in the distribution of the third division of the left fifth cranial nerve.

Radiologic examination showed extensive pneumatization of both temporal bones with mucoperiosteal disease on the left. It also demonstrated a widespread destruction of the left anterior pyramid and petrous ridge (Fig. 30.16A and B). The anteroposterior polytomograms revealed a destructive process involving the petrous apex with erosion of the tegmen tympani, cochlea, vestibule, internal auditory canal, and anterior wall of the middle ear (Fig. 30.16C and D).

At *operation,* an epidermoid was found that had destroyed about 2.5 cm of the left anterosuperior petrous pyramid, completely exposed the horizontal segment of the internal carotid artery, and elevated the overlying dura of the middle cranial fossa about 1 cm. It appeared to have originated in the area of the geniculate ganglion (Fig. 30.17). It had eroded the anterior and superior walls of the internal auditory canal and the medial wall of the vestibule, had extended into the epitympanum, and had partially eroded the malleus and incus. It was totally removed. The patient made an uneventful recovery except for a transient aggravation of the preexisting facial paresis.

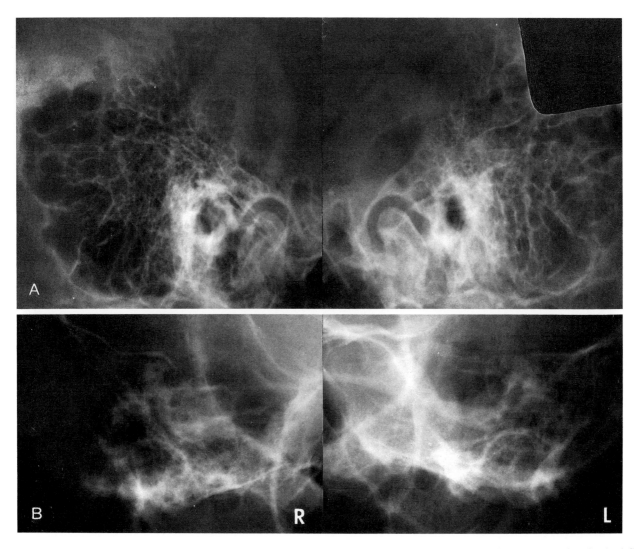

Figure 30.16.   A. Lateral (Schüller) projection of left temporal bone displays an extensive pneumatization of the mastoid process and evidence of a mild diffuse mucoperiosteal disease. **B.** Longitudinal (Stenvers) projection of the left petrous pyramid demonstrates the clearly defined destruction of the petrous apex and overlying petrous ridge.

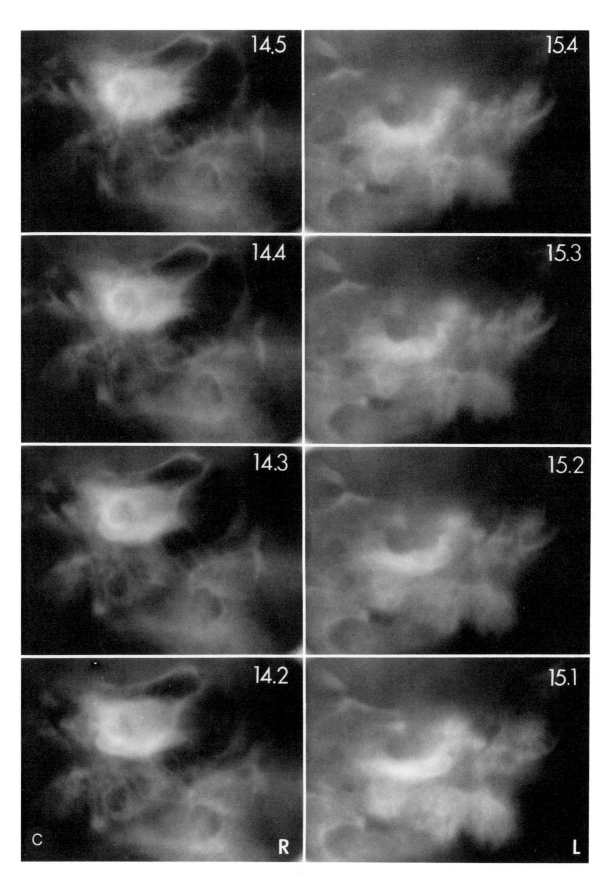

Figure 30.16. **C** and **D.** In the multidirectional coronal tomograms, the anterior and superior erosion of the cochlea and internal auditory canal (15.2), the destruction of the tegmen (15.3), and the erosion of the medial wall of the vestibule (14.9) are well recognized.

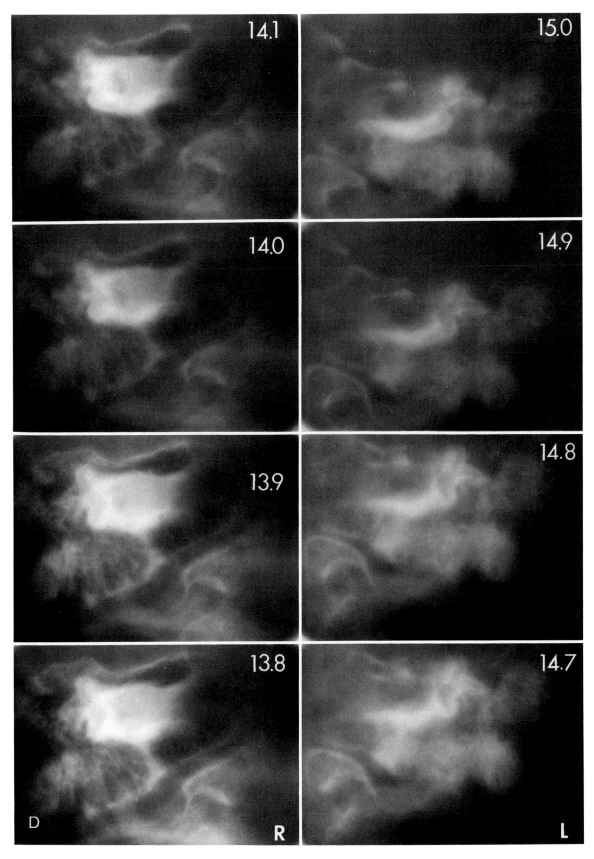

Figure 30.16.   D.

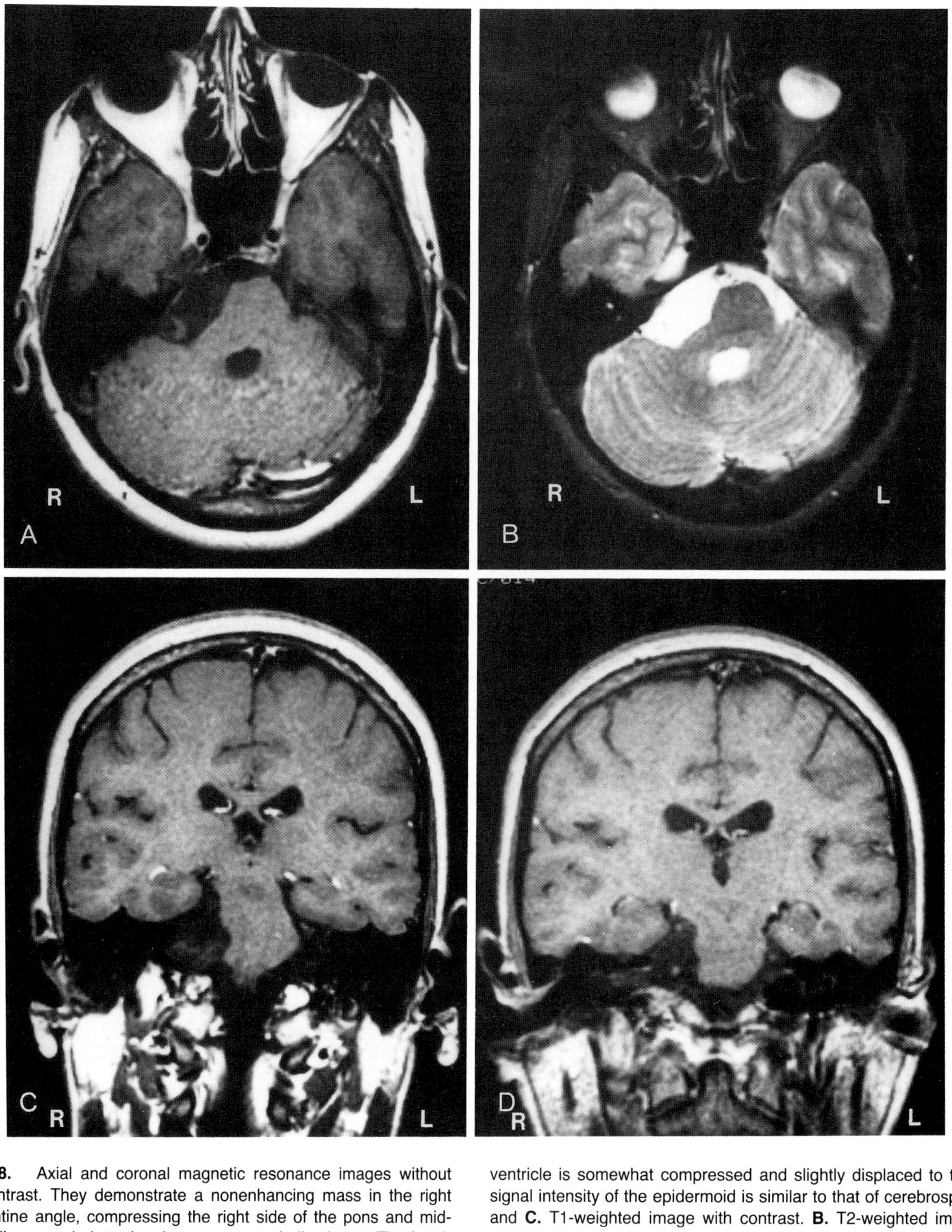

Figure 30.18.   Axial and coronal magnetic resonance images without and with contrast. They demonstrate a nonenhancing mass in the right cerebellopontine angle, compressing the right side of the pons and mid-brain, extending superiorly to the circummesencephalic cistern. The fourth ventricle is somewhat compressed and slightly displaced to the left. The signal intensity of the epidermoid is similar to that of cerebrospinal fluid. **A** and **C.** T1-weighted image with contrast. **B.** T2-weighted image. **D.** T1-weighted image without contrast.

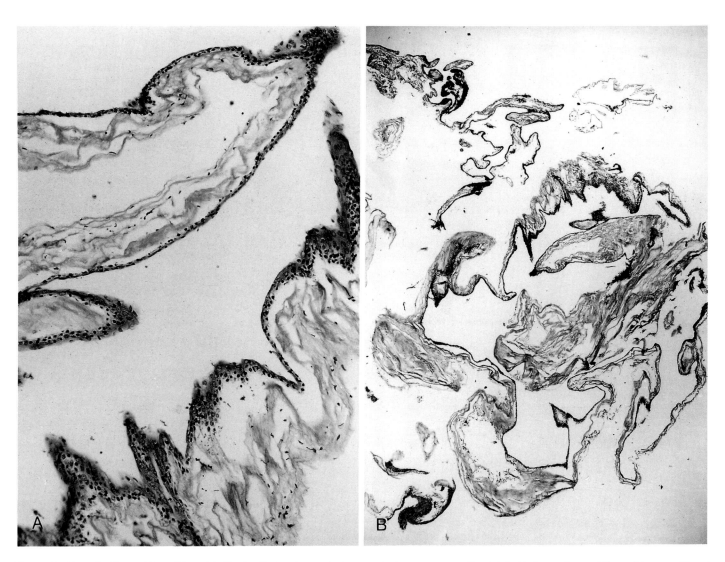

Figure 30.19. **A.** The epidermoid cyst is lined with keratin-producing squamous epithelium and contains keratinous debris in a concentric lamellar arrangement. **B.** The delicate capsule consists of the three normal layers of the epidermis: stratum germinativum, stratum granulosum, and stratum corneum, with a total of between two and five cell layers, although occasionally there are up to ten cell layers. (Hematoxylin and eosin, ×35 and ×200, respectively.)

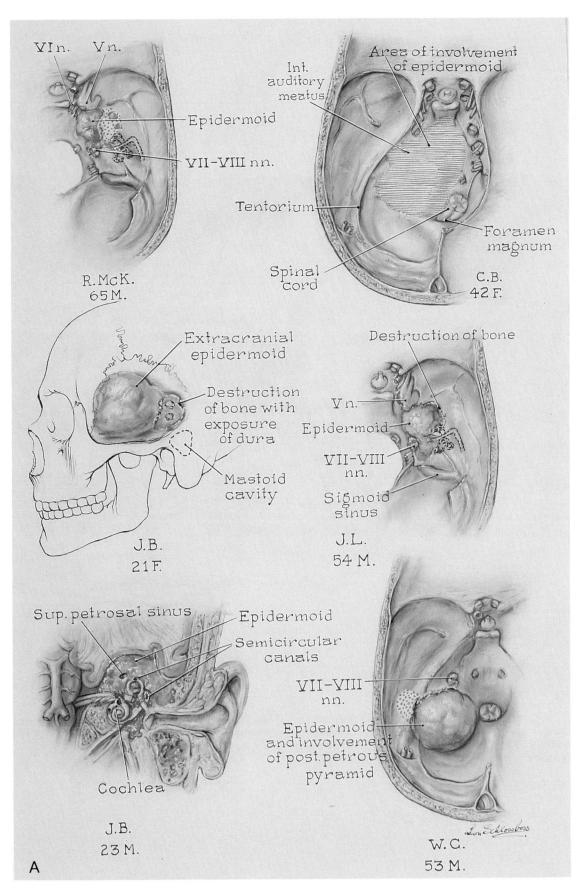

Figure 30.20. **A** and **B.** Location, extent, and regional behavior of 11 selected epidermoids observed by the author, 5 of which are discussed in the text in greater detail.

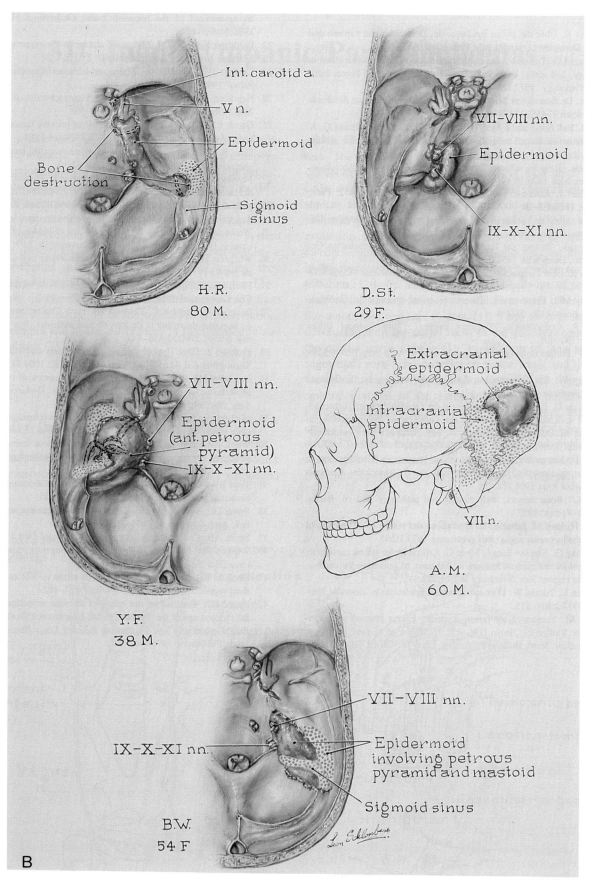

Figure 30.20.   B.

the development of paragangliomas in locations where paraganglia have not routinely been observed in the adult (1).

Microscopic Anatomy

The paraganglia reveal a typical morphologic structure. Lobules of parenchymal cells arranged in a loose or compact fashion are separated by strands of connective and adipose tissue and occasionally intermingled with other autonomic elements including ganglion and paraganglion cells of the aorticosympathetic type and with numerous mast cells (Figs. 31.2–31.6). These lobules consist of chief cells (type I cells) congregated in compact cell nests and of sustentacular or satellite cells (type II cells) (1). Two kinds of chief cells are distinguished: the clear form, with a lucid cytoplasm and uniform spherical granules; and the dark form, with a more condensed cytoplasm and more irregular, angular granules (Figs. 31.2–31.6). The clear form of chief cells predominates. These clear cells are often surrounded by dark cells. The satellite cells, by extending slender processes around and between the chief cells and separating small cell groups from neighboring cell groups and capillaries, create a typical cell-nest pattern that is well recognized histologically (Figs. 31.2–31.6) (1). A vast capillary network provides for the extraordinary perfusion of the paraganglia with blood. The blood flow through these structures, in comparison with their mass, exceeds that of all other tissues including the brain (Figs. 31.2–31.6) (6). Nonmyelinated nerve axons, accompanied by satellite cells, enter the chief cell nest. Catecholamines and certain esterases have been identified in the chief cells (1).

Jugulotympanic Paraganglia

The jugulotympanic paraganglia are found in several areas of the temporal bone. About 50% are located in the adventitia of the anterolateral region of the jugular dome, in close proximity to the tympanic branch of the glossopharyngeal nerve or nerve of Jacobson (paraganglion jugulare) (Figs. 31.2 and 31.4). The remaining 50% are situated in equal distribution within the tympanic canaliculus, leading from the jugular fossa to the middle ear cavity, or on the cochlear promontory along the nerve of Jacobson (paraganglion tympanicum) (Figs. 31.4 and 31.5) and within the mastoid canaliculus along the auricular branch of the vagus nerve or nerve of Arnold (Fig. 31.6) (9). They vary considerably in number, location, and bilateral distribution. Whereas up to 12 paraganglia may be found in each specimen of a pair of temporal bones, the average is about 2 or 3 (Fig. 31.5). They are ovoid and measure about 0.25–1.5 mm in diameter. They are intimately associated with the inferior tympanic artery (a branch of the ascending pharyngeal artery) and with the superior tympanic artery (a branch of the middle meningeal artery) (Figs. 31.3B, 31.4B, and 31.5B). Their location corresponds to the level of the first branchial pouch between the mandibular and hyoid arch. They may accompany the nerve of Arnold into the facial canal (Fig. 31.6A and B).

PARAGANGLIOMAS

Incidence, Age, and Sex Distribution

The distribution and relative frequency of neoplasms involving the paraganglia in the head and neck region vary somewhat in statistics from different series. Of the 69 patients observed at the Memorial Sloan Kettering Institute over a period of 38 years, there were 44 carotid body, 13 vagal body, 8 jugulotympanic, and 3 nasal tumors and 1 each of tumors of the orbit, larynx, and aortic arch (10). In another review there were, in order of decreasing frequency, carotid body, jugulotympanic, intravagal, nasal, nasopharyngeal, and orbital tumors (11). In a more recent series, the jugulotympanic paraganglioma was the predominant paraganglioma in the head and neck area, followed by the carotid body and vagal paragangliomas.

Jugular and tympanic paragangliomas represent the most common neoplasm of the temporal bone. Their absolute and relative incidence remain to be determined. They may manifest themselves at any age, but they occur most frequently in patients between ages 25 and 65, with an average age at onset of approximately 50 years. Three-fourths of jugular paragangliomas are found in women (1).

Macroscopic Appearance

In the middle ear cavity the tumor generally presents as a somewhat lobulated, soft, compressible, slightly pulsating, friable mass with a purplish-red and, occasionally, dark reddish color (Figs. 31.7 and 31.8). As the tumor arises from the cochlear promontory, it remains attached by a slender stalk (Figs. 31.9 and 31.30). In the absence of a prominent capsule, its delicate cover ruptures easily at the slightest trauma. Its enormous vascularity causes profuse arterial bleeding during segmental resection, which at times may be cumbersome to control as a result of lack of contractile elements in the walls of the vascular channels (Figs. 31.9, 31.10, 31.13E, and 31.28A and B). The tumor may be confused with a polyp, a pyogenic granuloma, or a rare aberrant internal carotid artery.

Microscopic Appearance

The tumor is generally readily identifiable, as it reflects the characteristic features of the paraganglion. Delicate strands of reticulin fibers form a network that separates groups of clear-staining cells into a variety of typical patterns. These patterns may resemble an alveolar formation, an epitheliomatous or a mesenchymal configuration of sheets, anastomosing cords, islands, and clusters. The alveolar pattern generally predominates (Figs. 31.13A, 31.18H, 31.22A, 31.23B, and 31.27A). The epitheliomatous pattern evolves in areas of hypercellularity with poor delineation between cell clusters, consisting of plump chief cells with abundant cytoplasm with pleomorphic vesicular nuclei. This creates the appearance of epithelial sheets with occasional pseudoacini (Fig. 31.9C). The mesenchymal pattern is less frequently found. It is made up of spindle-shaped or crescentic tumor cells arranged in cell nests (Figs. 31.20B, 31.22A, and 31.28B). Occasionally, the various cell patterns are found in the same tumor. In both the endotheliomatous and mesenchymatous cellular patterns, the demarcation of the cellular arrangement can be demonstrated by reticular stains. The tumor cells assume a polyhedral or ovoid shape. Their nuclei display a considerable pleomorphism and are round or ovoid, vesicular, and often hyperchromatic (Figs. 31.18H and I and 31.27C). Occasionally, 2 or more nuclei are found (Figs. 31.18H and I, 31.25C, and 31.27C). Mitotic figures are rare. The cytoplasm is pale, homo-

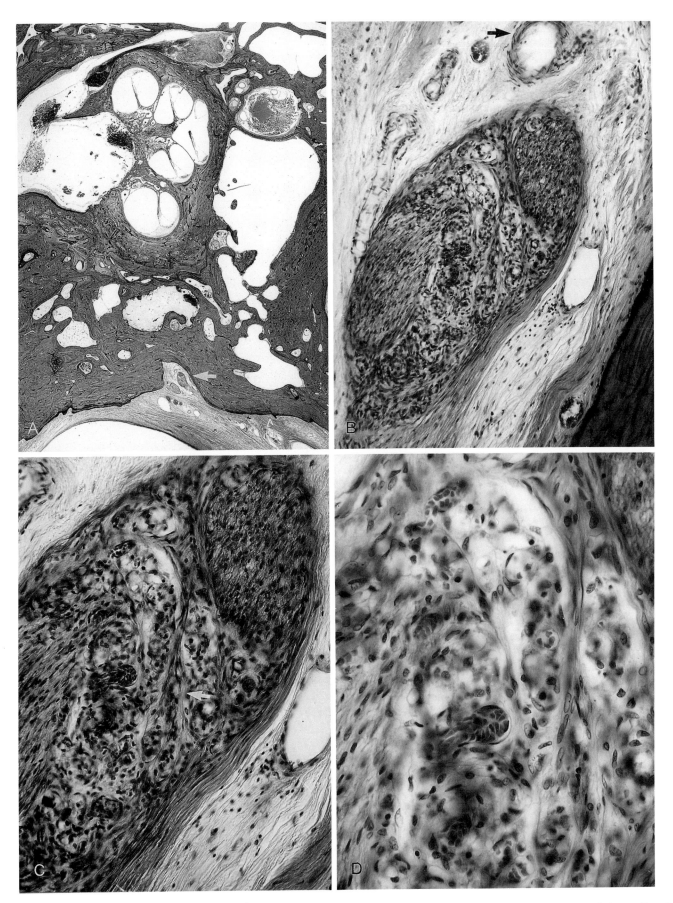

Figure 31.2. **A.** Midmodiolar section through left temporal bone with paraganglion in inferior aperture of tympanic canaliculus. The paraganglion is situated in the adventitia of the jugular bulb directly adjacent to the nerve of Jacobson *(arrow)*. **B.** The paraganglion forms a functional unit in a common capsule with the nerve of Jacobson and receives its large blood supply from the adjacent inferior tympanic artery *(arrow)*. **C.** Nerve fibers from the nerve of Jacobson can be seen entering the clusters of predominantly clear chief cells *(arrow)*. **D.** The cell clusters are surrounded by sinusoids and capillaries and intimately connected with nerve fibers. (Hematoxylin and eosin, ×6.4, ×140, ×225, and ×400, respectively.)

geneous, or vacuolated, although it is occasionally more dense and eosinophilic. The cell boundaries are poorly defined. Interdigitation of adjoining cells, giving the impression of embracement of one tumor cell by another, is a characteristic feature of these neoplasms (1). Cytoplasmic granules similar to those found in the chief cells of paraganglia are often observed in tumor cells. Examination of the ultrastructure of the tumor has identified these structures as neurosecretory granules of catecholamine (12). These findings are consistent with the observations that some paragangliomas contain considerable amounts of catecholamine or norepinephrine. Arylesterase activity has also been demonstrated in many of the chief cells. The tumor cells also have a tendency toward polymorphism and formation of syncytial and multinucleated giant cells (Figs. 31.18*I* and 31.25*C*). The rare occurrence of cellular elements resembling the sustentacular cells in paraganglia and the lack of the normal relationship of nerve fibers to chief cell clusters support a true neoplastic, rather than a hyperplastic or hamartomatous, origin of the chief cell element (1).

The proportion of parenchyma and stroma may vary greatly—from tumors consisting largely of the chief cell type in an alveolar arrangement, to neoplasms made up primarily of stroma with neural elements prevailing. Hyalinization and sclerosis are a frequent feature of the stroma (Figs. 31.20*B* and 31.23*B*). Vascularization is remarkably extensive (Figs. 31.13*E* and 31.28*B*). Blood vessels enter the parenchyma at the periphery, accompanying trabeculae of collagen tissue (Fig. 31.9). Their walls may be quite well developed or ill-defined. In general, they soon decrease to an endothelial lining, supported by fine reticulin fibers (1). The resulting vascular channels consist of wide capillaries and sinusoids with thin endothelial walls, varying greatly in size (Figs. 31.9*D* and *E*, 31.18*H* and *I*, and 31.25*C*). Occasionally, individual clusters of tumor cells have become separated into small islands of expanded sinusoids (Fig. 31.9*D*). The tumor cells frequently give the impression of lining the sinusoids directly (Figs. 31.9*E*, 31.13*C*, and 31.18*I*) (1). In some instances the tumor cells have become so numerous that they protrude into and obliterate the vascular lumen (Fig. 31.22*C*). Nonmyelinated nerve fibers can be observed in the hyalin and collagen framework of the stroma. When taking a biopsy the otologist should remember that a neoplasm presenting as an aural polyp in the external auditory canal is often covered by a considerably thick layer of squamous epithelium and underlying inflammatory granulation tissue, with the tumor tissue being localized in the center and around the stalk (Fig. 31.9).

Blood Supply

The paraganglioma that arises over the promontory derives its vast supply from the inferior and superior tympanic arteries, from one or, occasionally, two caroticotympanic arteries, as well as from the vascular network of the mucoperiosteum covering the promontory (Figs. 31.8 and 31.9). The principal contributing arteries are always remarkably enlarged. In a larger jugular tumor with extension into the neck, skull base, or posterior cranial fossa, the ascending pharyngeal artery, occipital artery, branches of the internal and external carotid and internal maxillary arteries, and occasionally a branch from the vertebral artery may be greatly enlarged (Figs. 31.17, 31.20*A* and *B*, and 31.21*A*).

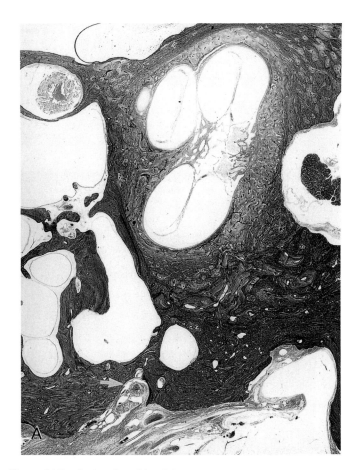

Figure 31.3. **A.** Anterior midmodiolar section through right temporal bone with paraganglion in inferior orifice of tympanic canaliculus. The paraganglion is located immediately below the floor of the middle ear in the adventitia of the jugular bulb *(arrow)*. (Hematoxylin and eosin, ×8.5.)

Multicentric and Familial Paragangliomas

The occasional multicentric and familial occurrence of jugulotympanic and other paragangliomas is well documented (1). Three to eight percent of jugular paragangliomas may be associated with ipsilateral, contralateral, and bilateral carotid body tumors (Fig. 31.21). The simultaneous occurrence of paragangliomas of the carotid body and neoplasms of the vagal, aortic, adrenal medulla, and bilateral para-aortic gangliomas (organs of Zuckerkandl) has been well established (13–16). The coexistence of other paragangliomas with ones in different anatomical locations has also been recorded (1). The detection of a paraganglioma in one anatomical location should, therefore, prompt the physician to look for concurrent or subsequent development of a paraganglioma in another site. Jugulotympanic paragangliomas, like carotid body tumors, are known to occur in families, affecting, for example, three sisters in one and several members through three generations in another (17). The association of a tympanic paraganglioma with multiple endocrine neoplasia type II (MEN II/A or Sipple syndrome), including pheochromocytoma, medullary carcinoma of the thyroid, and parathyroid hyperplasia, has recently been described (Figs. 31.10–31.14) (18).

Malignant Characteristics

The invasion of the middle ear cleft, the infiltration of the mastoid process and petrous pyramid, the erosion of the otic

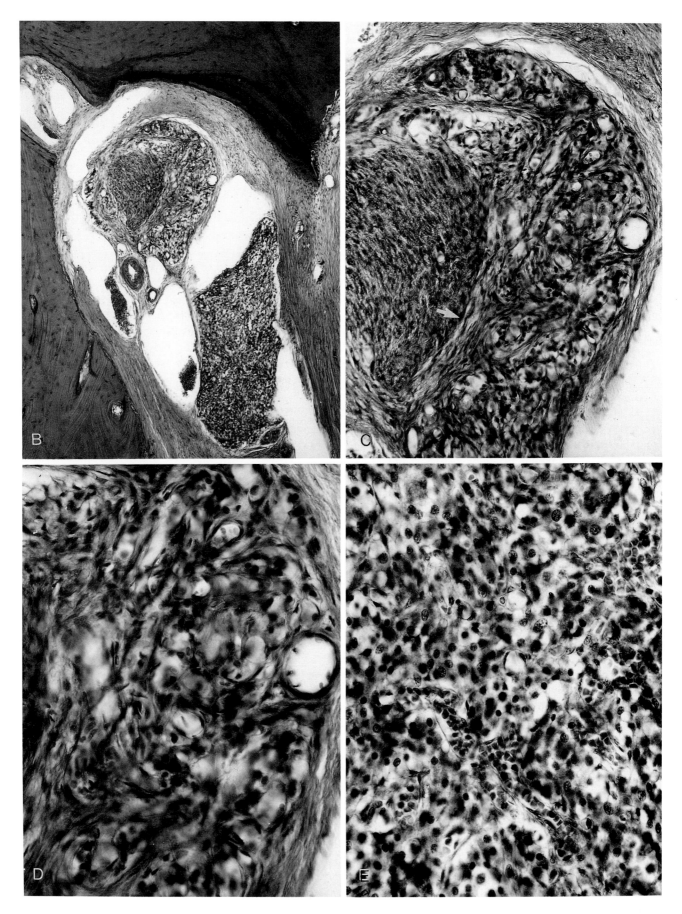

Figure 31.3. B. The paraganglion that partially envelops the nerve of Jacobson is accompanied by large feeding and draining blood vessels. In the upper portion of the paraganglion the clear form of chief cells predominates, whereas in the lower portion the dark form of chief cells prevails. **C.** Numerous afferent nerve fibers from cell clusters are seen joining the nerve of Jacobson *(arrow).* **D.** Capillaries and nerve fibers are closely related to the lobules of chief cells. **E.** This area from the lower portion of the paraganglion shown in *B* consists mainly of the dark form of chief cells. The cytoplasm of these cells is more condensed. ($\times$75, $\times$230, $\times$400, and $\times$400, respectively.)

capsule, jugular fossa, and canal for the internal carotid artery, the invasion of the jugular vein, and the extension of 40% of jugular paragangliomas through the jugular foramen into the posterior cranial fossa reflect the aggressive behavior of these neoplasms in spite of their benign histologic appearance. In rare instances, however, metastases to bone, cervical lymph nodes, and liver are known to occur (19–21).

Clinical Aspects

To assess the clinical manifestations of these tumors our clinical material of the past 30 years was reviewed. Thirty-four patients were selected for that study. All patients with incomplete long-term documentation or who were initially treated elsewhere and referred to us for evaluation and management were excluded. Of these 34 patients, 29 had tumors classified as jugular or tympanic paragangliomas, 3 had carotid body tumors, and 2 had vagal tumors. The ages of the patients ranged from 21 to 68 years for both jugular and tympanic tumors. The ratio of females to males was 9:1, higher than previously reported. The tumors affected both sides of the neck with equal frequency. The jugular paragangliomas showed a slight preponderance for the left side, whereas tympanic paragangliomas were somewhat more frequently located on the right. The initial symptoms in the 29 patients with jugular and tympanic paragangliomas are listed, in order of decreasing frequency, in Table 31.1.

On admission, tinnitus was the most common symptom, occurring in 93% of patients, followed by loss of hearing (80%) and pain (39%). Pain was a more frequent feature of tympanic tumors (75%) than of jugular paragangliomas (24%). Involvement of the cranial nerves was present in almost 25% of patients with jugular tumors. Vertigo, otorrhea, and aural bleeding were infrequent. The duration of symptoms varied from 5 months to 25 years. All patients had abnormal otoscopic findings. A reddish vascular mass behind an intact or bulging tympanic membrane was observed in 85%, and a polypoid tumor in the external auditory canal was present in 15%. Patients with jugular paragangliomas revealed an involvement of the seventh and tenth cranial nerves in 17% and of the twelfth cranial nerve in 24%. These figures are lower than the ones reported earlier.

Table 31.1. Initial Symptoms of 29 Patients with Jugular and Tympanic Paragangliomas

Symptom	Number of Patients	%
Tinnitus	14	93.5
Loss of hearing	12	80
Otalgia	6	39
Vertigo and dizziness	4	26
Otorrhea	3	20
Aural bleeding	2	13
Cranial nerve involvement		
VI	1	6.5
VII	1	6.5
VIII	?	?[a]
IX	2	13
X	2	13
XI	1	6.5
XII	2	13

[a] Not listed due to lack of accurate information.

All patients with jugular tumors had a hearing loss that was conductive in 40%, sensorineural in 33%, combined in 13%, and total in 13%. Nearly half of the patients with tympanic tumors had normal hearing. Of the remaining half, the majority had a conductive hearing loss. Eight patients with a jugular tumor had had electronystagmography, which revealed an ipsilateral decreased response in 6, a normal response in 1, and no response in 1. Of the 6 patients with a tympanic tumor, 3 had a normal and 3 had a decreased response to electronystagmography.

Slightly more than half of the patients with jugular tumors disclosed abnormal findings in conventional radiographs. Erosion of the jugular bulb or petrous bone was noted in 27%. A soft tissue mass could be identified with equal frequency. In 81% of the patients with jugular tumors, the tomograms were abnormal, with bone erosion being the most common manifestation.

Postoperative radiation therapy was used in 75% of patients with jugular tumors and in 33% of patients with tympanic lesions. Combination therapy yielded a 71% cure rate in patients on follow-up examinations averaging 43 months. The cure rate was equal for patients with tympanic (75%) and jugular tumors (70%). Patients with a more extensive resection had a slightly higher cure rate (83%).

Radiologic Aspects

Serial computed axial and coronal tomograms of the temporal bones provide the necessary information on the enlargement and destruction of the jugular bulb and jugular foramen and on erosion of the adjacent bony structures. They demonstrate the destruction of the floor of the tympanic cavity, inner ear capsule, neural compartment of the jugular foramen, and carotid and hypoglossal canals. They also show the invasion of the middle ear space, mastoid bone, and petrous pyramid, as well as the adjacent clivus and occipital bone (Figs. 31.19, 31.24, and 31.26).

Serial computed axial and coronal magnetic resonance images of the head and upper neck reveal the extension of the tumor into the posterior cranial fossa, foramen magnum, and upper neck. The jugular venogram demonstrates the invasion of the internal jugular vein by tumor and the extent of intravascular involvement. Carotid and vertebral angiography with digital subtraction outlines the tumor and identifies its abnormal vascularity and the main feeding vessels (Figs. 31.20, 31.21, and 31.28).

Classification and Management

Various classifications or stagings of jugulotympanic paragangliomas have been proposed. They are dependent on anatomical considerations, local behavior, invasion and degree of extension into the posterior cranial fossa and infratemporal fossa, and involvement of adjacent bony structures (clivus, occipital bone, etc.).

The surgical approach in the resection of these lesions depends on their size, location, and extension within and beyond the temporal bone. Larger tumors may require a mobilization of the seventh cranial nerve, exposure of the infratemporal fossa, or a two-staged combined otologic and neurosurgical procedure. Preoperative embolization of the major feeding vessels, ligation of the external carotid artery, and hypotensive anesthesia greatly reduce the blood loss during the operation.

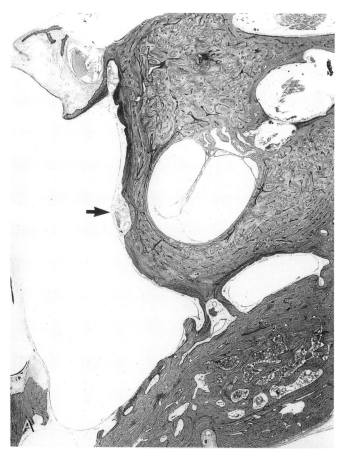

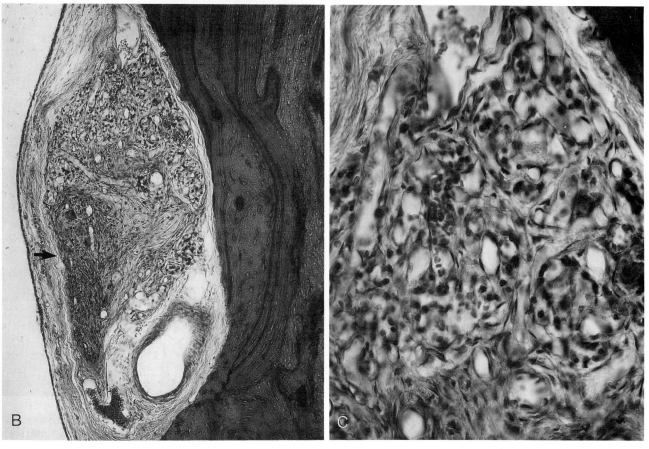

Figure 31.4.   A. Vertical section through right temporal bone anterior to oval window. The tympanic paraganglion is situated within the middle ear mucoperiosteum overlying the promontory *(arrow)*. **B.** The tympanic paraganglion is intimately associated with the tympanic branch of the glossopharyngeal nerve (nerve of Jacobson) *(arrow)*. The size of the afferent artery (tympanic branch of the ascending pharyngeal artery) and of the efferent vein reflect the unusually high blood flow through that structure. **C.** The chief cell clusters are embedded in a dense meshwork of sinusoids, capillaries, and nerve fibers. (Hematoxylin and eosin, ×10.5, ×110, and ×400, respectively.)

The role of radiation therapy continues to be a subject of debate. A response to radiation therapy with partial, sometimes transient reduction in tumor volume has been well recognized, and many reports have been concerned with the degree of responsiveness. Most of them document tumor shrinkage with or without improvement in cranial nerve palsies. The effect of radiation is primarily on small vessels, producing an obliterative endovasculitis. Endothelial hyperplasia and subendothelial hyalinization have been documented. The tumor cells, however, are believed to be rather insensitive to radiation. At present, radiation therapy is being used postoperatively for the control of unresectable residual disease. Surgical treatment appears to be the treatment of choice, with combination therapy providing an effective way to manage the remaining tumor.

Case Reports

Case 1. *Right tympanic paraganglioma arising from promontory at level of round window.*

The patient was a 49-year-old white woman who 18 months prior to admission developed occasional discomfort and pains in the right ear and, 6 months later, a low-pitched humming tinnitus that in the ensuing months assumed a pulse synchronous character. Shortly before admission she developed a sensation of fullness and tightness in that ear. She never had any impairment of hearing or equilibrium, facial weakness or paresthesias, or discharge or bleeding from that ear.

On examination the right ear revealed a bright red, slightly pulsating mass behind an intact tympanic membrane (Fig. 31.7). The tumor, which appeared to have originated in the lower half of the tympanic cavity, was impinging on the adjacent portion of the eardrum (Fig. 31.8). The audiogram showed normal hearing, and the function of all cranial nerves was intact. Routine radiographs and tomograms of the temporal bones revealed no abnormalities. The opposite middle ear cavity was unremarkable, and there were no palpable masses in the area of the carotid bifurcation on either side.

The tumor was removed through a hypotympanotomy approach. It had the size of a large cherry stone and extended from the jugular dome to the tympanic portion of the Fallopian canal (Fig. 31.8). It received its blood supply from the markedly enlarged inferior and superior tympanic arteries and from an extended caroticotympanic branch of the internal carotid artery. The histologic examination confirmed the diagnosis of a tympanic paraganglioma (Fig. 31.9).

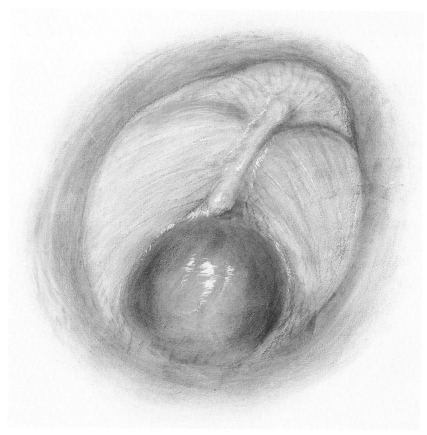

Figure 31.7. Drawing of right tympanic paraganglioma impinging on undersurface of intact tympanic membrane and displacing it laterally.

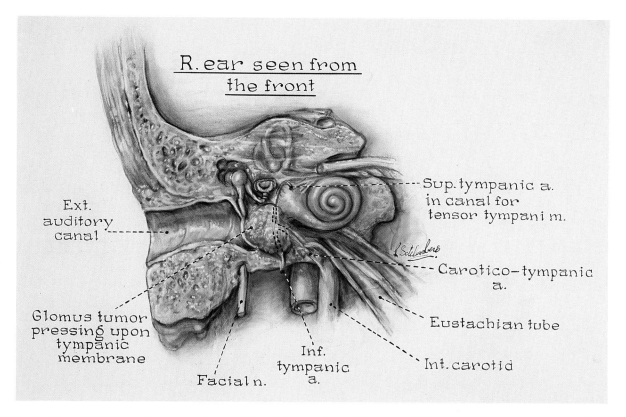

Figure 31.8. Drawing of right tympanic paraganglioma originated from the promontory. It receives its blood supply from the inferior and superior tympanic artery and from the caroticotympanic branch of the internal carotid artery. All three feeding vessels are remarkably enlarged.

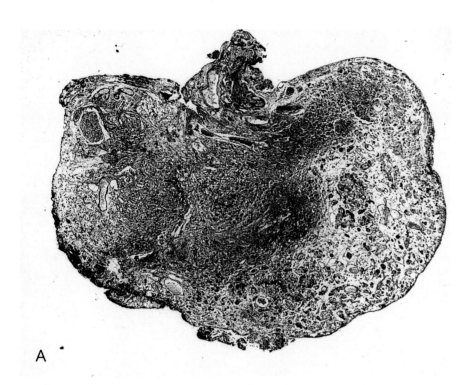

A

Figure 31.9. A. Cross-section through right tympanic paraganglioma, removed in one piece. It shows the delicacy of the capsule, the variation of the tumor cell pattern, and the remarkable vascularization. (Hematoxylin and eosin, ×35.)

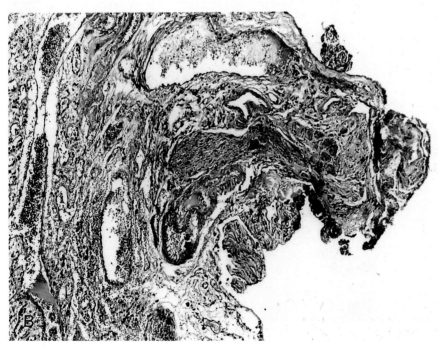

B

Figure 31.9. B. The stalk by which the tumor was attached to the promontory includes cross-sections through the greatly enlarged inferior tympanic artery and vein and through the nerve of Jacobson. Note the large blood channels in the adjacent tumor. (×125.)

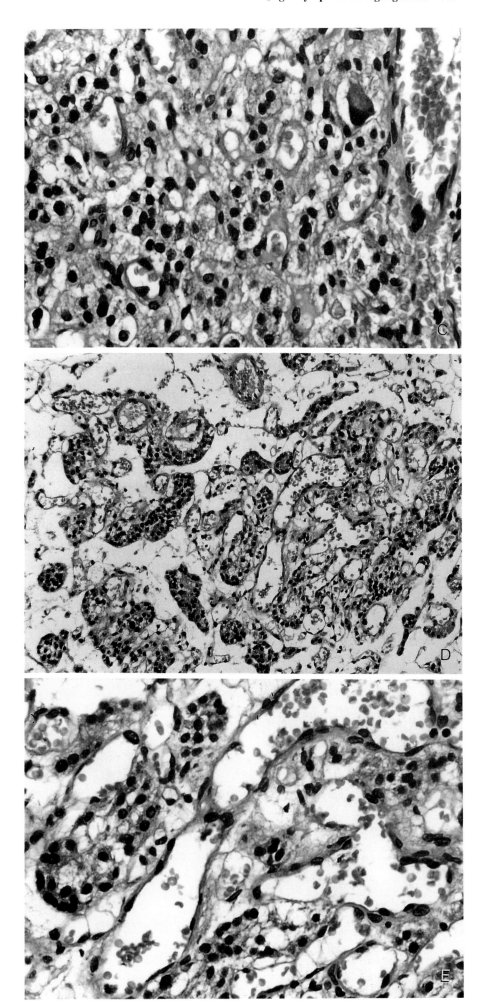

Figure 31.9. C. In the epitheliomatous pattern of tumor cells, the cell clusters are poorly defined, the cells are densely packed, the cytoplasm is abundant, and the nuclei are pleomorphic. (×500.)

Figure 31.9. D. In this section of the paraganglioma the individual clusters of tumor cells have become separated into small islands by the large numbers of expanded sinusoids. (×200.)

Figure 31.9. E. The distended capillaries and sinusoids are generally lined by endothelial cells but in some instances by tumor cells directly. (×500.)

Case 2. *Right tympanic paraganglioma associated with multifocal medullary carcinoma of thyroid, metastasizing to several regional lymph nodes. Parathyroid hyperplasia. Bilateral pheochromocytomas (multiple endocrine neoplasia type II/A).*

A 37-year-old woman with a history of discomfort in the right ear, intermittent hearing loss for 18 months, and a more recently manifest right-sided pulsatile tinnitus was seen on referral. The referring otolaryngologist had noted a vascular mass in the right middle ear that on polytomography appeared as a soft tissue density with no evidence of adjacent bone erosion (Fig. 31.10A). A right external carotid angiogram had demonstrated a small vascular lesion confined to the middle ear (Fig. 31.10B).

On *admission,* her family history revealed that her grandfather had had a thyroid tumor and had died of a stroke. Her father had died from metastases from a thyroid tumor at age 42. Her past medical history disclosed that she had a neurinoma removed from the right foot at age 22 and had suffered from occasional very severe headaches following exercise and exposure to the sun. She gave no history of hypertension.

Otolaryngologic examination showed (a) a pulsatile vascular mass in the right middle ear, displacing the tympanic membrane slightly outward, (b) a diffuse enlargement of the thyroid gland with a 1–2-cm nodule in the right upper pole, and (c) an enlarged adjacent lymph node. Vocal cord function was normal, and the oral examination revealed no evidence of mucosal neurinomas. The audiogram exhibited a mild low-frequency conductive hearing loss on the right but normal hearing on the left.

During hospitalization, blood pressure fluctuated between 120/80 and 140/92 without significant elevations. A 24-hour urine collection for metanephrines showed a marked elevation in creatinine to 6.2 mg/g (normal of 0.21–1.28 mg/g). The thyroid scan showed a cold nodule in the right upper pole that on sonography appeared as a nonhomogeneous solid lesion (Fig. 31.11A and B). The serum calcitonin level was 4.2 mg/ml (normal of 0.2 mg/ml), indicating the presence of a medullary thyroid carcinoma (Fig. 31.11C). A serum calcium level of 9.9 mg/100 ml was normal. An abdominal computed tomography (CT) scan demonstrated a right adrenal mass displacing the kidney downward, histologically identified pheochromocytoma and a smaller tumor on the opposite side (Fig. 31.12). This confirmed the diagnosis of MEN-II/A. After removal of bilateral pheochromocytomas her metanephrine levels returned to normal (0.7 mg/g/24 hr). The patient then underwent a total thyroidectomy and bilateral modified neck dissections. The histologic examination exhibited (a) a medullary carcinoma, with multifocal involvement and C-cell hyperplasia (Fig. 31.11C), and (b) metastases in several of the regional lymph nodes. Two of the parathyroid glands that were removed showed evidence of hyperplasia. Subsequent removal of the right middle ear tumor confirmed the clinical impression of a paraganglioma and restored normal hearing in that ear (Fig. 31.13).

Evaluation of all 28 available family members for MEN-II/A, with provocative testing for the disease by calcium gluconate and pentagastrin infusion with calcitonin estimation, identified 11 additional cases of medullary carcinoma of the thyroid (Fig. 31.14). Persons with a positive calcitonin stimulation also underwent metanephrine estimation, but there were no other living family members with pheochromocytoma.

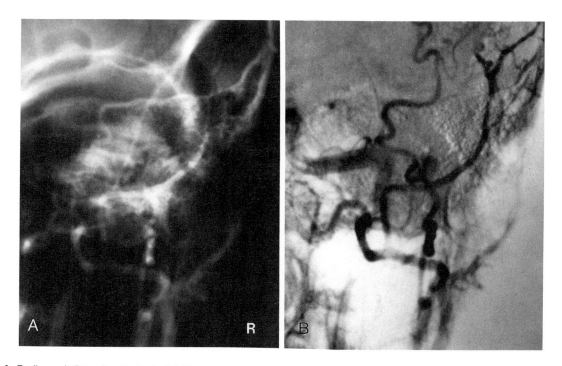

Figure 31.10. **A.** Radiograph (lateral projection) of right petrous pyramid and mastoid process. **B.** The carotid angiogram outlines the size of the right tympanic paraganglioma and its confinement to the middle ear cavity. It identifies the principal, notably enlarged feeding vessels.

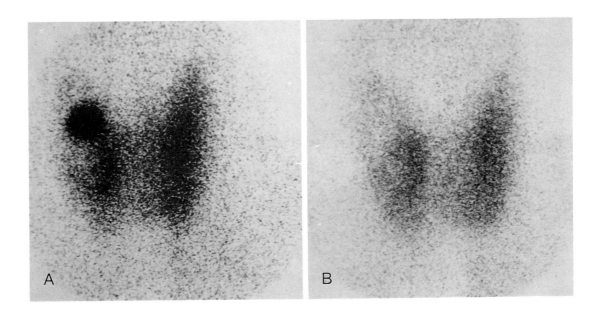

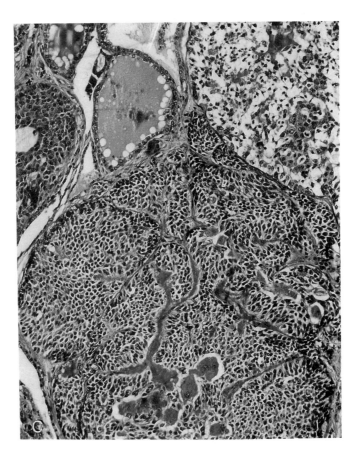

Figure 31.11. Technetium pertechnetate scan of thyroid gland with **(A)** and without **(B)** marker over tumor in right upper lobe. **C.** The neoplasm in the right upper thyroid lobe is a medullary carcinoma, a form of undif-ferentiated carcinoma. It is composed of relatively large cells divided by distinct fibrous bands. (Hematoxylin and eosin, ×100.)

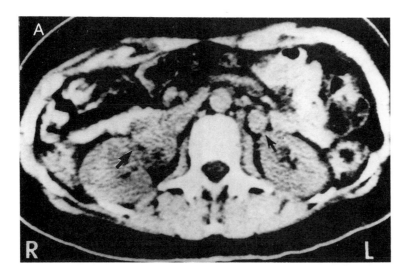

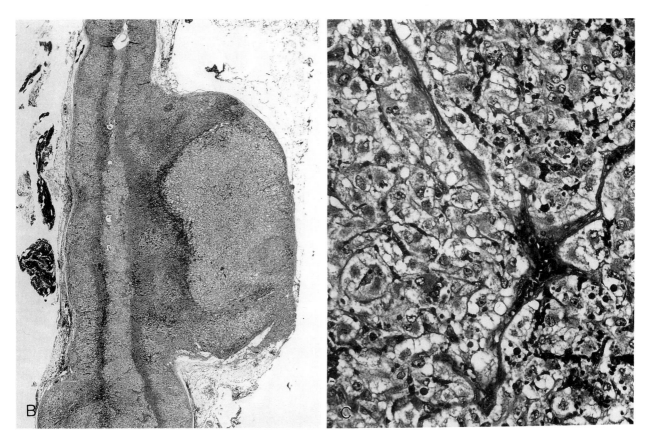

Figure 31.12. **A.** Abdominal CT scan showing the bilateral adrenal tumors *(arrows).* **B.** Left adrenal gland with pheochromocytoma measuring about 1.5 cm in diameter. **C.** The cellular arrangement of the adrenal medullary pheochromocytoma resembles that of the paraganglioma. There is a noticeable variability of cell and nuclear size and arrangement as well as of cytoplasmic volume and basophilic and acidophilic staining property. The cell cords are separated by a dense network of small blood vessels. (Hematoxylin and eosin, ×11 and ×250 for *B* and *C,* respectively.)

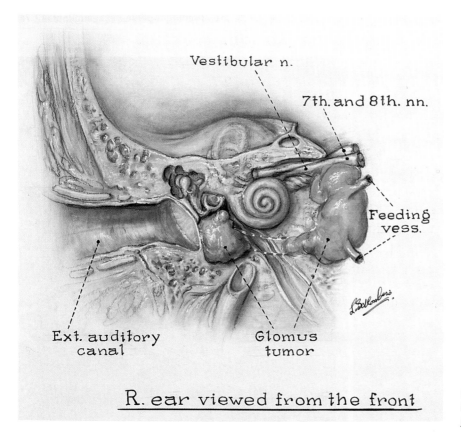

Vestibular n.

7th. and 8th. nn.

Feeding vess.

Ext. auditory canal

Glomus tumor

R. ear viewed from the front

Figure 31.15. Drawing of right jugular paraganglioma involving the tympanic cavity and extending through the jugular foramen into the posterior cranial fossa.

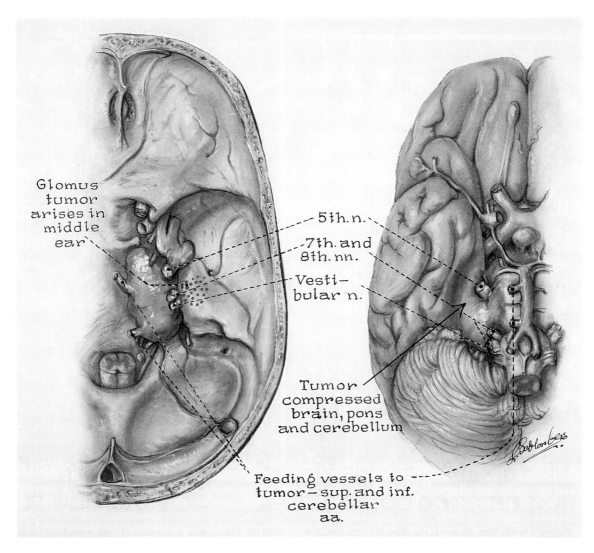

Glomus tumor arises in middle ear

5th. n.

7th. and 8th. nn.

Vesti-bular n.

Tumor compressed brain, pons and cerebellum

Feeding vessels to tumor—sup. and inf. cerebellar aa.

Figure 31.16. Drawing of intracranial portion of right jugular paraganglion impinging on the brain stem, indenting the right cerebellar hemisphere, and compressing the facial nerve at the porus acusticus.

Case 3. *Right jugular paraganglioma with erosion and enlarge-ment of jugular bulb and foramen. Invasion of middle ear, mas-toid process, and perilabyrinthine marrow spaces. Infiltration of inferior petrosal sinus. Extension through jugular foramen into posterior cranial fossa with formation of a cerebellopontine angle tumor measuring about 2.5×2×2 cm, indenting the cerebellum. Involvement of right cranial nerves VII and X.*

The patient was an 84-year-old white woman who at age 58 had noticed tinnitus and loss of hearing in the right ear, at age 65 became hoarse with a right vocal cord paralysis, and at age 67 developed right deep-seated otalgia. The otologic examination revealed a bright red, pulsating vascular tumor occupying the lower two-thirds of the right middle ear cavity, impinging on and pushing the eardrum out-ward (Fig. 31.15). The audiogram showed a 60-dB conductive hear-ing loss in the right ear, with normal hearing in the left ear. A lateral radiograph of the right temporal bone showed alternating areas of radiolucency and increased density throughout the mastoid process. At age 70 the patient developed episodic lightheadedness, unsteadi-ness, and a tendency to fall. She also noticed numbness in the left leg and a sensation of fullness in the back of her head and neck. A neurologic examination then showed: *(a)* a positive Romberg phe-nomenon, *(b)* increased deep tendon reflexes and a positive Babin-sky sign on the left side, *(c)* loss of position sense in the right great toe, and *(d)* a spontaneous nystagmus to the left side. At age 71 she developed right facial twitching, and at age 74 she developed a right-sided palatal weakness. Between ages 60 and 71 the patient had received a total of 5 radiation treatments to the right temporal bone, totaling about 4000 rads. After each treatment there was a very no-ticeable but temporary decrease in the size of the middle ear tumor. After a period of repeated pulmonary emboli, death occurred at age 84 from cerebral arteriosclerosis.

Postmortem examination of the brain revealed: *(a)* a spherical tumor in the right cerebellopontine angle, arising from the jugular foramen (Figs. 31.15–31.17); *(b)* small contusions of the right fron-tal and temporal lobes; *(c)* a small subdural hematoma over the right parieto-occipital area; and *(d)* disseminated plaques of demyeliniza-tion.

Examination of the right temporal bone reveals a very extensive jugular paraganglioma that had invaded the entire middle ear cavity and mastoid process, the perilabyrinthine cells and marrow spaces, the jugular bulb, and the inferior petrosal sinus (Fig. 31.18). There is massive bone destruction throughout the petrous pyramid and jug-ular foramen (Fig. 31.18*C, D,* and *F*). The neoplasm extends along the enlarged and eroded jugular foramen into the right cerebellopon-tine angle to form a spherical tumor measuring about 2.5×2×2 cm (Figs. 31.15–31.17 and 31.18*A*) This intracranial extension of the tumor partially obliterates the porus to the internal acoustic meatus compressing the right facial nerve and indenting the cerebellar hem-isphere (Figs. 31.17 and 31.18*B*). The neoplasm displays all the characteristics of a paraganglioma with remarkable cellular pleo-morphism and evidence of old and recent hemorrhages but very little necrosis (Fig. 31.18*H* and *I*).

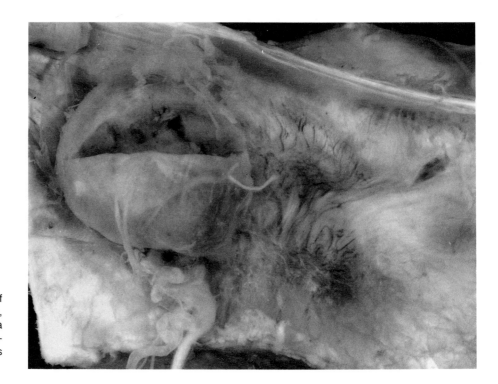

Figure 31.17. Photograph of medial aspect of right temporal bone, showing the extratemporal, intracranial portion of the jugular paraganglioma with its enlarged feeding and draining blood ves-sels. It covers the anterior pyramid and the porus of the internal auditory canal.

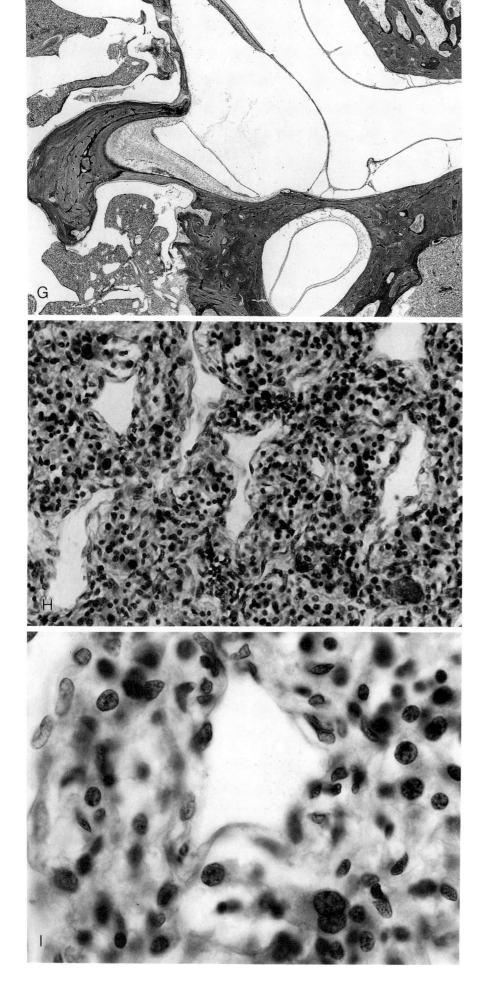

Figure 31.18.   G. Vertical section through right otic capsule at level of oval and round windows. The tumor occupies the entire middle ear cavity, obliterates both window niches, but does not affect the stapes, annular ligament, or round window membrane. (Hematoxylin and eosin, ×15.)

Figure 31.18.   H. The jugular paraganglioma is made up of clear staining cells arranged in an epitheliomatous pattern of sheets, anastomosing cords, and clusters with poor demarcation between cell groups. The cells have an ovoid or polyhedral shape and contain abundant cytoplasm. Their nuclei are spherical, ovoid, vesicular, and frequently hyperchromatic and exhibit remarkable pleomorphism. (×300.)

Figure 31.18.   I. The tumor includes an extraordinary number of blood vessels, enlarged capillaries, and sinusoids. The tumor cells frequently give the impression of lining the sinusoids. (×850.)

Case 4. *Massive left jugular paraglioma with involvement of entire petrous pyramid, invasion of left posterior cranial fossa, left clivus, and basiocciput, and extension through foramen magnum into upper cervical canal. Paralysis of left cranial nerves V and VII–XII. Two-stage subtotal resection of tumor with placement of "false" dural barrier through left suboccipital craniotomy, followed by partial resection of temporal bone and exploration of infratemporal fossa. Postoperative external beam radiation (4000 rads). Subsequent reexploration for removal of residual tumor.*

A 43-year-old white woman had developed pulse synchronous tinnitus and progressive loss of hearing in the left ear for 5 years, occasional unsteadiness, hoarseness, left-sided periocular facial twitching, and left aural fullness and discomfort for 4–5 months. The initial otologic examination revealed a reddish vascular mass behind an intact, laterally bulging, left tympanic membrane. This tumor subsequently perforated through the tympanic membrane and presented as a polypoid tumor in the external auditory canal. There was no visible or palpable mass in the left nasopharynx or neck. The facial twitching involved the temporal and zygomatic branches. The episodes were intermittent with contractions occurring 30–60 times/min. Lacrimation was not decreased in the left eye. Cochlear and vestibular function studies showed total loss of hearing on the left side and a spontaneous, horizontal first-degree nystagmus to the right side that increased during the head-hanging position with eyes open and closed. There was a left lateral canal paresis and involvement of left cranial nerves V and VII–XII. A CT scan of the head showed a uniformly enhancing soft tissue lesion involving the entire temporal bone but destroying mainly the inferior and apical portions of the left petrous pyramid (Fig. 31.19). It occupied the middle ear and extensively involved the posterior cranial fossa. It had eroded and enlarged the jugular foramen, the left side of the clivus, and the basiocciput and extended inferiorly to the level of C1. The angiograms demonstrated the remarkable size and vascularity of the tumor and the patency of the left internal jugular vein (Fig. 31.20). It also identified the greatly enlarged ascending pharyngeal and occipital arteries as the principal sources of the tumor's blood supply. The patient underwent a left suboccipital craniotomy for tumor removal and placement of the fascia layer to provide an additional dural barrier, followed by a left temporal bone resection and exploration of the infratemporal fossa. The tumor had extended into the foramen magnum and the upper neck. Most of the tumor was resected. It proved to be a paraglioma (Fig. 31.20). The three small areas of residual tumor tissue were on the brain stem, in the wall of the carotid artery in its horizontal section, and in the neural compartment of the jugular foramen. Because of a recurrent left facial paralysis, the infratemporal fossa was reexplored 14 months later, and most of the residual tumor tissue could be removed. There has been no clinical evidence of tumor regrowth during the past 4 years.

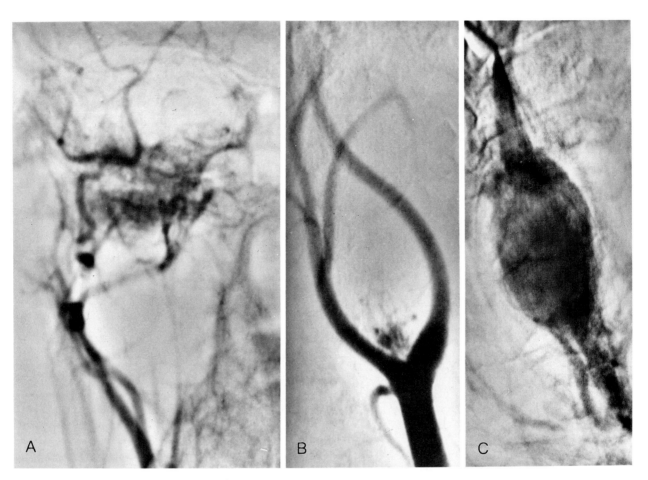

Figure 31.21. A. The right external carotid angiogram reveals a vascular mass in the area of the jugular fossa, measuring about 4×3×2 cm in the frontal view. The tumor receives its major blood supply from an enlarged ascending pharyngeal artery. **B** and **C.** The left common carotid angio- grams demonstrate a 4×3×2-cm vascular mass in the carotid bifurcation. The tumor separates the two carotid arteries and is supplied by several branches from the proximal external carotid artery.

Case 5. *Right jugular paraganglioma with extension to middle and posterior cranial fossa and upper cervical region of neck. Left intercarotid paraganglioma (carotid body tumor).*

The patient was a 34-year-old white man who at age 21 had received radiation therapy (5000 rads) to the left temporal bone for an extensive, then-considered-inoperable jugular paraganglioma that had widely eroded the jugular fossa, partially occluded the jugular vein and sigmoid sinus, destroyed the petrous pyramid in an area measuring about 4×5 cm, and invaded the entire middle ear cleft and cellular system (Figs. 31.21 and 31.22). It extended through the tegmen into the middle cranial fossa and through the posterior cortex of the pyramid into the posterior cranial fossa. It had grown through the jugular foramen and mastoid tip into the jugulodigestive region where it had created a sizeable extratemporal tumor mass. Since age 18 he had noticed pulsatile tinnitus, fullness, and a progressive con- ductive hearing loss in his right ear. Because of "promontorial hy- peremia" he had been treated repeatedly for "otitis media" for 3 years. At age 27 a left intercarotid paraganglioma measuring 4×3×2.5 cm was removed from the carotid bifurcation (Figs. 31.21 and 31.22). By that time the right jugular paraganglioma according to the angiogram had decreased considerably in size to about 3×2 cm. Meanwhile, the patient had lost all cochlear and vestibular func- tion in that ear. A CT scan with contrast of the head and neck and a cerebral angiogram done several years later no longer showed any evidence of bone erosion, enhancement, hypervascularity, or a tu- mor mass in the right temporal bone or base of the skull. The mas- toid air cells, middle ear structures, and internal auditory canals ap- peared radiologically normal bilaterally, and no abnormal soft tissue structures were found in either neck. The patient's situation has re- mained stable for the past several years.

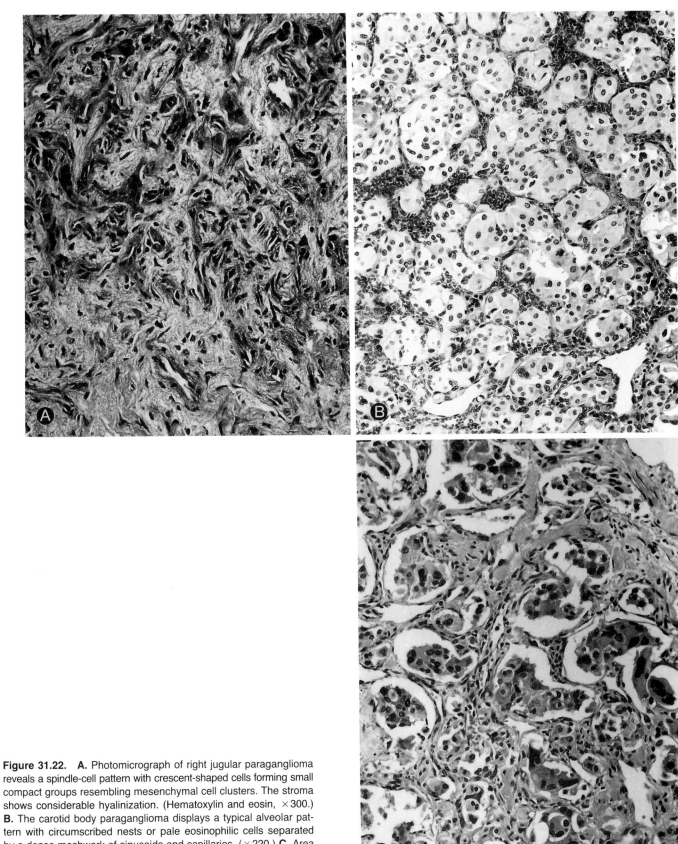

Figure 31.22. **A.** Photomicrograph of right jugular paraganglioma reveals a spindle-cell pattern with crescent-shaped cells forming small compact groups resembling mesenchymal cell clusters. The stroma shows considerable hyalinization. (Hematoxylin and eosin, ×300.) **B.** The carotid body paraganglioma displays a typical alveolar pattern with circumscribed nests or pale eosinophilic cells separated by a dense meshwork of sinusoids and capillaries. (×220.) **C.** Area of remarkable cellular and nuclear pleomorphism and multinucleation. (×220.)

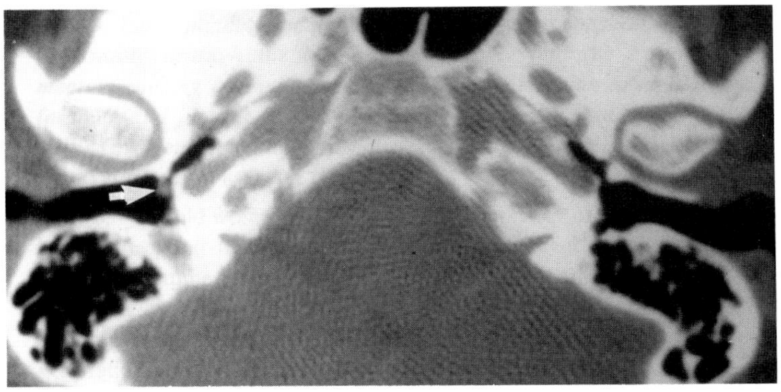

Figure 31.30. Axial CT scan of head with small, asymptomatic tympanic paraganglioma of right middle ear *(arrow)* in an adult woman. The tumor, which arose at the superior aperture of the tympanic canaliculus, was an incidental observation.

References

1. Glenner GG, Grimley PM. Tumors of the extra-adrenal paraganglion system (including chemo-receptors). In: Atlas of tumor pathology. 2nd series, Fascicle 9. Washington, DC: Armed Forces Institute of Pathology, 1974.
2. Bock P, Lassmann H. Histochemische Untersuchungen über die Reserpinwirkung am glomus caroticum (Ratte). Verh Anat 1972;67:20–24.
3. Chiocchio SR, King MP, Angelakos ET. Carotid body catecholamines. Histochemical studies on the effects of drug treatments. Histochemie 1971;25:52–59.
4. Comroe JH Jr. The peripheral chemoreceptors. In: Fenn WO, Rahn H, eds. Handbook of physiology: respiration, Section 3. Washington, DC: American Physiological Society, 1964;1:557.
5. Williams THW. Electron microscopic evidence for an autonomic interneuron. Nature 1967;214:309–310.
6. Heymans C, Neil E. Reflexogenic areas of the cardiovascular system. Boston: Little, Brown, 1958.
7. Hollinshead WH. A comparative study of the glomus coccygeum and the carotid body. Anat Rec 1942;84:1–16.
8. Venkatachalam MA, Greally JG. Fine structure of glomus tumor: similarity of glomus cells to smooth muscle. Cancer 1969;23:1176–84.
9. Guild SR. The glomus jugulare, a nonchromaffin ganglion in man. Ann Otolaryngol 1953;62:1045–1071.
10. Lack EE, et al. Paragangliomas of the head and neck region: a clinical study of 69 patients. Cancer 1977;39:397.
11. Batsakis JG. Tumors of the head and neck. 2nd ed. Baltimore: Williams & Wilkins, 1979.
12. Hamberger B. Catecholamines in glomus tumors. In: Disorders of the skull base region. Proceedings of the 10th Nobel Symposium. Stockholm: Almquist & Wiksell, 1968:269–272.
13. Lattes R. Nonchromaffin paraganglioma of ganglion nodosum, carotid body, and aortic-arch bodies. Cancer 1950;3:667–694.
14. Lattes R, McDonald JJ, Sproul E. Non-chromaffin paraganglioma of carotid body and orbit. Report of case. Ann Surg 1954;139:282–284.
15. Cave TE Jr. Recurrent pheochromocytoma. Report of a case in a previously treated child. Pediatrics 1958;21:994–999.
16. Cragg RW. Concurrent tumors of the left carotid body and both Zuckerkandl bodies. Arch Pathol 1934;18:635–645.
17. Ladenheim JC, Sachs E Jr. Familial tumors of the ''glomus jugulare.'' Report of 2 cases, with a note on the vascular origin of the glomera. Neurology 1961;11:303–309.
18. Kennedy DW, Nager GT. Glomus tumors and multiple endocrine neoplasia. Otolaryngol Head Neck Surg 1986;94:644–648.
19. Taylor DM, Alford BR, Greenberg SD. Metastases of glomus jugulare tumors. Arch Otolaryngol 1965;82:5–13.
20. Windship T, Klopp CT, Jenkins WH. Glomus jugulare tumors. Cancer 1948;1:441–448.
21. Lattes R, Waltner JG. Non-chromaffin paraganglioma of the middle ear. (Carotid body-like tumor; glomus jugulare tumor). Cancer 1949;2:447–468.
22. Spector GJ, Maisel RH, Ogura JH. Glomus tumor in the middle ear. I. An analysis of 46 patients. Laryngoscope 1973;83:1652–1670.

32/ Lipomas of the Cerebellopontine Angle and Internal Auditory Canal

The recognition and the identification of a space-occupying lesion in the cerebellopontine angle have become considerably easier with the availability of modern imaging techniques. Occasionally, however, there may still be a problem. The more frequent neoplasms and cystic processes in that region, i.e., the schwannomas of the acoustic and other cranial nerves, the meningiomas, gliomas, paragangliomas, epidermoids, cholesterol granulomas, arachnoid cysts, etc., are being discussed in separate chapters. There remains, however, a group of less common space-occupying lesions that have to be included in the differential diagnosis because of their very similar or identical clinical manifestations.

To gain a clearer understanding of the lipomas in the cerebellopontine angle, it is advantageous to briefly review the pertinent data on the origin, location, nature, and regional behavior of all forms of intracranial lipomas.

CHARACTERISTICS OF INTRACRANIAL LIPOMAS

Definition and Origin

Intracranial lipomas should be regarded as true, dysgenetic lesions affecting both the cerebral ectomesenchyma and brain parenchyma. They arise primarily from a developmental anomaly of the primitive meninges during the ingrowth of vascular connective tissue. They should be classified correctly as true hamartomas, i.e., as tumor-like but primarily nonneoplastic malformations (1–6).

Localization

Small accumulations of fat cells have been observed in many sites of the primitive meninges (7), in the pia of the corpus callosum (8), and in the central area at the base of the brain (9). Intracranial lipomas arise in the subarachnoid cisterns and choroid plexus. The cisterns are expansions of the subarachnoid space over the ventral and dorsal aspects of the brain. Lipomas may be located along the midline or in a lateral position along the midsagittal plane. The majority, about 50–65%, are situated in the pericallosal cistern along the upper surface of the corpus callosum (10–12). Other locations include the quadrigeminal (superior), cerebellomedullary (cisterna magna), pontine, interpeduncular (basal cistern), infundibular, and chiasmatic cisterns and sites of attachment to the choroid plexus and tela choroidea. Although less frequent (13, 14), laterally located lipomas have been found in the middle cranial fossa, insula, and Sylvian region (13, 15–17). Intracranial lipomas of the cerebellopontine cistern are very rare (18); so far, only about 26 have been reported.

Intracranial lipomas tend to occur at junctions between segments of the central nervous system: the cerebellopontine angle, the pontomesencephalic junction, the mesencephalic-diencephalic junction, and the telencephalic junction (corpus callosum). They present as sites of flexion of the neural tube and, therefore, areas of redundancy of arachnoid tissue (18).

According to their development within the subarachnoid cisterns, intracranial lipomas occur predominantly in the following five areas:

1. Above the site of the corpus callosum, associated with partial or total agenesis of the corpus callosum (the general form and size of a bean, sausage, or plaque of a few millimeters).
2. At the infundibulum (pea size).
3. On the quadrigeminal plate or between the mammillary bodies (pea size).
4. Attached to the choroid plexus of the lateral or third ventricles (bean to egg size).
5. In the cerebellopontine angle or in other cisterns over the convexity (bean to walnut size) (4).

Incidence, Age, and Sex Distribution

The earliest observations of intracranial lipomas were made by neuroanatomists and pathologists in 1818, 1856, and 1897 (7, 18–20). During the past six decades, excellent reports, reviews, and critical discussions have provided all the pertinent data (5, 6, 16, 21). Intracranial lipomas are rare in comparison with extracranial subcutaneous lipomas, which are the most common benign tumors. A number of intracranial lipomas were reported as incidental observations during postmortem examinations and computed tomography (CT) scans of the brain performed for other reasons (6, 21). By 1974, more than 200 cases had been reported (6). All age groups are affected, although the lesion appears to show a preference for patients in their second and fourth decades (4). Both sexes appear to be equally affected (14).

Association of Multiple Intracranial Lipomas with Other Malformations

The association of certain intracranial lipomas with malformations of the skull and brain is well recognized. Callosal lipomas may occur jointly with cranium bifidum, spina bifida, polymicrogyria, microcephaly, hypoplasia of the cerebellum, agenesis of the cerebellar vermis, meningomyeloencephalocele, hypoplasia or aplasia of the corpus callosum or septum pellucidum, and other malformations (6, 22). This further supports the concept of the dysgenetic origin of intracranial lipomas (23).

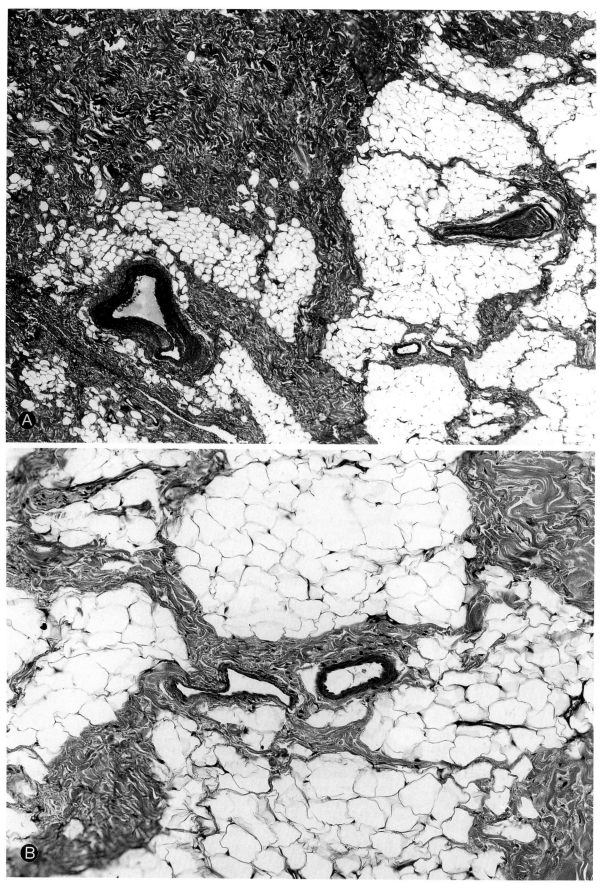

Figure 32.5.   The tumor consists of mature adipose tissue with the eighth nerve splayed apart into medium-sized nerve fascicles and individual nerve fibers. (Hematoxylin and eosin, ×65 and ×190, respectively).

Case 4. *Walnut-sized, surprisingly vascular lipoma occupying the left cerebellopontine angle, completely incorporating cranial nerves VII and VIII and compressing and displacing cranial nerve V anteriorly and inferiorly. Moderate compression and displacement of brain stem.*

A 38-year-old man with a history of total loss of hearing in the left ear following an infection in childhood was admitted for a neurologic evaluation after a sudden loss of hearing in the opposite right ear that was associated with persistent tinnitus.

Neurologic examination is said to have been otherwise unremarkable.

Radiologic examination demonstrated, on the axial CT scan, a clearly defined, hypodense (−100 HU), nonenhancing lesion in the left cerebellopontine angle, identical with fat tissue. It measured about 2.5 cm in diameter (Fig. 32.6). The internal auditory canal was not

enlarged. The area of the right cerebellopontine angle was unremarkable. The lipoma displayed a high signal intensity on the T1-weighted magnetic resonance image but only a moderate signal intensity on the T2-weighted image (Fig. 32.7). The arterial and venous vertebral angiograms disclosed a displacement of the vascular structures that resulted from a space-occupying process in the left cerebellopontine angle, a displacement of the left labyrinthine artery, and a vascular stain of the lesion in the venous phase (Fig. 32.8).

At *operation,* a remarkably vascular lipoma was found in the left cerebellopontine angle. It had completely incorporated the seventh and eighth cranial nerves and compressed and displaced the fifth cranial nerve anteriorly and inferiorly. The lipoma was not adherent to the brain stem. A partial resection with decompression of the brain stem and fifth nerve was carried out. Histologic diagnosis was a vascular lipoma.

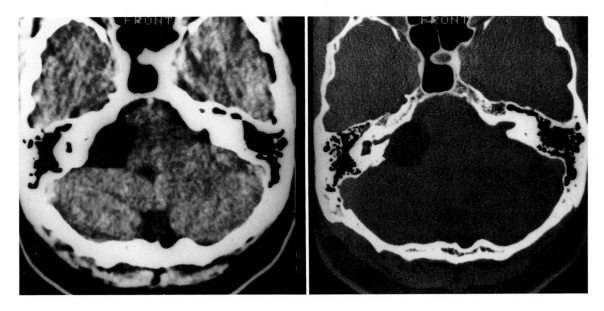

Figure 32.6. Axial CT scans demonstrate a smooth, homogeneous, hypodense (−100 HU), and nonenhancing lesion in the left cerebellopontine angle but a normal internal auditory canal. (Courtesy of Dr. E. Heiss.)

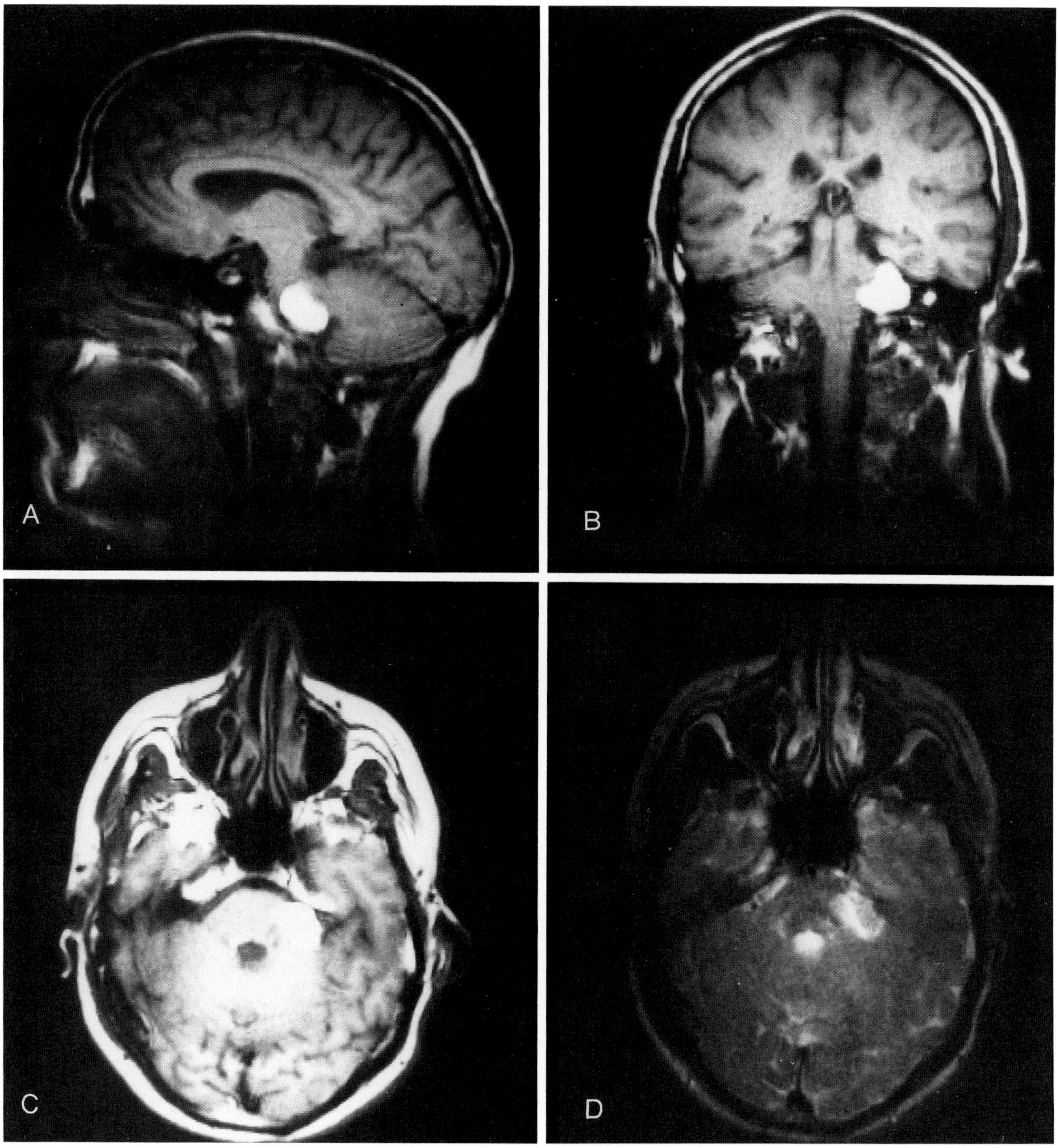

Figure 32.7. The lipoma in the left cerebellopontine angle exhibits a high signal intensity in the T1-weighted images **(A–C)** but only a moderately high signal intensity in the T2-weighted image **(D).** (Courtesy of Dr. E. Heiss.)

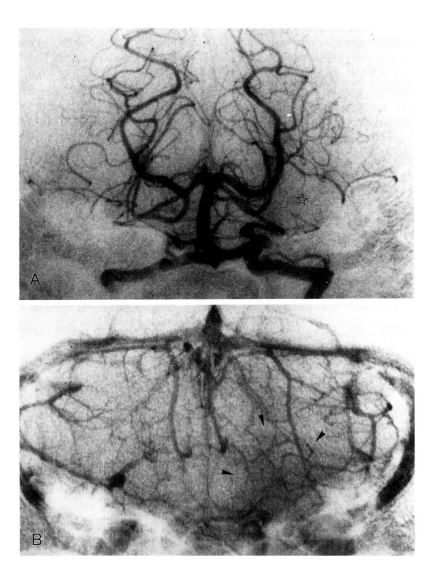

Figure 32.8. Arterial **(A)** and venous **(B)** vertebral angiograms show displacement of the vascular structure related to a space-occupying process in the left cerebellopontine angle. The left labyrinthine artery is displaced, and the lipoma takes up a vascular stain in the venous phase. (Courtesy of Dr. E. Heiss.)

34/ Chordomas

Origin

Chordomas are relatively uncommon neoplasms, as they account for only 3–4% of all primary tumors of bone (1). They arise in all likelihood from aberrant remnants of the notocord and are therefore considered of dysontogenic origin. They are found anywhere along the chorda, occasionally lateral to the midline, but are most frequently observed in the sacrococcygeal area (51%), in the spheno-occipital region of the skull (37%), and in the vertebral regions (2).

INTRACRANIAL CHORDOMAS

Location and Regional Behavior

Intracranial chordomas develop at the skull base, within or below the pituitary fossa, in the clivus, or in the petrous apex (3, 4). As the tumor extends laterally, it may invade the cavernous sinus and petrous pyramid. Extending forward, it may enter the middle cranial fossa through the tentorium, invade the sphenoid and posterior ethmoid sinuses, infiltrate the posterior orbit, and expand into the nasopharynx, nasal cavity, and maxillary sinus (Figs. 34.11 and 34.12). Or it may spread posteriorly into the posterior cranial fossa and become a cerebellopontine angle lesion, compressing the pons and medulla (4). Growing inferiorly and posteriorly, it may invade the infratemporal fossa. In so doing, it destroys (and honeycombs) the adjacent bony structures.

Depending on the site of origin and direction of growth, different forms, i.e., sellar, parasellar, and clival chordomas, may be distinguished clinically. Chordomas are generally slow-growing lesions that recur locally following excision, and they can metastasize (5–7).

Incidence, Age, and Sex Distribution

Chordomas account for about 0.2% of all intracranial tumors (2). They may occur at any age, but they most frequently occur in the 20–40-year-old age group (2, 8, 9). The mean age at diagnosis is approximately 45 years.

Variant Forms

Chondroid chordomas were first described in 1973 (10) and are considered to be variants of conventional chordomas (11). They tend to occur in younger individuals and have generally been limited to the spheno-occipital region (10). They are distinguished by the presence of a considerable chondroid component, which may mimic either a chondroma or a chondrosarcoma, combined with areas more characteristic of a conventional chordoma (10, 11).

Macroscopic and Microscopic Appearance

Chordomas vary considerably in size and may range from that of a millet grain to that of an apple. Their surface is nodular or lobulated with a whitish-pink color. Their consistency is soft or elastic. On cross-section the surface appears gelatinous, translucent, and occasionally brownish-red, resulting from a recent hemorrhage (Fig. 34.11). It may include cysts filled with tenacious mucoid material and granular calcium deposits (2).

On light microscopic examination the tumor resembles the pattern of notochordal tissue (Fig. 34.3). It displays a lobular arrangement created by ingrowth of vascular connective tissue strands from the capsule, intersecting and surrounding compact masses and bands of clear cells with a regular pattern (Fig. 34.7). Sheets and cords of cells with abundant eosinophilic cytoplasm are mixed with physaliphorous cells and embedded in a mucinous stroma (Figs. 34.1, 34.5, 34.8, and 34.11). The cells are well demarcated and polyhedral, with a fairly large, round and dark chromatin-dense nucleus and a fair-sized, characteristic, intracytoplasmic bubble-like vacuole (Figs. 34.1, 34.5, 34.8, and 3.11) (4). In the presence of a chondroid chondroma, directly adjacent to these areas of conventional chordoma, are islands of cells with clear-cut cartilaginous differentiation (Figs. 34.1, 34.5, and 34.10) (12). This second, smaller tissue component consists of a basophilic stroma that resembles hyaline cartilage that includes lacunae containing stellate cells. These cells within the lacunae lack the abundant eosinophilic cytoplasm and vacuoles found in cells of areas of conventional chordoma (11). Occasionally, small foci of necrosis, calcifications, and cysts may be seen, as well as aggregations of hemosiderin-laden macrophages indicating former hemorrhages (Figs. 34.11 and 34.12). The cytologic features are usually benign, and mitotically active cells are generally absent (11).

Chordomas often cause considerable bone destruction. Malignant degeneration has been observed in spheno-occipital chordomas. It is characterized by hypercellularity, cell pleomorphism and anaplasia, and increased mitoses.

Case Reports

Case 1. *Chordoma originating from dorsal aspect of clivus with widespread destruction and replacement of bone. Compression of midbrain and posterior hypothalamus. Involvement of left cavernous sinus and extension into left cerebellopontine angle. Postoperative left suboccipital craniectomy and left lateral transtemporal sphenoid approach to clivus with subtotal removal of original and recurrent tumor. Progressive involvement of left cranial nerves II and IV–XII and right cranial nerves II and V.*

The patient was a 69-year-old white woman with a 6-month history of unsteadiness, staggering, veering to the left and several falls, difficulties with writing, swallowing, and slurred speech, and left retro-orbital pain. Evaluation following a fall disclosed a 2-cm lesion in the anterior portion of the left posterior cranial fossa. A vertebral angiogram demonstrated a shift of the basilar artery to the right.

Neurologic examination on admission revealed involvement of left cranial nerves V, VII, IX, and X and of the left cerebellum.

Operation consisted of a left suboccipital craniectomy that exposed a grayish tumor underneath left cranial nerves V, VII, and XII. A generous partial resection across the midline with decompression of all cranial nerves involved in the tumor capsule was performed. Postoperatively the patient required a tracheostomy and gastrostomy. During the ensuing 4 years, the patient developed increasing loss of function of left cranial nerves II–XII, including paralysis of VII and VIII, and progressive difficulties with swallowing. Magnetic resonance imaging (MRI) showed a large tumor mass arising from the dorsal surface of the clivus, widely destroying and replacing it, compressing the midbrain and posterior hypothalamus, and extending into the left cerebellopontine angle. The mass appeared hypodense in the T1-weighted image and hyperdense in the T2-weighted image.

During a *second operation,* a left lateral transtemporal sphenoid approach, the left clivus and parasellar regions were exposed, and most of the tumor was resected. Histologically, it proved to be a recurrent chordoma (Fig. 34.1). The postoperative course has been characterized by slowly progressive loss of multiple cranial nerve function and involvement of the brain stem.

Case 2. *Chordoma originating in left lacerated foramen with destruction of posterior portion of left sphenoid bone and petrous apex. Extension to left cavernous sinus, anterior portion of left brain stem, and medial portion of temporal lobe. Extension into left cerebellopontine angle. Postoperative left modified transtemporal sphenoid approach to left petrous apex and parasellar region for subtotal resection.*

The patient was a 75-year-old white woman with a 3-year history of double vision on left lateral gaze and left temporofrontal headaches. During the 6 months prior to admission she developed some staggering with a tendency to fall to the left, difficulties with swallowing, slurred speech, and left retro-orbital pain.

Neurologic examination on admission revealed involvement of left cranial nerves V–VII and IX–XII.

A computed tomography (CT) scan showed an irregularly enhancing mass with destruction of the posterior portion of the left sphenoid bone and petrous apex. The tumor extended into the anterior portion of the left brain stem, medial portion of the left temporal lobe, and left cavernous sinus (Fig. 34.2). The cerebral angiogram showed an anterior displacement and straightening of the ascending portion of the left cavernous carotid artery but no hypervascularity of the mass nor significant contributory vessels.

Operation consisted of a left, modified, transtemporal sphenoid approach to the left petrous apex for subtotal resection of a histologically confirmed chordoma. The tumor had eroded the left petrous apex and the adjacent clivus and extended into the cerebellopontine angle, compressing the midbrain. Histologically, the tumor proved to be a chordoma (Fig. 34.3). Postoperatively, the patient received a course of proton beam radiation at the Massachusetts General Hospital with a tumor bed dose of 6488 rads.

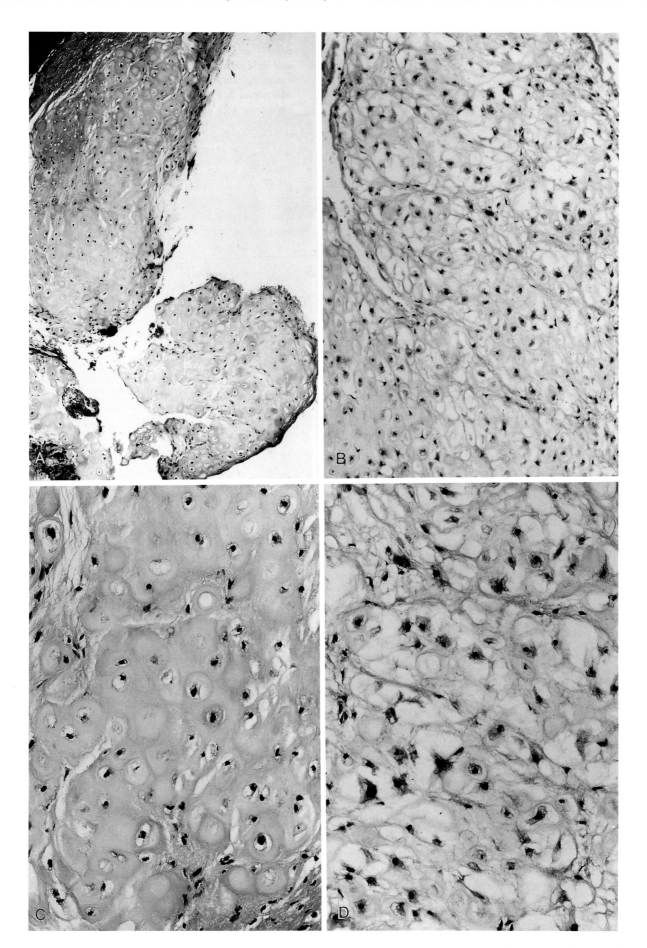

Figure 34.5. A. Low-power photomicrograph of low-grade chondrosarcoma. **B.** The major component of the tumor consists of a slightly basophilic stroma including lacunae containing stellate cells. **C.** The stroma displays a tendency toward hyaline degeneration. **D.** The tumor cells exhibit some pleomorphic chromatin-dense nuclei. Some cells have assumed a more spindle-cell form, and they occasionally show evidence of mitotic activity. (Hematoxylin and eosin, ×90, ×100, ×300, and ×300, respectively.)

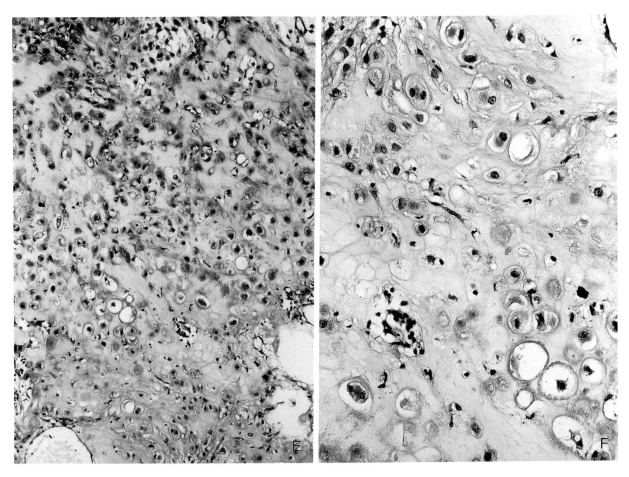

Figure 34.5. **E.** Some areas of the tumor show evidence of cartilaginous differentiation. **F.** Some lacunae contain cells with two or more pleomorphic nuclei. (Hematoxylin and eosin, ×200 and ×300, respectively.)

Case 4. *Large, recurrent chondroid chordoma originating from left clivus. Extensive destruction of left skull base in middle cranial fossa. Partial destruction of left pterygoid plate and clinoid processes. Erosion of pituitary fossa and left sphenoid wing. Massive invasion of left posterior ethmoid, left maxillary, and left and right sphenoid sinuses, and left posterior orbit. Extension toward right optic nerve. Involvement of left cranial nerves II–VI. Postoperative facial degloving, partial resection of left maxillary, ethmoid, and sphenoid sinuses, with section of chordoma from left posterior paranasal sinuses, nasal and nasopharyngeal cavity, and left pituitary and left infratemporal fossa (9/24/85). Extensive tumor recurrence in infratemporal fossa, petrous apex, and sellar and premesencephalic cistern regions.*

A 46-year-old man at age 36 had developed progressive diplopia on left lateral gaze, loss of vision in the left eye, numbness of the left face, and occipital headaches. Two years later, a CT scan of the head revealed a large skull base lesion that on biopsy proved to be a chordoma. The patient was treated with 10 MEV x-rays from the linear accelerator for a total dose of 5360 rads, which resulted in resolution of dysfunction of cranial nerves V and VI and of the headaches.

Neuro-otologic examination on admission revealed, via MRI, a very large skull base lesion involving the left middle cranial fossa, almost the entire left maxillary sinus, the left posterior ethmoid sinus, and both sphenoid sinuses. It had partially destroyed the left pterygoid plate and left sphenoid wing and had eroded the left pituitary fossa and clinoid processes (Figs. 34.6 and 34.7). The patient underwent a facial degloving and partial resection of the left maxillary sinus, exploration of the posterior nasal sinuses and posterior orbit, and resection of the chordoma from the nose, paranasal sinuses, nasopharynx, posterior orbit, pituitary, and left infratemporal fossa (9/24/85). On follow-up examination 4 years later, there was evidence of massive tumor recurrence in the areas of the left infratemporal fossa, left petrous apex, tentorium, sella, and premesencephalic cistern.

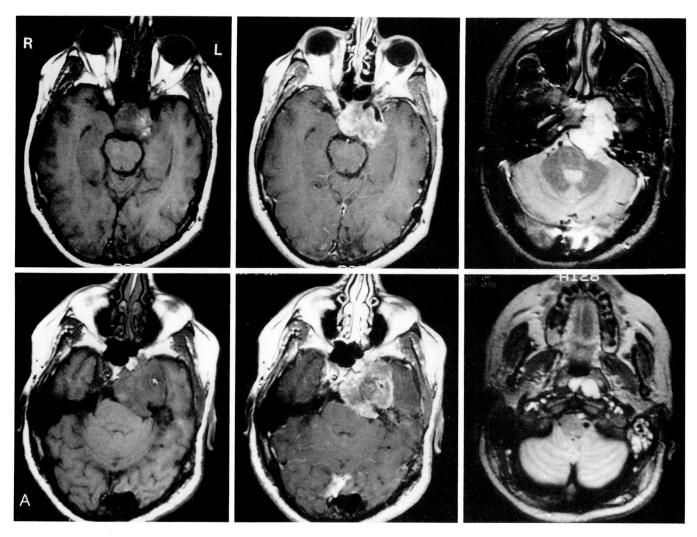

Figure 34.9. Axial and sagittal T1-weighted serial magnetic resonance images **(A** and **B)** of head before and after intravenous gadolinium injection. A large heterogeneously enhancing soft tissue mass involves the left side of the clivus and extends posteriorly into the posterior cranial fossa including the pontomesencephalic cistern, compressing and displacing the brain stem to the opposite side. It also involves the left cavernous sinus and has eroded the posterior clinoid processes. Extending downward, it has eroded the pterygoid processes and invaded the infratemporal fossa. The mass extends superiorly into the suprasellar cistern and encircles the left internal carotid artery. Anteriorly, it extends into the left optic canal and superior orbital fissure, sphenoid sinus, and middle cranial fossa, destroying the floor. Inferiorly, it extends along the submucosal plane into the nasopharynx down to the level of the uvula. Postoperative changes involving the nose, left maxillary sinus, and sphenoid sinus reflect a preceding midfacial approach for tumor removal. The three-dimensional reconstruction **(C)** demonstrates the erosive process affecting the left middle cranial fossa, left petrous apex, clivus, pterygoid plate, sella, and posterior wall of the sphenoid sinus. (Courtesy of Dr. M. J. Holliday.)

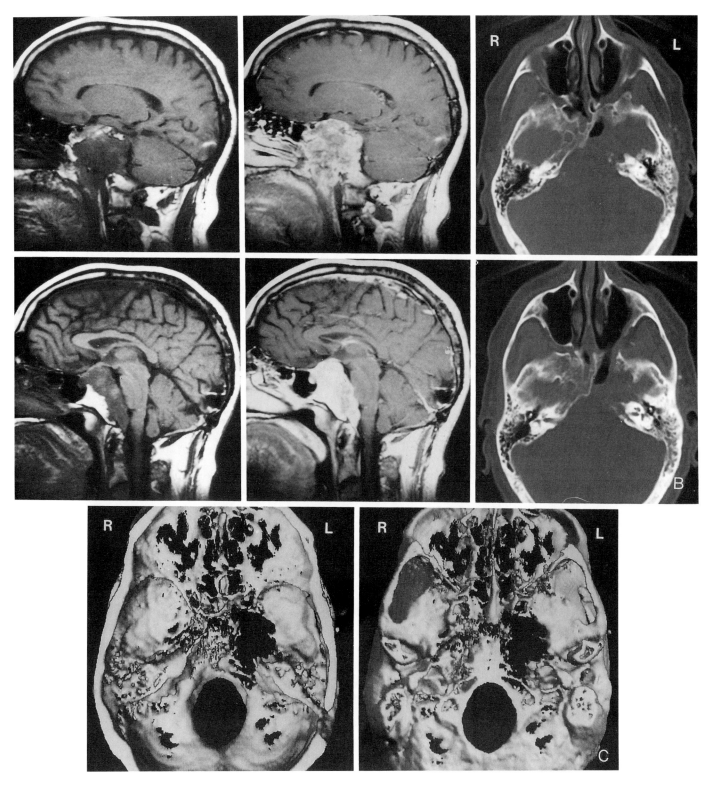

Figure 34.9. B and C.

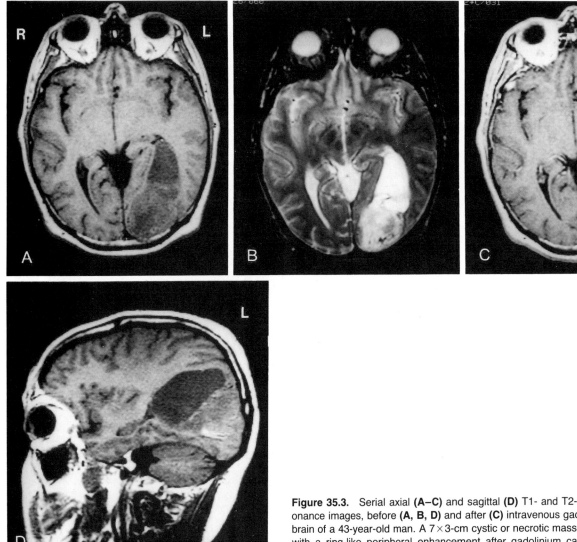

Figure 35.3.   Serial axial **(A–C)** and sagittal **(D)** T1- and T2-weighted magnetic resonance images, before **(A, B, D)** and after **(C)** intravenous gadolinium contrast, of the brain of a 43-year-old man. A 7×3-cm cystic or necrotic mass in the left occipital lobe with a ring-like peripheral enhancement after gadolinium can be seen. There is a 1-cm midline shift to the right, and the brain stem is deviated anteriorly to the right.

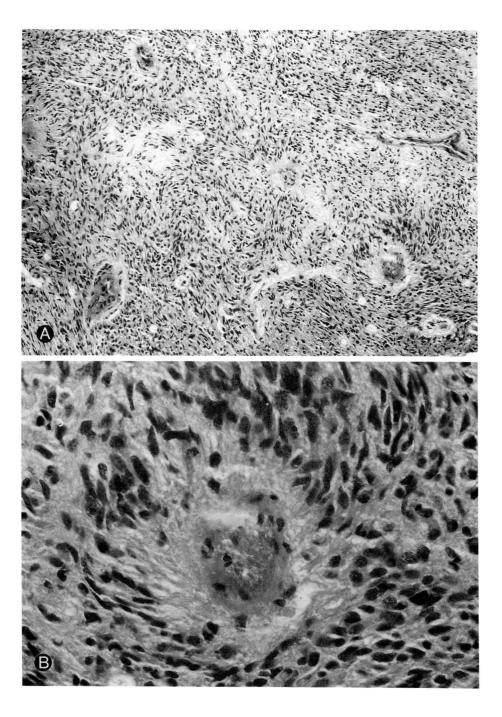

Figure 35.4. A and **B.** The cytoarchitecture of the tumor is disorderly. It consists of closely packed spindle cells varying in size and form. The chromatin density of the nuclei varies considerably. There are occasional giant cells and multinucleated cell forms. Mitotic figures are numerous. (Hematoxylin and eosin, ×65 and ×200, respectively.)

36/ Cerebral Herniations and Ectopic Brain Tissue

Cerebral tissue may be found in the middle ear cleft and internal auditory canal under a variety of conditions. In the middle ear cleft it may be present as a meningoencephalocele or a cephalocele or as a small herniation of brain tissue from the overlying temporal lobe, with or without a meningeal cover. The two forms may be congenital, idiopathic, or acquired. The predisposing condition for both is a dehiscence in the tegmental bone and overlying dura. Whereas in the congenital herniation the defect is present at birth, in the acquired form it develops or occurs at the later time in life. The congenital form is rare; the acquired herniation, on the other hand, is observed more often.

Brain herniations were first recognized in 1870 (1), and shortly thereafter were observed to be associated often with arachnoid granulations. The first detailed description appeared in 1919 (2) when they were regarded as pathologic changes resulting from a long-standing increase in intracranial pressure. Even a transient period of intracranial hypertension during nephritis, a migraine attack, or an infectious disease was considered a possible contributing factor, based on histologic observations of bone resorption and new bone formation in the immediate vicinity of the herniations in these patients (2).

Since cerebral herniations are generally associated with arachnoid granulations, they share several of their predilective locations. Arachnoid granulations or villi are concentrated in the walls of the major venous sinuses and along their contributory veins. With regard to the temporal bone, they are found in the immediate vicinity, on the lateral and medial aspect of the pyramid, and in four locations inside the petrous portion. They are distributed along the cavernous, sphenoparietal, superior and inferior petrosal, sigmoid, and transverse sinuses. They are also observed in the Gasserian envelopes, at the entrance and within the internal auditory canal, and in the neural compartment of the jugular foramen. They may also be found in the labyrinthine segment of the facial canal, at the geniculate ganglion, in the roof of the Eustachian tube, and occasionally along a petrosquamous sinus (Fig. 36.1) (3). The space contained within an arachnoid granulation is continuous with the subarachnoid space and contains cerebrospinal fluid (CSF) on its way to be absorbed into the venous sinus.

Cerebral herniations are generally embedded or partially covered by arachnoid granulations (Fig. 36.2). They are regularly associated with a defect in the bone and dura of the middle cranial fossa. In that area the dura separates into two layers, an outer layer lining the excavation in the tegmental bone and an inner layer continuing in the original plane. A dehiscence in the inner layer, similar to the opening in the diaphragm of the sella, represents the hernial opening into the underlying intradural cavity. The gradual extension of cerebral tissue through that aperture results in the formation of a brain herniation or a small encephalocele (4).

Brain herniations are located mostly in the tegmental area (Figs. 36.2 and 36.3), predominantly above the tensor tympanic muscle, and only rarely on the posterior aspect of the pyramid in the vicinity of the porus acusticus, superior petrosal, and lateral sinus. As the surrounding bone undergoes progressive resorption, a cerebral herniation may come in apposition with the mucosa lining a tegmental cell or with the middle ear mucosa (Fig. 36.2). This contiguity predisposes to direct extension of an inflammatory process from the middle ear to the meninges and brain. The pathway may be by direct extension following necrosis of the dura or, more frequently, via vascular channels. This route for an otogenic endocranial complication has long been documented (4–7). Another clinically significant route occurs when a cerebral herniation is torn and the arachnoid space is opened incidentally during resection of the tegmental bone or exposure of the posterior fossa dura. An arachnoid villus protruding into a petrosal sinus may provide a pathway for the extension of a thrombophlebitis or bacteremia to the subarachnoid space and meninges (4).

Cerebral herniations are infrequently observed under normal circumstances (4, 8). Under certain pathologic conditions, however, they are found more often. Several decades ago, cerebral herniations were frequently found in young children with vitamin D deficiency and occasionally found in adults with histologic evidence of healed rickets (7). The frequent occurrence of arachnoid granulations and cerebral herniation in the temporal bone after long-standing elevation of intracranial pressure in patients with larger posterior fossa tumors, especially acoustic schwannomas, or hydrocephalus has been well documented (4–7). In the preantibiotic era, the acquired cerebral herniation was a common complication following mastoid surgery, especially after transmastoid drainage of a temporal lobe or cerebellar abscess. Among 147 brain herniations of the middle ear cleft reported during the past 43 years (9–12), 30 (21%) were congenital in origin. Ten of the 30 patients had multiple herniations, and 1 patient had bilateral herniations. The congenital form may remain asymptomatic but can manifest itself by recurrent CSF otorrhea and rhinorrhea, "serous otitis," and recurrent meningitis. The acquired brain herniation may result from destruction of the tegmental bone by an osteitic process, a cholesteatoma, or both. Far more often, however, it arises as a complication of an iatrogenic injury of the tegmental bone and dura during a surgical procedure for removal of an inflammatory process (13).

The acquired brain herniation when covered by arachnoid may manifest itself by a CSF otorrhea or rhinorrhea, by the presence of a clear middle ear fluid, occasionally by recurrent meningitis, and by a conductive loss. In a patient with a history of a preceding radical mastoidectomy, it usually presents itself as a soft, grayish, pulsating mass protruding from the tegmental region. The congenital and acquired cerebral herniations vary considerably in size from 2 mm to 2 cm in diameter (11). A larger herniation may impinge on the ossicular chain and the walls of the middle ear. It may be lined by middle ear mucosa or modified glial tissue. On histologic examination it generally reveals

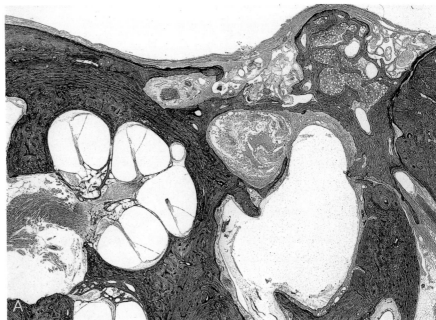

Figure 36.1. **A.** Vertical midmodiolar section through left temporal bone of an adult male with two arachnoid granulations located in the tegmen tympani above the tensor tympani muscle. (Hematoxylin and eosin, × 10.)

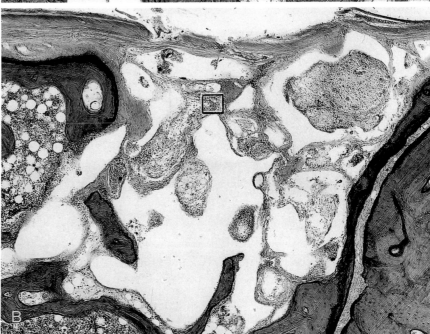

Figure 36.1. **B.** Adjacent section. This arachnoid villus is near the sphenopetrosal suture and well covered by dura. (× 50.)

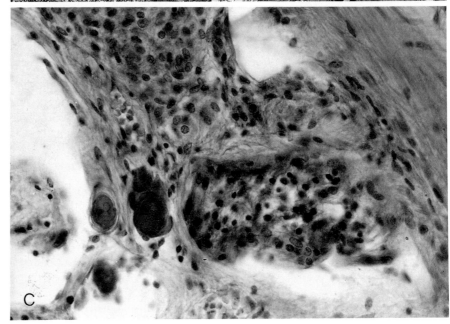

Figure 36.1. **C.** Same section as *B*. The arachnoid lining cells tend to collect in clusters around the tips of the arachnoid granulations. The concentric calcifications represent psammoma bodies. (× 400.)

References

1. Von Recklinghausen FD. Über multiple Hirnhernien. Sitzungsberichte der Würzburger Physik Med Gesellsch, N.F. 11, 1872 (6. Sitzung v 12.3.1870).

2. Erdheim J. Über die Folgen des gesteigerten Hirndruckes. Jahrb Psychiatr Neurol 1919;39:322.

3. Nager GT. Cerebral herniations in the temporal bone. In: Nager GT, ed. Meningiomas involving the temporal bone. Clinical and pathological aspects. Springfield, Illinois: Charles C Thomas, 1964.

4. Mayer O. Zwei Fälle von Frühmeningitis bei akuter Mittelohrentzündung. Arch Ohrenheilkd 1930;64:271.

5. Brunner H. Zur Pathogenese der Meningitis bei akuter Otitis. Monatsschr Ohrenheilkd 1930;64:271.

6. Mehler L, Satz L. Zur klinischen Bedeutung der Hirnhernien und pacchionischen Granulationen im Bereiche des Schläfenbeines. Gesamte Neurol 1934;151:441.

7. Ruttin E. Zur Klinik und Pathologie der Hirnhernien im Bereiche des Schläfenbeines. Monatsschr Ohrenheilkd 1938;72:197.

8. Wojno S: Über physiologische Hirnhernien. Frankf Z Pathol 1912;9:279.

9. Iurato S, Ettorre GC, Selvini C. Brain herniation into the middle ear: two idiopathic cases treated by a combined intracranial-mastoid approach. Laryngoscope 1989;99(9):950–954.

10. Golding-Wood DG, Williams HO, Brookes GB. Tegmental dehiscence and brain herniation into the middle ear cleft. J Laryngol Otol 1991;105(6):477–480.

11. Iurato S, Bux G, Collucci S, Davidson C, Ettore GC, Mazzarella L, Mevoli S, Selvini C, Zallone AZ. Histopathology of spontaneous brain herniations into the middle ear. Acta Otolaryngol (Stockh) 1992;112(2):328–333.

12. Provedano RV, Iurato RA, Seco Pinero MI, Lopez Villarejo P. Idiopathic cerebral hernia in the middle ear. Ann Otorhinolaryngol Ibero Am 1992;19(2)217–223.

13. Grossenbacher R. Mastoid brain herniation following a cholesteatoma operation. HNO 1988;36(1):40–44.

14. Suyama K, Horimoto C, Tsutsumi K, Yasunaga A, Asou H, Okamoto K. A case of cerebrospinal fluid otorrhea 6 years after temporal bone fracture. No Shinkei Geka 1989;17(5):473–476.

15. Kuwata T, Kamei I, Uematsu Y, Iwamoto M, Kuriyama T. Growing skull fracture with rapid growth: a case report. No Shinkei Geka 1988;16(Suppl 5) 677–681.

16. Thompson JW. Transmastoid encephaloceles. A case report. Int J Pediatr Otorhinolaryngol 1988;15(2):179–84.

17. Klein MV, Schwaighofer BW, Sobel DF, Fantozzi RD, Hesselink JR. Heterotopic brain in the middle ear. J Comput Assist Tomogr 1989;13(6):1058–1060.

37/ Metastasis to the Temporal Bone and Cerebellopontine Angle

Temporal bone metastases have come to our attention more frequently in recent decades. That they no longer represent a rare entity is reflected by the 200 case reports in the literature (1–14). Recent reviews have shown that primary carcinomas are located, in order of decreasing frequency, in the breast, lung, kidney, prostate, stomach, pharynx, larynx, thyroid, cervix, and uterus (4–8). Other, less frequent primary sites are the salivary gland, colon, testis, bladder, carotid body, esophagus, gallbladder, ovary, pancreas, rectum, paranasal sinus, and scalp. Very rarely does a sarcoma of the meninges, neck, lung, liver, parotid, synovia, or bone or a melanoma in the head, neck and thoracic area, choroid, nasopharynx (9–13), spinal cord, or heel metastasize to the temporal bone. Leukemia, lymphoma, and myeloma may also involve the temporal bone. Metastases have been observed in all age groups. The incidence of bilateral involvement may exceed 50%. Females and males seem to be equally affected. The tumor may spread to the temporal bone through the bloodstream or the subarachnoid space, whereby the primary tumor may invade the subarachnoid compartment directly or after hematogenous dissemination to the meninges. The preferential location of the hematogenous metastases is the petrous apex, but they are also found in other regions of the petrous pyramid, in the mucoperiosteum of the middle ear cleft, in the tympanic membrane, and in the skin and periosteum of the external canal. A metastatic lesion in the middle ear cavity can manifest itself as a polypoid mass protruding through a perforation of the eardrum into the outer ear canal. Occasionally, a major portion of the temporal bone may show metastatic involvement. A metastasis of the petrous apex may remain asymptomatic for a long time, only to be detected incidentally or by involvement of adjacent structures, such as the hypotympanum, middle ear, Eustachian tube, facial nerve, and lower cranial nerves. By contrast, a secondary tumor in the internal auditory canal is most often associated with impairment of cochlear, vestibular, and facial nerve function. The metastasis may infiltrate and destroy the cranial nerves and extend along the perineural spaces to the cochlear modiolus and endolymphatic and perilymphatic compartments of the semicircular canals, vestibule, and cochlea. Invasion of the cochlea may or may not be associated with partial or total atrophy of the respective sensory end organs, ganglion cells, and nerve fibers. The location of a secondary tumor in the cerebellopontine angle can produce an identical neurologic deficit. A metastasis in the neural compartment of the jugular foramen may give rise to impairment of ninth, tenth, eleventh, and occasionally twelfth cranial nerve function. If a secondary tumor in the middle ear becomes superinfected or interferes with sound transmission, then otorrhea, loss of hearing, and otalgia may develop. Extension of a metastasis beyond the confines of the temporal bone can proceed across the mastoid cortex and tegmen, in the direction of the posterior cranial fossa, or into the infratemporal fossa. The neuro-otologic manifestations may, in a rare situation, herald the presence of a previously undiagnosed metastatic disease of the temporal bone.

A metastasis manifests itself radiographically as an irregular osteolytic defect with poorly defined margins. Gross bone destruction is usually a late phenomenon if the process is not accompanied by infection. The computed tomography (CT) scan may show tumor and secretions with equal density and can result in overestimation of the extent of tumor invasion. Magnetic resonance imaging (MRI) clearly defines the edges of the neoplasms and is superior in the identification and demarcation of soft tissue (2). Whereas a metastasis that manifests itself early and without erosion of bone may be missed on CT and MRI without intravenous contrast, it usually becomes recognizable with gadolinium enhancement.

Case Reports

Case 1. *Epidermoid carcinoma of nasopharynx with extension to sphenoid sinus, sella turcica, hypophysis, middle and posterior cranial fossa, and subarachnoid space. Minimal invasion of meninges and ventral brain stem. Metastasis to right internal auditory canal with involvement of facial, cochlear, and vestibular nerves. Paralysis of right cranial nerves V–XII.*

The patient was a 54-year-old woman who 16 months prior to her last hospital admission developed progressive loss of hearing in the right ear with a sensation of fullness and occipital headaches. Two months later she developed progressive paresis of right cranial nerves IX–XII and was found to have an epidermoid carcinoma of the nasopharynx. After a course of radiation therapy (4500 rads), she developed progressive palsies of cranial nerves V–VIII and diabetes.

Otolaryngologic examination revealed an extensive exophytic ulcerating tumor in the nasopharynx that extended inferiorly in the submucosal plane somewhat below the level of the soft palate. The right ear showed signs of serous otitis media resulting from the nasopharyngeal obstruction of the Eustachian tube. The posterior cervical lymph nodes were enlarged bilaterally. There was a complete loss of function of right cranial nerves V–XII and bilateral papilledema.

Death occurred, after a left posterior myocardial infarct, from aspiration pneumonia and brain stem involvement.

Postmortem examination revealed that the nasopharyngeal carcinoma had invaded the sphenoid sinuses, sella turcica, and hypophysis and had extended into the middle and posterior cranial fossae. There was minimal involvement of the basal meninges and ventral surfaces of the pons, medulla, and upper cervical cord.

Microscopic examination of the temporal bones reveals tumor metastasis in the subarachnoid compartment that occupies the entire right internal auditory canal (Fig. 37.1). It has infiltrated and partially destroyed the seventh and eighth cranial nerves but has not extended beyond the spiral foraminous tract into the modiolus.

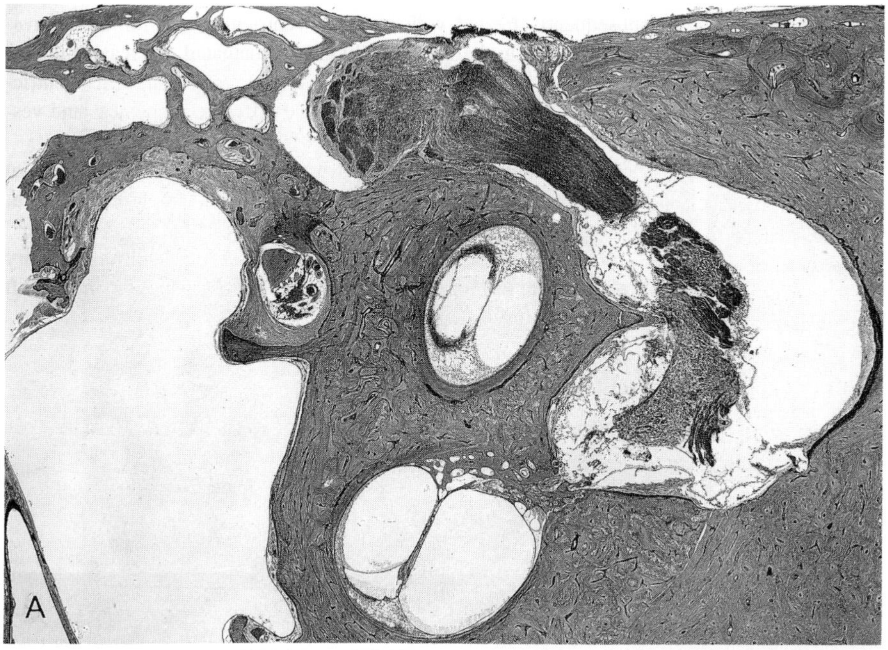

Figure 37.6. A. Vertical section through right petrous pyramid at level of labyrinthine segment of facial canal and geniculate ganglion. The metastasis is within the subarachnoid space of the internal auditory canal and infiltrates the facial nerve. The primary tumor was a cutaneous melanoma located on the posterior bony wall of the left external auditory canal. (Hematoxylin and eosin, ×10.)

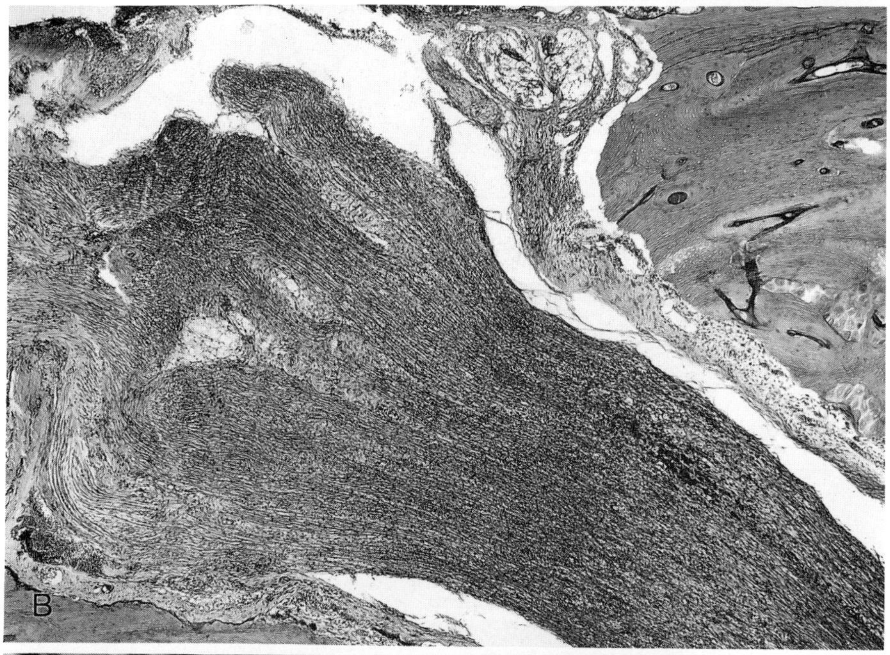

Figure 37.6. B. Strands of tumor cells are situated between the bundles of the facial nerve near the geniculate ganglion. (×230.)

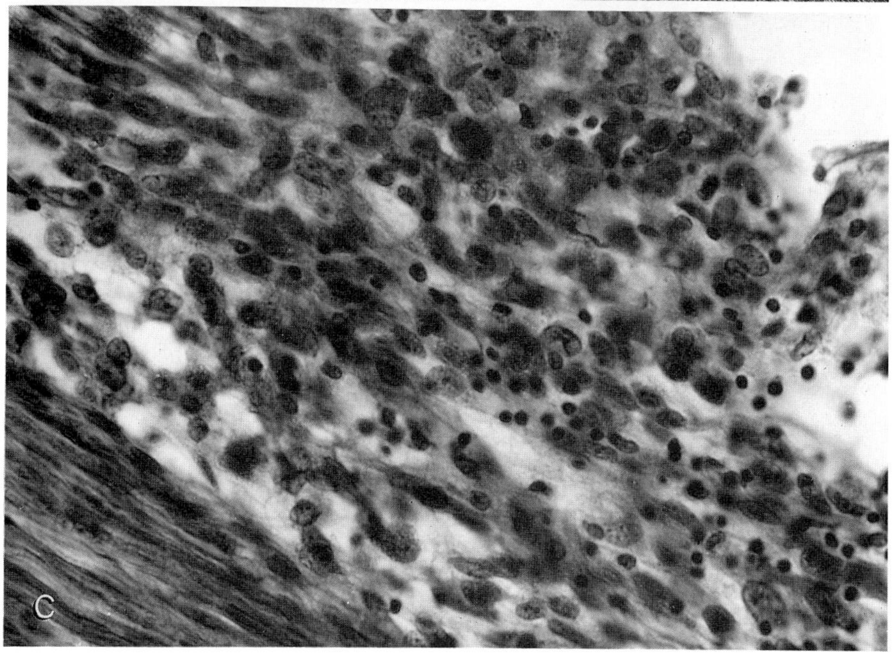

Figure 37.6. C. The tumor cells between the nerve fibers reveal a marked polymorphia and polychromesia and contain melanin granules. (×500.)

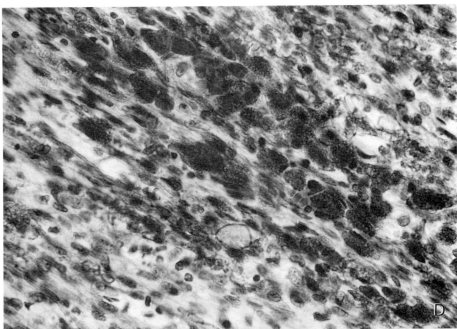

Figure 37.6.   D. The variation in size and form of the tumor cells and their content of melanin is clearly evident. (×500.)

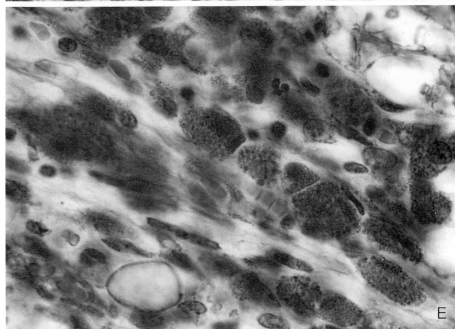

Figure 37.6.   E. The melanoma cells in the perineural spaces include a dense conglomerate of fine melanin granules. (×1000.)

Case 4. *Melanoma originating in left external auditory canal initially, metastasizing to left auxillary lymph nodes and, subsequently, to subarachnoid space, internal auditory canals, meninges, and brain and throughout the skeleton. Invasion and destruction of cranial nerves VII and VIII bilaterally.*

A 62-year-old man was admitted for evaluation of a left axillary lymphadenopathy and excisional biopsy of what proved to be a metastatic melanoma. He underwent a radical dissection of the left axilla and received a transfusion from a donor who apparently was considered to be cured from melanoma. He underwent three additional excisions of recurrent axillary tumors. One year later, a biopsy from a bleeding dark bluish mass in the left external auditory canal arising from the posterior bony canal wall proved to be a primary melanoma. This was followed by a partial resection of the left temporal bone and radical neck dissection. There was no evidence of tumor tissue in the portion of the temporal bone and neck structures re-

moved except for the area of the external meatus. His health deteriorated rapidly as he developed multiple metastases in the bones and intracranially, along with bilateral progressive loss of cochlear and vestibular function and tinnitus.

Postmortem examination showed multiple metastases throughout the brain.

Histologic examination of the temporal bones shows no evidence of residual tumor tissue in the osseous structures of the remaining, partially resected left temporal bone. However, there is extensive metastatic tumor tissue throughout the subarachnoid space and along the meninges of both internal auditory canals (Figs. 37.6 and 37.7). There is massive involvement and destruction of cranial nerves VII and VIII (Figs. 37.6 and 37.7), and strands of tumor cells extend along the perineural spaces into the cochlear modiolus and to the geniculate ganglion (Fig. 37.6), but there is no atrophy of the cochlear or vestibular end organs.

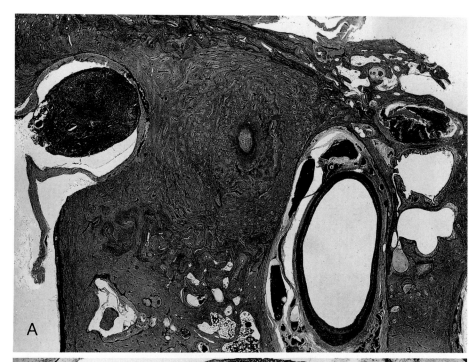

Figure 37.7. A. Vertical section through left petrous pyramid near anterior wall of internal auditory canal with cross-section through horizontal segment of internal carotid artery. A spherical metastasis of the melanoma occupies the subarachnoid space of the internal meatus. (Hematoxylin and eosin, ×10.)

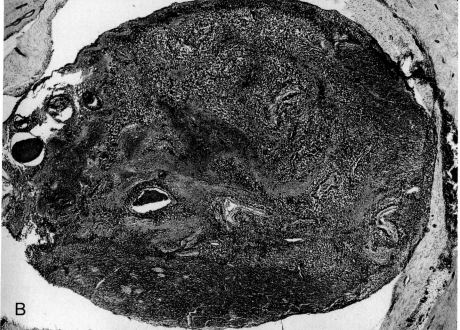

Figure 37.7. B. The metastasis includes the facial nerve superiorly and the cochlear nerve inferiorly. (×40.)

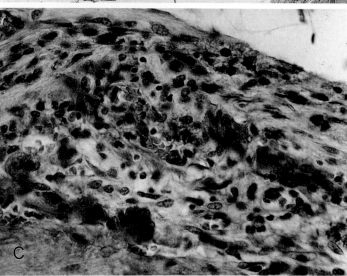

Figure 37.7. C. The melanoma, in infiltrating and extending within the periosteum of the canal, has begun to erode the underlying periosteal bone of the otic capsule. (×500.)

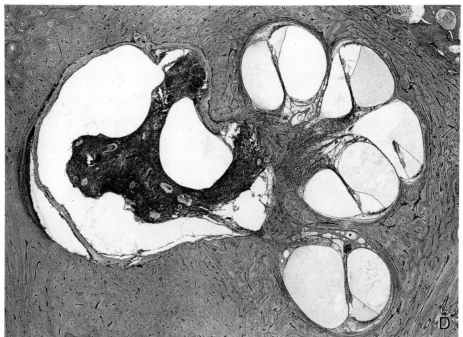

Figure 37.7. D. Vertical midmodiolar section through left temporal bone with extensive metastasis infiltrating and completely destroying the left facial, cochlear, and vestibular nerves. (×16.)

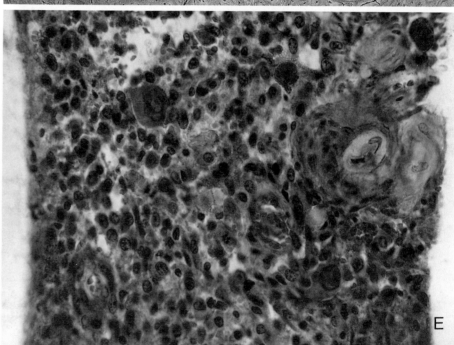

Figure 37.7. E. The tumor cells are arranged in compact sheets. They vary markedly in size, shape, and chromatin content. Giant cells and mitotic figures are numerous. (×500.)

Case 5. *Carcinoma of prostate with metastases to lymph nodes, pleura, lungs, vertebrae, and occipital, sphenoid, and left temporal bones. Chronic perforative left otitis media (secondary). Marginal papillary immigration of meatal epithelium at posteroinferior annulus with beginning development of papillary cholesteatoma induced by adjacent tumor tissue from metastasis to mucoperiosteum of hypotympanum.*

A 63-year-old man with a 5-months history of urinary frequency, nocturia, dysuria, weight loss, loss of muscular strength, ankle edema, anemia, and intermittent bleeding from the left ear was admitted for evaluation.

Physical examination revealed a paralysis of the right lateral rectus muscle and right hypoglossal nerve and advanced peripheral and cerebral arteriosclerosis. The prostate was enlarged and hard with a nodular surface. Several left axillary lymph nodes were enlarged and firm. In his confusion he constantly removed his retention catheter. He expired shortly after a suprapubic cystostomy from cardiac insufficiency.

Microscopic examination of the temporal bones reveals a chronic left tympanomastoiditis with an inferior pars tensa perforation (Fig. 37.8A–D). It is associated with an extensive granular tumor growth that involves the mucoperiosteum outlining the lower mesotympanum and hypotympanum, that extends into the round window niche, and that involves the inferior annulus and tympanic membrane (Fig. 37.8B–D). The meatal skin at the inferior tympanic annulus shows a papillary immigration of squamous epithelium into the underlying connective tissue, heavily infiltrated with metastatic tumor tissue (Fig. 37.8E and F). This papillary invasion reflects a very early stage of papillary cholesteatoma induced by the adjacent tumor tissue, as documented in other instances.

Case 6. Adenocarcinomatous metastasis in apical portion of left petrous pyramid with unknown origin of primary tumor. Generalized arteriosclerosis with severe involvement of aorta and coronary and cerebral arteries. Encapsulated tubercles in apical region of both lungs. History of apoplexy. Bilateral hypostatic pneumonia. Death from recurrent cerebral hemorrhage.

A 72-year-old man was admitted for evaluation of progressive multiinfarct dementia resulting from generalized arteriosclerosis and a history of a recent paralytic stroke with left hemiplegia. He expired shortly thereafter from a second severe cerebral hemorrhage.

Microscopic examination of the left temporal bone displays a localized metastasis in the left petrous apex just inferior and lateral to the horizontal segment of the intratemporal carotid artery (Fig. 37.9A and B). The petrous apex consisted of spongy bone that included a hematopoietic and fatty marrow. The metastasis (Fig. 37.9B and C) exhibits all the characteristics of an adenocarcinomatous primary tumor. The most likely locations for the unknown primary lesion were the lung, kidney, prostate, or stomach.

Case 7. Adenocarcinoma arising in lower pole of right kidney, metastasizing to heart, lungs, both adrenals, preaortic lymph nodes, thoracic, lumbar, and sacral vertebrae, and right petrous pyramid. Tumor thrombus in pulmonary artery. Thrombosis of left adrenal, renal, and both iliac arteries and inferior vena cava. Diabetes mellitus. Hyalinization of islets of Langhans.

A 55-year-old man had been admitted for evaluation because of increasingly severe pains and muscular weakness of the legs and intermittent claudication, progressive weight loss, and regulation of diabetes mellitus.

On *admission,* the patient was somewhat obese in spite of a recent very severe loss of weight, febrile, dehydrated, hypertensive, and chronically ill.

On *physical examination,* his chest was barrel shaped, his respiratory excursions were restricted, and his lungs were hypersonant on percussion. There was abdominal tenderness in the right flank with a palpable, round, firm mass the size of an apple, suspected to be a cortical tumor of the right kidney.

Neurologic examination disclosed *(a)* severe, generalized muscular weakness and atrophy of the extremities, including the small muscles of the hands, *(b)* chronic polyneuropathy, *(c)* dysphagia, *(d)* atrophy of the left side of the tongue, and *(e)* retinal arteriosclerosis.

The peripheral vessels were tortuous and quite thickened. *Intravenous pyelography* disclosed a filling defect in the right kidney, suggesting a cortical tumor.

Radiography revealed a destructive lesion in the right pelvis with beginning central dislocation of the acetabulum and several osteolytic lesions in the vertebrae with collapse of a thoracic vertebra.

Fasting blood sugar was 230 mg/100 ml, and the urine was 4+ for glucose and positive for albumin, acetone, and acetoacetic acid. The patient's further course in the hospital was characterized by progressive muscular weakness, atrophy and weight loss, dysphagia, generalized weakness, and cardiac decompensation, resulting in bilateral pleural effusion and death.

Postmortem examination disclosed a rounded, firm tumor measuring 7–8 cm in diameter, projecting from the lower pole of the right kidney. On cross-section, it consisted of a whitish tissue with a few areas of hemorrhage and necrosis that, on histologic examination, proved to be a renal adenocarcinoma. It had metastasized to the left ventricle of the heart, lungs, adrenals, preaortic lymph nodes, the thoracic, lumbar, and sacral vertebrae, pelvis, and left temporal bone, with every metastasis showing the adenocarcinomatous characteristics of the primary tumor.

Examination of the left temporal bone reveals an unusually extensive pneumatization of the petrous pyramid and mastoid bone (Fig. 37.10A). Within the neural compartment of the jugular foramen a metastatic tumor occupies the entire foramen, involving the superior ganglion of the glossopharyngeal nerve and the jugular ganglion of the vagus nerve (Fig. 37.10B). The metastasis extends medially and caudally toward the hypoglossal canal, where in all likelihood it also involved the twelfth cranial nerve, as evidenced by the atrophy of the left half of the tongue. This tumor has all the characteristics of an adenocarcinoma (Fig. 37.10C).

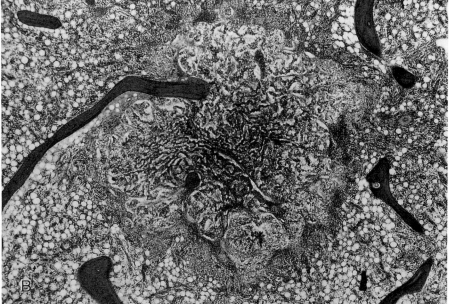

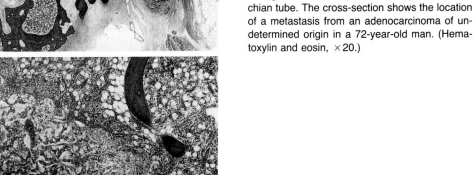

Figure 37.9.   A. Vertical section through left temporal bone in apical region with cross-section through carotid artery and cartilaginous Eustachian tube. The cross-section shows the location of a metastasis from an adenocarcinoma of undetermined origin in a 72-year-old man. (Hematoxylin and eosin, ×20.)

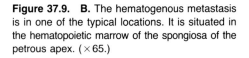

Figure 37.9.   B. The hematogenous metastasis is in one of the typical locations. It is situated in the hematopoietic marrow of the spongiosa of the petrous apex. (×65.)

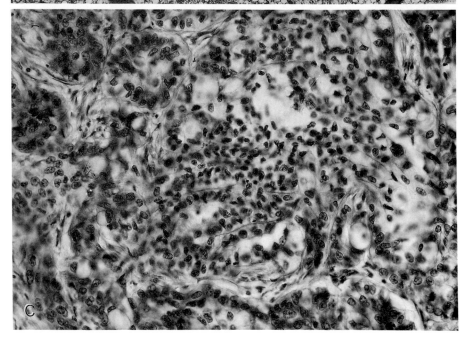

Figure 37.9.   C. The metastasis displays a limited degree of glandular differentiation. The primary tumor could have been localized in the lung. (×300.)

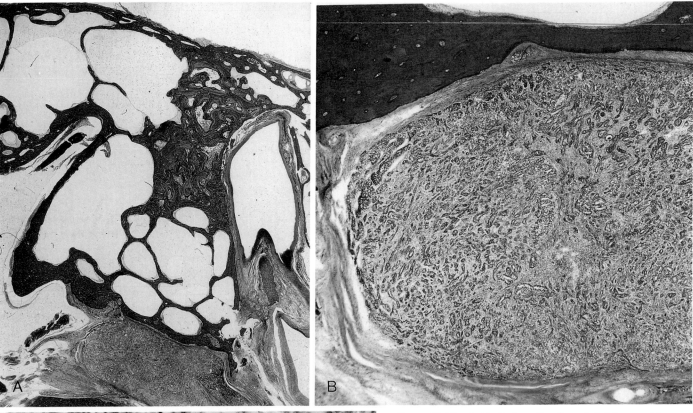

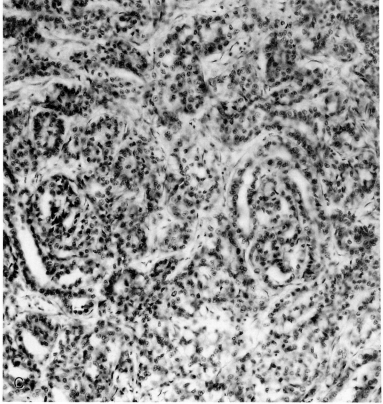

Figure 37.10. **A.** Vertical section through left temporal bone at level near anterior wall of internal auditory canal and of neural compartment of jugular foramen in a 55-year-old man. The patient died from an adenocarcinoma that originated in the right kidney and had metastasized to the heart, lungs, both adrenal glands, preaortic lymph nodes, and sacral and thoracic lymph nodes. A large metastasis completely occupies the jugular foramen at that level. **B.** The metastasis involves the superior ganglion of the glossopharyngeal nerve and the jugular ganglion of the vagus nerve. (Hematoxylin and eosin, ×6.5 and ×25, respectively.)

Figure 37.10. **C.** The tumor reveals primarily an adenomatous structure but includes a few nodular areas composed of clear cells with recognizable cell borders and relatively regular nuclei arranged in sheets, tubules, and cords. (×300.)

Case 8. *Renal adenocarcinoma of right kidney with solitary metastasis to right mastoid process and middle ear. History of chronic tympanomastoiditis and facial nerve palsy of right ear of 2 months duration, followed by acute onset of total loss of hearing, pulsating tinnitus in right ear, and unsteadiness. History of urinary tract infection and hematuria. Abnormal sonogram and intravenous pyelogram showing cortical mass in lateral portion of right kidney. CT scan of skull and cerebral angiogram revealing lytic lesion in right mastoid and middle ear with biopsy disclosing metastatic adenocarcinoma of kidney. Subsequent right nephrectomy for removal of primary tumor, confirming renal adenocarcinoma. History of exposure to asbestos and noise, miliary tuberculosis, and sideroblastic anemia.*

A 67-year-old man was admitted for evaluation of a right chronic perforative tympanomastoiditis of 8 weeks duration, associated with rapidly progressive loss of hearing, tinnitus, unsteadiness, and facial weakness, resulting in total loss of cochlear, vestibular, and peripheral facial nerve function. Multidirectional coronal tomograms of the temporal bones showed a large erosive lytic lesion involving the right petrous pyramid and mastoid region (Fig. 37.11A–C), which on subsequent CT scans proved to be an enhancing soft tissue mass involving primarily the jugular foramen and extending into the posterior cranial fossa. A jugular paraganglioma was suspected (Fig. 37.11D–F).

Operation consisted of an exploration of the right temporal bone, during which a reddish-blue pulsatile mass abutting the sigmoid sinus was found and removed.

Histologic examination of the metastasis shows some areas of poorly cohesive large cells with hyperchromatic nuclei and abundant slightly vacuolated to dense eosinophilic cytoplasm set in a background of thin-walled vessels (Fig. 37.12A). In other areas there are nests of atypical cells with clear to coarsely vacuolated cytoplasm, separated by a similar vascular plexus (Fig. 37.12B) Special stains demonstrated intracytoplasmic glycogen.

Electron microscopy demonstrates occasional lipid deposits and focal collections of densely arranged microvilli at the intercellular spaces or long, free surfaces of the plasma membranes (Fig. 37.13). Basal lamina and intercellular junctions are inconspicuous, and dense-core granules are absent.

A postoperative intravenous pyelogram demonstrated a 6-cm tumor mass in the right kidney that was subsequently removed and showed to be a typical renal adenocarcinoma. No other metastatic foci were identified macroscopically.

Microscopic examination of the temporal bones reveals an extensive osteolytic defect in the base of the petrous pyramid of the right temporal bone (Figs. 37.14 and 37.15). It extends vertically from the round window down through the skull base into the soft tissues of the infratemporal fossa. It stretches medially from the hypotympanum to the dura of the posterior cranial fossa and reaches posteriorly from the neural compartment of the jugular foramen beyond the sigmoid sinus (Figs. 37.14 and 37.15). The destruction, which resulted from the combined action of tumor erosion and superinfection (osteitis), includes the floor of the hypotympanum, lower bony canals of the internal carotid and facial nerves, jugular fossa, and jugular dome (Fig. 37.15). The bony margins of the lesion are irregular, jagged, and moth eaten (Fig. 37.15). The defect has been filled in with partially necrotic fibrous connective tissue that encompasses islands of devitalized bone, remnants of the original otic capsule, and foci metaplastic bone. In that scar tissue are also embedded the descending portion of the facial nerve and the stapedius muscle. The same tissue also partially obliterates the round window niche and occupies the lower half of the tympanic cavity (Fig. 37.15B and C). The osteolytic process has eroded the ampullated end of the posterior semicircular canal and given rise to a diffuse labyrinthitis with inflammatory exudate in the perilymphatic and endolymphatic compartments of the vestibular labyrinth and cochlea (Fig. 37.15A–D).

The labyrinthitis has resulted in complete atrophy of the cochlea and vestibular sensory end organs, to total atrophy of the spiral ganglion and cochlear nerve fibers, and to partial destruction of the first vestibular neurons (Figs. 37.14 and 37.15). There appears to be involvement of facial nerve in the vicinity of the stylomastoid foramen. Chronic inflammatory changes are seen in the middle ear cleft and with an occasional perilabyrinthine marrow space. The osteolytic process has also partially exposed the endolymphatic sac and destroyed the jugular vein (Fig. 37.15D). The metastasis has obviously extended beyond the skull base into the upper neck. Although the biopsy taken from the metastasis shows all the characteristics of an adenomatous carcinoma, no tumor cells can be identified within the bony defect included in our serial sections.

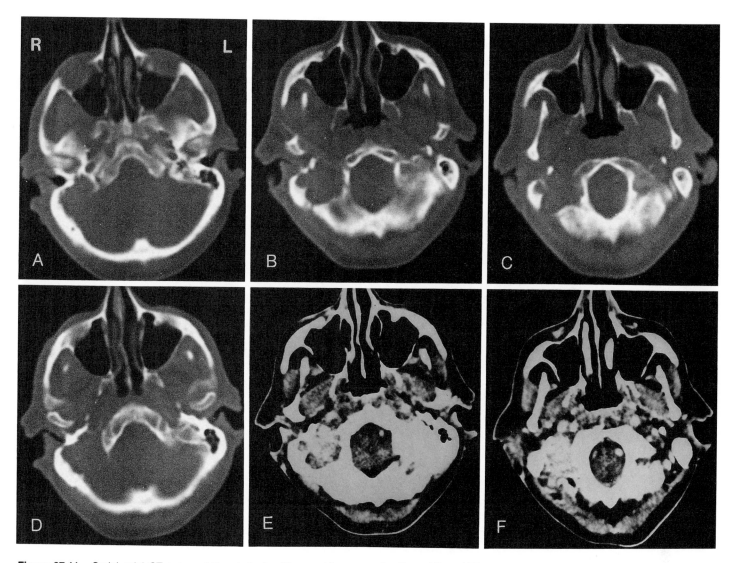

Figure 37.11. Serial axial CT scans of the skull of a 55-year-old man with adenomatous carcinoma of right kidney, with multiple metastases to lymph nodes, several organs, bones, and right petrous pyramid. It totally destroyed the infralabyrinthine portion of the petrous bone, eroded through the floor of the middle ear, and eroded the labyrinthine capsule and the Fallopian canal. It destroyed the jugular foramen and jugular vein and extended into the infratemporal fossa. The soft tissue lesion enhanced following intravenous contrast **(E** and **F).**

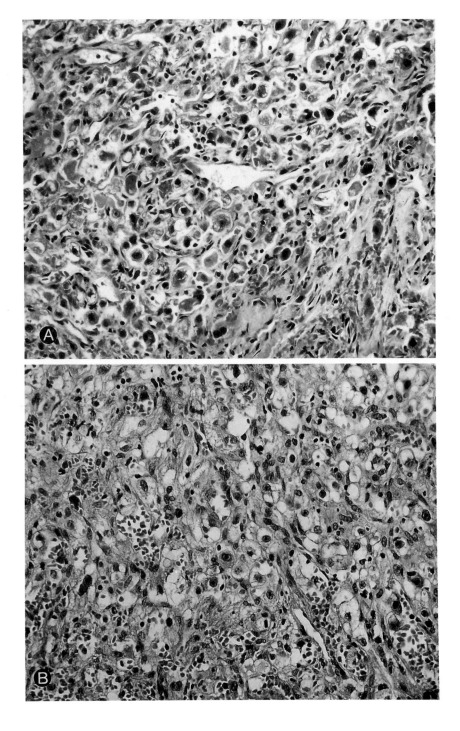

Figure 37.12. A. A major component of the metastasis consists of poorly cohesive cells with large, hyperchromatous nuclei and abundant granular cytoplasm invested by numerous thin-walled blood vessels. (Hematoxylin and eosin, ×175.)

Figure 37.12. B. Other areas of the tumor reveal nests of atypical cells with coarsely vacuolated to clear cytoplasm. (×175.)

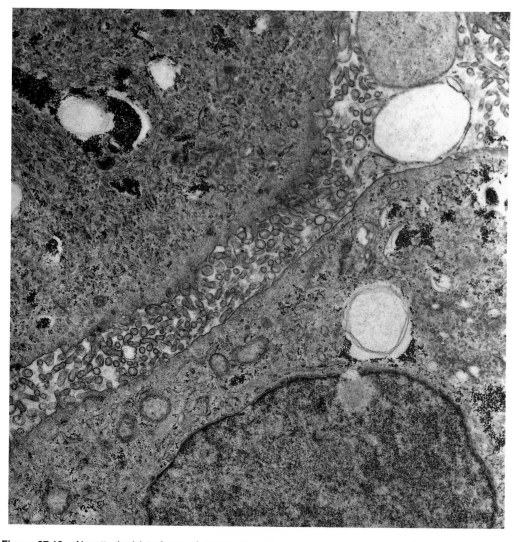

Figure 37.13. Nonattached interfaces of tumor cells with plasma membranes covered by a dense array of microvilli. Glycogen granules are prominent in the cytoplasm. (Hematoxylin and eosin, ×12,000.)

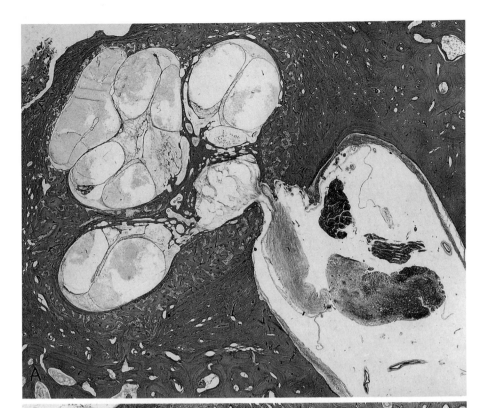

Figure 37.14.   A. Vertical midmodiolar section through right temporal bone. Erosion of the posterior semicircular canal resulted in a chronic labyrinthitis. The perilymphatic and endolymphatic compartments of the cochlea contain an inflammatory exudate. There is complete atrophy of the organ of Corti, spiral ganglion cells, and cochlear nerve fibers. (Hematoxylin and eosin, ×10.)

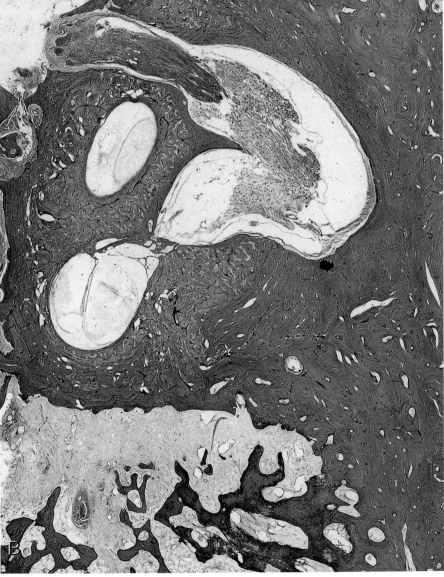

Figure 37.14.   B. Vertical section through right temporal bone at level of labyrinthine segment of facial nerve and geniculate ganglion. The chronic inflammation of the vestibular labyrinth resulted in a marked atrophy of the vestibular nerve fibers and cell bodies of Scarpa's ganglion. The anterior margin of the osteolytic defect is recognized just below the lower turn of the cochlea. (×10.)

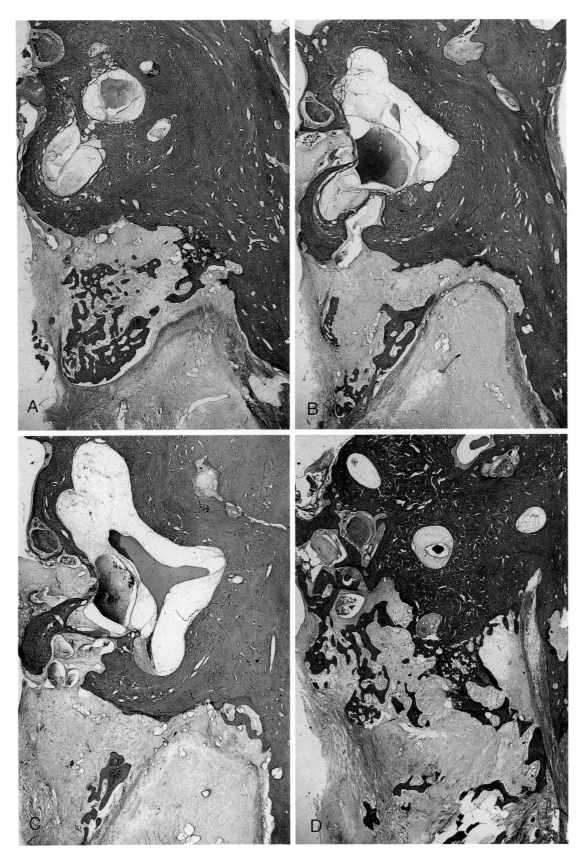

Figure 37.15.   A. Vertical section through right temporal bone at level just anterior to oval window. The osteolytic defect involves the infralabyrinthine portion of the otic capsule and the neural and the vascular compartments of the jugular foramen. The lower basal turn and saccule display evidence of labyrinthitis. **B.** Vertical section at level of oval and round windows. A partially necrotic fibrous scar tissue occupies the osteolytic defect, the jugular foramen, and the middle ear cavity. It includes remnants from the original otic capsule and obliterates both window areas. **C.** Vertical section through right temporal bone at center of vestibular fenestra. The utricle and the perilymphatic compartment of the vestibule contain a chronic inflammatory exudate. **D.** Vertical section through right temporal bone with cross-sections through lateral and posterior semicircular canals. The osteolytic defect is the result of tumor destruction and subsequent superinfection with osteitis. Erosion of the ampullated end of the posterior canal led to the development of labyrinthitis. The endolymphatic sac has become partially exposed. (Hematoxylin and eosin, ×7, ×7, ×8, and ×7.5, respectively.)

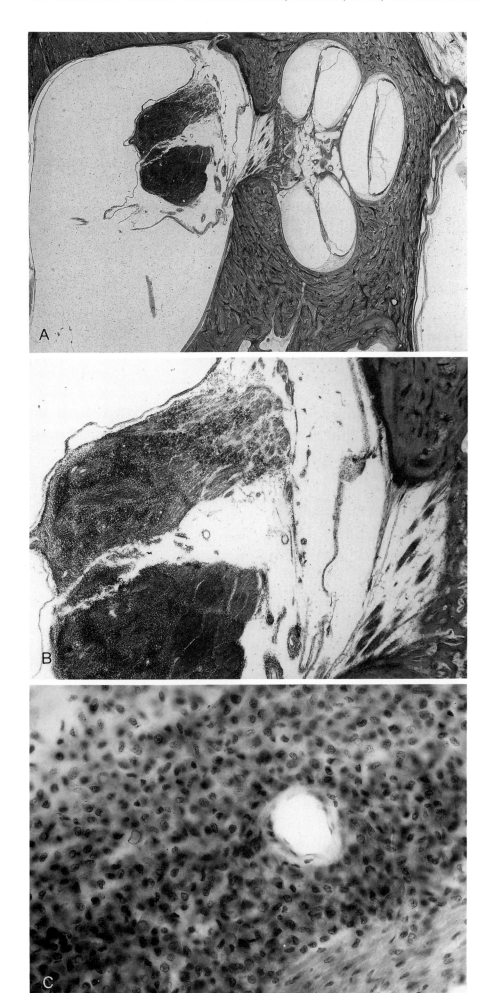

Figure 37.16. **A.** Vertical, anterior paramodiolar section through left temporal bone with sarcomatous metastasis in subarachnoid space of internal auditory canal near fundus. (Hematoxylin and eosin, ×12.)

Figure 37.16. **B** and **C.** The metastasis involved and subtotally destroyed the facial, cochlear, and vestibular nerves. (×25 and × 300, respectively.)

Case 9. *Large metastasis involving the left parieto-occipital region of the brain from a sarcoma of undetermined origin. Multiple metastases throughout brain, meninges, lungs, bronchi, pleura, liver, spleen, pancreas, mesentery, retroperitoneal lymph nodes, left ovary, uterus, and right adrenal gland. Metastasis in subarachnoid space of left internal auditory canal, involving cranial nerves VII and VIII.*

A 34-year-old woman with a 1-year history of intermittent occipital headaches associated with occasional dizziness, blurred vision, and diplopia was admitted for evaluation. Three months prior to admission she had experienced an episode of loss of consciousness, followed by an increase in headaches, nausea, vomiting, transient episode of aphasia, and difficulties with swallowing, ataxia, and motor weakness.

Death occurred 9 days after a left parieto-occipital craniectomy with total removal of a large metastatic lesion.

Microscopic examination of the left temporal bone reveals a metastasis in the subarachnoid space of the left internal auditory canal, involving cranial nerves VII and VIII, from a sarcoma of undetermined origin (Fig. 37.16).

References

1. Kobayashi K, Igarashi M, Ohashi K, McBride R. Metastatic sarcoma of the temporal bone. Arch Otolaryngol 1986;112:102–105.
2. Morton AL, Butler SA, Khan A, Johnson A, Middleton P. Temporal bone metastases—pathophysiology and imaging. Otolaryngol Head Neck Surg 1987;97(6):583–587.
3. Nelson EG, Hinojosa R. Histopathology of metastatic temporal bone tumors. Arch Otolaryngol Head Neck Surg 1991;117:189–93.
4. Schuknecht HF, Allan AF, Murakam Y. Pathology of secondary malignant tumors of the temporal bone. Ann Otol Rhinol Laryngol 1968;77:5–22.
5. Greer JA, Code TR, Weiland LH. Neoplasms of the temporal bone. J. Otolaryngol 1976;5:391–398.
6. Maddox HE III. Metastatic tumors of the temporal bone. Ann Otol Rhinol Laryngol 1976;76:149–163.
7. Jahn AF, Farkashidy J, Berman JM. Metastatic tumors in the temporal bone—a pathophysiologic study. J Otolaryngol 1979;8(1):1–95.
8. Graf K. Geschwülste des Ohres und des Kleinhirnbrückenwinkels. Stuttgart: Georg Thieme, 1952:247–250.
9. Saldanka CB, Bennett JD, Evans JN, Panebakian H. Metastasis to the temporal bone secondary to carcinoma of the bladder. J Laryngol Otol 1989;103(6):599–601.
10. Ruah CB, Bohigian RK, Vincent ME, Vaughan CW. Metastatic sigmoid colon adenocarcinoma to the temporal bone. Otolaryngol Head Neck Surg 1987;97(5):500–503.
11. Rapoport Y, Ruben RJ. Malignant ependymoma involving the temporal bone with remote metastasis. Can J Otolaryngol 1974;3(4):611–617.
12. Harbert F, Lin JC, Berry RG. Metastatic malignant melanoma to both VIIIth nerves. J Laryngol Otol 1969;83(9):889–898.
13. Jungreis CA, Seklar LN, Martinez AJ, Hirsch BE. Cardiac myxoma metastatic to the temporal bone. Radiology 1989;170(1 Pt 1):244.
14. Taxy JB. Renal adenocarcinoma presenting as a solitary metastasis. Cancer 1981;48(9):2056–2062.

38/ Hemangiomas and Vascular Malformations

Vascular tumors involving the temporal bone include: hemangiomas, vascular malformations, angiosarcomas, jugulotympanic paragangliomas, and certain other disease entities, such as the hereditary hemorrhagic telangiectasia and diffuse hemangiomatous lesions. They may arise in the immediate vicinity or, more commonly, within certain regions of the temporal bone. The differentiation between the various proliferative vascular lesions, including hamartomas and true vascular neoplasms, can be very difficult and can result in errors in terminology and classification (1).

HEMANGIOMAS

Definition

Hemangiomas are regarded by most pathologists as vascular hamartomas or hamartoblastomas, not as true neoplasms. A hamartoma represents a local malformation that resembles a neoplasm, both macroscopically and microscopically. It is an abnormal combination and proliferation of tissue elements normally present in the area, varying in amount, arrangement, and level of differentiation. Its growth rate is identical with that of normal tissue components. It may compress, involve, and destroy adjacent tissue structures including bone. The frequent observation of hemangiomas at birth, their occurrence in single or multiple form, and the fact that they are often indistinguishable from vascular malformations strongly support their hamartomatous origin.

Classification

Hemangiomas may be classified on the basis of their vascular caliber into capillary, cavernous, and combined forms. They characteristically originate from capillaries but may also develop from arterioles and venules. They may occur anywhere and can affect any organ, but their predilective site is the skin, especially the facial skin. Many are present at birth. About one-third of infants are born with one or another form of hemangioma (2). They vary in appearance, depending on the caliber and concentration of their tangled vessels, the amount of arteriovenous shunts, endothelial proliferation, thrombosis or fibrosis, and the structures involved (1).

The capillary hemangioma represents the most common form (3, 4). It may be present at birth or appear between the third and fifth week of life. It may increase in size during the course of several weeks, regress spontaneously by thrombosis or fibrosis, and undergo complete involution within a few years. Morphologically, it consists of thin-walled vessels of capillary size, is lined by a single layer of flat or plump endothelial cells, and, as a rule, is surrounded by an interrupted layer of pericytes and reticular fibers (Figs. 38.5 and 38.11) (1). It corresponds clinically to the port-wine lesion of the face and neck and to the small vascular nevus or birthmark. It often extends from the dermis into the subcutaneous tissue and in infants may be composed of capillary masses in which the vascular lumina can be obscured in many areas (Fig. 38.11D). In older children and adults, especially when inflamed and ulcerated, the capillary hemangioma has to be differentiated from the pyogenic granuloma, which has a polypoid appearance, bleeds easily, and has generally been present for less than 3 months. It is histologically indistinguishable from the so-called pregnancy tumor of the oral mucosa that is observed during gestation (5).

The cavernous hemangioma occurs most commonly within or beneath the skin of the face, neck, and extremities. It is also found in the mucosa of the oral cavity, stomach, and small intestines and in the liver and bone. It may present as a purple, globular, or multilobular well-circumscribed tumor or as a flat or slightly elevated, diffusely arranged strawberry-like lesion. It may manifest itself as a single lesion or as multiple lesions. Morphologically, it consists of convolutions of thin-walled cavernous blood vessels and vascular channels separated by a scanty connective tissue stroma (Figs. 38.3, 38.4, 38.7, 38.9). Spontaneous involution rarely occurs, however (1).

The combined capillary and cavernous hemangioma includes, by definition, areas of pure capillary and pure cavernous vessels with areas of transitional vascular calibers. Clinically, it resembles the cavernous hemangioma and in children (6) is often found in the head and facial region. It tends to recur after incomplete resection, is characterized histologically by its nuclear pleomorphism, and never metastasizes (1, 7).

Locations

Hemangiomas involving the temporal bone may arise in the immediate vicinity or within its structure. The two locations in the immediate vicinity are the cerebellopontine angle and the floor of the middle cranial fossa. Hemangiomas of the cerebellopontine angle tend to hug the lateroventral aspect of the brain stem. They may involve adjacent cranial nerves and extend into the internal auditory canal. Minor extensions may occasionally penetrate into adjacent brain tissue. They generally manifest themselves by subarachnoid hemorrhages of varying severity. Alteration of consciousness, contralateral hemiparesis, ipsilateral cranial nerve palsies, and headaches are the most frequent neurologic signs after hemorrhages. Exploration is advisable, provided that the lesion is located on the surface rather than within the brain stem (8, 9).

Hemangiomas that arise in the middle cranial fossa and involve the temporal bone are less common. Until 4 years ago, only 11 cases had been reported (10, 11). These tumors may manifest themselves by insidious loss of vision, multiple cranial nerve involvement, proptosis, papilledema, and bilateral hemianopsia. Involvement of pituitary function was observed in a more advanced case. There was a 4:1 female-to-male preponderance (10). In another instance, a cavernous hemangioma of the dura lining the middle cranial fossa had eroded the underlying tegmen tympani and caused an isolated seventh nerve palsy (11).

Hemangiomas originating within the temporal bone may develop in several locations. One of the predilective sites is within the internal acoustic meatus (12, 13), where they most likely arise from the small vascular convolutions frequently found in the area of Scarpa's ganglion (Figs. 38.1 and 38.2). They tend to infiltrate the seventh and eighth cranial nerves and in their clinical manifestations imitate an acoustic schwannoma. As their size increases, the auditory canal may become enlarged. They are most accurately demonstrated with magnetic resonance imaging (MRI) (Figs. 38.6 and 38.8).

Another predilective site is the area of the geniculate ganglion (12, 14). The hemangioma in that location manifests itself initially by a progressive facial paresis. In contrast to the intracanalicular hemangioma, which is best visualized with MRI, the hemangioma of the geniculate ganglion region is best recognized by a high-resolution computed tomography (CT) scan.

Few cases have been reported of hemangiomas arising in the hypotympanic region, where they may infiltrate the floor and extend to and involve the lower pars tensa of the tympanic membrane. They have been observed in a child and in adults. They may manifest themselves as intermittent or persistent hemorrhagic aural discharge (15).

Another preferred location is the intratemporal segment of the facial canal, where a number of hemangiomas have been found (14, 16). In contrast to the schwannoma of the facial nerve in that location, hemangiomas develop extraneurally and by compression produce symptoms at an early stage when they are still relatively small. As the hemangioma increases in size, the mastoid portion of the Fallopian canal becomes enlarged, and the canal wall loses its demarcation. Invasion of the perifacial cells and marrow spaces results in secondary infection and development of a purulent otorrhea. As the tumor usually develops outside the nerve and involves it by extrinsic compression, early exploration with resection, if called for, is the treatment of choice to preserve facial nerve function (14). An ossifying hemangioma occasionally found in that area may be identified by the presence of intratumoral bone spicules (16).

Hemangiomas are occasionally found in the mastoid, petrous, and squamous portions of the temporal bone (Fig. 38.3). In a few patients we have observed them subcortically near the tegmen, and in one patient, near the stylomastoid foramen. As the vascular tumor extends into adjacent air cells and marrow spaces, it may take on a honeycomb appearance on the CT scan and during exploration. Ossifying hemangiomas tend to give that appearance (16, 17).

The external auditory canal is another, but less frequent, location for the development of a hemangioma, where it may present as a red, soft, micronodular mass that blanches and decreases in size under the pneumatic otoscope with positive pressure. It may originate from the posterior bony canal wall and involve the adjacent tympanic membrane (Fig. 38.4) (18). In a rare instance, the hemangioma may develop bilaterally and present as pedunculated, soft, polypoid masses arising from the meatal wall, completely obliterating the lumen of both canals (Fig. 38.5). In one infant they were associated with recurrent bleeding and, on one side, with necrosis and spontaneous extrusion. The hemangiomas involving the pinna are discussed in Chapter 15 under vascular lesions of the external ear.

Finally, hemangiomas may also arise in the cerebellopontine angle and within any of the four portions of the temporal bone (Figs. 38.12).

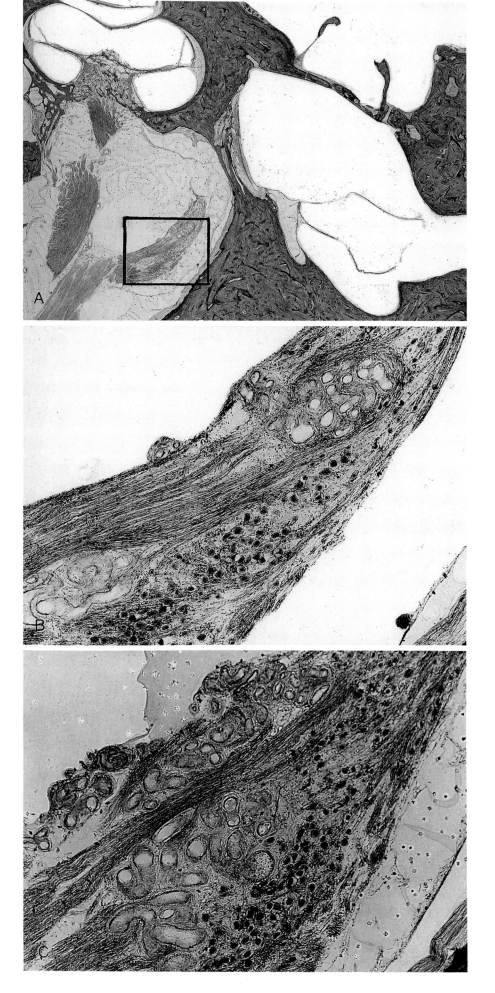

Figure 38.1. **A.** Horizontal section through right temporal bone at level of oval window in a 63-year-old man with bilaterally normal hearing and no history of tinnitus or vertigo. This section shows the location of an angiomatous formation within the vestibular nerve. (Hematoxylin and eosin, ×12.)

Figure 38.1. **B.** The formation is located between the superior and inferior division of Scarpa's ganglion. (×75.)

Figure 38.1. **C.** These vascular formations, which consist of a convolution of capillaries and are frequently found in that location, represent in all likelihood the site of origin for hemangiomas arising within the internal auditory canal. (×75.)

VASCULAR MALFORMATIONS

Whereas arteriovenous malformations account for about 0.5–1.5% of all intracranial space-occupying lesions and may selectively involve the intracranial dura, the temporal bone is an exceptional site. In one instance the vascular lesion involved the mastoid segment of the Fallopian canal (Figs. 38.13–38.15). It had eroded the osseous canal wall, extended into the perifacial cells, and gradually destroyed the facial nerve. The stylomastoid artery was the feeding vessel and drained into the veins of the facial canal. There was no history or clinical evidence of recurrent bleeding or of vascular malformations elsewhere in the skin, central nervous system, retina, lungs, or liver. The vascular anomaly occupied almost the entire length of the mastoid segment of the nerve (Figs. 38.13–38.15). It was made up of a convolution of predominantly arterial vessels with arteriovenous shunts larger than arterioles (Fig. 38.14).

The microscopic examination of these lesions confirms the obvious increase in both the number and the size of the blood vessels in the area involved. Their structure is often strikingly abnormal, in that the usual lamination of elastic and muscle fibers in the arteries is altered.

The treatment of choice is resection with replacement by a nerve graft.

Case Reports

Case 1. *Bilateral, multilobulated, pedunculated, congenital capillary hemangioma of external auditory canals, arising in meatal skin and occluding the external meatus. History of spontaneous necrosis and extrusion of right vascular lesion at age 6 months.*

A 2½-year-old girl was born with a soft, reddish-pink, slightly lobulated, pedunculated, epithelialized mass in the left external auditory canal. A similar, somewhat smaller lesion in the right ear canal had undergone necrosis and was spontaneously extruded at age 6 months. She had had intermittent bleeding from both ear canals.

Otoscopic examination revealed a bluish-black, pedunculated, somewhat lobulated mass measuring 1.5 cm in length, occupying the left external auditory canal. The previously reddish-pink tumor was soft, epithelialized, and attached to the skin of the posterior cartilaginous canal wall by a small stalk that had become twisted and had led to an infarction of the tumor. There was a chronic left external otitis, but the underlying tympanic membrane was normal.

At *operation,* a vascular tumor was excised under local anesthesia.

Histologic examination reveals a capillary hemangioma (Fig. 38.5).

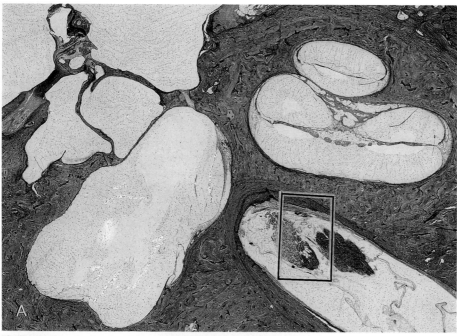

Figure 38.2. A. Horizontal section through left temporal bone at level of oval window in a 68-year-old man who 5 years prior to death had an episode of severe dizziness while his blood pressure was elevated. This section demonstrates the site of an angiomatous formation within the vestibular nerve. (Hematoxylin and eosin, ×10.)

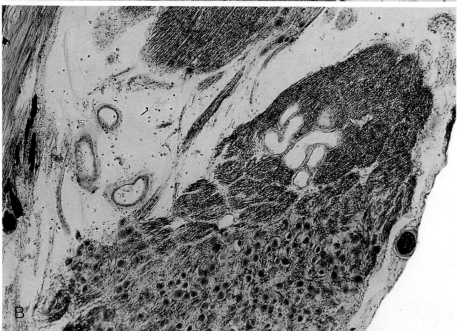

Figure 38.2. B. The formation is located in the inferior division of the vestibular nerve at the lateral border of Scarpa's ganglion. (×75.)

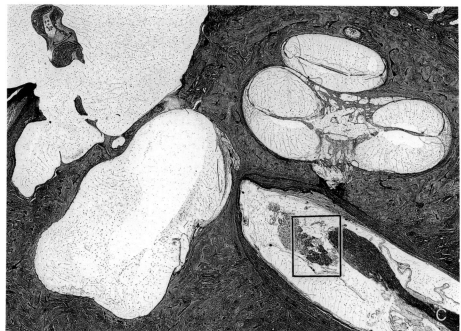

Figure 38.2.   C. Ten sections closer to mid-modiolar plane. A major portion of the angioma is located within the vestibular nerve. (×10.)

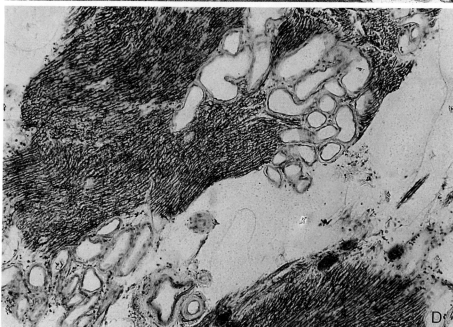

Figure 38.2.   D. The small hemangioma is of the capillary form. (×125.)

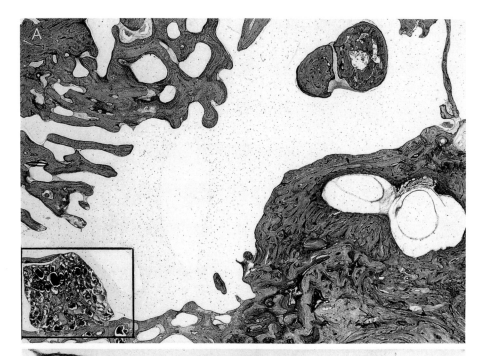

Figure 38.3. A. Horizontal section of left temporal bone at level of incudomalleolar articulation in a 76-year-old man with multiple telangiectasias and hemangiomas involving the facial skin, with a hemangioma in the mastoid antrum *(inset).* (Hematoxylin and eosin, ×8.)

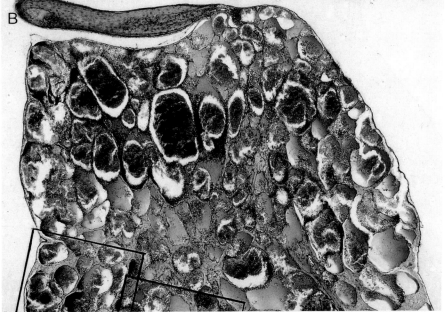

Figure 38.3. B. The hemangioma arises with a broad base from the upper medial wall of the antrum near the tegmen and measures about 3 × 4 × 3 mm. It is fed by branches from the nearby stylomastoid artery and drains into the perifacial veins *(inset).* (×40.)

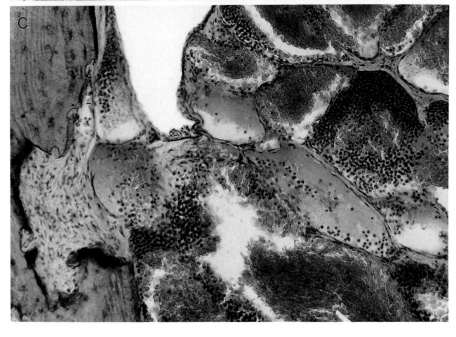

Figure 38.3. C. The hemangioma is of the cavernous variety. It consists of multiple, large, dilated, thin-walled and blood-filled vessels and vascular channels lined by a flattened endothelial layer. (×150.)

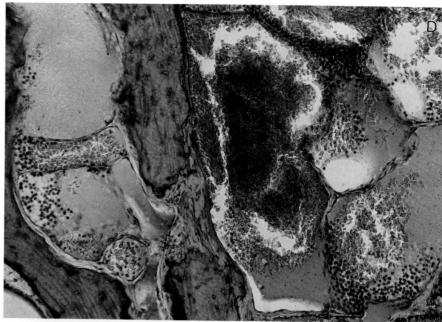

Figure 38.3. D. Some of the larger vascular channels extend into the adjacent cortical bone. (×150.)

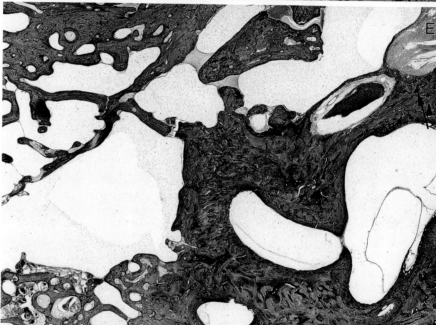

Figure 38.3. E. Sixty sections lower, at level of posterior attachment of incus. The cavernous hemangioma, although extending to the mucoperiosteum of the antrum, at that level involves the adjacent bony structures primarily. (×8.)

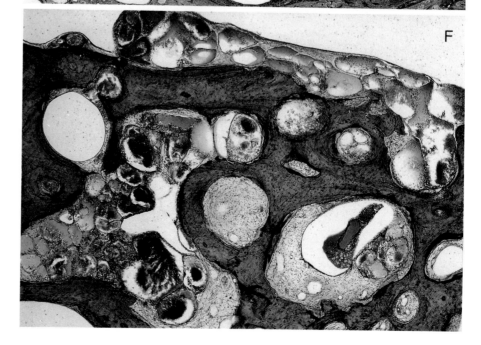

Figure 38.3. F. The cavernous hemangioma is invading air cells and marrow spaces of the cortical bone. (×40.)

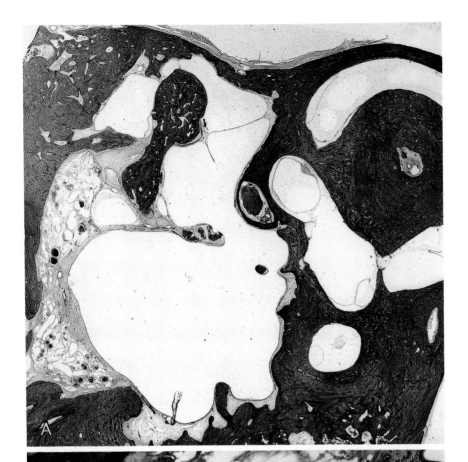

Figure 38.4. **A.** Vertical section through right temporal bone at level of head of malleus in a 42-year-old white man. This section shows a cavernous hemangioma that had originated in the external auditory canal and involves the tympanic membrane. (Hematoxylin and eosin, ×7.)

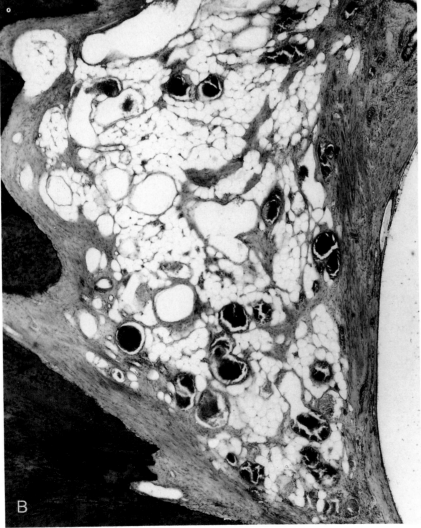

Figure 38.4. **B.** The hemangioma is of the cavernous variety. It consists of tangles of thin-walled cavernous blood vessels and vascular channels embedded in an adipose tissue. (×65.)

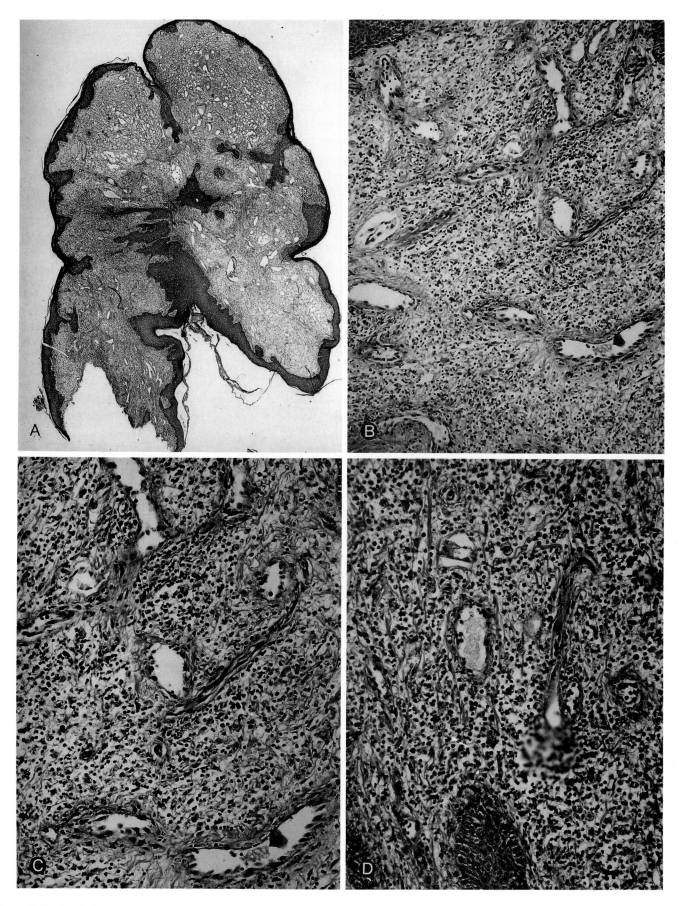

Figure 38.5. A. The hemangioma of the left external auditory canal is a polypoid pedunculated nodular mass with a lobulated, smooth surface covered by a keratinizing squamous epithelium. **B.** The structure of this hemangioma suggests a larger, centrally located vessel surrounded by a group of smaller feeding vascular channels. **C** and **D.** At higher magnification, the intervascular stroma displays plump spindle cells oriented around the vessel walls. (Hematoxylin and eosin, ×16, ×150, ×200 and ×200, respectively.)

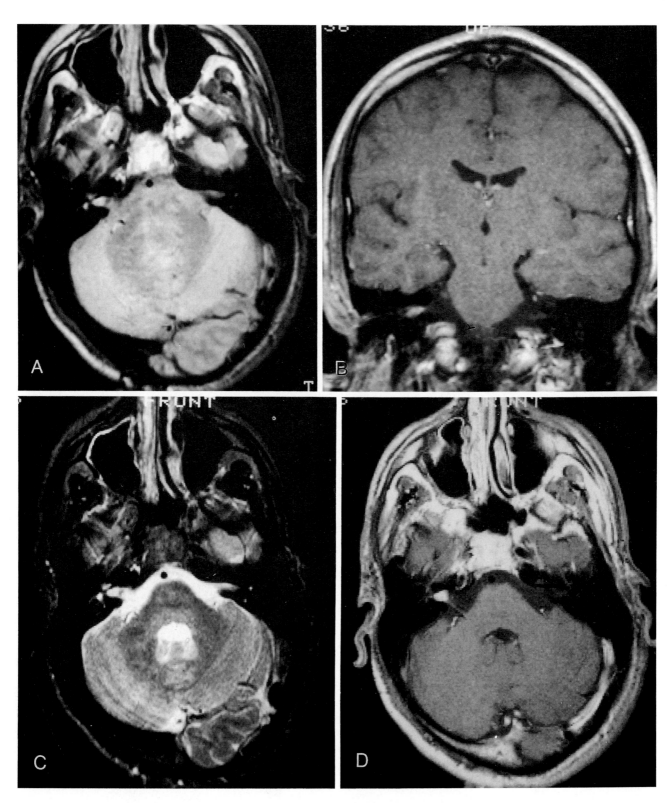

Figure 38.6. Axial and coronal magnetic resonance images of brain. There is a small focus of increased signal intensity in the right internal acoustic meatus **(A** and **B)** that shows homogeneous enhancement after gadolinium administration **(C** and **D).**

Case 2. *Intracanalicular cavernous hemangioma in right internal auditory meatus. Sudden onset of partial, moderately severe sensorineural hearing loss with no serviceable discrimination in right ear and some unsteadiness 4–5 months prior to admission. No history of tinnitus, vertigo, or involvement of facial nerve function.*

A 37-year-old man with a 4–6 month history of an abrupt-onset, moderately severe, low-tone sensorineural hearing loss in the right ear, associated with some unsteadiness but with no vertigo or impairment of facial nerve function, was admitted for examination.

Neuro-otologic examination revealed a moderately severe, low-tone sensorineural hearing loss in the right ear with a speech re-

sponse threshold (SRT) of 45 dB and 0% discrimination. MRI of the brain disclosed a small focus of increased proton density within the right internal auditory canal that showed a homogeneous enhancement following intravenous gadolinium administration that is consistent with an acoustic schwannoma (Fig. 38.6). The porus of the right internal auditory canal was widened.

At *operation,* the right auditory canal was explored through a translabyrinthine approach. The intracanalicular tumor was totally removed.

Histologic examination reveals a cavernous hemangioma (Fig. 38.7).

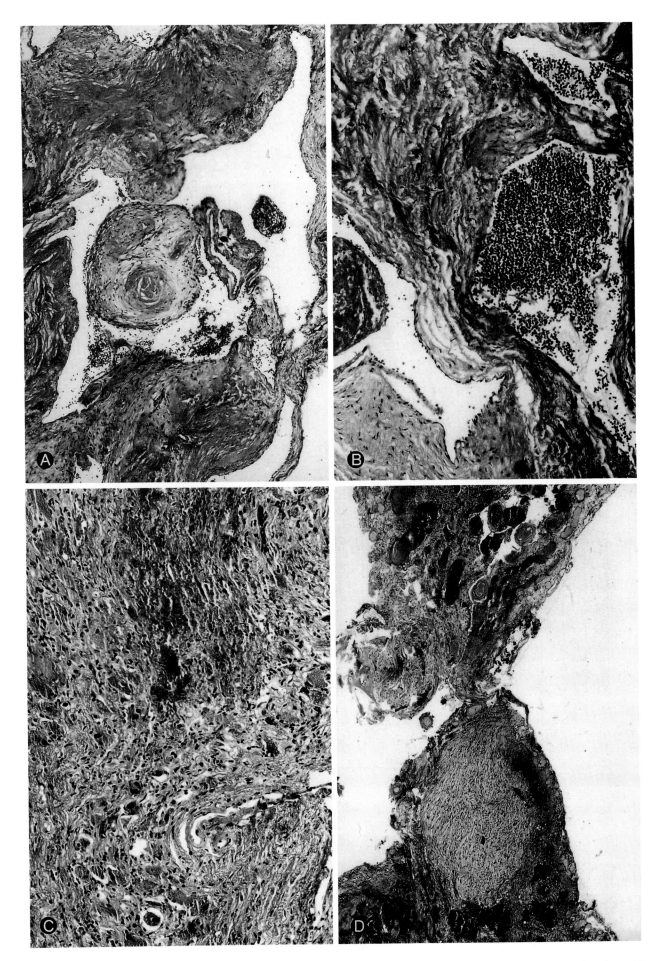

Figure 38.7. **A** and **B.** The hemangioma of the right internal auditory canal is of the cavernous variety. **C** and **D.** The eighth cranial nerve has been partially destroyed by the hemangioma and has been replaced in places by a fibrovascular tissue. (Hematoxylin and eosin, ×85, ×145, ×100, and ×70, respectively.)

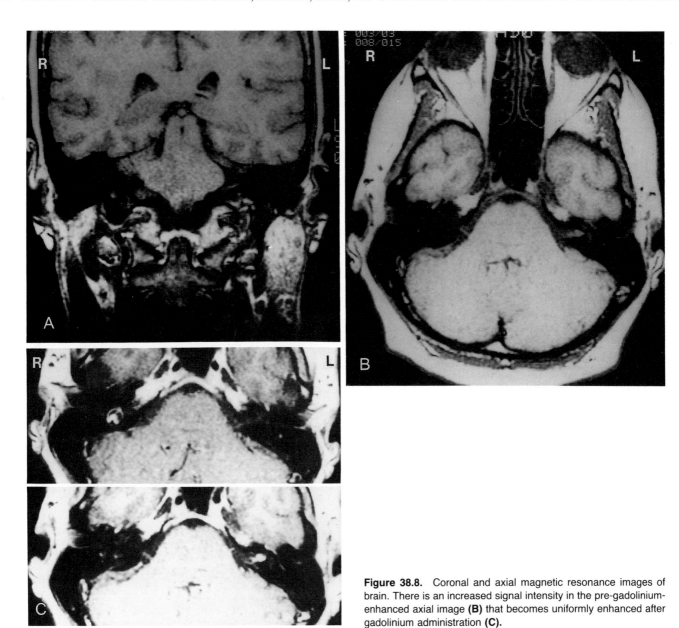

Figure 38.8. Coronal and axial magnetic resonance images of brain. There is an increased signal intensity in the pre-gadolinium-enhanced axial image **(B)** that becomes uniformly enhanced after gadolinium administration **(C)**.

Case 3. *Cavernous hemangioma of left internal auditory canal, arising in dura lining the superior portion of the meatus.*

A 41-year-old woman with a 5-month history of intermittent episodes of vertigo and dizziness, two transient episodes of tinnitus in the left ear, but normal hearing and facial nerve function bilaterally was admitted for examination. The onset of vertigo was generally sudden, although it was occasionally gradual, often associated with a sensation of spinning, nausea, and headaches brought on or aggravated by change of position and sudden head movements. Her past history was remarkable, in that 12 years ago she had had a lipoma removed from her right flank and was found to have several intrahepatic hemangiomas.

Neuro-otologic examination revealed normal cochlear function bilaterally with a SRT of 5 dB and a discimination of 100% in the left ear. The auditory evoked brain stem responses (ABR) were nor-

mal bilaterally. The vestibular tests showed a 31% reduction of the caloric responses in the left ear.

CT scan suggested a widening of the left internal auditory canal. *MRI* of the brain revealed an enhancing mass in the left internal auditory canal that is consistent with an intracanalicular schwannoma (Fig. 38.8).

At *operation*, the left internal auditory canal was explored via a middle cranial fossa approach. The dura lining the superior portion of the internal auditory canal appeared abnormal, greatly thickened, and heavily infiltrated by a tangle of blood vessels. The tumorous portion of the dura, which had partially compressed the superior division of the vestibular nerve, and the superior vestibular nerve and ganglion, which had become involved by the vascular lesion, were totally removed.

Microscopic examination of the intracanalicular mass displays a cavernous hemangioma (Fig. 38.9).

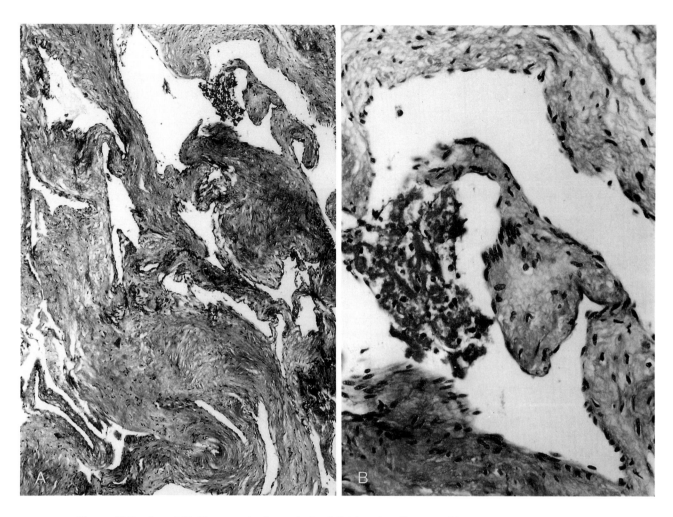

Figure 38.9. **A** and **B.** The vascular tumor in the left internal auditory canal is a cavernous hemangioma. (Hematoxylin and eosin, ×120 and ×320, respectively.)

Case 4. *Cellular infantile hemangioma involving the right middle ear, mastoid process, perilabyrinthine marrow spaces, and external auditory canal. Uniform bone resorption of middle ear walls extending anteriorly to bony canal of carotid artery, posteriorly to lateral sinus, and medially and inferiorly to posterior fossa dura and jugular bulb. Enlargement of tympanic annulus to twice the normal diameter. Extension underneath tympanic annulus to posterior meatal skin and underlying bone. Massive infiltration of entire mastoid process and infralabyrinthine marrow spaces.*

A 24-month-old infant boy with a 9-month history of recurrent episodes of right "acute mastoiditis" and serous middle ear effusion had developed a right pulsatile tinnitus 6 weeks prior to admission. Elsewhere, he had undergone an attempt at a right aspiration myringotomy with placement of a ventilation tube when a vascular tumor was discovered in the middle ear. There was no previous history of otalgia or discharge, especially bleeding, unsteadiness, facial weakness, hoarseness, or aspiration.

Otologic examination revealed a dark, purple pulsatile tumor in the right middle ear in apposition to the undersurface of the tympanic membrane. It had extended below the tympanic annulus to the meatal skin of the floor and posterior external ear canal wall and had enlarged the tympanic annulus to twice its original diameter. Cochlear function studies showed a 40-dB average air conduction puretone loss and normal bone conduction in the right ear. Hearing was normal on the left, and there was no facial weakness or spontaneous nystagmus. There was a vascular bruit over the carotid artery on either side. There was no evidence of a neoplastic lesion in the opposite ear and nasopharynx, and there was no mass or node in the neck.

Radiologic examination with routine mastoid films and axial views of the skull base revealed a generalized haziness of the right mastoid process and a uniform, smooth enlargement of the middle ear cavity without obvious bone destruction, suggesting a slow-growing, benign, space-occupying process extending to the carotid canal, lateral sinus, posterior fossa dura, and jugular bulb. Selective angiography failed to show any abnormality in position of the carotid artery, lateral sinus, or jugular bulb. There was no visible vascular connection to either the arterial or the venous system. The venous flow through the right lateral sinus was normal, and there was no evidence of an extrinsic or intrinsic narrowing of the jugular bulb or upper internal jugular vein. In the posterior projection there was no evidence of an abnormality of cerebral blood flow. Multidirectional tomograms of the right temporal bone in the lateral projection showed enlargement of the tympanic annulus to double its normal diameter (Fig. 38.10).

At *operation* (extended right radical mastoidectomy), the vascular tumor occupied the entire middle ear cleft. It had enlarged the tympanic cavity and annulus to the landmarks previously described. It had grown around and solidly embedded the ossicular chain, separating the incudomalleolar joint and displacing the outer two ossicles anteriorly and laterally. It had invaded extensively the perifacial cells, posterior bony canal wall, tympanic orifice of the Eustachian tube, and inferior perilabyrinthine cells. In the mastoid the tumor had infiltrated every air cell and marrow space, and it had exposed the lateral sinus and dura of the middle fossa without invading either structure. It had extended into the hypotympanum and exposed the vertical segment of the facial nerve, leaving the perineurium intact.

Histologic examination reveals cellular capillary hemangioma of childhood (Fig. 38.11).

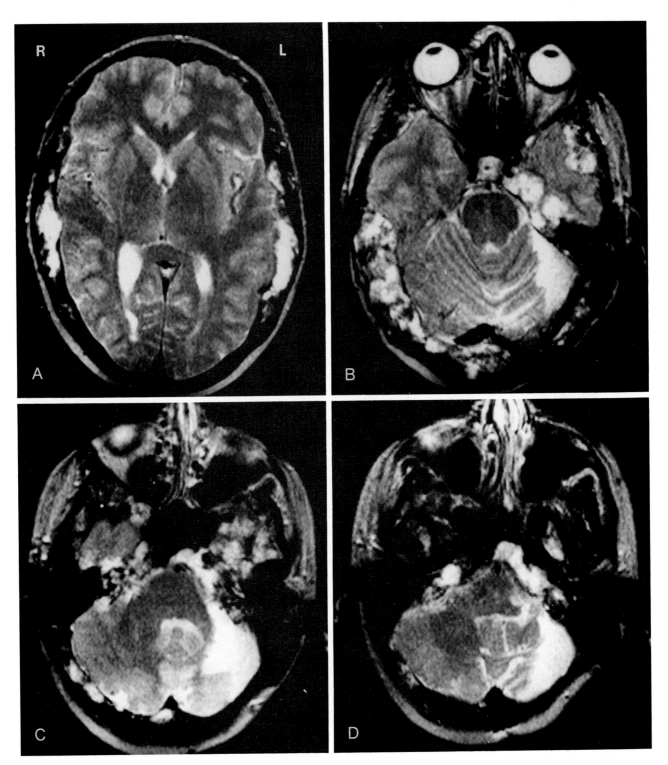

Figure 38.12. Nonenhanced axial cranial MRI reveals thick sheet-like areas of bony thickening involving the calvaria and skull base. These areas involve the frontal, parietal, temporal, occipital, and sphenoid bones. They are located predominantly in the diploë, within and above both petrous apices **(C** and **D)**. When the previous biopsy from the posterior cranial fossa revealing a cavernous hemangioma is taken into consideration, the bony abnormalities probably represent diffuse bony hemangiomatosis. (Courtesy of Dr. J. Gaare, Frederick, Maryland.)

Case 5. *Diffuse ossifying hemangiomatosis of calvaria and skull base involving primarily the diploic space with extrinsic impression on cerebral hemispheres. Involvement of both petrous apices. Biopsy from posterior fossa, showing a cavernous hemangioma. History of progressive bilateral loss of hearing, resulting in anacusis of the right ear and severe sensorineural loss in left ear.*

A 54-year-old woman with a history of bilateral progressive loss of hearing over several years, resulting in anacusis of the right ear and a severe sensorineural hearing loss in the left ear, was seen. In 1977 she had had an exploration of the posterior fossa with a biopsy that revealed a hemangiomatous tumor.

Neuro-otologic examination disclosed an anacoustic right ear and a severe sensorineural hearing loss in the left ear with a SRT of 45 dB and a discrimination score of only 64%.

Cranial MRI showed extensive pronounced bony abnormalities of the calvaria and skull base involving primarily the diploë. Widespread irregular globular, vascular, and new bone formations were recognized within and above both petrous apices (Fig. 38.12). In view of the patient's past history of cavernous hemangiomas, the consulting neuroradiologist concluded that these changes presumably represented a diffuse bony hemangiomatosis.

Case 6. *Vascular malformation involving the vertical segment of the right Fallopian canal and facial nerve. One-year history of right facial twitching progressing to facial paresis. Loss of taste involving the right side of the tongue. Hyperacusis of right ear.*

A 47-year-old woman who, 12 months earlier, developed right facial twitching involving primarily the lateral ocular region, occasional sharp pains in the same area, and hyperacusis in the right ear was admitted for examination.

Neuro-otologic examination disclosed a normal right external ear canal, tympanic membrane, and middle ear. Cochlear and vestibular function were normal except for evidence of hyperacusis in the right ear. There was an almost complete right peripheral facial nerve palsy with fibrillation involving the right orbicularis oculi muscle. Taste was severely impaired over the right anterior two-thirds of the tongue. Secretions from the right submandibular gland and tearing in the right eye were reduced by 50%, compared with that of the opposite side.

At *radiologic examination,* lateral, multidirectional tomograms of the right temporal bone showed a somewhat irregular radiolucency just anterior to the descending portion of the Fallopian canal, contiguous with its course, suggesting an erosive process adjacent to and involving the facial canal (Fig. 38.13). A neoplastic lesion was suspected, and the differential diagnosis included a schwannoma, paraganglioma, and a metastasis.

At *operation,* the right middle ear was explored, and the tympanic segment of the facial nerve appeared essentially normal. As the vertical segment of the Fallopian canal was approached, the bone became increasingly more soft and began to bleed profusely, and as the bone was thinned over the facial canal and removed, a purple, polypoid, vascular mass began to protrude. Halfway below the junction of the tympanic and mastoid segment, the facial nerve had become completely replaced by a polypoid, angiomatous mass that measured about 12 × 4 mm in diameter. It extended within and replaced the nerve for a distance of about 12 mm, tapering off slightly toward the stylomastoid foramen (Fig. 38.14). The vertical segment of the nerve containing the tumor was resected and replaced by an autograft from the greater auricular nerve. The adjacent bone, which had become softened by invading vascular channels, was also removed.

Microscopic examination of the vascular tumor in serial sections reveals that almost the entire facial nerve had been replaced by a convolution of blood vessels, vascular channels, and fibrous tissue containing myelinated nerve fibers and a proliferation of Schwann cells (Fig. 38.15). The vascular malformation, the connective tissue reaction, and Schwann cell proliferation clearly represent a primary lesion. The ultimate result of the facial reinnervation was quite satisfactory.

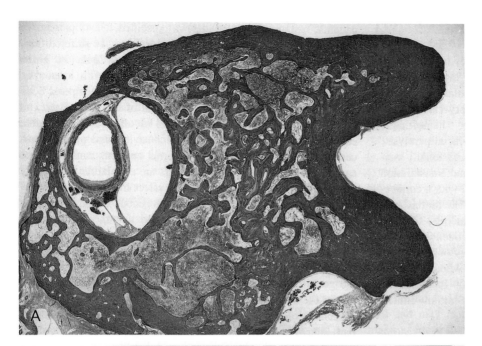

Figure 39.1. A. Vertical section through right petrous apex near anterior wall of internal auditory canal. Most of the apical marrow spaces contain leukemic infiltrations. (Hematoxylin and eosin, ×7.)

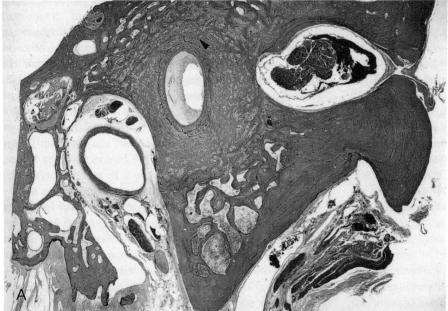

Figure 39.2. A. Vertical section through right petrous apex at neural compartment level of jugular foramen. Leukemic infiltrations are present in the infracochlear marrow spaces, in the subarachnoid space of the internal auditory canal, and between the tenth and eleventh cranial nerves. (Hematoxylin and eosin, ×7).

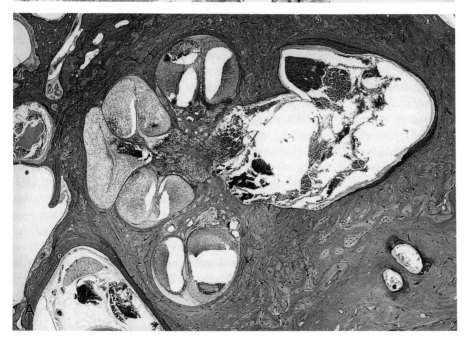

Figure 39.3. A. Vertical midmodiolar section of right cochlea. Leukemic infiltrations surround the cranial nerves in the subarachnoid space of the internal auditory canal. Masses of myeloblasts and erythrocytes completely fill the scala tympani, scala vestibuli, and scala media throughout the entire cochlea. (Hematoxylin and eosin, ×10.)

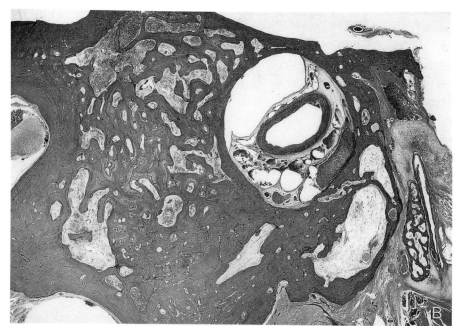

Figure 39.1. B. Vertical section through left petrous apex of the same patient as in Figure 39.1A *(opposite page)* at corresponding level. The distribution and extent of the leukemic infiltrations in the apex are similar. Many veins of the pericarotid plexus show accumulation of myeloblasts. (×7.)

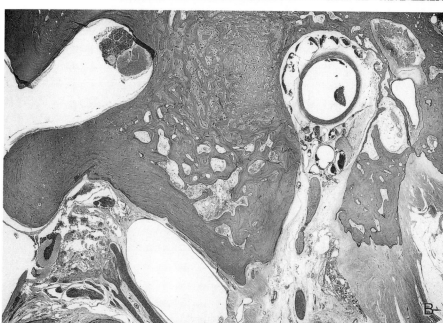

Figure 39.2 B. Vertical section through left petrous apex of the same patient as in Figure 39.2A *(opposite page)* at corresponding level. A noticeable leukemic infiltration is separating the ninth and tenth cranial nerves near the entrance to the jugular foramen. (×7.)

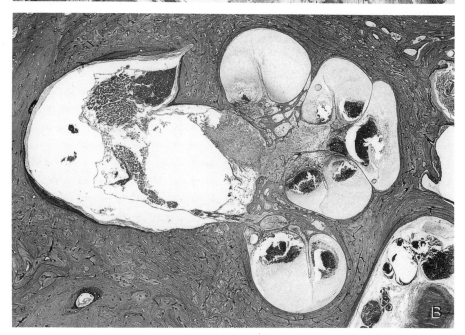

Figure 39.3 B. Vertical midmodiolar section through left cochlea of the same patient as in Figure 39.3A *(opposite page)* at corresponding level. In the subarachnoid space at the fundus of the internal auditory canal and in the cochlear modiolus, the cochlear nerve is densely infiltrated by white and red blood cells. The same cellular elements also fully occupy the three membranous compartments of the entire cochlea. (×10.)

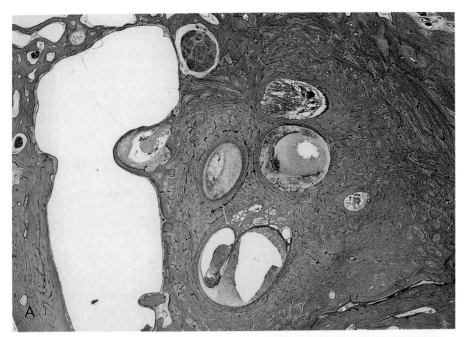

Figure 39.4. A. Vertical section through right petrous pyramid near anterior wall of vestibule. The saccule, the middle and basal turns of the cochlea, and the space around the superior division of the vestibular nerve are totally occupied by white and red blood cells. (Hematoxylin and eosin, ×10.)

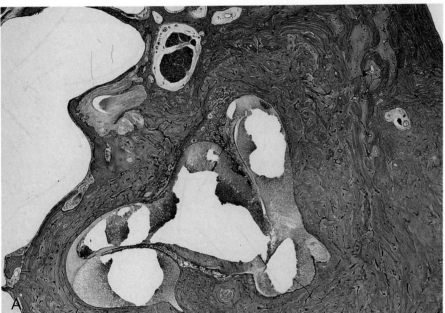

Figure 39.5. A. Vertical section through right petrous pyramid near lower end of cochlea. The utricle, the saccule, the vestibular end of the endolymphatic duct, the perilymph space of the vestibule, the lower end of the membranous cochlea, and the cochlear end of the cochlear aqueduct are packed with white and red blood cells. (Hematoxylin and eosin, ×12.)

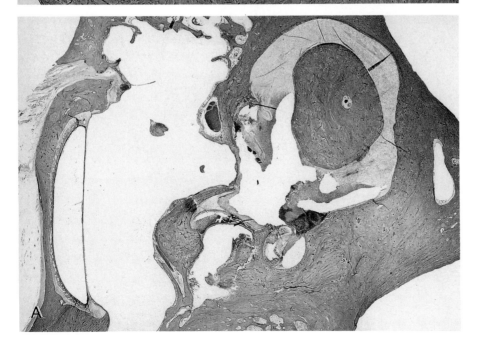

Figure 39.6. A. Vertical section through right petrous pyramid at level of oval and round windows. Masses of white and red blood cells occupy the endolymphatic and perilymphatic compartments of the vestibule, the superior and posterior semicircular canals, and the vestibular cecum of the lower basal turn. (Hematoxylin and eosin, ×7.)

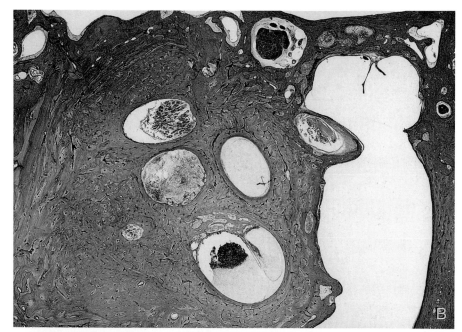

Figure 39.4. B. Vertical section through left petrous pyramid of the same patient as in Figure 39.4A *(opposite page)* at corresponding level. The macula of the saccule has been disrupted by the mass of myeloblasts and erythrocytes that also are present within the three scalae of the lower basal turn. (×10.)

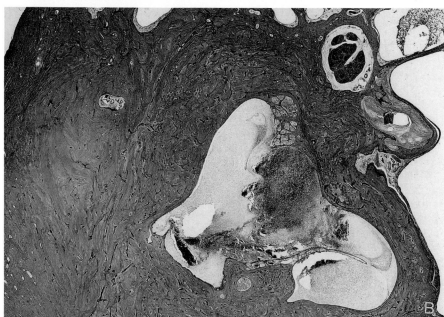

Figure 39.5. B. Vertical section through left petrous pyramid of the same patient as in Figure 39.5A *(opposite page)* at corresponding level. The perilymphatic and endolymphatic compartments of the cochlea and labyrinth and their connections to the subarachnoid space and endolymphatic sac are entirely occupied by myeloblasts and erythrocytes. (×12.)

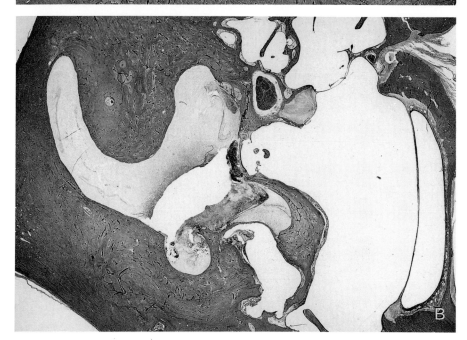

Figure 39.6. B. Vertical section through left petrous pyramid of the same patient as in Figure 39.6A *(opposite page)* at corresponding level. The extent and involvement of the cellular infiltration of the labyrinth and cochlea are the same as those of the right petrous pyramid. (×7.)

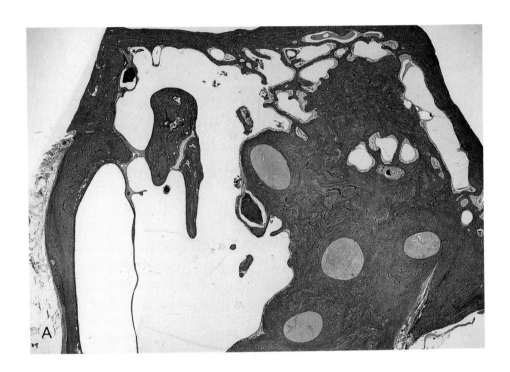

Figure 39.7. A. Vertical section through right petrous pyramid at level of incudomalleolar articulation. Cross-sections through the lateral and posterior semicircular canals display complete obliteration of their perilymphatic and partial obliteration or collapse of their endolymphatic compartments by white and red blood cells. (Hematoxylin and eosin, ×7.)

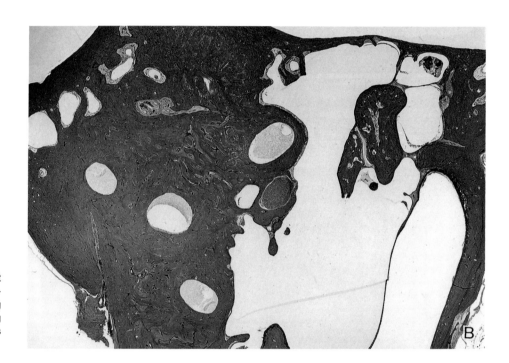

Figure 39.7. **B.** Vertical section through left petrous pyramid of the same patient as in Figure 39.7A *(opposite page)* at corresponding level. The pattern of cellular infiltration involving the lateral and posterior semicircular canals is the same as that on the right. (×7.)

SOLITARY PLASMACYTOMA OF THE CEREBELLOPONTINE ANGLE

Whereas plasmacytomas involving the calvaria are common, plasmacytomas involving the skull base and cranial nerves are rare (9, 15, 16). A typical example of such a lesion in the base of the skull (Case 3) was reported in 1980 (12).

Case Report

Case 3.

A 28-year-old man with an 8-month history of occipital headaches, unsteadiness of gait, and dysphagia of 2 months duration was seen.

Neurologic examination revealed involvement of the right fifth, eighth, and tenth cranial nerves and increased tendon reflexes in the left upper and lower extremities. Protein electrophoresis of serum and urine was initially normal. Plain cranial tomograms showed a destruction of the clivus and a soft tissue density in the right posterior cranial fossa. In the vertebral angiogram, the basilar artery was displaced posteriorly, and the right anterior and posterior meningeal branches of the vertebral artery were enlarged. The CT scan showed a high-density mass extending from the right cerebellopontine angle to the foramen magnum with a slight and irregular enhancement.

At *operation* (right suboccipital craniectomy), a well-encapsulated, smooth tumor mass was found in the right cerebellopontine angle, lateral to the brain stem displacing the right cranial nerves VII–XII. On histologic examination it proved to be a plasmacytoma. Repeat immunoelectrophoresis demonstrated an abnormal protein of the λ-type light chain in the CSF, serum, and urine. A skeletal survey showed no abnormality beside the skull base, and a bone marrow aspiration revealed no increase in plasma cells.

SOLITARY INTRACRANIAL PLASMACYTOMA

SIPs are also rare and less frequent than the extracranial lesions. They may arise in the meninges or the brain. Case 4, from the literature (3), is a pertinent example of a SIP extending from the tentorium into the right middle and posterior cranial fossa.

Case Report

Case 4.

A 62-year-old man with a 27-year history of right facial paresis, who 5 years before had begun to experience episodes of headaches, dizziness, vertigo, and blurred vision, was admitted for evaluation. Three weeks prior to admission he had developed severe headaches, numbness over the entire right side of his face, and progressive loss of hearing in the right ear.

Neurologic examination revealed involvement of the right fifth, seventh, and eighth cranial nerves. The CT scan showed an area of increased, enhancing density in the posterior part of the right middle cranial fossa and in the posterior cranial fossa.

Operation (a right temporal craniotomy) disclosed a brownish-pink tumor under the temporal lobe, extending from the tentorial surface into the middle cranial fossa and medially toward the edge of the incisura. The tumor was partially resected; histologically, it proved to be a plasmacytoma.

Subsequent tomograms of the base of the skull showed a destruction of the right petrous apex. A complete extracranial skeletal survey displayed no lytic lesions, and a bone marrow aspirate and biopsy were unremarkable. No Bence-Jones protein was present in the urine, and urine protein electrophoresis was normal. A peculiar clinical finding was the presence of an abnormal IgG λ-type protein in the CSF and blood serum.

Peculiar deposits of amyloid with a crystalloid plaque-like morphology were scattered throughout the tumor tissue. The tumor vessels also showed amyloid infiltrations. The immunohistochemical study confirmed that the tumor was composed of a population of plasma cells producing a single monoclonal immunoglobulin.

The lesion was considered to be a solitary one, and the residual tumor was treated with radiation (4500 rads) over a period of 4½ weeks.

Until 1983, 15 cases of SIPs involving the brain, cranial nerves, and meninges had been published (3, 17–30). Patient ages varied from 18 to 72 years, with a peak incidence in the fourth and fifth decades and a 4:1 female-to-male preponderance. Of 8 cases that were subsequently reviewed, only 3 were considered to be true SIPs. In the remaining 5, the possibility of multiple myeloma could not be excluded with sufficient certainty, as either the skull was involved or the morphology was suggestive of a granulomatous process (3, 27).

Consideration must be given to the possibility of a plasmacytoma originating in the nasopharynx, penetrating the endocranium across the skull base, extending into the middle and/or posterior cranial fossa, and producing very similar neurologic manifestations to a plasmacytoma with primary origin within the cranial cavity (23, 31–33). Conversely, a SIP may secondarily invade the nasopharynx, infratemporal fossa, and lateral parapharyngeal space. Similarly, a plasmacytoma originating in the mucosa of the sphenoid sinus may secondarily invade the sphenoid bone and skull base, and vice versa or a plasmacytoma originating in the sphenoid bone and skull base may secondarily invade the mucosa of the sphenoid sinus.

In a plasmacytoma involving the middle and/or the posterior cranial fossa, the tentorium, or the petrous apex, it is difficult and, in an advanced stage, impossible to determine the site of origin. A large tumor with only limited erosion of the petrous apex would suggest that the neoplasm arose, for instance, in the tentorium and that the erosion of the pyramid was most likely secondary to the compression of the tumor mass of meningeal origin (3).

DIFFERENTIAL DIAGNOSIS

In the differential diagnosis of plasmacytomas in these locations, four categories of pathologic processes have to be considered: *(a)* primary lesions in the skull base, *(b)* extracranial lesions with intracranial extension, *(c)* intracranial lesions with extracranial extension, and *(d)* metastatic lesions (1). Among the extracranial lesions with intracranial extension, malignant tumors of the sphenoid have to be included: undifferentiated, squamous cell, and minor salivary gland carcinomas including adenocarcinomas and adenocystic carcinomas. Other tumors of the sphenoid sinus that need to be considered include: lymphoma, melanoma, esthesioneuroblastoma, chondrosarcoma, fibrosarcoma, rhabdomyosarcoma, hemangiopericytoma, and chordoma. Many of these neoplasms, although developing in the paranasal sinuses, arise more frequently in adjacent areas including the nasal cavity and nasopharynx. Epidermoids, which are congenital tumors, may also arise in the suprasellar and parasellar regions and in the posterior cranial fossa. Angiofibromas and several other benign lesions of the nasal cavity and paranasal sinuses can extend intracranially but generally to a lesser extent. A sphenoid sinus mucocele, fibrous dysplasia, and ossifying fibroma are benign progressive lesions with tumor-like expansion and impingement on adjacent structures. Among the intracranial lesions extending extracranially, benign and malignant pituitary neoplasms, craniopharyngiomas, and meningiomas are to be considered. Meningiomas with a conspicuous plasma cell lymphocytic component have to be distinguished from intracranial plasma cell granulomas. Meningiomas with plasma cell and lymphocytic infiltrates consist of a mixed population of meningothelial cells, mature plasma cells with few Russell bodies, and lymphocytes (33). Plasma cell granulomas, on the other hand, are composed of, in addition to plasma cells, epithelioid-like cells, histocytes, histocytic giant cells, xanthomatous cells, and lymphoctyes disseminated throughout a collagenous stroma (34). The differential diagnosis based solely on morphologic criteria can be difficult. The definite identification can be made only by immunohistochemical analysis. More aggressive meningiomas of the globoid and en plaque variety, arising from the outer surface of the petrous pyramid, from the sphenoid wing, in the parasellar region, in the cavernous sinus, and in the middle and posterior cranial fossa, may infiltrate the skull base and extend beyond. They may invade the sphenoid sinus, nasal cavity, orbit, nasopharynx, oropharynx, hypopharynx, infratemporal fossa, and lateral neck. Benign and malignant schwannomas arising in the middle and posterior fossae and, in rare instances, in the paranasal sinuses can appear as intracranial and extracranial neoplasms with involvement of the skull base. Paragangliomas occur more often in the temporal bone and neck regions but as they destroy the petrous pyramid and extend along the carotid artery and through the jugular foramen, they can destroy the skull base and present as a tumor extension in the middle and posterior cranial fossa. Rhabdomyosarcomas, which presumably arise from primitive mesenchymal tissues, may arise in the sphenoid sinus and parasellar region and aggressively destroy the skull base. Intracranial vascular anomalies including carotid aneurysms, arteriovenous malformations, and vascular tumors, i.e., hemangiomas and hemangiopericytomas, have to be considered. Finally, tumor-like inflammatory or other granulomatous processes associated with tuberculosis, syphilis, and fungal infections must be included. Metastatic lesions involving the sphenoid sinus, sphenoid bone, or clivus are uncommon and more often found in the temporal bone; they are discussed in Chapter 37 on metastases of that region. As in the temporal bone, the lungs, prostate, and breast are the most common primary sites. Cholesterol granulomatous cysts that can develop in any portion of the temporal bone but are more frequently found in the petrous apex can expand into the posterior and middle cranial fossae but very rarely penetrate deeply into the cranial cavity.

MULTIPLE MYELOMA

The multiple plasma cell myeloma represents the disseminated form of the progressive malignant neoplastic disease of plasma cells. It is characterized by the proliferation of a clone of transformed plasma cells, resulting in tumor formation in the bone marrow and by an overproduction of a monoclonal immunoglobulin or Bence-Jones protein. It is frequently associated with extensive skeletal destruction, hypercalcemia, anemia, renal failure, immunodeficiency, and an increased susceptibility to bacterial infection. The skeletal areas most frequently involved are the skull, spine, ribs, and pelvis (35, 36). Skeletal x-rays may show multiple, punched-out, osteolytic lesions resulting from replacement by expanding plasma cell tumors or from the secretion of an osteoclast-activating factor by the malignant plasma cells (37). The radiographs may occasionally show a diffuse osteopenia but only extremely rarely show an osteosclerosis. The disseminated, nonosteolytic form of myeloma is very rarely seen. Renal failure

is observed in about 20% of patients. It may result from hypercalcemia, resulting in nephrocalcinosis, Bence-Jones proteinuria with extensive cast formation in the renal tubules, amyloidosis, pyelonephritis, etc. The anemia is probably a consequence of a tumor-related inhibition of erythropoiesis and disturbance of the bone marrow architecture. The immunodeficiency is related to a severely depressed serum level of normal immunoglobulins and a compromised normal humoral immune response, factors that increase the susceptibility to infection from common encapsulated organisms (37).

Multiple myeloma is most frequently found in the middle-aged and elderly patient, with a median age at onset of 60. Its annual incidence is 3/100,000 population, and men are affected somewhat more frequently than women. It accounts for about 10% of the malignant hematologic tumors and for 1% of all forms of cancer. Although certain predisposing factors and conditions are recognized, the etiology of the disease in humans has so far remained obscure (37).

The clinical manifestations include persistent unexplained skeletal pains, especially in the back or thorax, often associated with a spontaneous fracture of the spine and ribs, weakness from anemia, renal failure, and recurrent infections. Vertebral collapse resulting in spinal cord compression and paraplegia, bleeding disorders, proteinuria, and a marked elevation of the sedimentation rate are common.

The diagnosis of myeloma includes protein electrophoresis and immunoelectrophoresis of serum and urine, a skeletal x-ray survey, and a bone marrow aspiration.

The temporal bone lesion in multiple myeloma shares the same clinical and radiographic manifestations and features in CT and MRI as in solitary plasmacytoma of that region. Depending on the location and extent of the osteolytic process and the involvement of bone and soft tissues, it can be associated with impairment of sound transmission, loss of cochlear, vestibular, and facial nerve functions, and involvement of additional cranial nerves.

References

1. Norris CM Jr. Multiple myeloma presenting as plasmacytoma of bone extending into sphenoid sinus. Case records of the Massachusetts General Hosptial. Case 21-1922. N Engl J Med 1992;326(21):1417–1424.
2. Abemayor E, Canalis RF, Greenberg P, Worthan DG, Rowland JP, Sun NCJ. Plasma cell tumors of the head and neck. J Otolaryngol 1988;17:376–381.
3. Mancardi GL, Mandybur TI. Solitary intracranial plasmacytoma. Cancer 1983;51:2226–2233.
4. Cappel DF, Mathers RP. Plasmacytoma of the petrous temporal bone and base of skull. J Laryngol Otol 1935;50:340–349.
5. Cristophe L, Divry P. Deux cas de plasmocytomes nodulaires a hauteur d'une petite aile du sphenoide. J Belg Neurol Psychiatr 1940;40:281.
6. Gros JC. Plasmacytoma of the temporal bone. Arch Otol 1945;42:188–190.
7. Sparling HJ Jr, Adams RD, Parker F. Involvement of the nervous system by malignant lymphoma. Medicine 1947;26:285–332.
8. Calvet J, Claux J, Gayral E, Rascol C, Cadenat F. Syndrome de Garcin aigu par plasmocytome de la base du crane. Rev Otoneuroophthalmol 1950;22:481–484.
9. Herrmann E. Das Plasmacytom der Schädelbasis. Beitrag zu seiner Neurologie und Radiologie. Arch Psychol Z Gesamte Neurol 1963;204:262–270.
10. Schulz-Coulon HJ, Vogelsang H. Solitäres Plasmocytom der Mittelohrräume und der Schädelbasis. HNO 1974;22:267–271.
11. Iob I, Rigobello L, Andrioli GC, Salar G. Plasmocytoma solitario della rocca petrosa. Pathologica 1979;71:543–547.

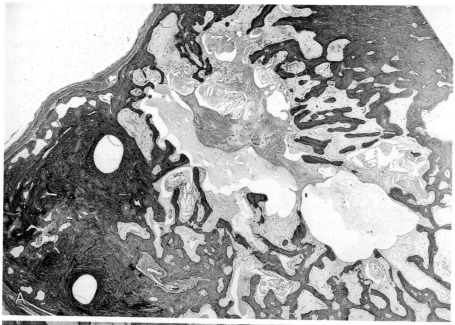

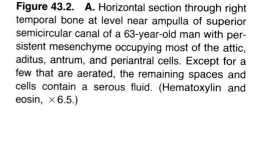

Figure 43.2. **A.** Horizontal section through right temporal bone at level near ampulla of superior semicircular canal of a 63-year-old man with persistent mesenchyme occupying most of the attic, aditus, antrum, and periantral cells. Except for a few that are aerated, the remaining spaces and cells contain a serous fluid. (Hematoxylin and eosin, ×6.5.)

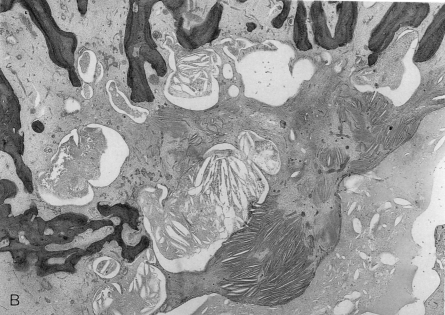

Figure 43.2. **B.** Aggregation of clefts, representing spaces formerly occupied by cholesterol crystals dissolved during the processing of temporal bones for histologic examination, are found in the mesenchyme and cystic spaces occupying the periantral cells and in the fluid of the middle ear cleft. (×17.)

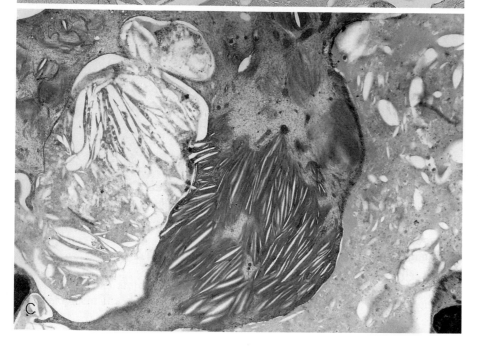

Figure 43.2. **C.** Cholesterol crystals may display a parallel or star-like arrangement or may be irregularly dispersed regardless of their surrounding media. (×35.)

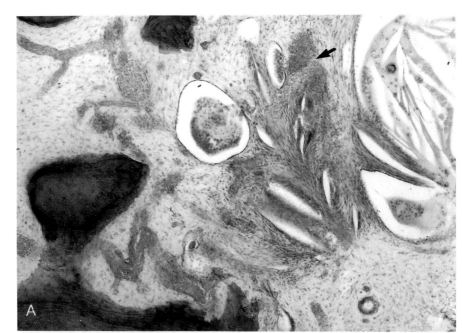

Figure 43.3. A. Same specimen as in Figure 43.2. The mesenchyme occupying the right mastoid process in this patient displays a very dense vascularization. (Hematoxylin and eosin, ×90.)

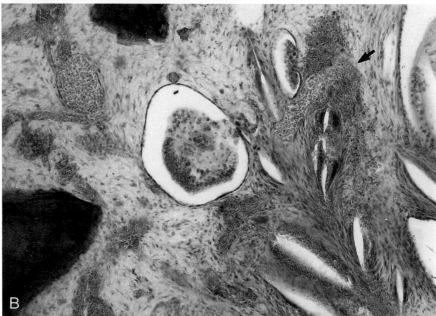

Figure 43.3. B. Many of these smaller blood vessels have become remarkably engorged and distended or have ruptured *(arrow)* and produced interstitial hemorrhages. (×130.)

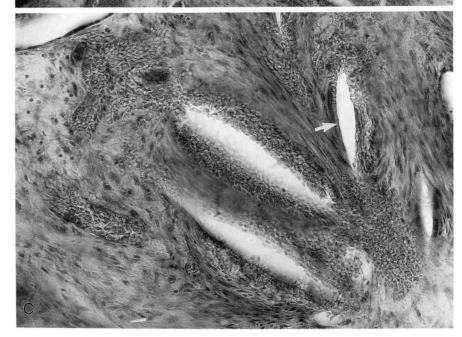

Figure 43.3. C. In these interstitial hemorrhages degradation of hemoglobin led to formation and crystallization of cholesterol *(arrow).* (×260.)

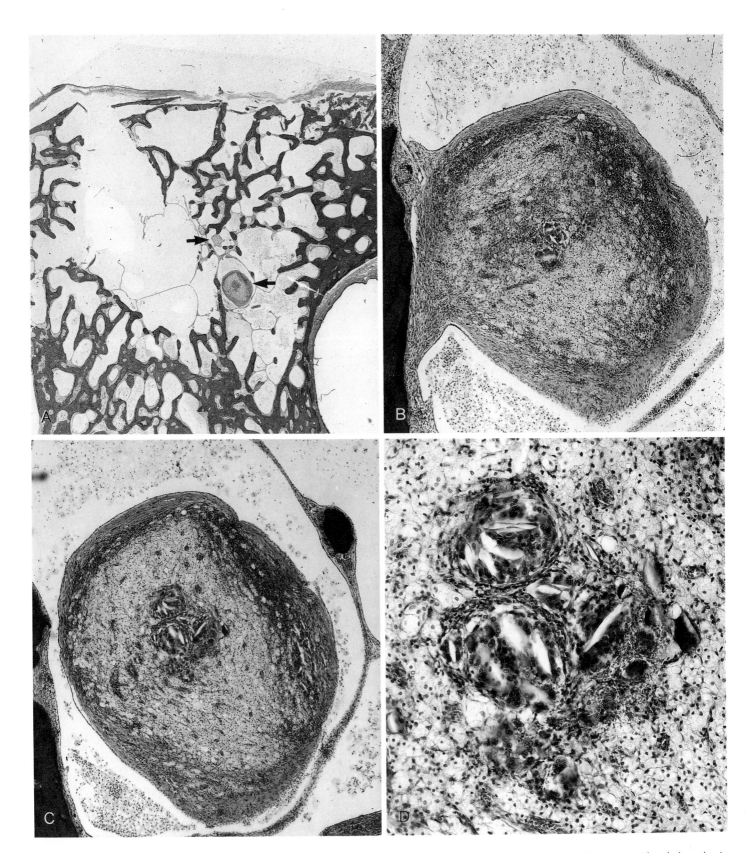

Figure 43.6. **A.** Vertical section through left temporal bone at level of mastoid antrum in adult male with no past history of otitis media. It shows the location of two polypoid changes *(arrow)* within a group of periantral cells that contain a cellular exudate and are sealed off from the air-containing antral cavity. **B.** The polyp is surrounded by cellular fluid and covered by a single layer of cuboidal epithelium; it includes a large number of small, engorged blood vessels. **C.** Different section of same specimen. A few of the distended vessels in the center have ruptured and given rise to interstitial hemorrhages with aggregations of cholesterol crystals. **D.** Same section as **C.** Deposition of cholesterol crystals incited a foreign body tissue reaction with histocytes, foreign body multinucleated giant cells, round cells, and localized areas of recent hemorrhages. (Hematoxylin and eosin, ×6, ×60, ×60, and ×185, respectively.)

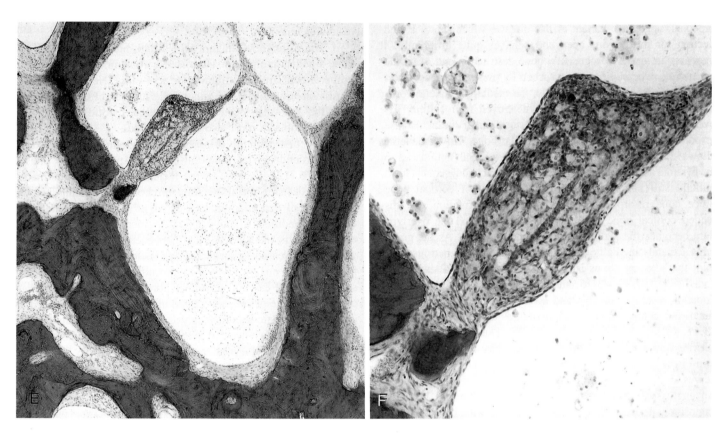

Figure 43.6.   E and **F.** The smaller of the two polyps shows the very beginning of a capillary rupture and blood extravasation. (×65 and ×145, respectively.)

Case 3. *Expansile cystic cholesterol granuloma with erosion of medial and posterior portions of left pyramid. Erosion of internal auditory canal, cochlea, and jugular foramen. Involvement of middle ear cavity and mastoid process and extension into diploic portion of occipital bone. Localized destruction of bony wall of lateral sinus.*

The patient was a 19-year-old man with a history of recurrent left tympanomastoiditis since infancy, progressive loss of hearing and tinnitus of the left ear since age 10, and persistent left serous otitis media for the past 5 years.

Otologic examination disclosed a pulsating soft tissue mass in the left middle ear surrounded by amber fluid. There was total loss of cochlear and vestibular function and minimal involvement of left cranial nerves V and VII. After an initial attempt to exteriorize the left apical cyst, the symptoms recurred.

CT scanning revealed an extensive cholesterol granuloma that had widely eroded the medial portion of the left petrous apex, the internal auditory canal, cochlea, undersurface of the pyramid, and jugular foramen. It had involved the middle ear cavity and mastoid bone and had extended into the diploic portion of the occipital bone (Fig. 43.13A).

At *operation*, the patient underwent a transcochlear exploration with a wide exteriorization of the granuloma. Histologic examination confirmed the clinical and surgical diagnosis of a cholesterol granuloma (Fig. 43.13B).

Case 4. *Expansile cystic cholesterol granuloma of right petrous apex with extension into posterior cranial fossa, impingement on brain stem, and massive destruction of internal acoustic meatus. Involvement of right cranial nerves V, VI, VII, and VIII.*

A 39-year-old woman was seen with a 20-year history of progressive hearing loss and tinnitus in her right ear, vertigo, recurrent right facial palsy, right facial numbness, diplopia on right lateral gaze, and occipital headaches. She had undergone a right posterior fossa exploration elsewhere 15 years earlier for removal of an "epidermoid" from the right petrous apex and experienced temporary improvement.

Otologic examination disclosed a normal right tympanic membrane, total loss of cochlear and vestibular function, and right fifth, sixth, seventh, and eighth cranial nerve involvement.

CT scanning disclosed a large cystic, isodense lesion in the right

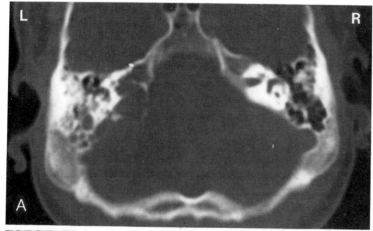

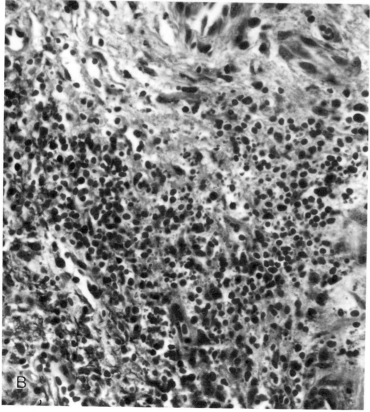

Figure 43.13. **A.** Axial CT scan of extensive cholesterol granuloma involving middle and posterior third of left petrous pyramid. It had destroyed the internal auditory canal, cochlea, and vestibule, occupied the middle ear and mastoid, eroded the jugular foramen, and extended into the diploic portion of the occipital bone. (Courtesy of Dr. M. J. Holliday.) **B.** Granuloma displaying areas of old and recent hemorrhages with numerous macrophages including hemosiderin. (Hematoxylin and eosin, ×400.)

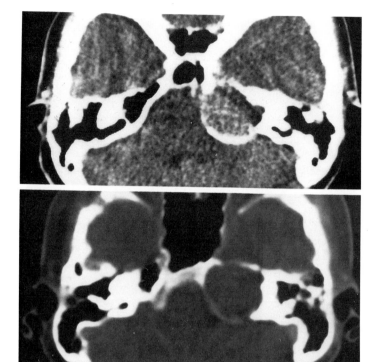

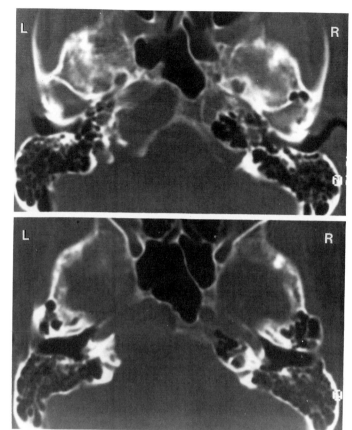

Figure 43.14. Enhanced axial CT scans of large cholesterol granuloma involving the right petrous apex with massive destruction of internal auditory canal, cochlea, and vestibule. It extends into the posterior cranial fossa, has eroded the *lateral* clivus, and is impinging on the brain stem. It is isodense and does not enhance. (Courtesy of Dr. M. J. Holliday.)

Figure 43.15. Enhanced axial CT scans of large cholesterol granuloma involving the left petrous apex. It protruded into the left sphenoid sinus and posterior nasopharynx, eroded the lateral clivus, and extended into the middle and posterior cranial fossae. It impinged on the left cavernous sinus and pons and eroded the infracochlear capsule and through the skull base. (Courtesy of Dr. M. J. Holliday.)

petrous apex that extended into the posterior cranial fossa, impinged on the brain stem, and caused massive destruction of the internal acoustic meatus (Fig. 43.14).

At *operation,* a transcochlear exteriorization of the cholesterol granuloma resulted in a remarkable restoration of function to cranial nerves V, VI, and VII. The surgical diagnosis was confirmed histologically.

Case 5. *Large expansile cystic cholesterol granuloma involving the left petrous apex with erosion of adjacent lateral clivus. Extension to left sphenoid sinus, posterior nasopharynx, and medial and posterior cranial fossae. Erosion of infracochlear otic capsule below internal auditory canal and through base of skull. Impingement on pons and left cavernous sinus.*

The patient was a 74-year-old man with a history of severe headaches 26 years prior to admission, double vision for 5 years, and episodes of rotatory vertigo and symptoms of vertebrobasilar insufficiency, with blackout spells and blurred vision, for the past 3 years. He had no history of otitis media or allergies.

Otologic examination revealed normal eardrums, mild bilateral sensorineural high-tone loss, and findings suggestive of a paretic type lesion involving the opposite right peripheral (nerve or labyrinth) vestibular mechanism.

CT scanning showed extensive erosion of the left petrous apex with destruction of the left lateral clivus, the region below the internal auditory canal, and the adjacent skull base. It extended to the left sphenoid sinus, posterior nasopharynx, and medial and posterior

cranial fossa and impinged on the pons and left cavernous sinus (Fig. 43.15).

At *operation,* Transsphenoidal marsupialization of the cholesterol granuloma in the left petrous apex was attempted. However, the local anatomical situation made this procedure impossible. Rescheduling for a different approach had to be postponed because of the patient's subsequent neurologic and intestinal problems. Meanwhile, repeated CT scans showed no increase in the size of the cystic lesion in the left petrous apex, and regular neurologic examinations revealed no further deterioration.

Case 6. *Large expansile cystic cholesterol granuloma of left petrous apex with extension into middle and posterior cranial fossae. Erosion of lateral clivus and internal acoustic meatus and impingement on brain stem. Involvement of left cranial nerves V–X and left cerebellar infarct.*

A 34-year-old man was seen with a several-year history of progressive hearing loss and tinnitus in the left ear, left-sided facial weakness, numbness, and headaches, diplopia on left lateral gaze, left vocal cord palsy, and left upper motor neuron weakness, spasticity, and ataxia in the left arm.

Otoneurologic examination revealed involvement of left cranial nerves V–X, a left hemiparesis, and left cerebellar ataxia.

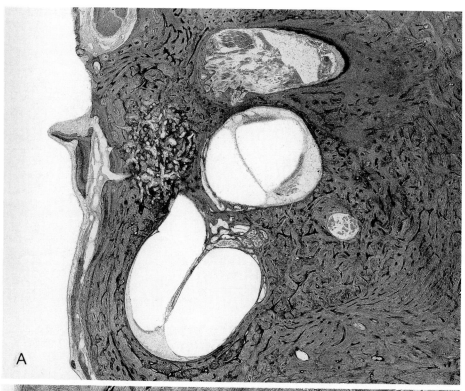

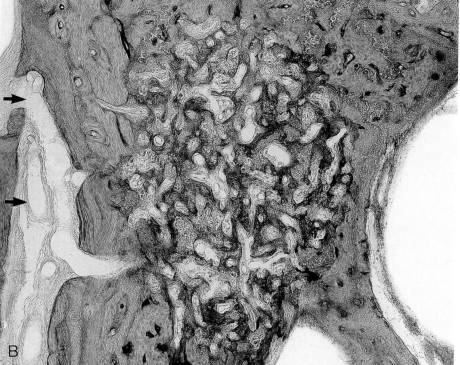

Figure 44.3. **A.** Vertical section through right pyramid of an 8½-year-old girl with essentially normal hearing bilaterally despite an active otosclerotic process involving the oval window (see also Fig. 44.6). (Hematoxylin and eosin, ×14.)

Figure 44.3. **B.** The superficial petrosal and superior tympanic arteries (*arrows*), branches of the middle meningeal artery, supply most of the blood to the otosclerotic lesion at the oval window. The vascular network within the otic capsule and the mucoperiosteum over the promontory supplies the rest of the blood. The inferior tympanic artery, through anastomosis with the superior tympanic artery, contributes blood; occasionally, the cochleovestibular branch from the internal auditory artery contributes to the vascular supply of the lesion. (×45.)

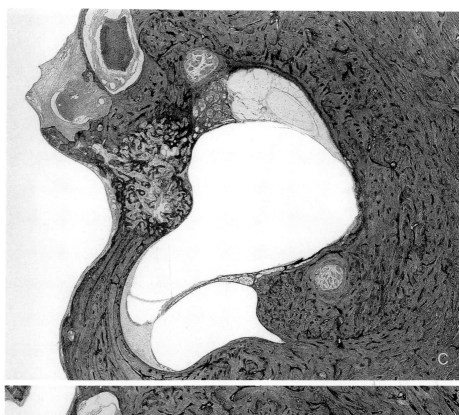

Figure 44.3. C. Vertical section through right pyramid anterior to vestibular fenestra. A second, independent, active otosclerotic lesion affects the lateral margin of both round windows. (×14.)

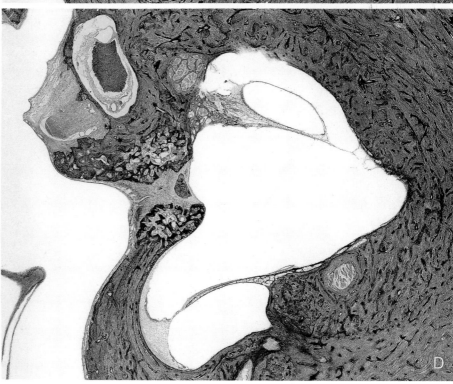

Figure 44.3. D. Vertical section through right oval window near anterior end of stapes footplate. The otosclerotic process extensively involves the superior and inferior oval window margins. (×14.)

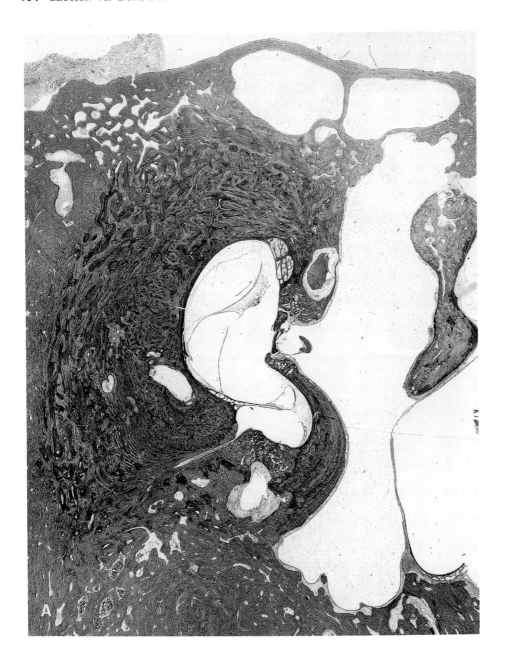

Figure 44.6. **A.** Vertical section through left petrous pyramid at level of oval window and lateral aperture of cochlear aqueduct. The oval and round windows are involved in two separate, active otosclerotic processes. Hematoxylin and eosin, ×7.)

44.19, 44.21, and 44.22) (16, 17). Very seldom are they found beyond the confines of the otic capsule; then they involve the carotid canal (35), tegmen (36), cochleariform process (16), malleus (Fig. 44.7) (37), or incus (38). A primary isolated lesion in the footplate of the stapes occurs in about 5–12% of cases (Figs. 44.8 and 44.9) (16, 32).

Whereas the otosclerotic process manifests itself in most instances in a well-demarcated, isolated form with one, often two, but rarely three or more independent lesions (Figs. 44.18 and 44.30), it rarely develops as a diffuse process involving vast areas of the labyrinthine capsule (35, 39). The diffuse manifestation can develop as such or may result from the confluence of multiple, initially independent lesions (Figs. 44.18 and 44.25). Diffuse otosclerosis often results in total obliteration of one or both windows (Figs. 44.30 and 44.33) (40). From the margins

of the oval window, the otosclerotic process can extend deeply into the vestibule and may involve all three turns of the cochlea, a situation commonly referred to as cochlear otosclerosis (Fig. 44.19). Involvement of the basal turn of the cochlea can stimulate formation of new lamellar bone in the scalae. Extensive otosclerotic bone remodeling of the cochlear capsule can cause marked distortion of the contours of the cochlea and radial and axial distortion of the cochlear modiolus and can result in numerous spontaneous fractures of the modiolar septa (Figs. 44.26–44.28 and 44.31) (41).

In about 70–80% of patients, both temporal bones are affected, and the otosclerotic lesions, more often than not, display a striking similarity in localization, extent, and direction of growth. Unilateral otosclerosis occurs only in about 10–20% of cases (16, 34, 42).

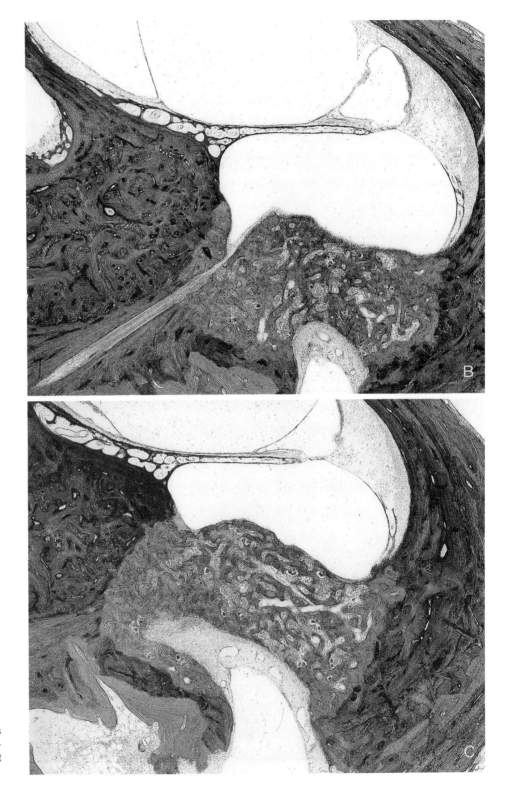

Figure 44.6. **B** and **C.** Otosclerotic process involving the round window niche has constricted the opening of the cochlear aqueduct **(B)** and the cochlear fenestra **(C).** (×30.)

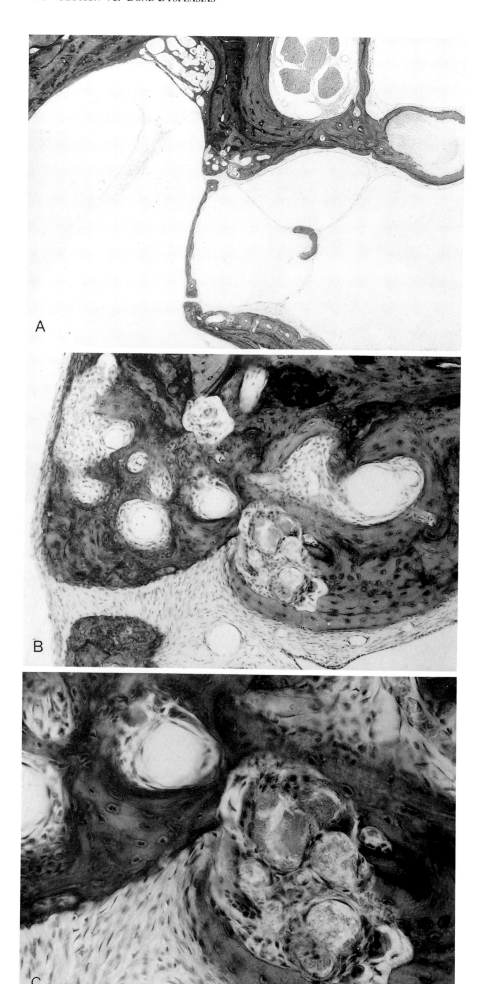

Figure 44.15.   A. Vertical section through left petrous pyramid at center of vestibular fenestra of a 4-year-old black girl who died from tuberculous meningitis. The superior and inferior oval window margins each display a very tiny otosclerotic lesion in the initial stage. (Hematoxylin and eosin, ×22.)

Figure 44.15.   B. Lesion in the superior window margin exhibits an increased number and size of regional blood vessels of the bone and the presence of several multinucleated osteoclastic giant cells in a characteristic perivascular distribution. (×160.)

Figure 44.15.   C. Process of osteoclastic bone resorption is clearly visible. (×350.)

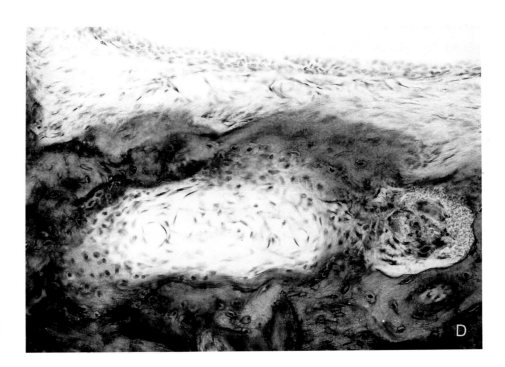

Figure 44.15. D. This very early otosclerotic lesion is located in the inferior oval window margin. ($\times$250.)

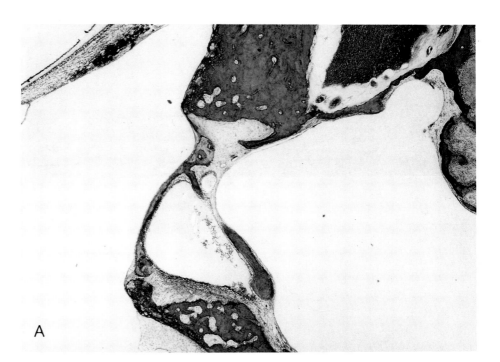

Figure 44.16. A. Vertical section through left petrous pyramid near center of stapes footplate of a 61-year-old man with bilateral clinical otosclerosis. The cartilage cover and a portion of the immediately underlying endochondral bone of the oval window margin have been resorbed. (Hematoxylin and eosin, $\times$25.)

SENSORINEURAL HEARING LOSS IN OTOSCLEROSIS

That otosclerosis may cause sensorineural hearing loss is an old conjecture, and the structural changes thought to be responsible have been discussed and debated for years. Although there is general agreement on the histopathologic changes found in such instances, opinions are divided as to their effect on the peripheral cochlear neuron. A quarter of a century ago, we were invited to present before the American Otological Society personally collected cases of clinical otosclerosis associated with an undisputable sensorineural loss in an attempt to correlate specific morphologic changes with the recorded sensorineural hearing impairment. Two of the cases presented at the time are discussed here briefly.

Case Reports

Case 1. *Extremely extensive otosclerosis with multiple small independent and large confluent lesions involving large areas of the cochlear and labyrinthine capsules representing all stages of bone transformation, but mainly the mature type of otosclerotic bone. Bilateral similarity of otosclerotic lesions in location, extent, and histologic appearance. Marked distortion of cochlear contours and compression and narrowing of upper cochlear turns. Axial and radial compression of cochlear modiolus and osseous spiral lamina resulting in multiple tiny fractures. Massive involvement of oval and round windows with partial obliteration, distortion, jamming, and ankylosis of the stapes. Protrusion of oval window margin into vestibule, and partial obliteration of scala tympani of lower basal turn. Involvement of membranous spiral lamina and spiral ligament, distortion of basilar membrane, and displacement of organ of Corti. Regional hyalin degeneration of spiral ligament and atrophy of stria vascularis in areas where otosclerotic lesions have replaced the endosteal capsule layer. Marked partial atrophy of cochlear nerve fibers and spiral ganglion cells. Nearly total loss of inner and outer hair cells. Independent otosclerotic lesions involving the ampullated end of the lateral semicircular canal as well as the walls and floor of the internal auditory meatus.*

The patient was a 95-year-old man with a history of bilateral progressive hearing loss since about age 20, resulting in a hearing impairment at age 50 and a profound loss at age 60. After age 75, the patient no longer had any measurable hearing in either ear. He gave no history of ear infections, head trauma, or ingestion of ototoxic drugs. The family history revealed that four of this patient's sons had bilateral progressive hearing impairment. Three had onset around age 30; the other, in whom it was associated with tinnitus, experienced onset at age 40. Three of the four sons were examined by the author, and the otologic examination in all revealed a bilateral symmetrical sensorineural hearing impairment. The remaining daughter had normal hearing.

Otologic examination revealed normal tympanic membranes and no response to any auditory stimuli by air or bone conduction in either ear. Caloric stimulation of both labyrinths elicited normal responses.

Eight months after the last otologic examination, death occurred from arteriosclerotic heart disease and terminal pneumonitis.

Histologic examination of the right temporal bone reveals multiple otosclerotic lesions involving the capsules of the cochlea and the vestibular labyrinth (Fig. 44.18). Some of the lesions are independent; others unite to form a conglomeration. Although the lesions represent all stages of bone transformation, the majority display the more mature type of otosclerotic bone. The lesions are most extensive around the apex of the cochlea, in the immediate vicinity of the middle and apical turns. Because of the growth of these foci, the

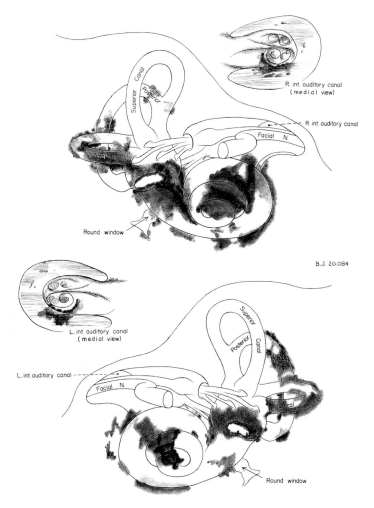

Figure 44.18. Schematic representation of site and extent of otosclerotic lesions involving the right and left otic capsules.

contours of the cochlea have become markedly distorted, so that the lumen of the upper cochlear turns is narrowed and the walls are irregular (Fig. 44.19). The change in configuration of these cochlear turns caused a compression of the modiolus and osseous spiral lamina resulting in multiple tiny fractures in the regions involved (Fig. 44.19B).

Other obvious changes involve the membranous portion of the spiral lamina and spiral ligament in the second and third cochlear turns. The decrease in radial diameter of the cochlea resulted in a foreshortening and distortion of the basilar membrane with an elevation and displacement of the organ of Corti. In the spiral ligament the fibrous tissue meshwork has almost disappeared except at the base where the ligament attaches to the otosclerotic bone. The base of the spiral ligament is further characterized by the presence of a translucent, homogeneous, structureless material arranged in bands between connective tissue fibers.

These hyalin "crescents" are present only in areas where an otosclerotic lesion has replaced the endosteal capsule layers and come in direct contact with the spiral ligament. Hyalin degeneration of the connective tissue most likely represents a reaction of the stroma to the invading otosclerotic process. The architecture of the stratum fibrosum is changed: the arrangement of the fibrous elements is no longer recognizable, and the cellular elements are greatly diminished. The stria vascularis no longer shows the differentiation into three distinct cell layers. The basal cells, intermediate capillary-bearing cells, and marginal cells are greatly diminished in number and reduced to small clusters of epithelial cells in a syncytium-like arrangement. These cell clusters may include a larger strial vessel. The external sulcus cells are noticeably flattened. The basal turn of the

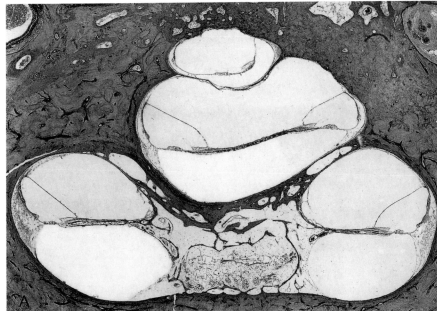

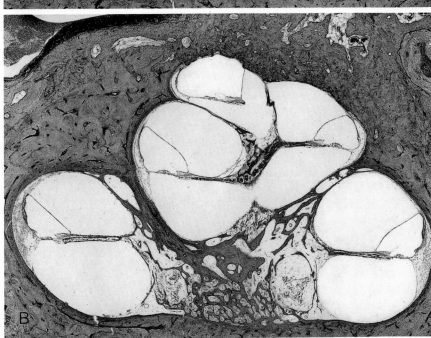

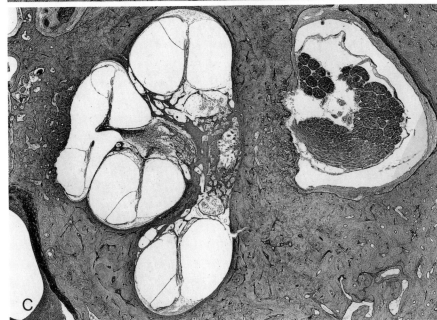

Figure 44.19. A. Vertical paramodiolar section through right cochlea. A large otosclerotic lesion involves the capsule of the middle and apical turns, compresses the modiolus in a radial direction, and causes multiple fractures of the horizontal septum between the middle and apical turns. (Hematoxylin and eosin, ×23.)

Figure 44.19. B. Vertical paramodiolar section through right cochlea. Compression of the modiolus by the same lesion in an axial direction causes several fractures of the vertical septum between the middle and apical turns. (×23.)

Figure 44.19. C. Vertical midmodiolar section through right pyramid nearby. A large otosclerotic lesion deforms the apex of the cochlea. One of the several other lesions is in the anterior wall of the internal acoustic meatus. Partial nerve atrophy is most prominent in the basal turn. (×15.)

cochlea is free from otosclerotic involvement, the spiral ligament is normal in appearance, and there are no hyalin crescents.

In the organ of Corti, the hair cells are absent within the turns involved in the otosclerotic process. In the remaining turns of the cochlea, an occasional hair cell is still present.

There is partial atrophy of the cochlear nerve fibers within the osseous spiral lamina and of the spiral ganglion cells, but this seems to be restricted to the basal turn of the cochlea.

Another extensive otosclerotic area involves the greater part of the promontory and the region of both windows. The niche of the oval window is greatly narrowed, and the window margins protrude into the vestibule. The footplate of the stapes is overgrown in addition to being ankylosed and replaced by otosclerotic bone. The niche of the round window is markedly distorted and narrowed (Fig. 44.20). The otosclerotic process involving the lateral margin of the cochlear fenestra protrudes widely into the scala tympani and partially obliterates its lumen. As a result, the round window membrane has become foreshortened and displaced, and the size of the window is obviously reduced (Fig. 44.20B).

Other otosclerotic lesions involve the region of the ampullated end of the lateral semicircular canal and the walls and floor of the internal auditory meatus.

The blood supply of the lesion at the oval window is principally from the superior tympanic artery and its branches in the overlying mucoperiosteum. In addition, the lesion receives blood from the vascular plexus normally present in the otic capsule. Very rarely, there is a small anastomosis connecting the vascular bed of the lesions with the capillaries in the spiral ligament.

The sections also reveal a terminal subacute otitis media and mastoiditis, probably associated with the pneumonitis (Fig. 44.20).

Histologic examination of the left temporal bone reveals lesions similar to those in the right ear, with otosclerotic foci of similar location, extent, and histologic appearance (Fig. 44.18). The lesions involving the cochlear capsule have distorted its contours. In the apical turn an active focus invades the spiral ligament, which exhibits morphologic changes similar to those in the corresponding regions of the opposite cochlea (Figs. 44.21 and 44.22). Hyalin crescents, for instance, are clearly visible.

The oval window is involved in a massive otosclerotic process (Fig. 44.23). This causes narrowing of the fenestra as well as protrusion of its margin into the vestibule (Fig. 44.24). A large focus in the anterior wall of the round window distorts the round window membrane and protrudes into the scala tympani, partially obliterating it.

Other areas of otosclerotic bone involve the ampullated end of the lateral semicircular canal and the walls and floor of the internal auditory meatus.

The vascular supply of the lesion at the oval window is from the superior tympanic artery and its branches, as well as from the vascular plexus within the otic capsule (Fig. 44.23). On occasion, a tiny vessel connects the vascular bed of the otosclerotic lesion and the spiral ligament.

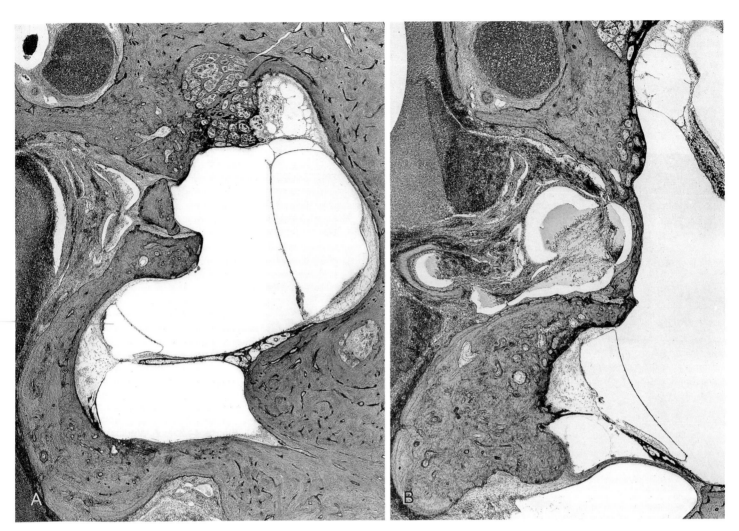

Figure 44.20.   A. Vertical section through right pyramid in anterior part of oval window. The otosclerotic process involves the entire window and stapedial footplate. The inferior window margin protrudes markedly into the vestibule. **B.** Vertical section through right pyramid at middle of oval win-dow. An extensive otosclerotic lesion involves both windows, ankyloses the stapedial footplate, and partially obliterates the scala tympani of the lower basal turn. (Hematoxylin and eosin, $\times 22$, respectively.)

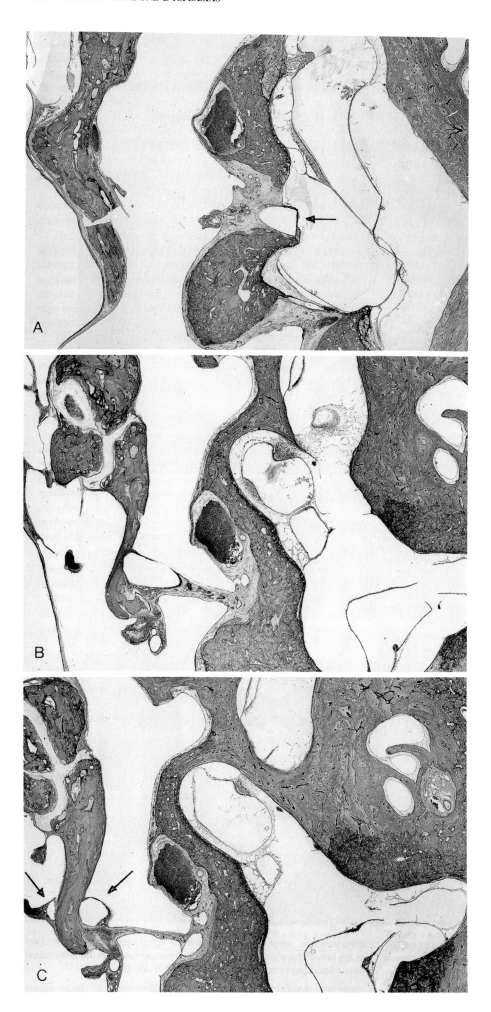

Figure 44.43. **A.** Vertical section through right petrous pyramid at level of oval and round windows. Extensive otosclerotic process produces marked constriction of both windows. Lower end of Teflon piston prosthesis *(arrow)* is firmly embedded in fibrous tissue. Its medial end, which does not protrude significantly into the vestibule, is covered by a few layers of connective tissue. (Hematoxylin and eosin, ×16.)

Figure 44.43. **B** and **C.** Vertical sections through right petrous pyramid posterior to oval window. Several large otosclerotic lesions involve the labyrinthine capsule. The lateral, ring-shaped end of the Teflon piston prosthesis *(arrow)* fits tightly around the lower end of the incus. There is no evidence of bone atrophy at the site of attachment. (×16 for both.)

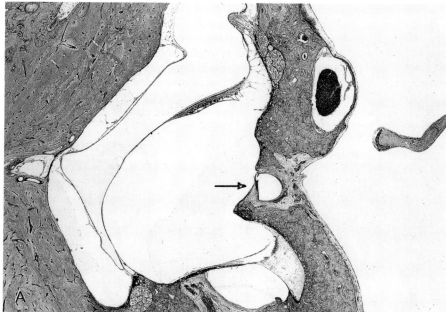

Figure 44.44. A. Vertical section through left petrous pyramid at level of oval and round windows, both of which are markedly narrowed by the otosclerotic process. The medial end of the Teflon piston prosthesis *(arrow)* is firmly embedded in scar tissue and aligns well with level of vestibular fenestra. (×16.)

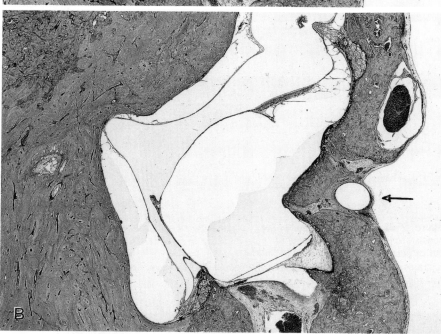

Figure 44.44. B. Vertical section through left petrous pyramid in plane of superior semicircular canal. Several large otosclerotic lesions involve the labyrinthine capsule. The cross-section through the lower half of the Teflon piston prosthesis *(arrow)* is clearly visible. (Hematoxylin and eosin, ×16.)

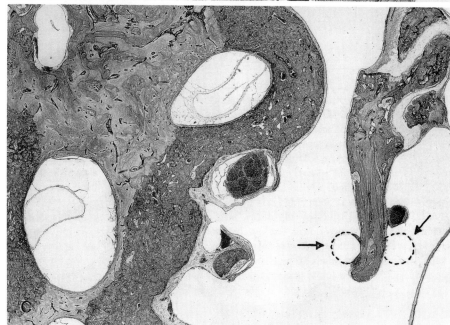

Figure 44.44. C. Vertical section through left petrous pyramid at level of incudomalleolar articulation. The Teflon ring *(arrows)*, which forms the lateral end of the prosthesis, has not produced incus atrophy at the site of its attachment. (×16.)

References

1. Valsalva AM. Valsalvae opera et morgagni epistolae. Venetiis: Francescus Pitteri, 1741:2.
2. Valsalva AM. Tractus de aure humana. Lugduna: Johannes Hasebroek, Chap II, 1742:24.
3. Toynbee J. Pathological and surgical observations on the diseases of the ear. Med Chir Trans 1824;24:190–205.
4. Toynbee J. Die Krankheiten des Gehörorgans: Ihre Natur, Diagnose und Behandlung. Würzburg: JM Richter, 1863.
5. Bezold F, Siebenmann F. Textbook of otology. 1894: lecture XXVI. (Holinger J, trans). Chicago: EH Colgrove, 1908.
6. Bezold F. Ein Fall von Stapesankylose und ein Fall von Nervöser Schwerhörigkeit mit den zugehörigen Sectionsbefunden und der manometrischen Untersuchung. Z Ohrenheilkd 1893;24(sect XIV):267–279.
7. Habermann JE. Zur Pathologie der sogenannten Otosklerose. Arch Ohrenheilkd 1894;60:37.
8. Siebenmann F. Über einen weiteren Fall von Spongiosierung der Labyrinthkapsel, mit dem klinischen Bilde der Stapesankylose beginnend und infolge Hinzutretens der Nervenveränderungen (ex cachexia carcinomatosa) mit Taubheit endigend. Z Ohrenheilkd 1900;36(sect XIV):291–300.
9. Gradenigo G. Trattato sulla patologia e terapia dell'orecchi e della prime vie aere. Otol Rhinol Laryngol R Acad di Medic (Torino) Jan 19, 1904.
10. Politzer A. Die Otosclerose. In: Politzer A, ed. Lehrbuch der Ohrenheilkunde für Praktische Ärzte und Studierende. 2nd ed. Stuttgart: Ferdinand Enke Verlag, 1889:233.
11. Politzer A. Über primäre Erkrankung der knöchernen Labyrinthkapsel. Z Ohrenheilkd 1894;25:309.
12. Brühl G. In: Denker A, Kahler O, eds. Handbuch der Hals-Nasen-Ohrenheilkunde, Vol 7: Gehörorgan. Wiesbaden: J Springer & GT Bergmann, 1926;7:410.
13. Manasse P. Die Otitis chronica metaplastica der menschlichen Labyrinthkapsel. Wiesbaden: Bergmann, 1912.
14. Mayer O. Untersuchengen über die Otosklerose. Wien: Holder, 1917.
15. Wittmaack K. Die Otosklerose auf Grund eigener Forschungen. Jena: Gustav Fischer Verlag, 1919.
16. Guild SR. Histologic otosclerosis. Ann Otol 1944;53:246–266.
17. Beickert P. Otosklerose. In: Berendes J, Link R, Zöllner T, eds. Hals-Nasen-Ohrenheilkunde, Ohr I. Stuttgart: Georg Thieme, Chap 19, 1979;5:1–64.
18. Nager FR. Pathology of the labyrinthine capsule and its clinical significance. In: Fowler EP Jr, ed. Medicine of the ear. New York: Thomas Nelson and Sons, Chap VII, 1947.
19. Lindsay JR. Otosclerosis. In: Paprella MM, Shumrich DA, eds. Otolaryngology. 2nd ed. Philadelphia: WB Saunders, Chap 25, 1980:II.
20. Cawthorne T. Otosclerosis (Dalby Memorial Lecture). J Laryngol Otol 1955;69:437–456.
21. Cawthorne T. Otosclerosis. In: Diseases of the ear, nose and throat. London: Butterworths, Chap 24, 1965;2:619–635.
22. Gray AA. Otosclerosis problem: including reports of 2 cases pathologically examined (Dalby Memorial Lecture). J Laryngol Otol 1934;49:629–663.
23. Nager FR. Zur Klinik und pathologischen Anatomie der Otosklerose. Acta Otolaryngol 1939;27(5):542–551.
24. Shambaugh GE Jr. Diagnosis and indications for surgery in otosclerosis. In: Shambaugh GE, ed. Surgery of the ear. Philadelphia: WB Saunders, Chap 17, 1959:437–460.
25. Schwarz M, Becker PE. Annomalien, Missbildungen v. Krankheiten der Ohren-, der Nase v. der Halses. In: Becker PE, ed Humangenetik. Stuttgart: Georg Thieme, 1964:IV:248–345.
26. Nager GT. Ein Paar weiblicher eineiiger Zwillinge mit klinisch sowie anatomisch konkordanter Otoskerose und ähnlichem Hörgewinn durch Fenestration. Acta Otolaryngol (Stockh) 1955;45:42–58.
27. Fowler EP. Otosclerosis in identical twins. Arch Otolaryngol 1966;83:324–331.
28. Larson A. Otosclerosis: a genetic and clinical study. Acta Otolaryngol (Stockh) 1960;5(Suppl 154):1–37.
29. Larson A. Genetic problems in otosclerosis. In: Henry Ford Hospital International Symposium on Otosclerosis. Boston: Little, Brown, 1962:109–117.
30. Nager GT, Nager M. The arteries of the human middle ear with particular regard to the blood supply of the auditory ossicles. Ann Otol Rhinol Laryngol 1953;62:923–949.
31. Nager GT. Origins and relations of the internal auditory artery and the subarcuate artery. Ann Otol Rhinol Laryngol 1954;63:51–61.
32. Ruedi L, Spöndlin H. Die Histologie der otosclerotischen Stapesankylose im Hinblick auf die chirugische Mobilisation des Steigbügels. Fortschr Hals-Nasen-Ohrenheilkd 1957;41:1–84.
33. Nylen B. Histopathological investigations on the localization, number, activity and extent of otosclerotic foci. J Laryngol Otol 1949;63:321–327.
34. Fleischer K. Die Formen otosclerotischer Fensterherde und ihre Auswirkungen auf das Operationsergebnis. Arch Ohren-Nasen-Kehlkopfheilkd 1958;171(2):176–184.
35. Nager FR. Über Labyrinthveränderungen bei Otosklerose. Schweiz Med Wochenschr 1938;68:85–91.
36. Kelemen G. Otosclerotic focus outside the inner ear capsule. Laryngoscope 1943;53:528–532.
37. Covell WP. The ossicles in otosclerosis. Acta Otolaryngol (Stockh) 1940;28(3):263–276.
38. Wustrow F. Die Knochenbildung in den Gehörknöchelchen. Z Laryngol Rhinol Otol Grenzgeb 1956;35:487–498.
39. Nylen CD, Nylen B. On the genesis of otosclerosis. J Laryngol Otol 1952;66:55–64.
40. Nager FR, Fraser JS. On bone formation in the scala tympani of otosclerotics. J Laryngol Otol 1938;53:173–180.
41. Nager GT. Sensorineural deafness and otosclerosis. Ann Otol Rhinol Laryngol 1966;75:481–511.
42. Lindsay Jr. Otosclerosis and fenestration. In: Kobrak HG, ed. The Middle Ear. Chicago: University of Chicago Press, Chap 7, 1959:123–140.
43. Guild SR. Early stages of otosclerosis. Arch Otolaryngol 1930;12:457–483.
44. Siebenmann F. Über die Anfangsstadien und über die Natur der progressiven Spongiosierung der Labyrinthkapsel. Verh Dtsch Otol Ges 1912;21:186–195.
45. Ruedi L. Histopathology of sensorineural degeneration and other inner ear changes in otosclerosis. In: Henry Ford Hospital International Symposium on Otosclerosis. Boston: Little, Brown, 1962:79–96.
46. Ruedi L. Histopathologic confirmation of labyrinthine otosclerosis. Laryngoscope 1965;75:1582–1609.
47. Ruedi L, Spöndlin H. Pathogenesis of sensorineural deafness in otosclerosis. Trans Am Otol Soc 1966;54:167–196.
48. Lindsay JR. Histopathologic findings following stapedectomy and polyethylene tube inserts in the human. Ann Otol Rhinol Laryngol 1961;70:785–807.
49. Baron SH, Lindsay Jr. Stapedectomy with fat graft and polyethylene strut. Arch Otolaryngol (Stockh) 1964;80:128–130.
50. Schuknecht H, McGee TM, Igarashi M, et al. Stapedectomy: post mortem studies. Arch Otolaryngol 1964;70:437–446.
51. Schuknecht H. Stapedectomy. Boston: Little, Brown, 1971:33–38.
52. Wolff D, Schuknecht H, Bellucci R. Otosclerosis and multiple surgery in the temporal bone. Ann Otol Rhinol Laryngol 1968;77:33–42.
53. Nager GT. Histopathology of otosclerosis. Arch Otolaryngol 1969;89:341–363.

45/ Osteitis Deformans Paget

DEFINITION

Osteitis deformans Paget is a fairly common, heritable, chronic, sometimes progressive and potentially deforming disease of bone affecting 3–4% of the population beyond age 40. The disease may present as a solitary, monostotic form, permanently asymptomatic, only to be discovered as an incidental finding; or it may evolve into a clinically manifest and obvious expression of Paget's disease. In its disseminated, polyostotic form, many bones in different regions of the skeleton may be affected. Occasionally, only a few bones are involved, a form referred to as oligostotic Paget's disease. In no instance, however, are all bones involved as in a generalized bone disorder, such as hyperparathyroidism. Cylindrical and flat bones are affected with equal frequency.

Paget's disease is morphologically characterized by an abnormal, accelerated remodeling of bone that results in a consolidation of fragmented osteons in a mosaic-like structure. Repeated episodes of bone resorption followed by exaggerated attempts at repair result in a structurally weakened and deformed skeleton with increased bone mass. Rebuilding of the cortical bone results in an exfoliation of the cortex, and the remodeling of the spongiosa results in atrophy and numeric reduction of the bony trabeculae and reinforcement and coarsening of the remaining trabeculae. The clinical manifestations with regard to the skeleton, therefore, include localized pain, deformation, and spontaneous fractures.

The susceptible sites commonly encountered in clinical practice are the long bones (tibia, femur, and humerus), whereas the most frequent sites from autopsy material are the spinal column, pelvis, and skull. Calcium and phosphorus metabolisms are not affected, but in better than half the patients, serum alkaline phosphatase is elevated and tends to fluctuate, with peaks up to 200 Bodansky units (1). In over 50% of instances the disease remains asymptomatic. It does not shorten the life span. The incidence of sarcomatous transformation of a pagetic process is less than 1%.

INCIDENCE, AGE, AND SEX DISTRIBUTION

The incidence of osteitis deformans in the general population is estimated at around 0.013% (2). Autopsy studies of unselected patients older than 40 years reveal an overall incidence of 3–3.7%, steadily increasing from 1% in the fifth decade to 5–10% in the ninth decade (3, 4). The disease is seldom found in patients under age 40. The actual incidence may well be higher, as asymptomatic and smaller lesions may never be detected. There is good evidence that in two of three cases the condition remains unrecognized. The disease is most common in England, Australia, and New Zealand, is somewhat less frequent in Central Europe, is rather infrequent in North and South America and in the Mediterranean countries, is only occasionally found in Af-

rica, China, and India, and is extremely rare in the Scandinavian countries (5). The reason for the differences in the geographic distribution is unknown.

Osteitis deformans is clearly a disease of the elderly, becoming more frequent with increasing age. Most clinical statistics reveal a slight male preponderance that is also confirmed by postmortem examinations. The actual male-to-female ratio is about 5:4.

LOCALIZATION

Osteitis deformans is principally a disease of the axial skeleton. The reliable information on localization is based on statistical analysis of autopsy material. Bones under particular mechanical stress are generally affected more often than bones that are not; thus the bones of the leg are involved more often than those of the arm. The bones most frequently affected are, in order of decreasing frequency, the sacrum (57%), spine (50%), pelvis (43%), and femur (35%). The incidence of vertebral involvement decreases steadily from the sacral (76%) to the lumbar (26%), thoracic (17%), and cervical (7%) regions of the spine. The right femur is involved about twice as often as the left (31% vs. 15%, respectively) (3). A similar observation was made of a brother and sister with Paget's disease, both with unilateral involvement of the radius. In the left-handed individual, the left radius was involved, whereas in the right-handed sibling, the right radius was affected (4). The structural changes tend to be most prominent at the attachments of tendons and ligaments. Although the involvement of the skeleton usually follows a pattern of localization consistent with the concept of stress and weight bearing, it should be remembered that this ''wear and tear'' is probably only one contributing factor and that a hereditary weakness possibly represents the primary factor.

CLINICAL MANIFESTATIONS

The symptomatology depends on the skeletal area involved. The most common complaints are musculoskeletal pain and skeletal deformity, particularly bowing, of the long cylindrical bones of the lower extremities. The symptoms associated with skull lesions include hearing loss, tinnitus, vertigo, and less commonly headaches. Widespread involvement of the calvarium may result in progressive enlargement of the neurocranium. Severe involvement of the skull base may result in basilar impression and compression of the spinal cord, brain stem, cerebellum, and vertebral and basal arteries, which, in turn, may result in impairment of swallowing and speech, diplopia, and loss of bladder control. Deformity of the facial bones resulting in leontiasis ossea is much less common in Paget's disease than in fibrous dysplasia, which is commonly recognized at a much earlier age (5). Occasionally, the course of the disease may be complicated by spontaneous fractures and development of a sarcoma in an area of active bone remodeling. Back pain can be severe and of complex origin and may reflect involvement of one or more vertebrae often associated with degenerative arthritis, with impingement on nerve roots. An abrupt onset of unbearable pain generally heralds a vertebral compression fracture. Involvement of the pelvis and proximal femur produces a recognizable pain syndrome that may be aggravated by the weight-bearing pain of the accompanying degenerative arthritis. Ambulation becomes impaired as progressive anterior and lateral bowing of the femur and tibia develops. Accelerated bone remodeling in the calvaria or a long bone is reflected by an increase in skin temperature over the affected skeleton area. This is the result of a significant increase in the cutaneous blood flow associated with the markedly augmented capillarization and arteriovenous shunting in the underlying bone (5). The increased vascularity associated with significant skeletal involvement, especially widespread involvement of the skull, may cause increased cardiac output, cardiac enlargement, and ultimately congestive heart failure.

Osteitis deformans appears in hospital practice more often as an incidental or subsidiary finding than as a principal cause of admission. Only about 15% of patients exhibit an advanced form of the disease with the well-known skeletal changes, striking deformities of the long bones, progressive kyphosis with shortening of stature, and enlargement of the skull (Fig. 45.1). The skull becomes involved in about 65–70% of patients (Fig. 45.2) (4). In most instances (about 70%), the skull shows evidence of an advanced stage of the disease. In only about one-third of instances, however, does the disease process eventually result in deformity and enlargement. The neurocranium is more often the site of involvement than the facial cranium, and of the facial bones the mandible is more frequently affected than the maxilla (Fig. 45.3) (3). Usually, the calvaria is involved in a diffuse and even manner, with the thickening and deformity varying greatly in different regions (Figs. 45.4–45.9). Occasionally, only one portion or only one-half of the calvaria is affected. At times, well-circumscribed lesions are scattered throughout the calvaria. In about 10% of cases, the disease presents as a sharply demarcated, predominantly osteolytic lesion recognized as osteoporosis circumscripta cranii (6, 7). The weight of the brain and enlarged skull may cause flattening of the softened bones constituting the base. Dorsal inclination of the plane of the foramen magnum and projection of the odontoid process into the posterior fossa result in bending of the brain stem over the odontoid and ventral margins of the foramen magnum, protrusion of the olivary processes of the cerebellum into the cervical canal, tension on the nerve roots, and compression of the basilar vessels. Reduction in volume of the neurocranium, invagination of the occipital condyle, and advanced changes in the cervical spine

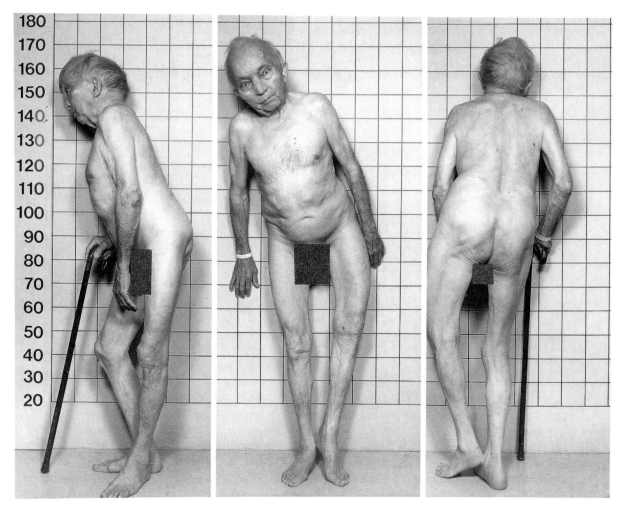

Figure 45.1. Patient KH, an 80-year-old man with polyostotic Paget's disease involving the entire skull, spine, sacrum, left pelvis and left femur and tibia. Anterior bowing of the left femur, short stature, kyphosis of the thoracic spine with forward thrust of the head, and skull enlargement are clearly recognizable.

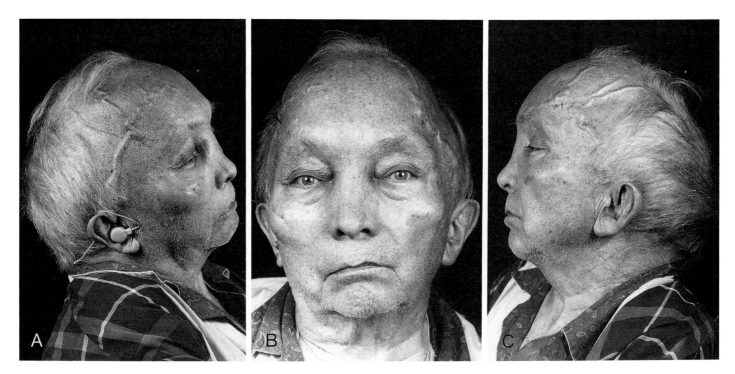

Figure 45.2. Enlargement of the neurocranium and the basilar impression with occipital overhang and enlargement and tortuosity of the super-ficial temporal artery and its parietal and frontal branches in patient KH are clearly recognizable.

can produce cerebral and cerebellar dysfunction and result in vertebrobasilar ischemia. Impingement on cranial and spinal nerves in their foramina of exit by periosteal new bone formation may result, as mentioned earlier, in impairment of hearing, equilibrium, and vision and produce motor and sensory disturbances. Impairment of hearing is the most common manifestation of cranial nerve involvement, being present in 30–50% of patients with skull involvement. It is predominantly sensorineural in nature, cochlear in origin, and often associated with low-frequency conductive loss with a peak of the air-bone gap at 500 cycles. Tinnitus is observed in about 20% of these patients, and vertigo and

unsteadiness occur in about 20–25% (8, 9). Decreased response to caloric stimulation is frequently observed in these patients (9). Once the skull becomes obviously involved, headaches become a prominent and constant symptom. Patients with widespread involvement of the calvaria often display an increase in skin temperature over the affected skull region and a conspicuous enlargement and tortuosity of the superficial temporal artery and its branches (Fig. 45.2). The enlargement of this vessel, when associated with a mixed hearing loss, should arouse suspicion of Paget's disease (9).

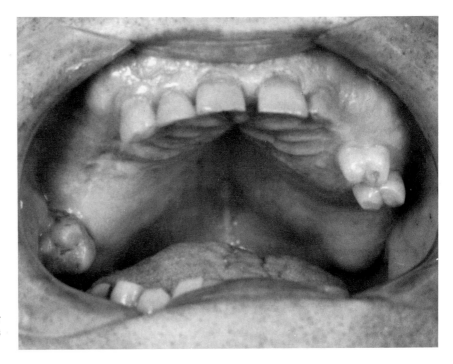

Figure 45.3. Enlargement and deformity of the alveolar process of the maxilla in patient KH, caused by Paget's disease, are evident.

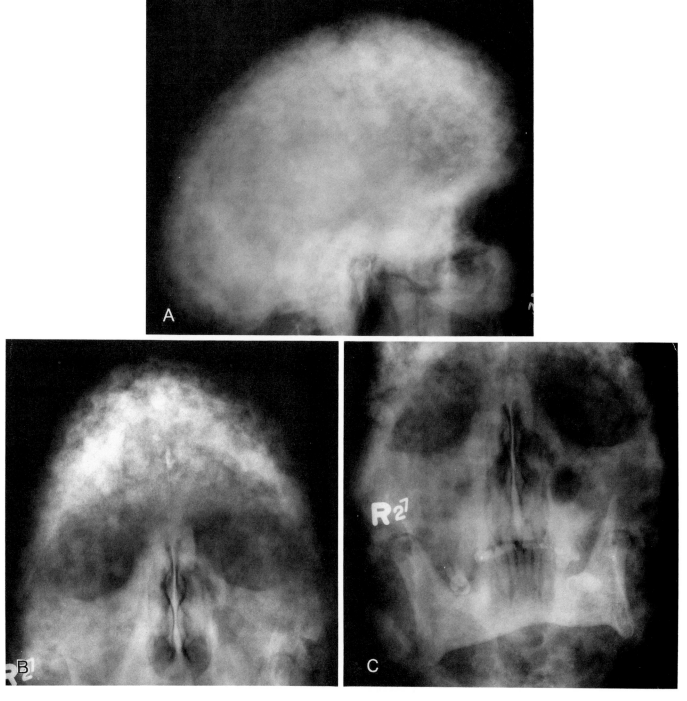

Figure 45.4. Extraordinary, diffuse sclerosis of the calvaria in patient KH resulted in complete effacement of the internal and external tables and obliteration of the calvarial diploë.

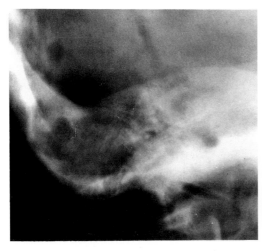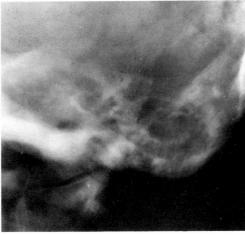

Figure 45.5. Longitudinal (Stenvers) view of petrous pyramids of patient KH. Extensive osteosclerosis of the perilabyrinthine bone, characteristic for the reconstructive phase and advanced stage of the disease, renders visualization of the vestibular labyrinth and cochlea more difficult. Note elevation of the petrous apices.

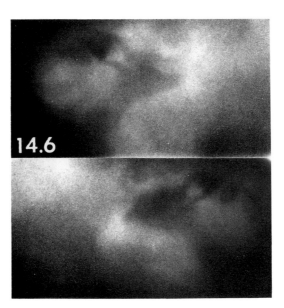

Figure 45.6. Anteroposterior multidirectional tomograms of petrous pyramids of patient KH, demonstrating sclerosis of the attic walls and constriction of the epitympanic space.

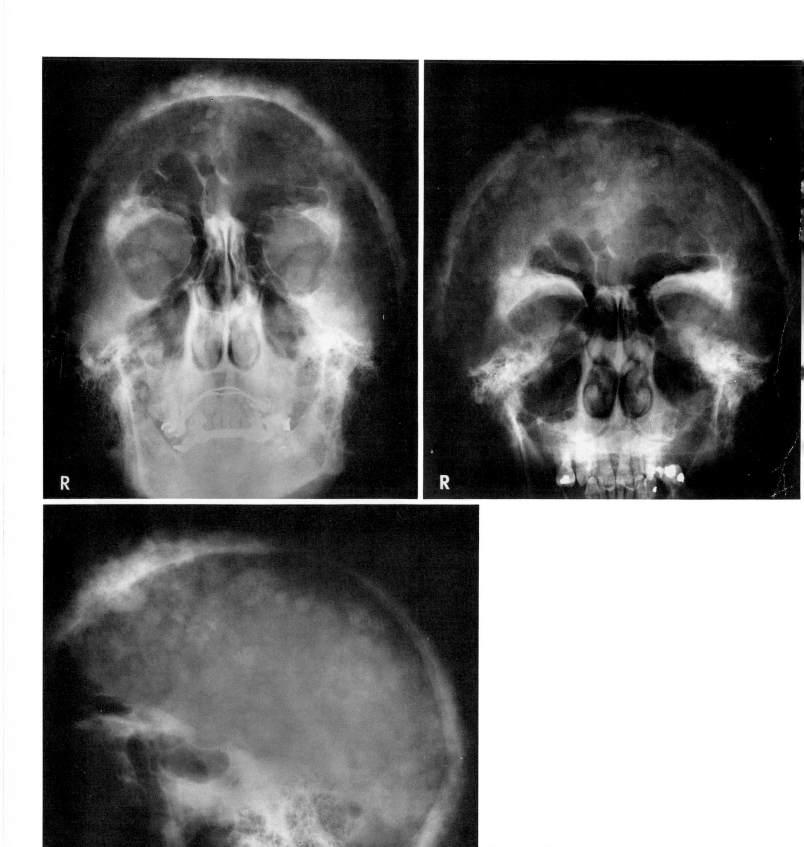

Figure 45.10. Patient TB, a 66-year-old woman with polyostotic Paget's disease involving the entire skull including temporal bones and mandible. The calvaria exhibits the characteristic "cotton-wool" pattern, basilar impression, and occipital overhang.

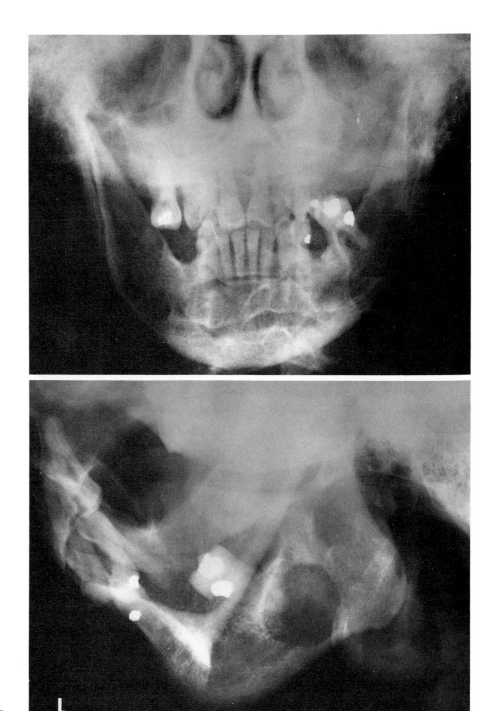

Figure 45.11. The mandible in patient TB reveals an osteolytic lesion on each side.

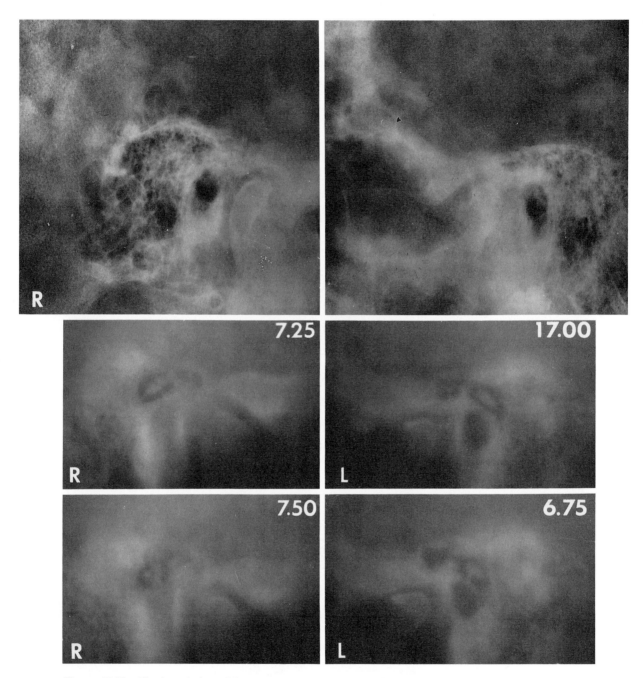

Figure 45.12. The lateral view of the temporal bones of patient TB displays the typical mottled pattern of pagetoid involvement. The multidirectional, lateral tomograms disclose constriction of the middle ear cleft.

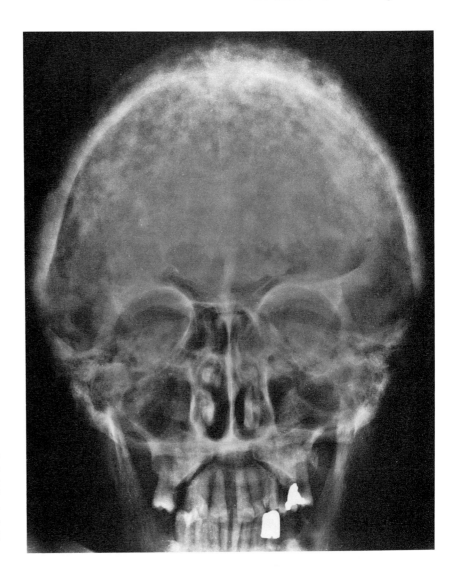

Figure 45.13. Posteroanterior view of the skull of a 63-year-old man. Involvement and enlargement of the calvaria are symmetrical. The outer table and diploë exhibit the most characteristic changes. Progressive softening of the base resulted in platybasia and convexobasia with elevation of petrous apices and downward slanting of the petrous crests. Note partial obliteration of the frontal sinuses.

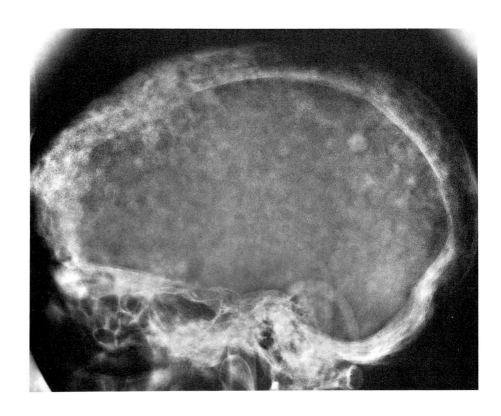

Figure 45.14. Lateral skull view of a 78-year-old man. Enlargement and change in configuration are the result of thickening of the diploë and outer table. The close association of areas of radiolucency (osteoporosis) and increased density (osteosclerosis) produces a "cotton-wool" pattern, most prominent in frontal and parietal regions. Alteration of the hypophyseal fossa and bulging of the skull base into the cranial cavity are apparent.

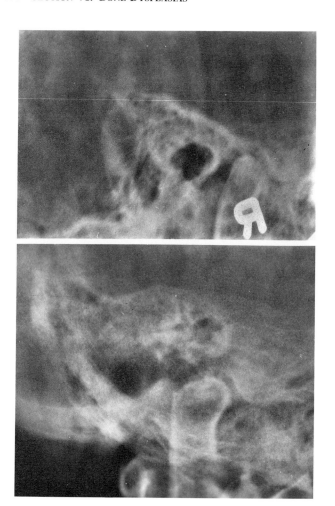

Figure 45.17. Schüller *(top)* and Stenvers *(lower)* views of right temporal bone of a 78-year-old man. In the terminal, sclerotic phase of the disease, the contours of the inner ear capsule become almost totally obscured.

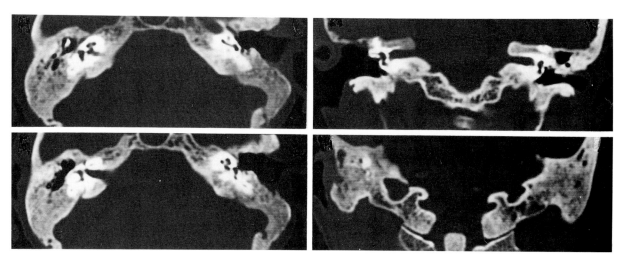

Figure 45.18. Axial *(L)* and coronal *(R)* CT scans of the temporal bones of 77-year-old woman with the predominantly reconstructive, sclerotic phase of osteitis deformans.

the amount of bone calcium in a given area before radiologic alterations become discernible, a patient can have Paget's disease without any radiologic evidence.

Involvement of an extremity long bone invariably begins with an osteolytic lesion at one end that usually progresses with a clearly delineated V-shaped form. Linear cortical radiolucencies may develop in the femur or tibia on the convex surface of a curved bone and subsequently can generate spontaneous fractures (5). The long bones may be thick and opaque, but pseudofractures, lateral bowing of the femur, and anterior bowing of the tibia show the influence of weight bearing and reflect their diminished strength (Fig. 45.9). The vertebral bodies affected by the disease may exhibit coarse trabeculation in a horizontal distribution, accentuating the margins of the bodies and producing a "picture frame" appearance, or they may simply reveal a homogeneous opacification. Compression fractures are not uncommon, resulting in anterior narrowing of the vertebral body and, occasionally, cord compression. Enlargement of the ischial and pubic bone is also characteristic of Paget's disease (Fig. 45.8). Pagetoid involvement of the maxilla and mandible is most prominent in areas adjacent to the tooth sockets (Fig. 45.11). Computed tomography is a useful way of evaluating the anatomic details of the bone remodeling process (Figs. 45.7, 45.15, 45.16, and 45.18). The bone scan, although not a specific diagnostic test, is the most sensitive means to identify an early-stage active lesion of Paget's disease when the bone transformation process may not yet be discernible radiographically (5).

COMPLICATIONS

Cardiovascular disease ranks as the most common cause of death in advanced, widespread Paget's disease, with several factors playing a contributory role. Restricted ventilatory capacity resulting from the deformity of the thorax may increase cardiac output, resulting in right-sided hypertrophy and, ultimately, right-sided heart failure. In Paget's disease the incidence of arteriosclerosis, valvular disease, and hypertension is increased. The augmentation of blood flow, the amount of arteriovenous shunting, and the large venous sinuses alone can account for the rise in cardiac output (10, 11).

One of the most tragic complications of osteitis deformans is the development of a sarcoma, usually an osteosarcoma, although in some instances fibrosarcomas, chondrosarcomas, and other varieties (malignant fibrous histiocytoma, reticulum cell sarcoma, and giant cell tumors) also have been reported (Fig. 45.38). It has been suggested that the exaggerated stromal and osseous activity observed in Paget's disease might serve as the precursor for this malignant group of mesenchymal neoplasms (12) or that there may be a common pathogenetic relationship between Paget's disease and sarcoma, with both processes possibly having a viral etiology (13). In patients with advanced polyostotic disease, the incidence of osteosarcoma may be about 6–10%. If all forms of Paget's disease are included, the frequency rate drops to 0.9% (14). Although sarcoma is usually found in patients beyond age 50 and with polyostotic disease, it can also occur in the monostotic form. Based on 250 observations of patients with osteitis deformans (15), the sites predisposed to sarcoma are, in decreasing frequency, the femur (31%), the humerus (20%), the pelvis (15%), the tibia (11.2%), and the skull and facial bones (10.8%). These observations were subsequently confirmed by a study of 987 Paget's disease patients (16). It is estimated that about 30% of patients eventually have sarcomatous involvement of multiple bones. Some investigators interpret these as metastases rather than multiple primary tumors. The prognosis of sarcoma arising in Paget's disease is very poor, with most patients dying within 2 years (15).

ETIOLOGY AND HEREDITY

For nearly a century since Sir James Paget's classic description of the disease in 1877 (16), little progress had been made in identification of an etiologic factor. During the past 15 years, however, electron microscope studies have provided evidence that the nuclei and, occasionally, the cytoplasm of the osteoclasts in Paget's disease often include abnormal inclusions resembling the nucleocapsides of viruses of the paramyxoviridae. Immunologic investigations revealed the presence of respiratory syncytial virus and measles virus antigens in the osteoclasts of these patients. These recent ultrastructural and immunologic studies support the concept that osteitis deformans Paget represents a "slow" virus infection (17–21). Genetic and environmental factors may be involved, favoring and modulating the expressivity of this slow virus infection.

The hereditary nature of the disease appears to be established. The malady has been reported repeatedly in identical twins, in several siblings, and in several generations of numerous families (22). While some investigators wonder whether or not hereditary plays a significant role in osteitis deformans (8), others are convinced that the disease is inherited either as a sex-linked recessive (22) or, more likely, as a simple, Mendelian autosomal dominant gene (23). Up to 25% of patients have been reported as having at least one relative with this disease (5). Pseudoxanthoma elasticum (PXE), a definite disorder of connective tissue, is regularly associated with angioid streaks of the retina. That PXE and angioid streaks, singly or in combination, are occasionally observed in patients with osteitis deformans suggests that Paget's disease may be a more or less generalized abiotrophy of connective tissue (23).

BIOCHEMICAL ASPECTS

Extent and activity of bone remodeling in osteitis deformans are reasonably well reflected by the serum alkaline phosphatase activity, which is an index of osteoblastic activity, and by the urinary excretion of hydroxyproline, which is an indicator of bone matrix resorption. Whereas these biochemical parameters are normal in locally limited active disease, they may be increased severalfold in patients with widespread polyostotic disease. Serum phosphorus and calcium concentrations are normal, however, in patients that are immobilized, and in those with a malignant process, the serum calcium level may be elevated. In such instances, hypercalcinuria precedes hypercalcemia (5).

OTOLOGIC HISTORY

The original, most comprehensive description of the morphologic changes in the temporal bones of patients with osteitis deformans was provided by Mayer (24) in 1917. Nager and Meyer (25) confirmed many of these earlier observations in 1932. In subsequent decades an extensive literature accumulated that was well summarized in the excellent clinical and pathologic review by Davis (9) in 1968. Lindsay and Lehman (26) and others (27, 28) since then have contributed additional valuable information.

Ruedi (29) in 1964 drew attention to the existence of shunts between the vascular network of an otosclerotic process and the vessels in the adjoining spiral ligament. Similar shunting was also observed between an otosclerotic lesion in the basal turn of the cochlea and the posterior spinal vein. The striking morphologic similarity between otosclerosis and osteitis deformans was first pointed out by Mayer (30) in 1913 and has puzzled investigators ever since. Ruedi (31) found the same shunts between the vascular network in pagetoid bone and vessels in the adjacent cochlear modiolus and internal auditory canal. These shunts, in his opinion, were causing a venous congestion, increasing damage to the cochlear end organ, and were probably responsible for the sensorineural hearing loss noted in otosclerosis and Paget's disease.

MEDICAL THERAPY

Most patients do not require medical therapy except for an occasional analgesic agent for control of musculoskeletal discomfort. Patients with severe bone pain and extensive osteolytic lesions of the skull and weight-bearing bones, however, may profit greatly from the administration of inhibitors of accelerated bone resorption and replacement. Calcitonin is particularly useful, as are the diphosphonates, with the latter binding to bone crystals and rendering them resistant to the action of osteoclasts (32, 33).

MICROSCOPIC APPEARANCE

The osseous lesions of advanced osteitis deformans reflect a long-standing and involved sequence of pathologic changes affecting both the osseous tissue and the marrow (Fig. 45.19). The disease is first manifest as osteoclastic resorption of bone. The original bone is dismantled by osteoclastic activity and replaced by densely packed, narrow trabeculae of coarse-fibered bone, which, in turn, may undergo resorption. The marrow is entirely replaced by cellular fibrovascular tissue. Waves of resorption and regeneration may ebb and flow over the same territory. The variation of osteoclastic and osteoblastic activity and the frequency of local exacerbations and remissions result in the simultaneous occurrence of different stages of bone formation in closely adjacent areas.

Areas of active bone transformation (Fig. 45.20) are recognized by the presence of a large number of osteoclasts and osteoblasts, often side by side and lining the same trabecula, and by a highly vascular, cellular, fibrous bone marrow. During remission there is neither osteoclastic nor osteoblastic activity. The trabeculae are surrounded by aplastic resting lines. The marrow has become aplastic and may revert to the adipose type. The process of bone transformation temporarily has come to a standstill. After a while the phase of inactivity is over, and resorption of the resting bone begins again (Fig. 45.21). The arrangement of fragments of newer bone, laid down on partially destroyed segments of older bone (which, in turn, may contain fragments of yet older, partially destroyed bone), all without recognizable orientation, constitutes the mosaic-like pattern of osteitis deformans (Fig. 45.21B).

MORPHOLOGIC CHANGES INVOLVING THE TEMPORAL BONE

In all of our 10 patients, the disease had involved both temporal bones. Whereas the extent of involvement varies to a certain degree with each case, the structural changes within a given pair of temporal bones are very similar (Fig. 45.22). In some instances, the periosteal and only part of the endochondral capsule layer are involved. In other instances, almost the entire endochondral and a considerable portion of the endosteal layer of the cochlear and vestibular capsules have been replaced by pagetoid bone. As the bone transformation steadily progresses, it may cause alteration of position, increase in size, and change in the architecture of the petrous pyramid and other areas of the temporal bone. The petrous pyramid may undergo an outward rotation around its long axis to the extent that the posterior, cerebellar aspect finally becomes the upper surface of the pyramid.

In instances of widespread petrous pyramid involvement, some distortion and narrowing of the internal acoustic meatus can be observed. This narrowing is generally not severe enough to exert pressure on the cranial nerves and blood vessels that the internal acoustic meatus contains. Occasionally, the tractus spiralis foraminosus, cochlear modiolus, and macula cribosa of the inferior and superior vestibular areas are involved in the bone disease (Fig. 45.23). The foramina and longitudinal canals of the modiolus and vestibular areas are lined with seams of hyalin and osteoid tissue. The nerve fibers in these areas appear crowded and even strangulated. The foramina and neural canals can also be invaded by connective tissue after preceding osteoclastic resorption of the endosteal bone. This process, which begins in an adjacent marrow space, can result in separation and even destruction of the nerve bundles. Separation of nerve bundles can occasionally enhance the formation of neuromas (24).

Remodeling of bone in the walls of the middle ear frequently results in obvious constriction of the tympanic cavity and its recesses (Fig. 45.24). Marked thickening of the tegmen tympani can cause impingement on the malleus and incus. Similarly, new bone formation in the lateral or medial wall of the epitympanic recess may jam the two outer ear ossicles and occasionally effect a fibrous or osseous union.

Concentric growth of the tympanic bone can cause a considerable decrease in diameter of the tympanic annulus with relaxation of the tympanic membrane (Figs. 45.25 and 45.26). It can also produce narrowing and tortuosity of the external auditory canal, form exotoses, induce chronic external otitis, and result in development of an external cholesteatoma.

Involvement of the oval window may produce marked distortion of its architecture (Fig. 45.26). This, in turn, will jam and immobilize the stapes. New bone formation in the region of the promontory can tilt the promontory upward, with protrusion of the inferior oval window margin into the vestibule.

The tympanic section of the Fallopian canal can be severely affected by the bone disease (Fig. 45.27). Concentric narrowing of the bony canal can result in partial extrusion of the facial nerve through a dehiscence in the floor of the canal. Such a displaced facial nerve can impinge on the posterior crus of the stapes and, by constant pressure, cause its partial destruction.

Ankylosis of the stapes has been described but has not been observed in our material. The mechanisms are as follows: Pagetoid bone in the oval window margin may grow across the annular ligament in the form of an osseous bridge and substitute

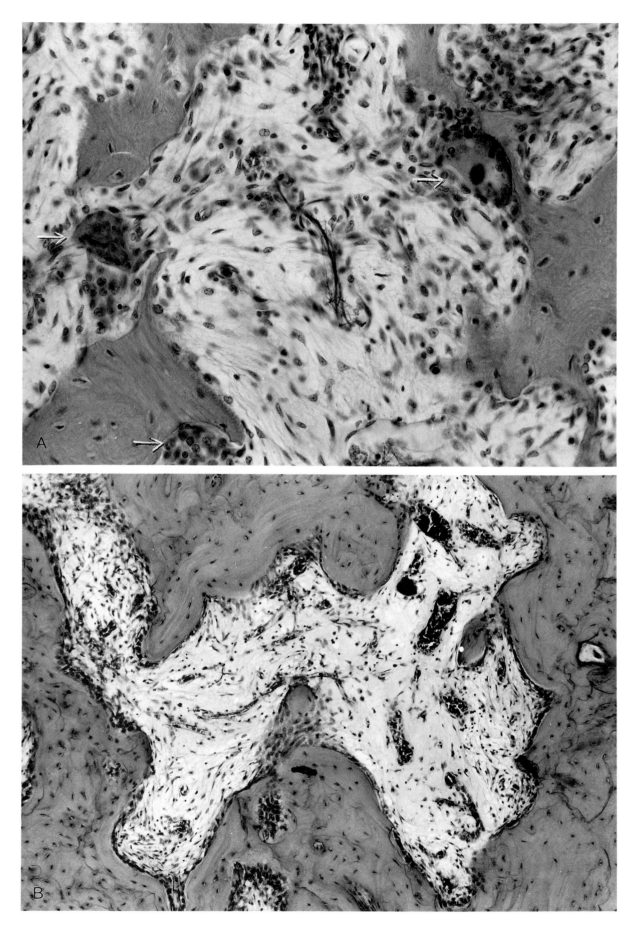

Figure 45.19.   A. Destruction of original bone begins in adjacent marrow spaces with lacunar erosion by osteoclasts *(arrows).* **B.** Marrow is replaced by vascular, cellular fibrous tissue. (Hematoxylin and eosin, ×350 and ×135, respectively.)

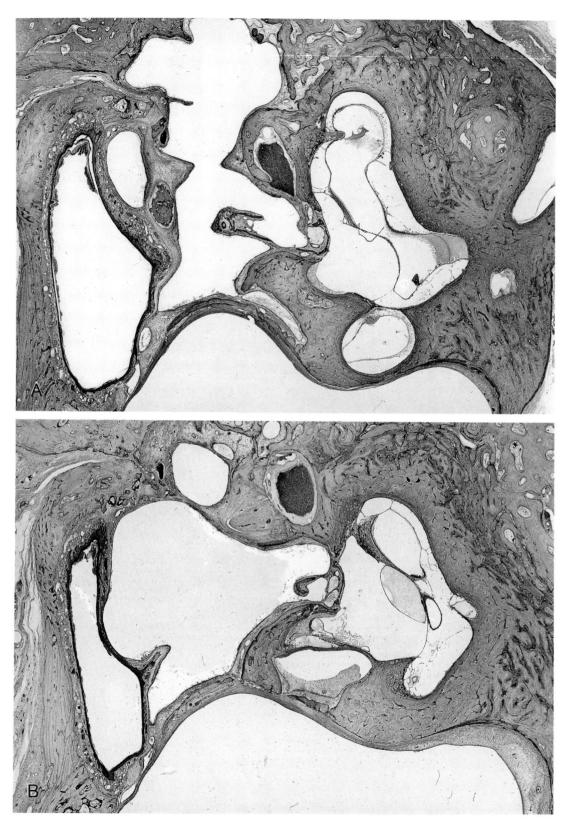

Figure 45.26. Vertical section through right petrous pyramid near posterior **(A)** and anterior **(B)** ends of oval window in patient KW. Concentric growth of the tympanic bone with decrease in diameter of the tympanic annulus resulted in relaxation of the tympanic membrane. New bone formation within the promontory caused it to tilt upward, with narrowing of the oval window niche and jamming of the stapes **(A).** The enormous enlargement of the jugular bulb caused marked elevation of the hypotympanum floor to almost the level of the umbo and total obliteration of the round window niche **(B).** (Hematoxylin and eosin, ×9½ and ×10, respectively.)

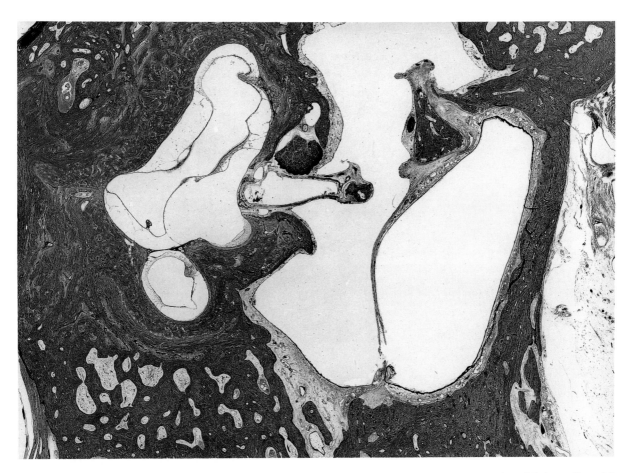

Figure 45.27. Patient KW. Vertical section through left petrous pyramid at level of oval window in patient KW. Intrinsic narrowing of the Fallopian canal produced partial extrusion of the facial nerve through a dehiscence in the floor and impingement on and partial destruction of the posterior crus of the stapes. (Hematoxylin and eosin, ×8½.)

an adjacent portion of the footplate; or the cartilaginous rim and the underlying bone of the stapedial footplate can be resorbed in a localized area. This area subsequently is replaced by pagetoid bone, which, in turn, becomes connected with pagetoid bone in the adjacent oval window margin. A predisposing factor to the development of stapedial ankylosis is the jamming of the stapes in the distorted oval window, which results in direct contact of two bony surfaces. Ossification of the annular ligament is another mechanism that can result in stapedial ankylosis (24, 25).

Involvement of the round window niche can cause marked distortion of its architecture, with constriction or even total obliteration of the niche. On the other hand, progressive enlargement of the jugular bulb with elevation of the floor of the hypotympanum can cause narrowing or total occlusion of the round window niche from below (Fig. 45.26B). Occasionally, the floor of the hypotympanum can rise to the level of the umbo where the jugular bulb may become widely exposed and covered only by mucosa of the middle ear. Similarly an enlargement of the jugular bulb in a more medial direction can result in distension

of this vessel until it reaches the dura lining the floor of the internal acoustic meatus. In all instances of widespread pagetoid bone transformation, the contributing arteries and arterioles and the corresponding venous blood vessels are markedly increased in size and number (Figs. 45.28 and 45.29). In addition to an enormous increase in blood flow, there is ample evidence of arteriovenous shunting, often across large venous lakes. All temporal bones with extensive, active bone transformation display an enormous enlargement of the jugular bulb (Figs. 45.26 and 45.30).

All auditory ossicles exhibit pagetoid changes, although to a lesser degree. Malleus and incus may show extensive areas of bone resorption and remodeling (Fig. 45.31A–C). Involvement of the osseous portion of the Eustachian tube can result in narrowing or collapse of its lumen.

An interesting observation is the occurrence of clefts or microfractures (Figs. 45.32 and 45.33). Some are filled with newly formed bone, whereas others contain connective tissue. They are found in certain regions of the labyrinth capsule and in areas

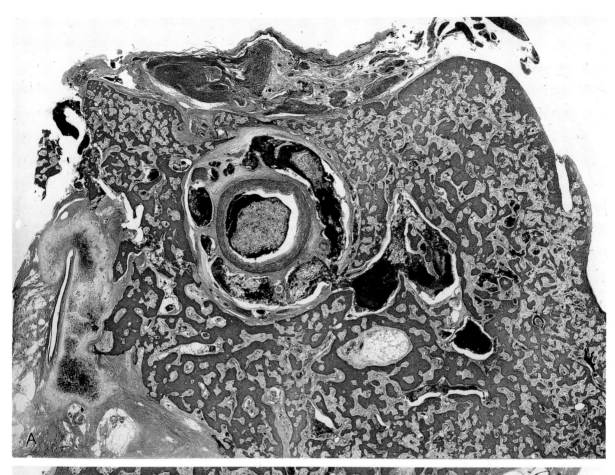

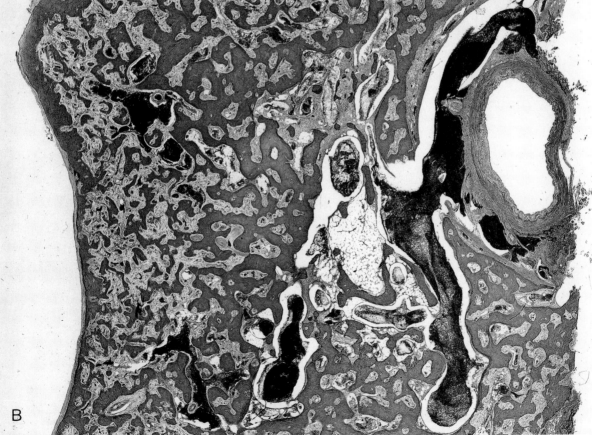

Figure 45.30. **A** and **B.** Vertical sections through right and left petrous apices of an 80-year-old woman with extensive, active pagetoid remodeling. Large venous channels and lakes collecting blood from many areas of the pyramid are seen emptying into a markedly distended pericarotid venous plexus, which, in turn, drains bilaterally into an enormously enlarged internal jugular vein. (Hematoxylin and eosin, ×8 and ×12, respectively.)

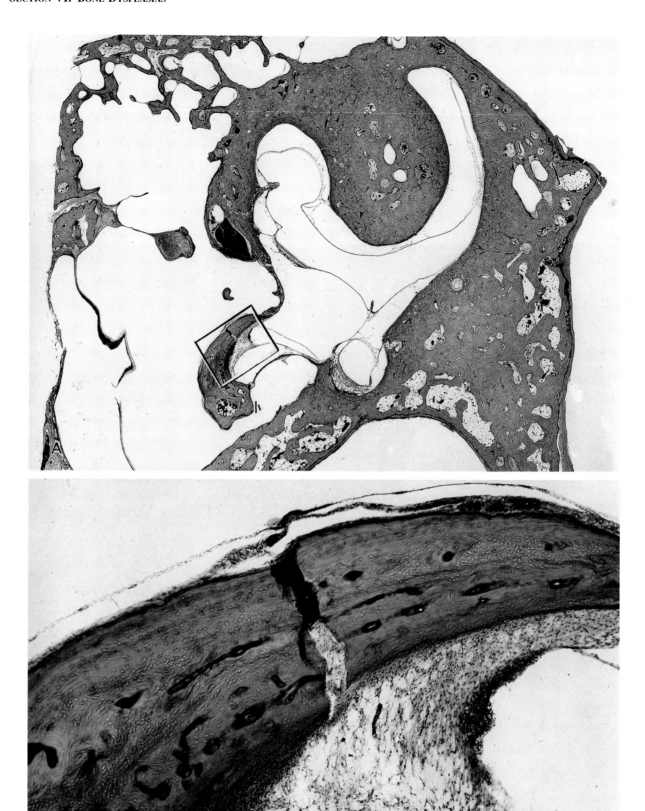

Figure 45.32. **A.** Vertical section through right pyramid at level of oval and round windows in 78-year-old man. An older radial microfracture traverses the promontory, extending from the middle ear surface to the base of the spiral ligament of the lower basal turn. **B.** *Inset* from *A.* Medial portion of cleft is filled with connective tissue. In the lateral portion a callus of calcified connective tissue unites the two bony surfaces. (Hematoxylin and eosin, ×8 and ×80, respectively.)

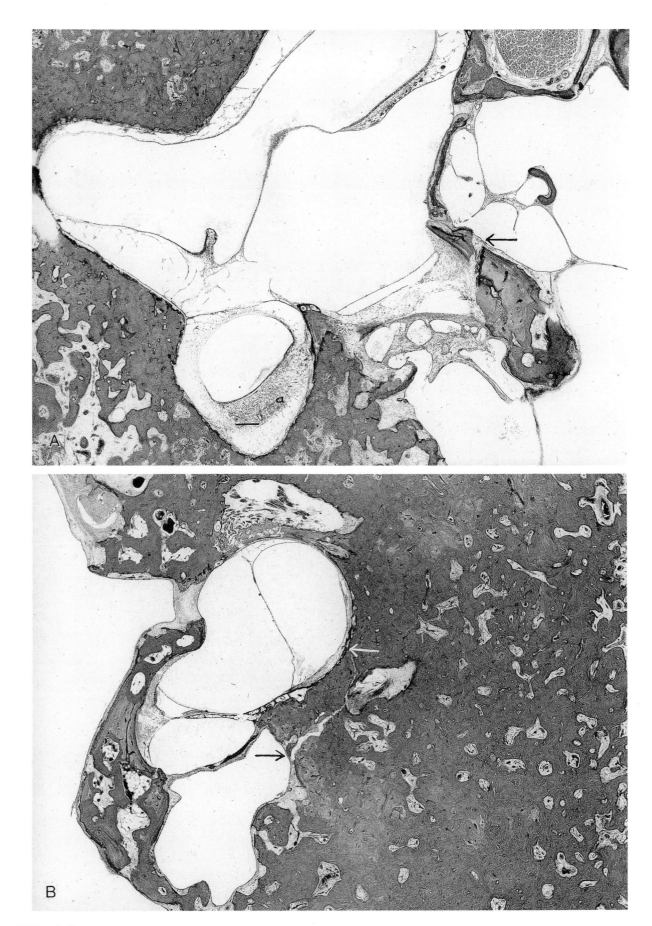

Figure 45.33. **A.** Vertical section through left pyramid at level of oval and round windows in patient SM. The radial microfracture below the inferior oval window margin is clearly recognizable *(arrow).* **B.** Vertical section through right pyramid at anterior end of oval window in patient D-GV. A microfracture extends from the medial wall of the round window niche to the macula cribrosa of the saccule and the anterior medial wall of the vestibule *(arrows).* (Hematoxylin and eosin, ×20 and ×14, respectively.)

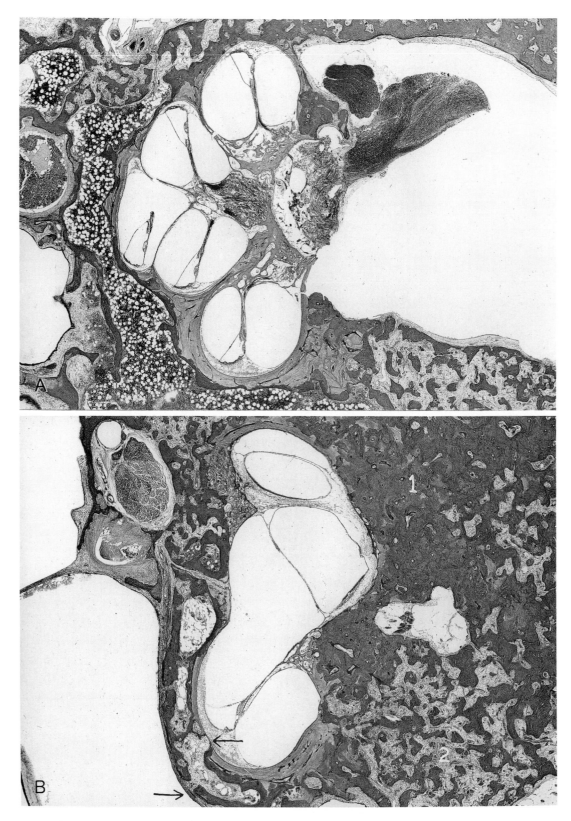

Figure 45.34. **A.** Vertical midmodiolar section through right pyramid of patient SM. In the cochlear capsule, bone resorption predominated over new bone formation. As a result, almost the entire endochondral capsule layer has been destroyed and replaced by hematopoietic marrow. **B.** Vertical section through same temporal bone as in *A* at level of fissula ante fenestram. Seen side by side are areas of osteosclerosis, made of dense, more regular, and mature lamellar bone *(1)* and areas of osteoporosis, consisting of a loose network of irregular trabeculae of web-like and lamellar bone. With bone resorption predominating in the cochlear capsule, the osteoclastic marrow extends in some areas from the mucoperiosteum of the middle ear to the base of the spiral ligament *(arrows).* (Hematoxylin and eosin, ×15 and ×16, respectively.)

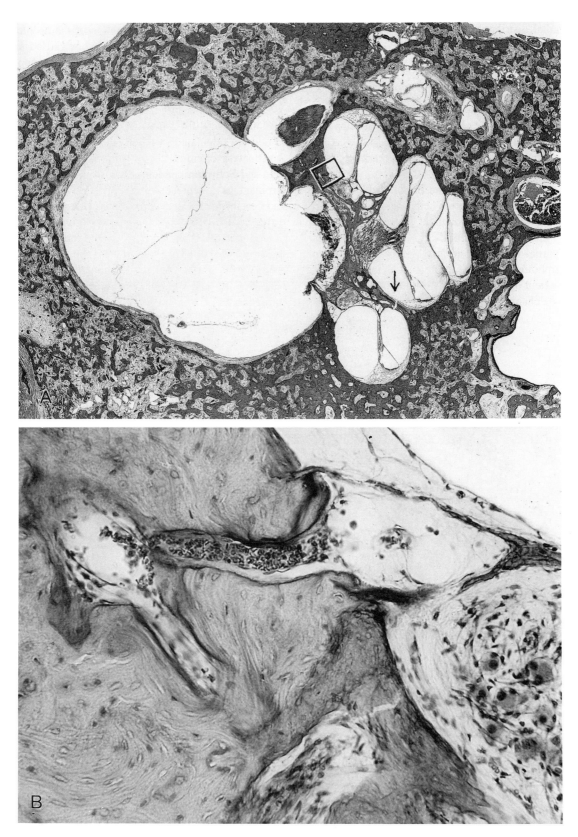

Figure 45.35.   A. Vertical midmodiolar section through left pyramid of patient SM. Extensive pagetoid remodeling caused obvious axial and radial distortion of the cochlear capsule and fracture of the osseous partition between the lower basal and middle cochlear turns *(arrow).* **B.** *Inset* from *A.* Vascular shunt between posterior spiral vein of upper basal turn and vein in adjacent pagetoid bone of cochlear capsule. (Hematoxylin and eosin, ×12 and ×300, respectively.)

blasts are surrounded by and embedded in immature osteoid bone (Fig. 46.7*B*). In areas representing a later, subsequent stage of the bone transformation process, the marrow spaces have become less numerous, smaller, and much less cellular and vascular, and the bone has taken a deeper reddish color (Fig.46.5*B*). In still other areas exemplifying an end stage of the bone remodeling process, the marrow spaces have filled in with bone, and the otosclerotic bone has become compact, with a mosaic structure and basophilic color (Figs. 46.8 and 46.9). The highly vascularized lesions receive their blood supply from the adjacent meningeal and periosteal arteries, and the venous blood drains into the respective veins (Figs. 46.7*A* and *C* and 46.14). Extensive arteriovenous shunting can be observed in numerous areas (Figs. 46.13 and 46.15).

In many places the periosteal, endochondral, and endosteal layers of the cochlear and vestibular capsules have been replaced by otosclerotic bone, with only a few small segments of the original bone remaining (Figs. 46.5*A*, 46.7*C*, and 46.11–46.15). The entire wall of the internal auditory canal has been replaced, but the spiral foraminous tract and the cochlear modiolus have remained unaffected. Localized areas of bone resorption in the internal auditory canal near the fundus have subsequently become occupied by an extension of the subarachnoid space (Figs. 46.5*A* and 46.7*C*).

The massive remodeling of bone involving the promontory and hypotympanum resulted in complete obliteration of the round window niches and in overgrowth, with concentric narrowing of the oval window niches (Figs. 46.8, 46.9, and 46.16). The entire footplate of the stapes and the base of the stapedial arch have been replaced by otosclerotic bone. The thickened footplate has become partially dislocated and jammed within the severely narrowed and distorted oval window frame. Bony ankyloses have developed between the footplate and the base of the stapedial arch and adjacent regions of the vestibular fenestra and wall of the oval window niche (Figs. 46.9 and 46.17). The lateral portion of the crural arch, which is not affected by otosclerosis, is severely atrophic and very thin. In some areas it is incomplete and replaced by fibrous tissue and has become distorted (Figs. 46.9, 46.10, and 46.17). Most of the stapedial superstructure is embedded in a greatly thickened and very vascular fibrous tissue of the mucoperiosteum. This fibrous tissue includes many small foci of metaplastic bone. Almost the entire Fallopian canal has been replaced by otosclerotic bone. The bone remodeling of the epitympanic walls has resulted in concentric narrowing of the attic and extensive, firm, fibrous ankylosis of the malleus head to the overlying tegmen tympani. The malleus displays a smaller otosclerotic focus; the incus, a larger one (Figs. 46.11 and 46.12). The bony walls of all semicircular canals reveal extensive remodeling which in several areas involves all three capsule layers (Figs. 46.11, 46.12, and 46.18).

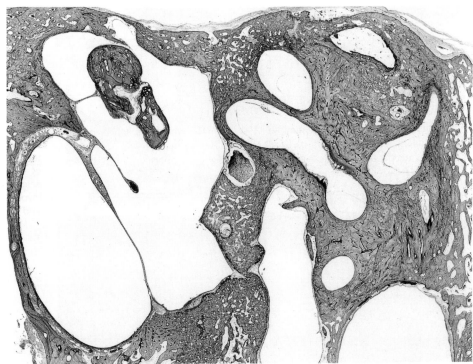

Figure 46.11. Vertical section through right temporal bone at level of incudomalleolar articulation. The otosclerotic involvement of all walls of the middle ear and Fallopian canal, osseous walls of the lateral and superior semicircular canals, and middle ear ossicles is well visualized. (Hematoxylin and eosin, ×7.2.)

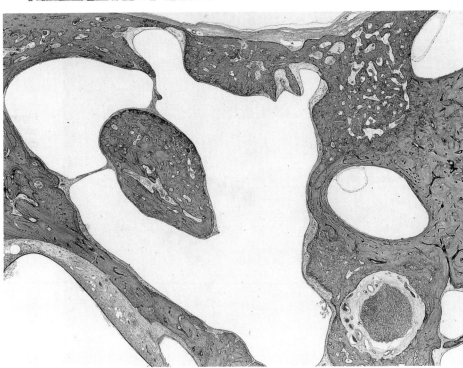

Figure 46.12. Vertical section through right temporal bone at level of incus body. The aditus walls and incus display otosclerotic involvement. (Hematoxylin and eosin, ×13.)

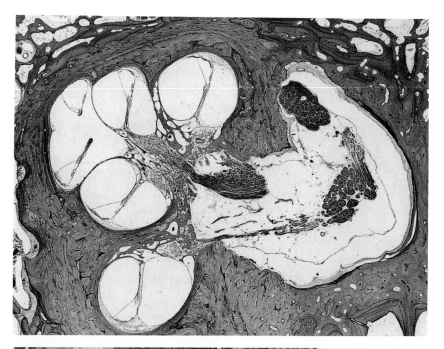

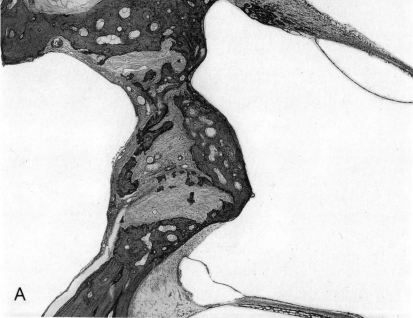

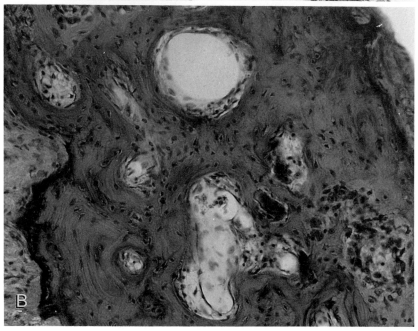

Figure 46.36. Vertical midmodiolar section of right cochlear capsule with well-demarcated three-layered structure and no evidence of abnormal ossification. (Hematoxylin and eosin, ×13.)

Figure 46.37. A. Vertical section through right vestibular capsule at level of oval window. An extensive otosclerotic process has involved and distorted the entire oval window margin and produced dislocation, jamming, and circumferential ankylosis of the stapedial footplate, which itself has been replaced by otosclerotic bone. Overlying mucoperiosteum is greatly thickened, is fibrosed, and includes metaplastic bone. (Hematoxylin and eosin, ×30.)

Figure 46.37. B. The otosclerotic process of the footplate displays extensive bone resorption with many multinucleated osteoclastic giant cells and bone remodeling. (×250.)

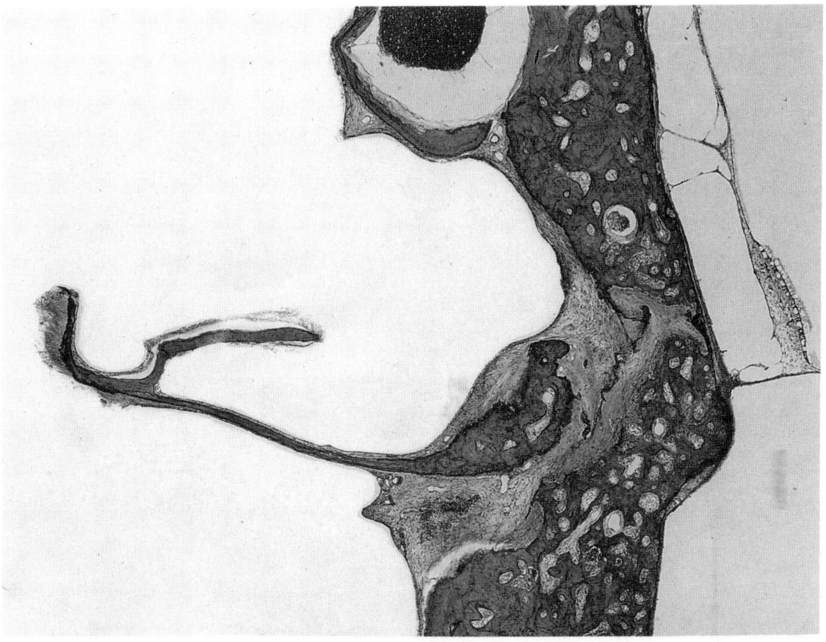

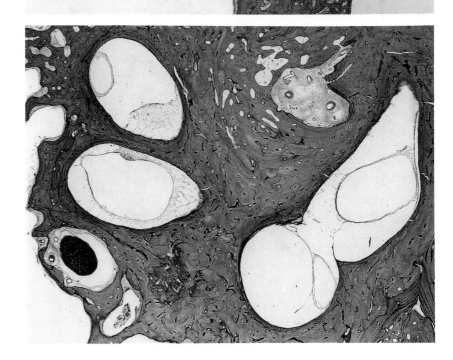

Figure 46.38.   Vertical section through right oval window at level of posterior crus of stapes. The lateral portion of the stapedial arch, which is not involved in the otosclerotic process, exhibits obviously abnormal osteoporosis. (Hematoxylin and eosin, ×30.)

Figure 46.39.   Vertical section through right petrous pyramid at level of lateral, superior semicircular canal and common crus. The otosclerotic process involving the oval window extends far posteriorly toward the center of the lateral semicircular canal. (Hematoxylin and eosin, ×15.)

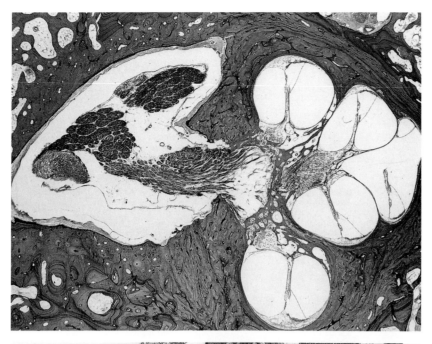

Figure 46.40. Vertical midmodiolar section through left cochlear capsule, showing essentially normal architecture and no evidence of abnormal ossification. (Hematoxylin and eosin, ×13.)

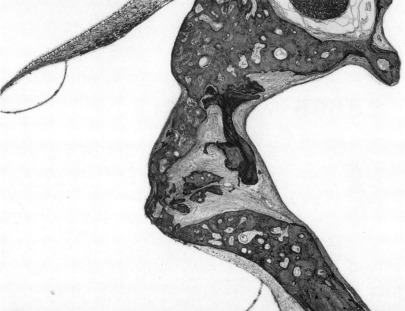

Figure 46.41. Vertical section through left vestibular capsule at level of oval window. The otosclerotic process involving the vestibular fenestra is identical in every respect with the one on the opposite side (see Fig. 46.36A). The extensive formation of metaplastic bone in the greatly thickened mucoperiosteum contributes further to the stapedial ankylosis. (Hematoxylin and eosin, ×30.)

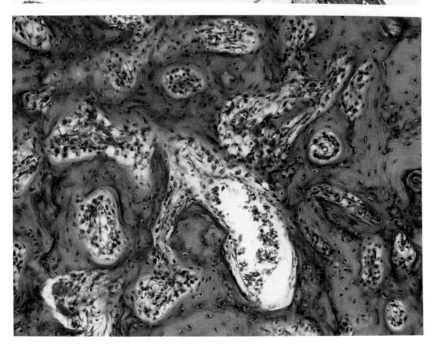

Figure 46.42. The otosclerotic process involving the left oval window shows every evidence of active bone remodeling. (Hematoxylin and eosin, ×175.)

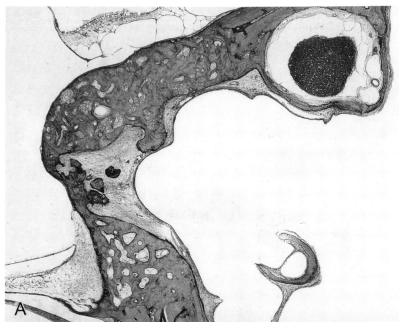

Figure 46.43. A. Vertical section through left oval window near its posterior margin. Massive otosclerotic involvement of the footplate resulted in a great increase in its diameter. The stapedial arch is abnormally thin. (Hematoxylin and eosin, ×30.)

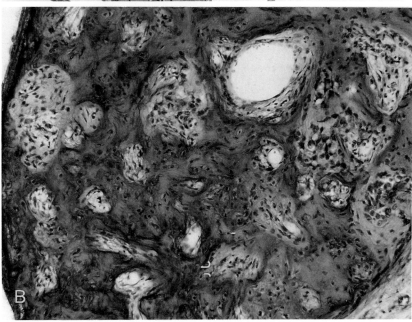

Figure 46.43. B. In several areas the otosclerotic process in the footplate displays osteoclastic bone destruction and replacement by new immature bone side by side. (×175.)

COMMENTS

Three of the six patients represent the most severe, lethal, perinatal form of the disease, type II OI. One was premature and stillborn, one died at birth, and another died at age 10 months. All had blue sclerae and abnormally thin skin, and two had documented disturbance of dentinogenesis. All had a negative family history. The three layers of their cochlear and vestibular capsule revealed evidence of deficient osteoid formation, with the periosteal and endochondral capsule layers being most severely affected. The periosteal layer was very thin and, in some areas, dehiscent. Many of the thin trabeculae were only partially covered by a single layer of osteoid bone. In the endochondral layer irregular spicules of cartilage were bordered by rugged, dark bluish cement lines and embedded in immature lamellar bone. In many places hardly any osteoid bone was deposited on these cartilaginous spicules. The marrow spaces were remarkably wide. Malleus and incus displayed a very thin shell of poorly developed periosteal and endochondral bone surrounding a large central space containing hematopoietic marrow. The stapedial arch was extremely thin; in one instance it was deformed, and in another it was fenestrated, and in every patient it was dehiscent.

Two of the remaining three adult patients represent the less severe, progressive and deforming form of the disease, type III OI. The third represents an expression of type IV OI, a mild to moderately severe form. All had blue sclerae. One had lost all of her teeth at an early age as a result of abnormal softness and caries. The second had normal teeth, and no mention was made about the dental status of the third patient. All had a negative family history of bone diseases and multiple fractures, but one had a sister and several children with blue sclerae. In the two adults with type III OI, the disease produced atrophy, thinning, and deficiency of the cortical bone of the petrous pyramid and of the lamellar bone in other regions of the temporal bone. These changes were best recognized in the petrous apex where the cortex was locally deficient, the osseous canal of the internal carotid artery was unusually thin, and the trabeculae of the spongiosa often appeared extremely delicate. This atrophy varied considerably in severity in different locations. The periosteal bone formation was severely affected in some areas and hardly affected in others. The periosteal layer of the cochlea was separated into a thin outer and a broader inner zone, separated by a sheer network of very slender trabeculae and bone marrow. The stapedial arch was abnormally thin and, in several areas, dehiscent.

In the type IV OI, the cochlear and vestibular capsule displayed their usual three-layered structure without a deficiency in ossification. Malleus and incus were unremarkable, but the stapedial arch exhibited the same delicate architecture with holes and dehiscences. In the petrous apex and in some perilabyrinthine and periantral regions, the trabeculae were unusually fine, delicate, and irregular and reflected a localized defect in osteoid formation. Although they exhibited osteoblastic rimming, there was no evidence of osteoid deposition. In the type IV OI, severe osteoporosis of the petrous apex and, to a lesser degree, mastoid bone and obvious atrophy of the stapedial arch were the sole evidence of the disease.

All three adult patients demonstrate the association of OI with otosclerosis. Our observations, therefore, have corresponded with those of other investigators (23–29). The otosclerotic lesions were extensive, multicentric, and exhibited every evidence of active bone remodeling. All patients showed two or more independent otosclerotic foci involving the inner ear capsule, walls of the middle ear, malleus and incus, and other areas. In one patient the otosclerotic process caused subtotal occlusion of the oval window and complete obliteration of the round window. In the two patients with progressive hypacusis, the otosclerosis was solely responsible for the hearing loss. It caused a marked distortion of the oval window, with jamming of the footplate in addition to ankylosis of the stapes.

Otosclerosis may be part of the OI syndrome. In instances in which the two coexist, their morphologic differences are clearly distinguishable. They represent different bone dysplasias. The relation of otosclerosis to OI is analogous to that of hereditary dentinogenesis imperfecta and OI. Both conditions may occur as part of OI or as isolated abnormalities. The hearing loss occurring in OI may be the result of OI or otosclerosis or of a combination of the two.

References

1. McKusick VA. Osteogenesis imperfecta. In: McKusick VA, ed. Heritable disorders of connective tissue. 4th ed. St Louis: CV Mosby, Chap 8, 1972:390–454.
2. Smars G. Osteogenesis imperfecta in Sweden. Clinical, genetic, epidemiological and sociomedical aspects. Stockholm: Scandinavian University Books, 1961.
3. Schröder G. Osteogenesis imperfecta. Z Menschl Vererbungs Konstitionsl 1964;37:632–676.
4. Sillence DO. Osteogenesis imperfecta: an expanding panorama of variants. Clin Orthop Relat Res 1981;159:11–25.
5. Riedner ED, Levin SL, Holliday MJ. Hearing patterns in dominant osteogenesis imperfecta. Arch Otolaryngol 1980;106:737–740.
6. Shapiro JR, Pikus A, Weiss G, Rowe DW. Hearing and middle ear function in osteogenesis imperfecta. JAMA 1982;247:2120–2126.
7. Sillence DO, Senn A, Danks DM. Genetic heterogeneity in osteogenesis imperfecta. J Med Genet 1979;16:101–116.
8. Byers PH, Bonadio JF. The molecular basis of clinical heterogeneity in osteogenesis imperfecta. Mutations in type I collagen genes have different effects on collagen processing. In: Lloyd JK, Scriver, CR, eds. Genetic and metabolic diseases in pediatrics. London: Butterworths, 1985:56–90.
9. Smith R, Francis MJO, Haughton JR. The brittle bone syndrome. London: Butterworths, 1983.
10. Levin LS. Osteogenesis imperfecta. In: Gorlin RJ, Cohen MM Jr, Levin LS, eds. Syndromes of head and neck. 3rd ed. Oxford: Oxford University Press, 1989.
11. Rubin P. Dynamic classification of bone dysplasias. Chicago: Year Book Medical Publishers, 1964.
12. Follis RH, Jr. Maldevelopment of the chorium in the osteogenesis imperfecta syndrome. Bull Johns Hopkins Hosp 1953;93:225.
13. Becks H. Histologic study of tooth structure in osteogenesis imperfecta. Dent Cosmos 1931;73:737.
14. Adair-Dighton CA. Four generations of blue sclerotics. Ophthalmoscope 1912;10:188.
15. Van der Hoeve J, de Kleyn A. Blaue Skleren, Knochenbrüchigkeit und Schwerhörigkeit. Arch Ophthalmol 1918;95:81.
16. Friedberg CK. Zur Kenntnis des vererbbaren Syndroms: Abnorme Knochenbrüchigkeit, blaue Skleren und Schwerhörigkeit. Klin Wochenschr 1931;10:830.
17. Opheim O. Loss of hearing following the syndrome of Van der Hoeve and de Kleyn. Acta Otolaryngol (Stockh) 1968;65:337.
18. Bergstrom L. Osteogenesis imperfecta: otologic and maxillo-facial aspects. Laryngoscope 1977;87(suppl 6):1–42.
19. Igarashi M, King AI, Schwenzfeier CW, Watanabe T, Alford BR. Inner ear pathology in osteogenesis imperfecta congenita. J Laryngol Otol 1980;94:697–705.
20. Sando I, Myers D, Hinojosa R, Harada T, Myers EN. Osteogenesis imperfecta tarda and otosclerosis. A temporal bone histopathology report. Ann Otol Rhinol Laryngol 1981;90:199–203.

21. Patterson CN, Stone HB III. Stapedectomy in Van der Hoeve's syndrome. Laryngoscope 1970;80:544.

22. Milgram JW, Flick MR, Engh CA. Osteogenesis imperfecta. A histopathological case report. J Bone Joint Surg [Am] 1973;55(A):506–515.

23. Nager FR. Die Labyrinthkapsel bei angeborenen Knochenerkrankungen. Arch Ohren-Nasen-Kehlkopfheilkd 1922;109:81–103.

24. Ruttin A. Osteopsathyrose und Otosclerose. Z Hals-Nasen-Ohrenheilkd 1922–1923;3–4:263–279.

25. Altmann F. The temporal bone in osteogenesis imperfecta congenita. Arch Otolaryngol 1962;75:486–497.

26. Altmann F, Kornfeld M. Osteogenesis imperfecta and otosclerosis, new investigations. Ann Otol Rhinol Laryngol 1967;76:89–104.

27. Bretlau P, Balslev-Jorgenson M. Otosclerosis and osteogenesis imperfecta. Acta Otolaryngol (Stockh) 1969;67:269–276.

28. Bretlau P, Balslev-Jorgenson M. Otosclerosis and osteogenesis imperfecta. Acta Otolaryngol (Stock) 1969;67:269–276.

28. Bretlau P, Balslev-Jorgenson M, Johansen H. Osteogenesis imperfecta. Acta Otolaryngol (Stockh) 1970;69:172–184.

29. Zajtchuk JT, Lindsay JR. Osteogenesis imperfecta congenita and tarda: a temporal bone report. Ann Otol Rhinol Laryngol 1975;84:350–358.

47/ Fibrous Dysplasia

Fibrous dysplasia of bone is a disorder of unknown etiology in which skeletal aberrations constitute the cardinal feature but in which certain endocrinopathies, abnormal pigmentation of skin and mucous membranes, and occasionally other abnormalities form part of the total disease process. Fibrous dysplasia is by no means a rare disorder. Although some of the clinical manifestations had been described earlier, the condition was not recognized as an independent disease entity until about four and a half decades ago. In fibrous dysplasia a single bone, a few bones, or many bones may be affected. The monostotic form is characterized by involvement of a single bone; a rib, femur, tibia, or facial bone, especially a jawbone, may be the site of a lesion. In the polyostotic form in which several bones are affected, one limb, more often a lower extremity, may be the site of multiple bone lesions. Involvement of an upper or lower limb is not uncommonly associated with lesions of the skull. Since the facial and cranial bones are among the preferred sites and since their involvement may produce symptoms of disturbance and dysfunction, fibrous dysplasia becomes of particular interest to the otolaryngologist.

Unfortunately, some of the more recent clinical information about the disease is scattered throughout the literature. Therefore, in the first part of this chapter, an attempt has been made to compile all pertinent data on the clinical and pathologic aspects of fibrous dysplasia. The second part discusses the clinical manifestations of fibrous dysplasia as it involves the temporal bone. This investigation is based on an intensive review of the literature and examination and long-term observation of our own patients.

DEFINITION

Fibrous dysplasia of bone is a locally circumscribed, slowly progressive, benign disorder of fibro-osseous tissue; its etiology is undetermined. Normal bone undergoing physiologic resorption is replaced by abnormal proliferation of an isomorphous fibrous tissue of spindle cells and poorly formed bony trabeculae of woven bone. The trabeculae have an irregular size, form, and distribution. They display no orientation or apparent relation to the function of the affected cylindrical or flat bone. Sooner or later this proliferation process may extend beyond normal boundaries and cause expansion, distortion, and structural weakness. Since it involves primarily the cancellous and seldom the cortical bone formation, a lesion replaces normal cortex by erosion from within, but in most instances it is always covered with a shell, however thin, of normal cortical bone.

Fibrous dysplasia may affect one, a few, or many bones but never all bones. Accordingly, monostotic, oligostotic, and polyostotic forms are distinguished. The preferred sites include the diaphyses and metaphyses of long bones, the ribs, pelvis, shoulder, and craniofacial skeleton. The lesions tend to be unilaterally distributed. The monostotic form may become arrested at puberty, whereas the polyostotic form may progress beyond the third and even later decades. The initial clinical symptoms usually appear during the first decade of life and include pain, deformity, and repeated spontaneous fractures.

The McCune-Albright syndrome represents a special category of polyostotic fibrous dysplasia. It is characterized by extensive, clearly defined, predominantly ipsilateral skin hyperpigmentation and precocious sexual development. Females primarily are affected. Fibrous dysplasia may be associated with additional endocrine disorders, particularly with hyperthyroidism.

Fibrous dysplasia may be observed in combination with nonendocrine diseases such as hypophosphatemic vitamin D-resistant rickets or osteomalacia (1), adamantinoma of the long bones (2, 3), paraosseous fibromas of the soft tissue (4, 5), and intraosseous and extraosseous arteriovenous aneurysms (6, 7).

Sarcomatous dedifferentiation is a rare complication. The estimated incidence is about 0.5% (8).

HISTORICAL BACKGROUND

The bone lesions were first described by von Recklinghausen (9) in 1891. Elmslie (10) in 1914 discussed the case of a 6-year-old boy with disseminated skeletal lesions and skin hyperpigmentation in the back of the neck. In 1922, Weil (11) reported on a 9-year-old girl with hyperpigmented skin patches and precocious skeletal and sexual development. During the following years there was increasing evidence that despite some apparently common features, essential differences existed between hyperparathyroidism or generalized osteitis fibrosa cystica (von Recklinghausen) and localized or disseminated osteitis fibrosa (12). Jaffe (13) in 1933 also acknowledged that the hitherto unrecognized disease entity differed from hyperparathyroidism and osteitis deformans Paget. Furthermore, it became obvious that this bone disease could sometimes be associated with certain extraskeletal manifestations (14). In 1937, McCune and Bruch (15) confirmed the separate entity and used the term "osteodystrophia fibrosa." Albright and coworkers in 1937 (16) reported 5 cases of bone involvement associated with endocrine disturbances and hyperpigmented patches in the skin, which they described as "osteitis fibrosa disseminata." The authors regarded it as a separate entity. The condition was thereafter known as "Albright's syndrome" or "Albright's triad" (i.e., polyostotic, predominantly unilateral bone lesions, precocious sexual development, and skin hyperpigmentation) and had already been mentioned earlier by several investigators (17–19). The polyostotic form of the disease associated with skin hyperpigmentation but not accompanied by precocious sexual development had been described before by Hummel (20) in 1934. In 1938, Lichtenstein (21) reported 8 cases with detailed studies of bone lesions. He proposed the term "fibrous dysplasia" or "polyostotic fibrous dysplasia'' in the presence of multiple bone involvement. In 1942, Lichtenstein and Jaffe (22) added 15 more cases. By 1947, Schlumberger (23) had collected 67 cases of monostotic fibrous dysplasia. Thus the study of a sufficiently large clinical population during the first half of this century led to the general recognition of fibrous dysplasia as an independent entity that, from the standpoint of the pathologist, should probably be termed more correctly ''fibro-osseous dysplasia'' or ''fibrous osteodysplasia''(24).

Fibrous dysplasia has affected the human skeleton for centuries. Several reports of the disease have appeared in the literature of paleopathology (25, 26).

INCIDENCE AND AGE DISTRIBUTION

By 1971, the number of reported cases exceeded 1500 (27), confirming the fact that fibrous dysplasia is not an uncommon disease. Available data seem to indicate that the monostotic form accounts for about 70% of cases, the polyostotic form without endocrine disturbances for about 27%, and the polyostotic form with endocrine disturbances (McCune-Albright syndrome) for about 3% (24). The actual incidence of each form, however, cannot be assessed precisely, since the monostotic form may remain asymptomatic only to be detected accidentally and thus can often escape clinical detection. Even the polyostotic form can occasionally exist unnoticed for decades and present as an incidental finding.

Fibrous dysplasia generally makes its appearance in late childhood. Some severe forms, however, may manifest themselves in infancy. Each form of the disease has a different average age of onset; figures vary slightly from clinic to clinic. One study based on 57 patients showed that the monostotic form manifests itself initially around age 14, the polyostotic form without endocrine disorders manifests itself around age 11, and the polyostotic form associated with endocrine disturbances manifests itself around age 8 (18). Two other studies indicate a slightly earlier onset for the monostotic and polyostotic forms of the disease (28, 29). Although it is not uncommon for certain lesions to be detected during later decades of life, there is good evidence that most, if not all, bone lesions develop during the period of skeletal growth (30).

According to Uehlinger (31), the monostotic and polyostotic forms of fibrous dysplasia without endocrine disorders have an even sex distribution. By contrast, polyostotic fibrous dysplasis *with* endocrine disorders (McCune-Albright syndrome) displays an obvious predilection for the female sex.

LOCALIZATION AND DISTRIBUTION OF BONE LESIONS

Fibrous dysplasia may present as a solitary lesion (monostotic form) or as multiple lesions in a single or several bones (polyostotic form). The term ''oligostotic'' is occasionally applied when there are a very small number of lesions. Polyostotic fibrous dysplasia may be limited to a single limb (monomelic distribution) or to one side of the skeleton (unilateral distribution), or involve both sides of the skeleton (bilateral distribution) (Fig. 47.1).

The skeletal locations of lesions from 269 patients with monostotic fibrous dysplasia (7, 8, 23, 28, 29, 32–34) are shown

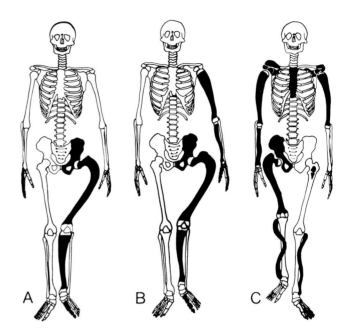

Figure 47.1. Distribution patterns of polyostotic fibrous dysplasia. **A.** Monomelic distribution. **B.** Unilateral distribution. **C.** Bilateral distribution.

in Figure 47.2*A* and Table 47.1 (35). A survey by Eversole et al. (36) of a large number of patients with monostotic fibrous dysplasia involving the jaws revealed that the maxilla was almost twice as frequently affected (64% of cases) as the mandible (36%).

The skeletal locations of lesions from 66 patients with polyostotic fibrous dysplasia unassociated with endocrine disturbances (7, 28, 37, 38–41) are shown in Figure 47.2*B* and Table 47.2. The polyostotic form is distinguished from the monostotic

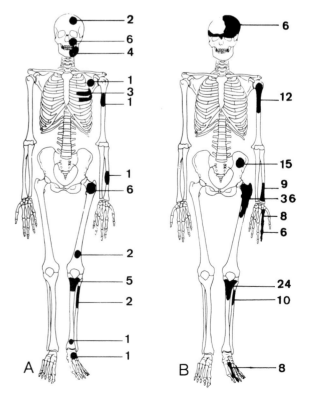

Figure 47.2. Localization of monostotic **(A)** and polyostotic **(B)** fibrous dysplasia in 35 cases of monostotic disease and 36 cases of polyostotic disease from the Institute of Pathology in Zürich.

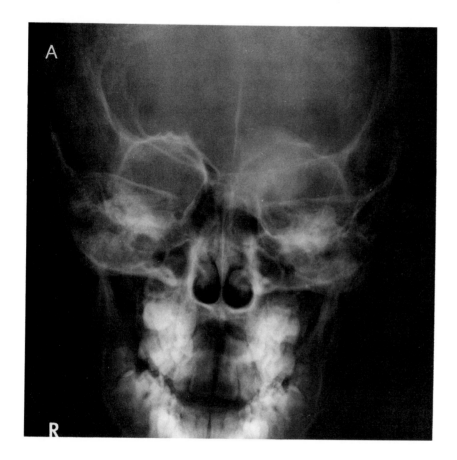

Figure 47.9. **A–C.** Unilateral polyostotic fibrous dyspla-sia of left frontal and ethmoid bones in a 9-year-old boy. The lesion has a uniform ground-glass appearance **(A).** It extends into the left anterior cranial fossa **(B),** left orbit, and left ethmoid sinus **(C)** and involves the cribriform plate. (Courtesy of Dr. John Dorst, Russell H. Morgan Depart-ment of Radiology, Johns Hopkins Hospital, Baltimore, Maryland.)

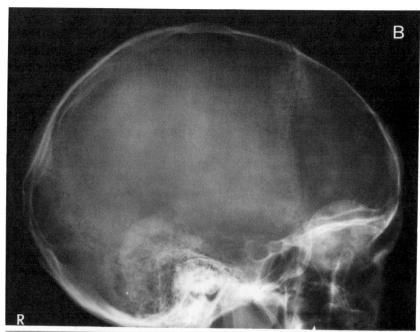

Figure 47.9.   B.

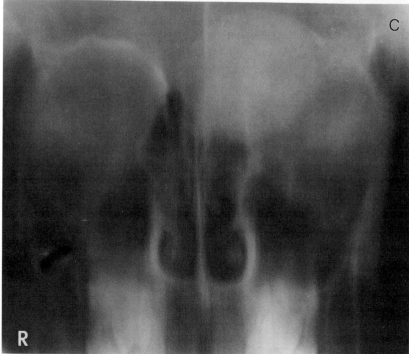

Figure 47.9.   C.

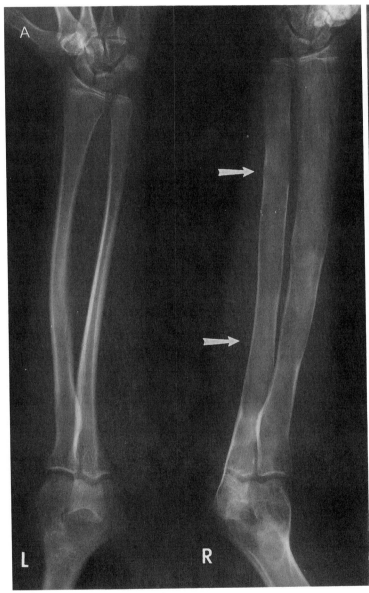

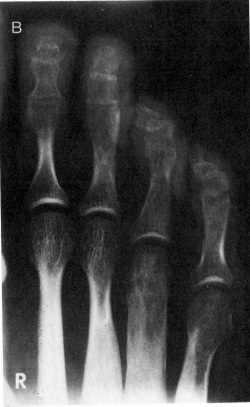

Figure 47.13. Predominantly unilateral polyostotic fibrous dysplasia in a 16-year-old girl. **A.** The involvement of the entire right radius and ulna, cortical thinning, "smoky" appearance of the fibrodysplastic process, and transverse zones and areas of radiolucency *(arrows)*, predisposing to pathologic fractures, are easily recognizable. **B.** Cylindrical expansion, alterations of the cortex, and fine granular texture characterize involvement of the right fourth and fifth metatarsi. (Courtesy of Dr. Jack Bowerman, Russell H. Morgan Department of Radiology, Johns Hopkins Hospital, Baltimore, Maryland, and Harford Memorial Hospital, Havre de Grace, Maryland.)

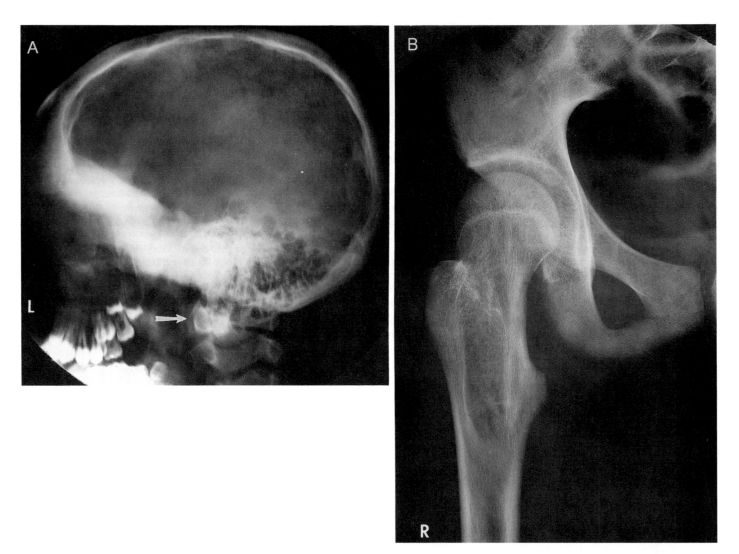

Figure 47.14. Polyostotic fibrous dysplasia in a 10-year-old Caucasian girl with the skeletal development of a 15–16-year-old. Epiphyseal fusion has already occurred in numerous areas, including the head and greater trochanter of the femur. The most striking features are: *(a)* enormous thickening and sclerosis of the anterior two-thirds of the base of the skull, involving the frontal and sphenoid region, *(b)* distortion and constriction of the sella turcica, and *(c)* sclerosis of the anterior portion of the first cervical vertebra *(arrow)* **(A).** Extensive "cystic" lesions involve the upper end and neck of the right femur and right ischiopubic junction **(B).** (Courtesy of Dr. John Dorst, Russell H. Morgan Department of Radiology, Johns Hopkins Hospital, Baltimore, Maryland.)

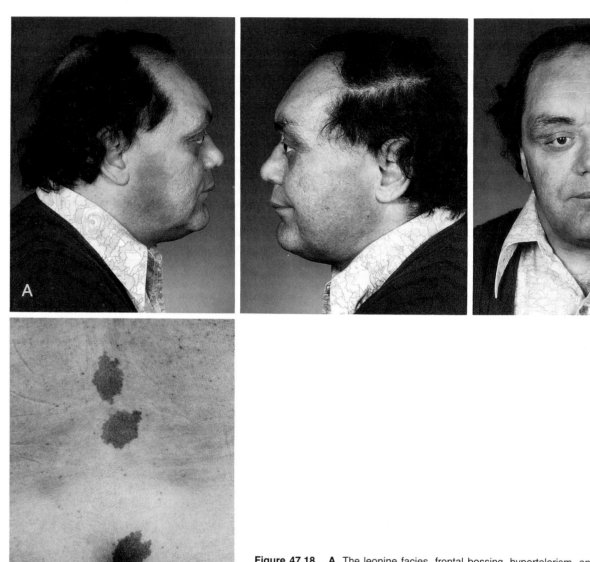

Figure 47.18. **A.** The leonine facies, frontal bossing, hypertelorism, and occipital prominence of the patient in Case 1 at age 45 are evident.

Figure 47.18. **B.** The irregular, nonelevated skin pigmentations in the lumbosacral area are distributed along the midline.

Laboratory studies indicated that serum alkaline phosphatase was elevated (44 IU/liter) and that calcium (8.8 mg/dl) and phosphates (3 mg/dl) were decreased.

At *operation,* the left external auditory canal was reconstructed, and a large external cholesteatoma was removed. The lesion involved all four portions of the temporal bone; it had the consistency of pumice stone, felt gritty, and was very vascular. The middle ear cavity was constricted, and several of the landmarks were distorted by new bone formation. The middle ear ossicles were also involved in the disease process. The histologic examination confirmed the diagnosis of fibrous dysplasia (Fig. 47.23).

The postoperative course was uneventful. A permanent Silastic stent was placed in the external canal for prevention of restenosis, to be exchanged and cleaned at regular intervals (Figs. 47.20*B* and 47.24). It has been tolerated very well for many years. The patient's most recent hearing test disclosed an SRT of 10 dB and a discrimination score of 100% in the operated ear. The patient was started on a course of antithyroid medication. His alkaline phosphatase level gradually decreased to almost normal levels, and so did his serum calcium and phosphate levels.

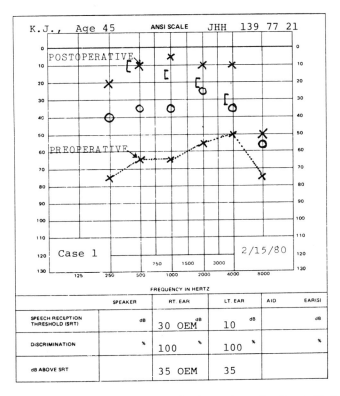

Figure 47.19. Case 1 audiogram reflecting postoperative thresholds for pure tones and speech in operated left ear.

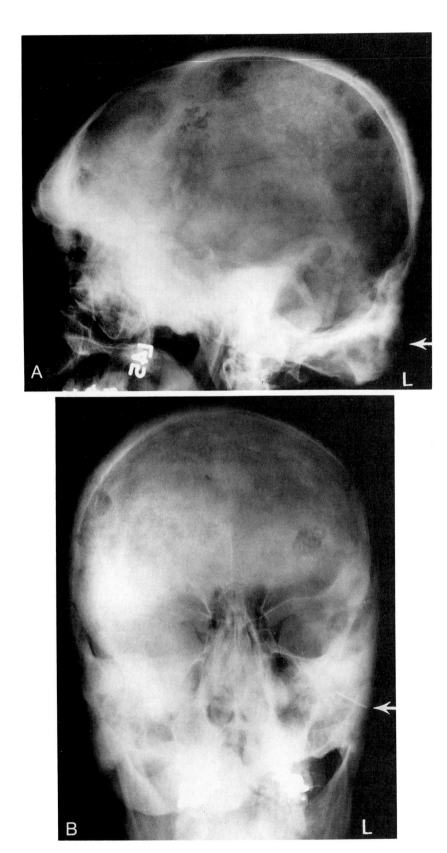

Figure 47.20. **A.** Marked overgrowth and sclerosis of bone in the frontal and occipital areas led to the development of the leonine facial structures and the occipital pug *(arrow)*. Together with thickening and sclerosis of the base of the skull, they exemplify the extensive skull involvement. **B.** Diffuse sclerosis characterizes the widespread involvement of the neural and facial cranium. The radiopaque thread-like marker *(arrow)* in the wall of the Silastic stent is clearly visible in the left external auditory canal.

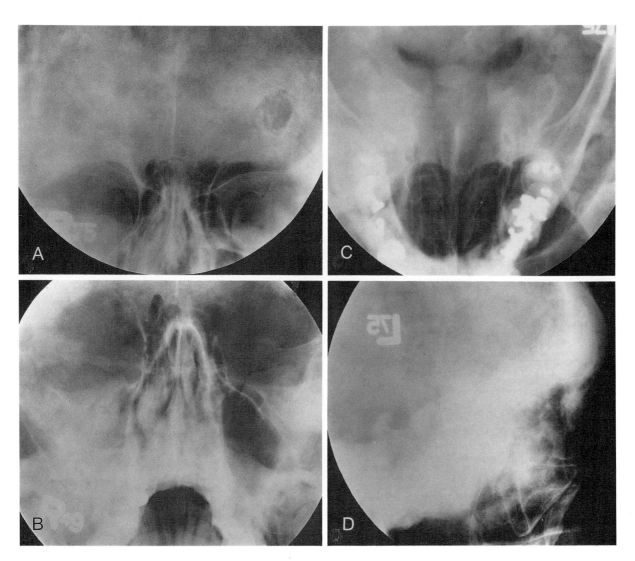

Figure 47.21. **A–D.** Both frontal **(A)** and sphenoid **(D)** sinuses and the right maxillary sinus **(B)** are completely obliterated by the disease process, whereas the ethmoid and left maxillary sinuses **(A–C)** display only partial involvement.

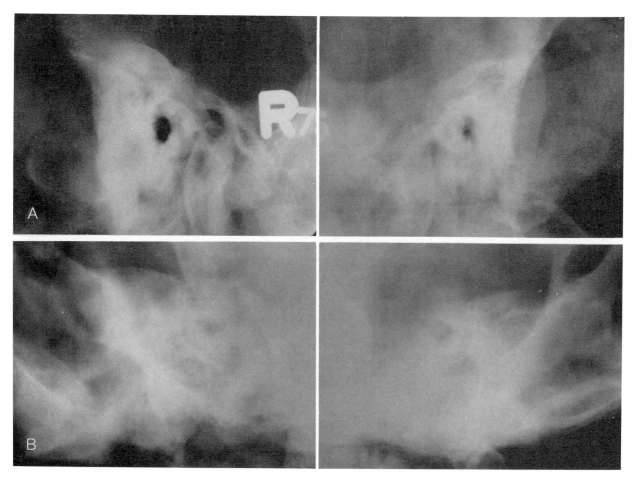

Figure 47.22.   Immense, dense sclerosis marks the severe involvement of the temporal bones as seen in the Schüller **(A)** and Stenvers **(B)** views. The narrowing of both external auditory canals, particularly the left one, is evident.

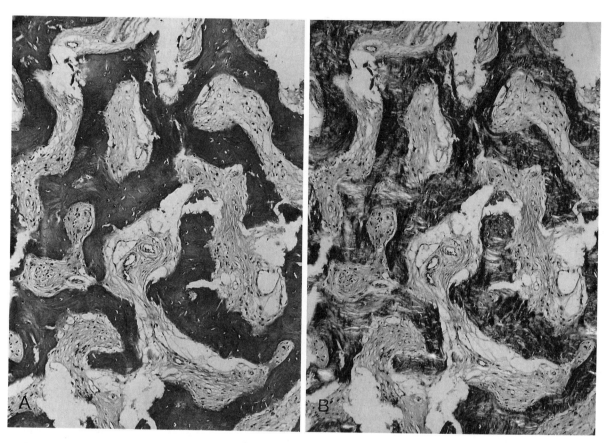

Figure 47.23. Group 1.   A. Biopsy from left tympanic bone. Proliferation of vascular fibrous connective tissue and trabeculae of woven bone characterize the fibrodysplastic process. **B.** The same section under polarized-light shows the random distribution of birefringent collagen fibers, typical for immature bone. (Hematoxylin and eosin, ×150 and ×150, respectively.)

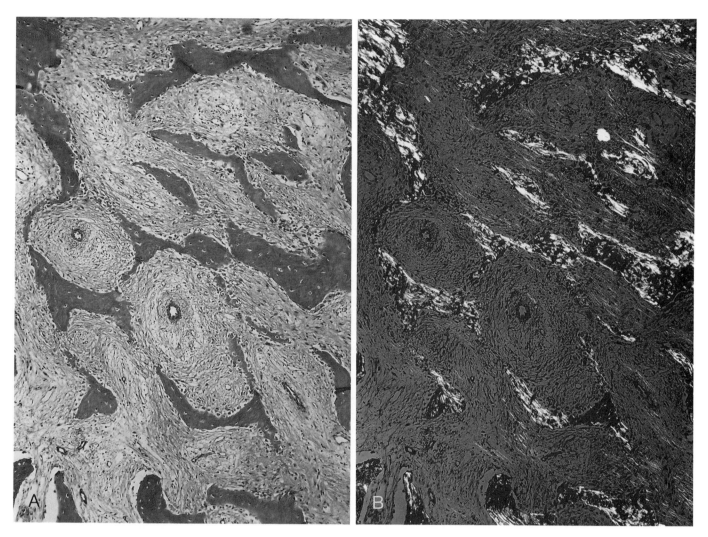

Figure 47.23. Group 2. Biopsy from right ear of an 11-year-old white girl with fibrous dysplasia, presenting as two spherical, pea-sized "osteomas" arising from the posterior bony canal wall. Patient had a 30-dB conductive hearing loss. The appearance, distribution, and orientation of the C-sha-ped bony trabeculae **(A)** and the nature of their immature bone, with disorderly distribution of the birefringent fibers **(B),** characterize the lesion as fibrous dysplasia. (Hematoxylin and eosin, ×120.)

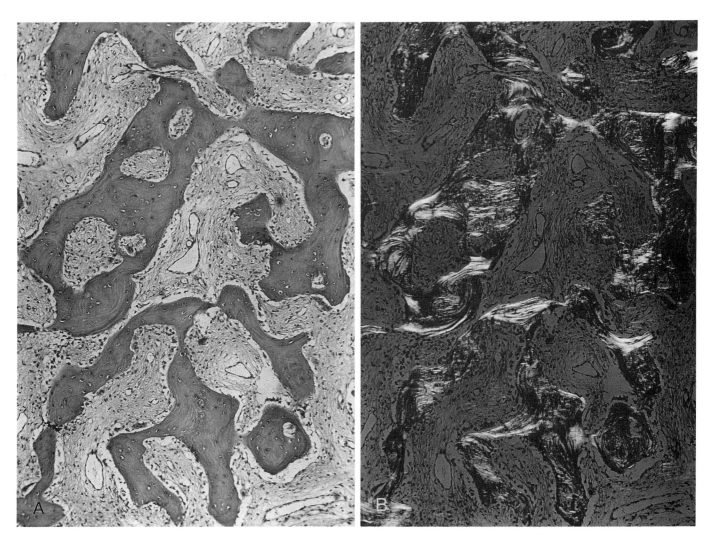

Figure 47.23. Group 3. Biopsy from left external auditory canal of a 12-year-old white boy with obliterative fibrous dysplasia of tympanic portion of temporal bone. Progressive hearing loss began at age 10. The patient had a 50-dB conductive hearing loss and a secondary external cholesteatoma that required three operative procedures. Irregular, poorly oriented, partly calcified trabeculae of immature bone **(A)**; irregular, randomly distributed birefringent fibers under polarized light **(B)**; and a fairly cellular and vascular stroma all identify this lesion as fibrous dysplasia. (Hematoxylin and eosin, ×120.) (Courtesy of Prof. E. Steinbach, ORL Clinic, Tübingen, Germany.)

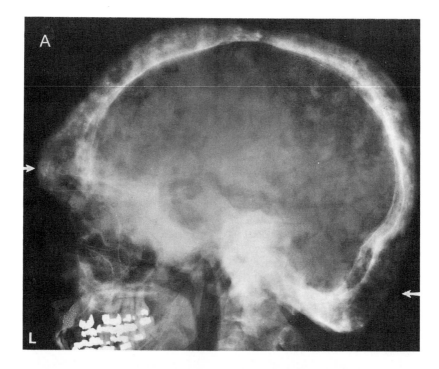

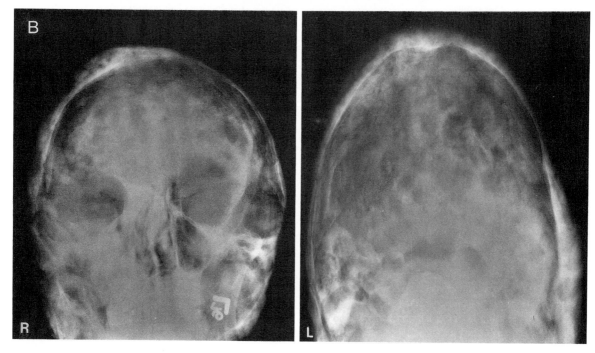

Figure 47.26. **A.** The frontal bossing *(arrow)*, occipital pug *(arrow)*, and basilar impression reflect massive involvement of the entire calvaria and base. The coexistence of localized lytic and diffuse sclerotic lesions strongly resembles pagetoid bone remodeling. **B.** Extensive involvement of the facial cranium resulted in obliteration of most paranasal sinuses.

a result of bone involvement (Fig. 47.28). Cochlear function studies revealed mild, bilateral conductive hearing loss with an SRT of 30 dB on the right side and 25 dB on the left side; discrimination was 100% bilaterally (Fig. 47.35). Vestibular function studies revealed rather feeble responses to caloric stimulation bilaterally, poor opto-kinetic nystagmus, positional nystagmus in the head-hanging posi-tion with Frenzel glasses, and bidirectional gaze nystagmus, sug-gesting the possibility of brain stem involvement.

An earlier biopsy from the right tibia had identified the bone lesion as fibrous dysplasia (Fig. 47.36). The patient has been fol-lowed regularly for the past 10 years. His gradually progressive skeletal deformity forced him to retire at age 40.

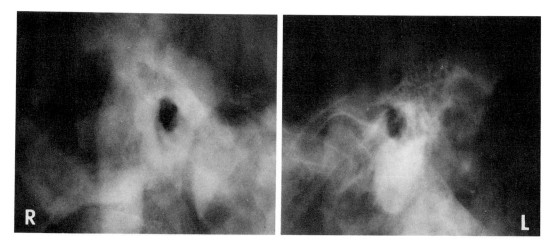

Figure 47.27. The lateral (Schüller) view displays diffuse sclerosis of the mastoid bone and slight narrowing of the external auditory canals.

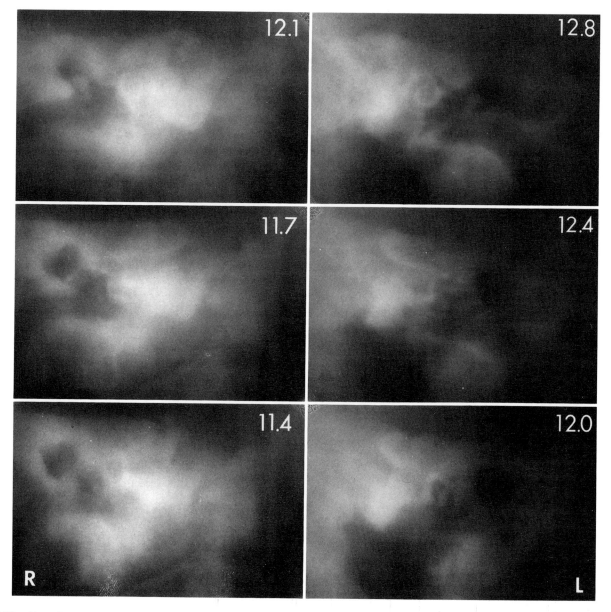

Figure 47.28. Frontal tomograms of the petrous pyramids reveal downward bending of the external auditory canal and upward slanting of the internal auditory canal, regularly seen in basilar invagination. The diffuse sclerosis tends to obscure the landmarks of the cochlear and vestibular capsules. The outer middle ear ossicles are enlarged, but there is no encroachment on the seventh and eighth cranial nerves.

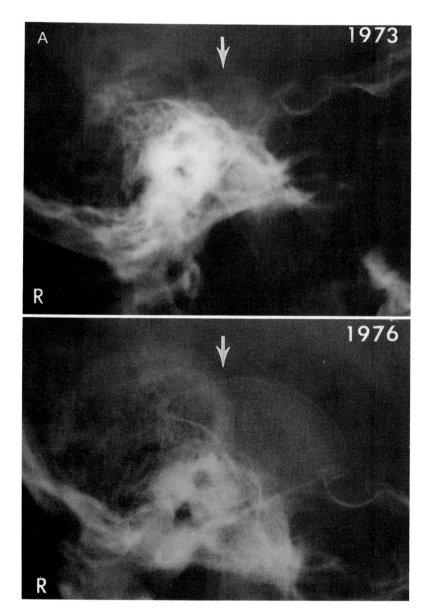

Figure 47.39. The lateral projection of the right temporal bone **(A)** and the anteroposterior (Town) projection of the skull **(B)** clearly show the increase in size of the dysplastic process over the 3-year period *(arrows)*.

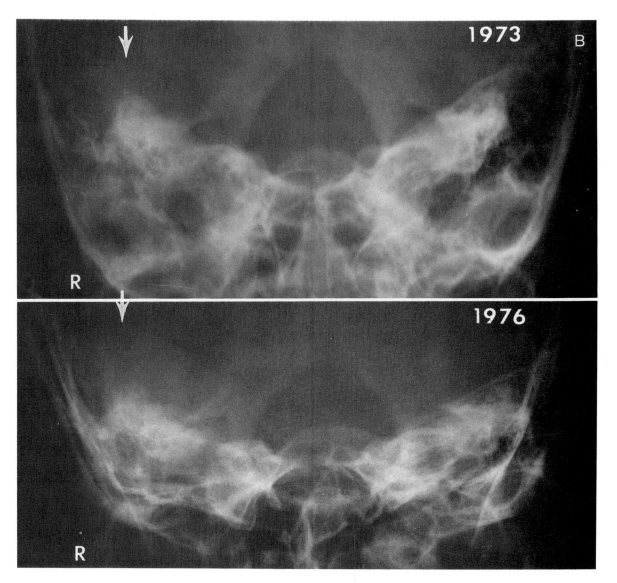

Figure 47.39.   B.

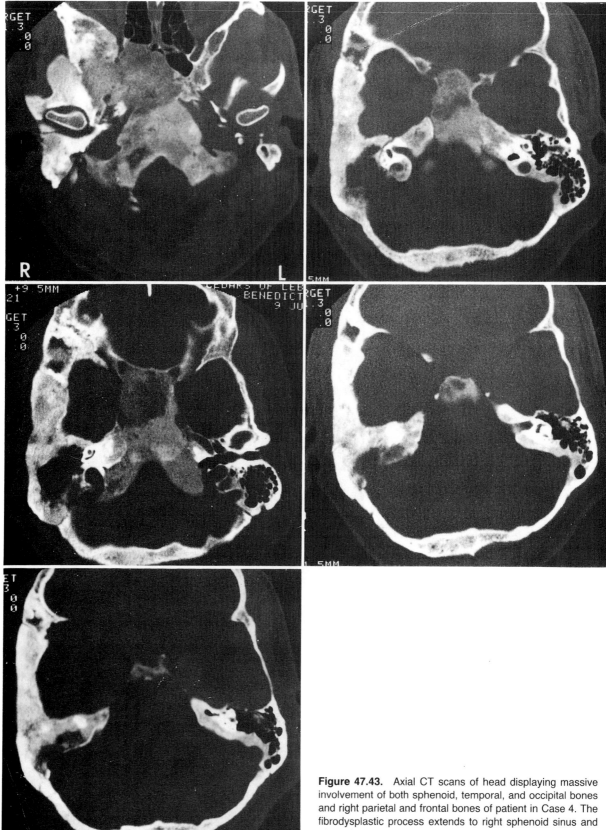

Figure 47.43. Axial CT scans of head displaying massive involvement of both sphenoid, temporal, and occipital bones and right parietal and frontal bones of patient in Case 4. The fibrodysplastic process extends to right sphenoid sinus and along the posterior aspect of the left pyramid. The posterior aspect of the right pyramid is widely eroded.

Case 5. *Oligostotic fibrous dysplasia involving the right temporal, sphenoid, and zygomatic bones. Operation for "chronic infection of mastoid," followed by progressive stenosis of right external auditory meatus.*

The patient was a 54-year-old man who at age 7 had undergone a right mastoidectomy for "chronic infection"; this was followed by gradually increasing constriction of the right outer ear canal. For the past year he had noticed progressive hearing loss and tinnitus in the right ear, enlargement and deformity in the area of the right temporal bone and temporal fossa, difficulties with adjustment of the right temple bar of his eyeglasses, and occlusion of the right external auditory canal.

Otologic examination revealed a uniform, spherical, hard, nontender enlargement of the right temporal and zygomatic bones. It extended from the right lateral canthus posteriorly over the entire squama temporalis, measuring about 7 × 6 × 5 cm. It fully occupied the temporal fossa, protruded beyond it, and had totally obliterated the right bony external auditory canal. Cochlear function studies disclosed severe, mixed, predominantly conductive hearing loss in the right ear with a SRT of 55 dB and a discrimination score of 92%. Hearing was normal in the left ear. With the exception of the eighth cranial nerve, cranial nerve function was normal on that side. Serum levels for alkaline phosphatase, calcium, and phosphate were normal.

Radiologic examination showed: diffuse enlargement of the right temporal, zygomatic, and sphenoid bones; thickening of the floor of the right middle cranial fossa; ballooning of the external and internal table; and cortical thinning (Fig. 47.44A). The lesion displayed a uniform ground-glass pattern. It occupied the entire right temporal fossa and extended laterally beyond it (Fig. 47.44B).

At *operation,* the right external ear canal was reconstructed, and an external cholesteatoma was removed. The tympanic membrane appeared normal. A permanent tubular Silastic stent was inserted. The dysplastic bone was very soft, crumbly, and very vascular. Histologic examination of the bone removed identified the process as fibrous dysplasia (Fig. 47.45).

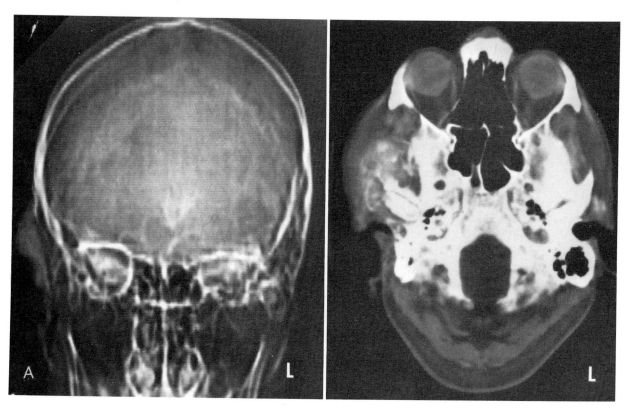

Figure 47.44. CT tomograms showing enlargement and distortion of right temporal, zygomatic, and sphenoid bones and thickening of floor of right middle cranial fossa of patient in Case 5. **A.** Anteroposterior and axial views. **B.** Anteroposterior and lateral views. Lesion has a uniform ground-glass appearance.

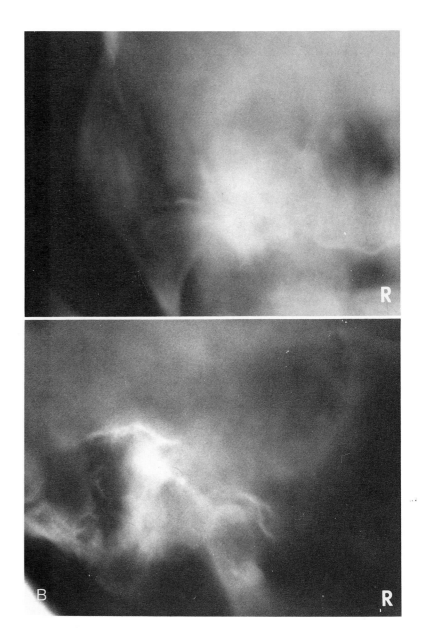

Figure 47.44. B.

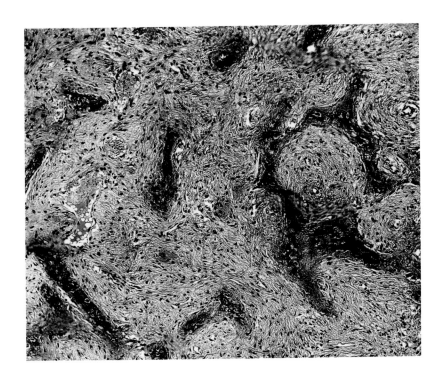

Figure 47.45. Biopsy from right temporal bone of patient in Case 5. The lesion is characterized as fibrous dysplasia by *(a)* the varying size, random distribution, and poor orientation of C-shaped bony trabeculae, *(b)* the nature of their immature bone, and *(c)* the surrounding proliferation of isomorphous, vascular, fibrous tissue of spindle cells. (Hematoxylin and eosin, ×125.)

Case 6. *Monostotic fibrous dysplasia involving all portions of left temporal bone, resulting in an overall increase in size and almost complete stenosis of the external auditory canal. No distortion of middle ear cleft or internal acoustic meatus. Normal hearing.*

The patient was a 9-year-old boy whose mother had noticed a bone growth in his left outer ear canal when cleaning the ear with a Q-tip. The pediatrician confirmed the finding, and the consulting otologist, while examining the left ear, noted diffuse concentric osseous stenosis with narrowing of the lumen to less than 1 mm in diameter. He suspected fibrous dysplasia. The patient had been asymptomatic with no history of external or middle ear infections, tinnitus, or impairment of cochlear, vestibular, or facial nerve function. His younger sister apparently had a form of osteochondrodysplasia.

Otologic examination disclosed extreme narrowing of the left external auditory canal, resulting from concentric growth of three diffuse hemispherical bone protrusions covered by normal meatal skin. The central portion of the tympanic membrane, as seen through the small opening, appeared normal. There was no distortion of the outer contours of the temporal bone. The opposite ear was essentially normal, and seventh and eighth cranial nerve function was normal bilaterally.

Radiologic examination included serial axial and coronal CT scans, which showed almost the entire left temporal bone involved in a diffuse osteodysplastic process that had increased overall dimensions without distorting the original landmarks. The tympanic bone and the base of the squamous portion of the temporal bone were most severely affected. The bone lesion had a uniform ground-glass appearance with a thin cortex (Fig. 47.46, *Groups 1 and 2*). Massive involvement of the tympanic bone resulted in severe longitudinal concentric stenosis of the external canal, leaving only a thread-like lumen. The middle ear cleft was slightly constricted, but there was no impingement on the middle ear ossicles, which were unaffected. The inner ear capsule and internal auditory canal had normal configurations. Extensive involvement of the mastoid process obliterated a considerable portion of the air cell system.

At *operation,* the patient underwent a reconstruction of the left external auditory meatus with placement of a Silastic stent for the prevention of future restenosis. The diagnosis was histologically confirmed (Fig. 47.47).

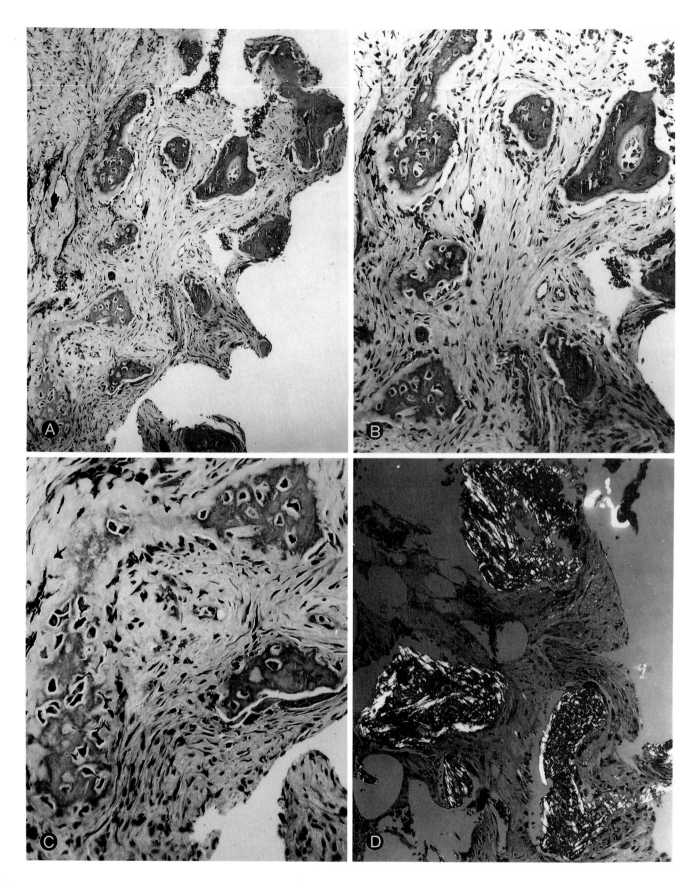

Figure 47.47. Biopsy from left temporal bone. **A.** Trabeculae of fibrous bone are interspersed in an area of fairly mature collagenous tissue. **B.** They are somewhat thicker than usual and, in some places, poorly calcified. **C.** There appears to be osteoblastic osteogenesis along the concave surface of a partially tangentially cut, sickle-shaped trabecula in the left upper and lateral field. **D.** Under polarized light the collagen fibers in the bony trabeculae are irregular, unevenly distributed, and arranged in a woven rather than lamellar pattern. (Hematoxylin and eosin, ×120, ×200, ×320, and ×320, respectively.)

Case 7. *Polyostotic fibrous dysplasia, slowly progressive, unilateral (left-sided), with extensive involvement of the left neural and facial cranium, entire cervical spine, left pelvis, and left leg. History of seven pathologic fractures involving left femoral neck and one fracture involving left tibia. Left femur nail fixation for recurrent subtrochanteric fracture with intertrochanteric osteotomy and cortical cadaver strut grafts. Right distal femoral osteotomy and shortening with blade plate fixation and left intramedullary tibial rod with cadaver cortical bone grafting. Involvement of left mandible, maxilla, orbit, frontal, ethmoid, sphenoid, parietal, occipital, and temporal bones. Scoliosis of thoracic spine. McCune-Albright syndrome according to history.*

A 16-year-old Oriental woman was seen who had a history of three orthopedic procedures for eight pathologic fractures of the left femoral neck and one involving the left tibia, all resulting from fibrous dysplasia (Figs. 47.49A and 47.50). The patient was referred for evaluation of an acute diffuse swelling of the left side of her face. She had noticed increasing throbbing pain over the left maxilla and around the left eye and a purulent postnasal discharge for the preceding 3 days. For some time she had been aware of a slight increase in the size of her left face and a mild hearing loss in the left ear.

Otolaryngologic examination revealed a tender inflammatory edema involving the left preseptal, premaxillary, and periorbital area over seemingly enlarged underlying bone structures. The left anterior cervical lymph nodes were enlarged, and there was purulent exudate in the left middle nasal meatus. The left temporal bone was somewhat extended, and the bony external auditory canal displayed irregular concentric narrowing. The tympanic membrane was dull and immobile, and the tympanogram was flat. The audiogram showed a low-tone conductive loss in the left ear with a SRT of 20 dB and a discrimination score of 100%.

Ophthalmologic examination disclosed an old optic neuropathy on the left that resulted from fibrous dysplasia involving the orbital apex.

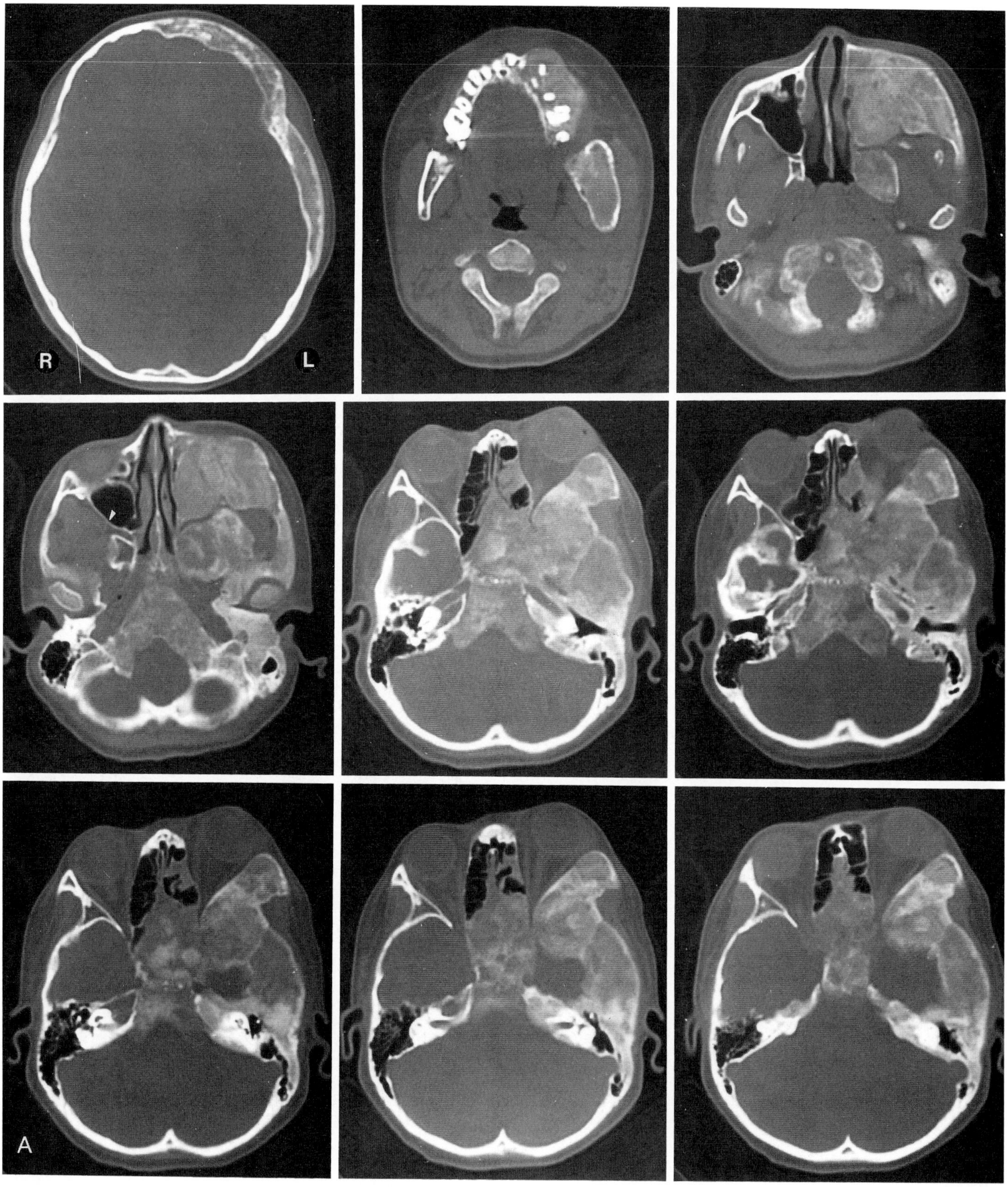

Figure 47.48. **A.** Axial CT scan of the head of the patient in Case 7 displays diffuse thickening of the left side of the calvaria, skull base, and facial bones, caused by fibrous dysplasia. The process involves the mandible, maxilla, frontal, parietal, ethmoid, sphenoid, zygoma, temporal, and occipital bones. As a result, the left frontal, ethmoid, and maxillary, and both sphenoid sinuses are obliterated, and the orbital apex, optic foramen, nasal cavity, middle ear cleft, and external auditory canal are constricted.

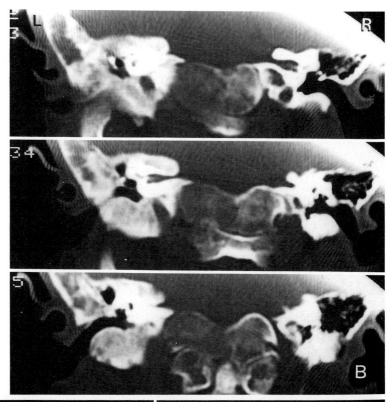

Figure 47.48.   B. Coronal CT scans reveal the overall increase in size, almost homogeneous sclerosis of the left temporal bone, and narrowing of the middle ear cleft.

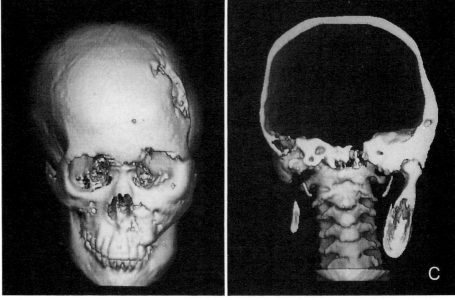

Figure 47.48.   C. Three-dimensional reconstruction from the CT scans demonstrates the augmentation and distortion of the left facial and temporal bones.

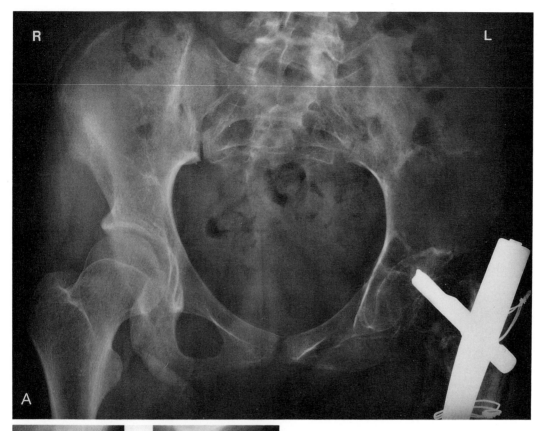

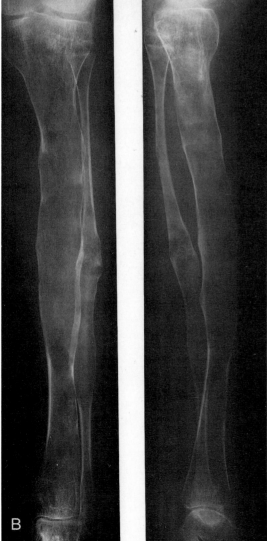

Figure 47.49. **A.** Left hemipelvis demonstrates extensive involvement with a large cystic lesion in the iliac wing and osteoporosis and deformation of the acetabulum, os pubis, and ischium. The left femoral head and neck, supported by a Zickel nail prosthesis, is severely osteoporotic and nearly totally resorbed. **B.** The left tibia and fibula display massive involvement and severe distortion of bone architecture, resulting from irregular widening, bending, and cortical thinning of the diaphyses. The process is characterized by areas of osteoporosis, diffuse sclerosis, and cystic radiolucencies.

Laboratory studies indicated a white blood cell count of 10,900/mm^3, with 30.2% lymphocytes, 63.1% granulocytes, and 6.7% monocytes. The erythrocyte sedimentation rate was 64 mm. Serum calcium was 8.4 mg/dl; phosphate, 2.0 mg/dl; and alkaline phosphatase, 364 U/liter (normal, 120–320 U/liter).

Radiologic examination via CT scans showed extensive changes in the left facial and neural cranium caused by fibrous dysplasia (Fig. 47.48). A three-phase bone scan with 15.2 mCi ^{99m}Tc methylene diphosphate revealed an increased uptake in the left mandible, maxilla, orbit, and frontal bone with superimposed inflammation compatible with either cellulitis or osteomyelitis. Subsequent leukocyte imaging with 364 nCi ^{111}In-labeled white blood cells showed a normal, even distribution of the labeled white blood cells within the bone marrow without abnormal accumulation on the left, thus ruling out osteomyelitis. The pelvis, femur, tibia, and fibula displayed extensive fibrous dysplasia.

The patient was treated with antibiotics for facial cellulitis and prevention of osteomyelitis and is being followed regularly for her progressive fibrous dysplasia and its manifestations in the temporal bone.

References

1. Dent CE, Gertner IM. Hypophosphataemic osteomalacia in fibrous dysplasia. Q J Med 1976;45:411–420.

2. Cohen DM, Dahlin DC, Pugh DG. Fibrous dysplasia associated with adamantinoma of the long bones. Cancer 1962;15:515–521.

3. Johnson LC. Congenital pseudarthrosis, adamantinoma of long bones and intracortical fibrous dysplasia of the tibia. J Bone Joint Surg [Am] 1972;54A:1355–1362.

4. Uehlinger E. Osteofibrosis deformans juvenilis. Polyostotische fibrose Dysplasie (Jaffe-Lichtenstein). Virchows Arch Pathol Anat Physiol 1940;306:255–299.

5. Wirth WA, Leavitt D, Enzinger FM. Multiple intramuscular myxomas. Cancer 1971;27:1167–1173.

6. McIntosh HD, Miller DE, Goldner JL. The circulatory dynamics of polyostotic fibrous dysplasia. Am J Med 1962;32:393–403.

7. Firat D, Stutzman L. Fibrous dysplasia of bone. Am J Med 1968;44:421–429.

8. Schwartz DT, Alpert M. The malignant transformation of fibrous dysplasia. Am J Med Sci 1964;247:35–74.

9. Von Recklinghausen F. Die Fibröse oder deformierende Ostitis, die Osteomalacie und die osteoplastische Carcinose in ihren gegenseitigen Beziehungen. Festschrift Rudolf Virchow zum 13 Oktober, Berlin, 1891.

10. Elmslie RC. Fibrocystic diseases of the bones. Br J Surg 1914;2:17–67.

11. Weil A. Pubertas praecox und Knochenbrüchigkeit. Klin Wochenschr 1922;1:2114–2115.

12. Hunter D, Turnbull HL. Hyperparathyroidism: generalized osteitis fibrosa. Br J Surg 1931;32:203–284.

13. Jaffé HL. Hyperparathyroidism. Arch Pathol 1933;16:63–67.

14. Freund E, Meffert CB. On the different forms of nongeneralized fibrous osteodystrophia. Surg Gynecol Obstet 1936;62:451–461.

15. McCune DJ, Bruch H. Osteodystrophia fibrosa: report of a case in which the condition was combined with precocious puberty, pathologic pigmentation of the skin and hyperthyroidism, with review of the literature. Am J Dis Child 1937;54:806–848.

16. Albright F, Butler MA, Hamptom AO, Smith P. Syndrome characterized by osteitis fibrosa disseminata, areas of pigmentation and endocrine dysfunction with precocious puberty in females. N Engl J Med 1937;216:727–746.

17. McCune DJ. Osteitis fibrosa cystica: the case of a nine year old girl who also exhibits precocious puberty, multiple pigmentation of the skin and hyperthyroidism. Am J Dis Child 1936;52:745–748.

18. Gaupp V. Pubertas praecox bei Osteodystrophia fibrosa. Monatsschr Kinderheilkd 1932;53:312–322.

19. Goldhammer K. Osteodystrophia fibrosa unilateralis. Fortschr Roentgenstr 1934;49:456–481.

20. Hummel R. Zwei Fälle von Ostitis deformans Paget juvenilis. Rontgen Laboratoriumspraxis (Stuttgart) 1934;6:513–519.

21. Lichtenstein L. Polyostotic fibrous dysplasia. Arch Surg 1938;36:874–898.

22. Lichtenstein L, Jaffé HL. Fibrous dysplasia of bone. Arch Pathol 1942;33:777–816.

23. Schlumberger HG. Fibrous dysplasia of single bones (monostotic fibrous dysplasia). Mil Surg 1947;99:504–527.

24. Van Tilburg W. Fibrous dysplasia. In: Vinken PJ, Bruyn GW, eds. Handbook of clinical neurology. Amsterdam: North Holland, 1972;14:163–212.

25. Wells C. Polyostotic fibrous dysplasia in a 7th century Anglo-Saxon. Br J Radiol 1963;36:925–926.

26. Gregg JB, Reed A. Monostotic fibrous dysplasia in the temporal bone: a late prehistoric occurrence. Am J Phys Anthropol 1980;52:587–593.

27. Slow IN, Stern D, Friedman EW. Osteogenic sarcoma arising in pre-existing fibrous dysplasia: report of case. J Oral Surg 1971;29:126–129.

28. Stewart MJ, Gilmer WS, Edmonton AS. Fibrous dysplasia of bone. J Bone Joint Surg [Am] 1962;44:302–318.

29. Harris WH, Dudley HR Jr, Barry JR. The natural history of fibrous dysplasia. J Bone Joint Surg [Am] 1962;44:207–233.

30. Aegerter EE, Kirkpatrick JA Jr. Orthopedic diseases. 3rd ed. Philadelphia: WB Saunders, 1968:182–192.

31. Uehlinger E, Fibröse Dysplasia (Jaffé-Lichtenstein): Osteofibrosis deformans juvenilis (Uehlinger); Albrightsches Syndrome. In: Schinz HR, Baensch WE, Frommhold W, Glauner R, Uehlinger E, Wellauer J, eds.

32. Hadders HN. Dysplasia fibrosa monostotica. Ned Tijdschr Geneeskd 1957;101:378–380.

33. Henry A. Monostotic fibrous dysplasia. J Bone Joint Surg [Br] 1969;51:300–316.

34. Talbot IC, Keith DA, Lord IJ. Fibrous dysplasia of the cranio-facial bones. A clinicopathological survey of seven cases. J Laryngol Otol 1974;88:429–443.

35. Becker MH. Fibrous dysplasia. In: Ranniger K, ed. Encyclopedia of medical radiology. New York: Springer-Verlag, 1977;5:488–512.

36. Eversole LR, Sabes WR, Rovin S. Fibrous dysplasia. A nosologic problem in the diagnosis of fibro-osseous lesions of the jaws. J Oral Pathol 1972;1:189–220.

37. Van Horn PE Jr, Dahlin DC, Bickel WH. Fibrous dysplasia: a clinical pathologic study of orthopedic surgical cases. Proc Mayo Clin 1963;38:175–189.

38. Furst NJ, Shapiro R. Polyostotic fibrous dysplasia: review of literature with two additional cases. Radiology 1943;40:501–515.

39. Hoboek A. Polyostotic fibrous dysplasia of bone. Acta Radiol 1951;36:145–153.

40. Reed RJ. Fibrous dysplasia of bone. Arch Pathol 1963;75:480–495.

41. Gibson MJ, Middlemiss JH. Fibrous dysplasia of bone. Br J Radiol 1971;44:1–13.

42. Hopf M. Zur Kenntnis der polyostotischen fibrösen Dysplasie. Radiol Clin 1949;28:129–159.

43. Windolz F. Cranial manifestations of fibrous dysplasia of bone. AJR 1947;58:51–63.

44. Fries JW. The roentgen features of fibrous dysplasia of the skull and facial bones: a critical analysis of thirty-nine pathologically proven cases. AJR 1957;77–88.

45. Hall R, Warrick CH. Hypersecretion of hypothalamic releasing hormones: a possible explanation of the endocrine manifestations of polyostotic fibrous dysplasia (Albright syndrome). Lancet 1972;1:1313–1316.

46. Pritchard JE. Fibrous dysplasia of the bones. Am J Med Sci 1951;22:313–332.

47. Ivimey M. Bone dystrophy with characteristics of leontiasis ossea, osteitis fibrosa cystica. Am J Dis Child 1929;38:348–369.

48. Revers FE. Albright's disease (osteitis fibrosa cystica). Ned Tijdschr Geneeskd 1947;91:1695–1704.

49. Spjut HJ, Dorfman HD, Fechner RE, Ackerman LV. Fibrous dysplasia. In: Atlas of tumor pathology. 2nd series, Fascicle 5. Washington, DC: Armed Forces Institute of Pathology, 1970:270–280.

50. Jaffé HL. Fibrous dysplasia of bone. Bull N Y Acad Med 1946;22:588–604.

51. Proffit JN, McSwain B, Kalmon FH. Fibrous dysplasia of bone. Ann Surg 1949;130:881–895.

52. Russell LW, Chandler FA. Fibrous dysplasia of bone. J Bone Joint Surg [Am] 1950;32:323–337.

53. Fairbank HAT. An atlas of general affections of the skeleton. Edinburgh: E & S Livingstone, 1951.

54. Benedict PH, Szabo G, Fitzpatrick TB, Sinesi SJ. Melanotic macules in Albright's syndrome and in neurofibromatosis. JAMA 1968;205:618–626.

55. Benedict PH. Sexual precocity and polyostotic fibrous dysplasia. Am J Dis Child 1966;111:426–431.

56. Scurry MT, Bichnell JM, Fajans SS. Polyostotic fibrous dysplasia and acromegaly. Arch Intern Med 1969;114:40–45.

57. Benjamin DR, McRoberts JW. Polyostotic fibrous dysplasia associated with Cushing syndrome. Arch Pathol 1973;96:175–178.

58. Aarskog D, Tveteraas E. McCune-Albright's syndrome following adrenalectomy for Cushing's syndrome in infancy. J Pediatr 1968;73:89–96.

59. Peck FB, Sage CV. Diabetes mellitus associated with Albright's syndrome. Am J Med Sci 1944;208:35–46.

60. Benedict PH. Endocrine features in Albright's syndrome (fibrous dysplasia of bone). Metabolism 1962;11:30–45.

61. Moldawer M, Rabin ER. Polyostotic fibrous dysplasia with thyrotoxicosis. Report of a complete autopsy and skeletal reconstruction. Arch Intern Med 1966;118:379–385.

62. Kim JP, Kbera SAK. Polyostotic fibrous dysplasia associated with hyperthyroidism. J Bone Joint Surg [Am] 1961;43:897–904.

63. Wortham JT, Hamblen EC. Polyostotic fibrous dysplasia with sexual precocity and pigmentation (Albright's syndrome) and associated non-neoplastic acromegaly. J Clin Endocrinol Metab 1952;12:975–976.

64. Albright F. Polyostotic fibrous dysplasia: a defense of the entity. J Clin Endocrinol Metab 1947;7:307–324.

65. Schally AV, Bowers CY. The nature of thyrotropin-releasing hormones (THR). In: Kenny AD, Anderson R, eds. Proceedings of the Sixth Midwestern Conference on the Thyroid and Endocrinology. Columbia, Missouri: University of Missouri, 1970:25.

66. Hamilton CR, Maloaf F. Unusual types of hyperthyroidism. Medicine 1973;53:195–215.

67. Faglia G, Ferrari C, Beck-Peroz P, Ambrosi B, Valantini F. High plasma thyrotropin levels in two patients with pituitary tumors. Acta Endocrinol (Copenh) 1972;69:649–658.

68. Sherman L, Kolodny HD. The hypothalamus, brain catecholamines and drug therapy for gigantism and acromegaly. Lancet 1972;1:682–685.

69. Mazabraud A, Toty L, Roze R, Semat P. Un nouveau cas d'association de dysplasie fibreuse des os avec un myxome des tissues mous. Sem Hop Paris 1969;45:862–868.

70. Daves ML, Yardley JH. Fibrous dysplasia of bone. Am J Med Sci 1957;234:590–606.

71. Gatewood OMB, Esterly JR. Coexistent polyostotic fibrous dysplasia and eosinophilic granuloma of bone. AJR 1966;97:110–117.

72. Stauffer HM, Arbukle RK, Aegerter EE. Polyostotic fibrous dysplasia with cutaneous pigmentation and congenital arteriovenous aneurysm. J Bone Joint Surg [Am] 1941;23:323–334.

73. Fischer JA, Bollinger A, Lichtlen P, Wellauer J. Fibrous dysplasia and high cardiac output. Am J Med 1970;49:140–146.

74. Moore RT. Fibrous dysplasia of the orbit. Surv Ophthalmol 1969;13:321–334.

75. Sassin JF, Rosenberg RN. Neurological complications of fibrous dysplasia of the skull. Arch Neurol 1968;18:363–369.

76. Feiring W, Feiring EH, Davidoff ML. Fibrous dysplasia of the skull. J Neurosurg 1951;8:377–397.

77. Falconer MA, Cope CL, Robb-Smith AHT. Fibrous dysplasia of bone with endocrine disorders and cutaneous pigmentation (Albright's disease). Q J Med 1942;11:121–154.

78. Dieckmann H, Tanzer A. Zur Klinik der fibrösen Dysplasie und des Albright Syndoms. Dtsch Z Nervenheilkd 1957;176:615–636.

79. Kanavel AB. Surgical intervention in leontiasis ossea. Surg Gynecol Obstet 1917;4:719–734.

80. Evans J. Leontiasis ossea. Critical review with reports of 4 original cases. J Bone Joint Surg [Br] 1953;35:229–234.

81. Teng P, Gross SW, Newman CM. Compression of the spinal cord by osteitis deformans (Paget's disease), giant cell tumor and polyostotic fibrous dysplasia (Albright's syndrome) of vertebrae. J Neurosurg 1951;8:482–493.

82. Jirout J, Lewit K. Cases of fibrous dysplasia with disturbances of the nervous system. Zentrbl Ges Radiol 1957;54:161.

83. Lecocq M. Un cas de localisation vertebrale de la dysplasie fibreuse de l'os ou maladie, Jaffe-Lichtenstein. J Belge Rhumatol Méd Phys 1956;11:17–24.

84. Rosandahl-Jensen SV. Fibrous dysplasia of the vertebral column. Acta Chir Scand 1956;6:490.

85. Vial A. De ziekte van Jaffé-Lichtenstein of "osteofibromatosis cystica." Ned Tijdschr Geneeskd 1948;92:1784–1787.

86. Jervis GA, Schein H. Polyostotic fibrous dysplasia (Albright's syndrome); case showing central nervous system changes. Arch Pathol 1951;51:640–650.

87. Cahill P. Fibrous dysplasia of the skull. Med J Aust 1963;50:843–847.

88. Coley RL, Stewart FW. Bone sarcoma in polyostotic fibrous dysplasia. Ann Surg 1945;121:872–881.

89. Huvos AG, Higinbotham NL, Miller TR. Bone sarcomas arising in fibrous dysplasia. J Bone Joint Surg [Am] 1972;54:1047–1056.

90. Fuchsbrunner E, Kolb E, Schoenwald A. Oberkiefersarkom bei polyostotischer fibröser Knochendysplasia (Morbus Jaffé-Lichtenstein). Zahnärzt Prax 1964;15:105–107.

91. Standish SM, Gorlin RJ. Bone disorders affecting the jaws. In: Gorlin RJ, Goldman HM, eds. Thoma's oral pathology. 6th ed. St Louis: CV Mosby, 1970;1:541.

92. Reitzik M, Lownie JF. Familial polyostotic fibrous dysplasia. Oral Surg 1975;40:769–774.

93. El Deeb M, Waite ED, Gorlin RJ. Congenital monostotic fibrous dysplasia—a new, possibly autosomal-recessive disorder. J Oral Surg 1979;37:520–525.

94. Lemli L. Fibrous dysplasia of bone. Report of female monozygotic twins with and without the McCune-Albright syndrome. J Pediatr 1977;91:347–349.

95. Dahlmann J. Zur Kenntnis des Albright's Disease. Fortschr Rontgenstr 1955;82:723–740.

96. Harris HW, Dudley R Jr, Barry RJ. The natural history of fibrous dysplasia. An orthopedic, pathological and roentgenographic study. J Bone Joint Surg [Am] 1962;44:207–233.

97. Ramsey HE, Strong EW, Frazell EL. Progressive fibrous dysplasia of the maxilla. J Am Dent Assoc 1970;81:1388–1391.

98. Berger R. Fibrome envahissant de la mastoide. Presse Méd 1947;55:202.

99. Cooke SL, Powers WH. Monostotic fibrous dysplasia. Report of two cases. Arch Otolaryngol 1949;50:319–329.

100. Towson CE. Monostotic fibrous dysplasia of the mastoid and the temporal bone. Arch Otolaryngol 1950;52:709–724.

101. Jezek K. Pripad fibrosni dysplasie kostni vyenelku soscoviteho. Cas Lek Ces 1951;90:1386–1388.

102. Brunner H. Fibrous dysplasia of facial bone and paranasal sinuses. Arch Otolaryngol 1952;55:43–54.

103. Skolnik EM, Perrelli SL, Pornoy RA. Fibrous dysplasia of the skull and temporal bone. Eye Ear Nose Throat Mon 1958;57:755–772.

104. Deuber JW. Dissertation. Zurich: University, 1958.

105. Kearney HL. Fibrous dysplasia of the temporal bone. Laryngoscope 1959;69:571–574.

106. Kleinsasser O, Friedmann G. Die fibröse Knochendysplasie des Gesichts und Hirnschädels. Laryngol Rhinol Oto Ihre Grenzgeb 1960;39:201–220.

107. Sussman HB. Monostotic fibrous dysplasia of the temporal bone. Report of a case. Laryngoscope 1961;71:68–77.

108. Clay A, Deguine C. Un cas de dysplasie fibreuse a localisation occipitomastoidienne. J Fr Oto-Rhino-Laryngol Chir Maxillo-Fac 1962;11:393–400.

109. Leeds N, Seaman WB. Fibrous dysplasia of the skull and its differential diagnosis. Radiology 1962;78:570–582.

110. Wong A, Vaughan CW, Strong StM. Fibrous dysplasia of temporal bone. Arch Otolaryngol 1965;81:131–133.

111. Flurr E, Soderberg G. Monostotic fibrous dysplasia (ossifying fibroma) of the mastoid. J Laryngol Otol 1966;80:678–685.

112. Shiffman F, Aengst FE. Fibrous dysplasia of temporal bone. Arch Otolaryngol 1967;86:528–534.

113. Basek M. Fibrous dysplasia of the middle ear. Arch Otolaryngol 1967;85:26–29.

114. Deshmukh SS, Gandhi RK, Mody SN, Deshmukh SM. Fibrous dysplasia of temporal bone. J Postgrad Med 1967;13:198–200.

115. Samy LL, Girgis IH, Wasef SA. Fibrous dysplasia in relation to the paranasal sinuses and the ear. J Laryngol Otol 1967;81:1357–1371.

116. Privara M, Cerny E. Osteodysplasia fibrosa kosti spankove. Cesk Otolaryngol 1968;17:141–144.

117. Antonova NA, Kosakova EI, Fostovsky JA. Fibrous dysplasia of the temporal bone. Vestn Otorinolaringol 1968;30:101–102.

118. Cohen A, Rosenwasser H. Fibrous dysplasia of the temporal bone. Arch Otolaryngol 1969;89:31–43.

119. Kinnman JEG, Hong CE, Lee EB, Shin HS. Fibrous dysplasia of the face and skull. Pract Oto-Rhino-Laryngol 1969;31:11–21.

120. Brusis T. Extensive deformation of the skull in fibrous dysplasia (Jaffé-Lichtenstein). J Laryngol Otol 1970;49:643–653.

121. Stecker RH. Ossifying fibroma of the middle ear. Arch Otolaryngol 1971;94:80–82.

122. Tembe D. Fibro-osseous dysplasia of temporal bone. J Laryngol Otol 1970;84:107–114.

123. Sharp M. Monostotic fibrous dysplasia of the temporal bone. J Laryngol Otol 1970;84:697–708.

124. Venker DH. Monostotische fibreuze dysplasie uitgaande van de mastoid. Ned Tijdsch Geneeskd 1971;115:327–329.

125. Bouche J, Freck D, Chaix G. Fibrous dysplasia in otorhinolaryngology. Apropos of 17 personal cases. Ann Otolaryngol Chir Cervicafac 1971;88:421–423.

126. Steinbach E. Die Gehörgangstenose als Folge der fibrösen Dysplasie. Arch Klin Exp Ohren-Nasen-Kehlkopfheilkd 1972;202:623–627.

127. Mündnich K. In: Discussion. Steinbach E. Die Gehörgangstenose als Folge der fibrösen Dysplasie. Arch Klin Exp Ohren-Nasen-Kehlkopfheilkd 1972;202:627.

128. Mathieu L, Martin C. Essential fibrous dysplasia: several uniosseous forms of the temporal bone and superior maxillary bone. Ann Odontostomatol (Lyon) 1972;29:87–105.

129. Deringuia BA. Fibrous dysplasia of the temporal bone. Vestn Otorinolaringol 1973;35:88–89.

130. Pokrajcic M. Ostitis fibrosa localisata of the temporal bone. Srp Arh Celok Lek 1972;10:419–421.

131. Sienkiewicz M. A case of fibrotic degeneration of temporal bone. Otolaryngol Pol 1971;25:241–243.

132. Mizuno M. Monostotic fibrous dysplasia. Otolaryngology (Tokyo) 1971;44:15–20.

133. Scott MJ. Nonprogressive calcified mass of the skull involving unilateral cranial nerves. J Neurosurg 1974;40:779–782.

134. Canigiani G, Ferreira CS, Czech W, Wickenhauser J. Beitrag zur fibrosen Dysplasie des Os temporale. Monatsschr Ohrenheilkd Laryngo-Rhinol 1974;108:285–293.

135. Schlumberger HG. Fibrous dysplasia (ossifying fibroma) of the maxilla and mandible. Am J Orthod Oral Surg 1946;32:579–587.

136. Ward PH, Foster CH. Monostotic fibrous dysplasia of the temporal bone. Trans Pac Coast Oto-ophthalmol Soc 1975;56:147–157.

137. Williams DML, Thomas RSA. Fibrous dysplasia. J Laryngol Otol 1975;88:359–374.

138. Ukleja J, Domawiewski J. Case of fibrous osteodysplasia of the temporal bone complicated by cholesteatoma. Otolaryngol Pol 1975;29:605–608.

139. Fernandez E, Calavita U. Fibrous dysplasia of the skull with complete unilateral cranial nerve involvement. Case report. J Neurosurg 1980;52:404–406.

140. Barrinuevo CE, Marcallo FA, Coelho A, Cruz AG, Mocellin M, Patrocinio JA. Fibrous dysplasia and the temporal bone. Arch Otolaryngol 1980;106:298–301.

141. Evans J. Leontiasis ossea. A critical review, with reports of four original cases. J Bone Joint Surg [Br] 1953;35:229–243.

142. Carpes LCF, Cardoso I, Kos AO. Displasia fibrosa monostotica do osso temporal. Rev Bras Otorhinolaryngol 1972;38:108–200.

143. Samant MC, Agarwai MK. Fibrous dysplasia of the mastoid. J Laryngol 1980;94:545–548.

144. Canigiani G, Wickenhauser J. Zur Diagnose und Aktivitätsbeurteilung der fibrösen dyssplasie des Gesichtsschädels und des Schläfenbeines. Radiologe 1982;22:253–259.

145. Nager GT, Kennedy WD, Kopstein E. Fibrous dysplasia. A review of the disease and its manifestations in the temporal bone. Ann Otol Rhinol Laryngol 1982;91(Suppl 92):1–52.

146. Schrimpf R, Karmody CS, Chasin WD, et al. Sclerosing lesions of the temporal bone. Laryngoscope 1982;92:116–119.

147. Nager GT, Holliday MJ. Fibrous dysplasia of the temporal bone. Update with case reports. Ann Otol Rhinol Laryngol 1984;93:630–633.

148. Lambert PR, Brackmann DE. Fibrous dysplasia of the temporal bone: the use of computerized tomography. Otolaryngol Head Neck Surg 1984;92:461–467.

149. Basset JM, Perrin A. Un faux osteom obstructive du canal auditive externa (dysplasie fibreus du temporal). J FORL 1984;33:353–356.

150. Despraux G, Kuffer R, de Roquantcourt A, et al. Quelques affections rare de l'oreille: dysplasie fibreuse du tympanal, rct. Ann Oto-Laryngol (Paris) 1985;102:255–261.

151. Younus M, Haleem A. Monostotic fibrous dysplasia of the temporal bone. J Laryngol 1987;101:1070–1074.

152. Samouha EE, Edelstein DR, Parisier SC. Fibrous dysplasia involving the temporal bone: report of three new cases. Am J Otol 1987;8:103–107.

153. Talmi YP, Zin JB, Shimberger R, et al. Monostotic fibrous dysplasia of the temporal bone. Radiological case of the month. Am J Dis Child 1989;143:1351–1352.

48/ Sclerosteosis

DEFINITION

Sclerosteosis is one of the rare, autosomal recessive, progressive, potentially lethal bone dysplasias in which a poorly understood intrinsic abnormality of bone development results in generalized hyperostosis and sclerosis of the cranium and cortex of the tubular bones. The condition generally manifests at birth as syndactyly, which is usually bilateral, but asymmetrical, and cutaneous, although it is seldom osseous; it involves the second and third fingers regularly, the third and fourth fingers frequently, and the first and second fingers only occasionally. One or more fingers may be reduced in length and distorted, and they may display a radial deviation of the terminal phalanges. The terminal phalanges may be kinked and exhibit various forms of dystrophy of the fingernails. There may be partial cutaneous webbing of the second and third toes. Accelerated skeletal development begins in early childhood, often leading to gigantism and characteristic enlargement and distortion of the calvaria, mandible, clavicles, ribs, and long bones. Hyperostosis and sclerosis are most prominent in the skull and tubular bones. The steep, high forehead, the ocular hypertelorism, the broad and flat root of the nose, the relative midfacial hypoplasia, and the square and prognathic mandible, frequently associated with bilateral facial weakness, are usually apparent at age 10, although in some instances they may manifest themselves earlier, and create an unmistakable facial expression. The complications arise *(a)* from overgrowth of the calvaria, resulting in progressive reduction of the capacity of the cranial cavity, *(b)* from narrowing of the canals for the cranial blood vessels and of the foramina for the cranial nerves, and *(c)* from elevation of the intracranial pressure. Progressive loss of hearing and facial nerve function, which generally appears in childhood, and impairment of vision are common complications. Severe headaches frequently develop in early adulthood, and death may result suddenly from acute compression of the medulla oblongata (1).

The clinical and radiologic features permit early recognition of the disorder and differentiation from similar cranial sclerosing bone dysplasias associated with generalized hyperostosis and sclerosis. The condition is very similar to the autosomal recessive form of endosteal hyperostosis (van Buchem's disease) (2–5). Some authors are of the opinion that the bony abnormalities tend to be more severe in sclerosteosis, but Cremin (6) believes that they are identical. Gorlin (7) has come to the conclusion that sclerosteosis and van Buchem's disease are the same disorder.

HISTORY

Sclerosteosis has been recognized for over half a century. The first description was, in all likelihood, by Hirsch (8). It was Hansen (9) who recognized it as a separate clinical entity, independent of osteopetrosis (10–15). During the past three decades, case reports have also been published by Klintworth (16), Witkop (17), and Sugiura and Yasuhara (18). Cremin, Beighton, Davidson, Durr, Epstein, and Hamersma (6, 19–25) provided the definitive description of the disease.

SKELETAL MANIFESTATIONS

In most patients the disease is evident at birth in the presence of a partial or, rarely, total syndactyly. The hands usually have bilateral but asymmetrical, cutaneous although occasionally osseous union. It involves the second and third fingers most often, the third and fourth fingers frequently, and the first and second fingers rarely (Fig. 48.10A). The cutaneous webbing most often extends only part way to the first interphalangeal articulation and occasionally extends to the distal articulation. Characteristically, one or more digits are foreshortened and deformed, with radial deviation of the terminal phalanges and with different forms of onychodysplasia to the point of total aplasia. The toes also may show cutaneous webbing.

Except for syndactyly and occasionally facial paralysis, patients appear normal at birth. Mandibular prognathism and frontal prominence become noticeable by age 5. The skeletal deformities thereafter progress steadily. Overgrowth of the calvaria, a steeply elevated forehead, ocular hypertelorism, proptosis, a flattened nasal root, relative midfacial hypoplasia, and a square and broadened mandible, together with the bilateral facial paralysis, lead in adulthood to a severe facial deformity marked by a somewhat bizarre expressionless countenance (Figs. 48.2 and 48.16). Children affected with the disease are tall for their age, and affected adults may have gigantism and excessive skeletal mass.

NEUROLOGIC MANIFESTATIONS

Impairment of hearing is frequently a presenting symptom. It is often preceded by recurrent otitis media. It may manifest in early childhood. As a rule, it is bilateral. In the beginning, it is an expression of impairment of sound conduction. Later, it may become associated with a loss of perception. A pure sensorineural hearing loss is an exception. The conductive loss is attributed to ossicular immobilization and jamming of the stapedial arch that resulted from concentric narrowing of the middle ear cavity and distortion of the vestibular fenestra (Figs. 48.22 and 48.23). The sensorineural loss is thought to result from narrowing of the internal acoustic meatus, resulting in cochlear nerve atrophy and degeneration. The loss of vestibular nerve function is explained on the same basis (Figs. 48.18–48.20).

Impairment of facial nerve function is another salient feature. It is observed almost as often as hearing loss. As a rule, it manifests initially as a recurrent unilateral paresis that eventually progresses to a permanent, in general partial, bilateral loss of facial nerve function. The progressive facial paresis is attributed to increasing constriction of the nerve within the Fallopian canal (Figs. 48.18–48.25).

Unilateral impairment and bilateral impairment of vision associated with optic nerve atrophy are infrequent. They generally represent a later complication that develops during the third decade of life.

Headaches are common and often begin in adolescence. They probably reflect a rise in intracranial pressure. Intracranial hypertension has been documented by lumbar puncture and papilledema. Several patients have died suddenly from impaction of the medulla oblongata in the foramen magnum.

Anosmia has been observed in several patients. One possible explanation is constriction of the foramina for the transmission of the olfactory nerves in the cribriform plate.

Involvement of the trigeminal nerve may be another manifestation of the disease. Corneal hypesthesia occurs less frequently. Constriction of the foramen rotundum has been documented by multidirectional tomography.

So far, there has been no report of lower cranial nerve involvement (Fig. 48.27). Constriction of the cervical intervertebral foramina may cause impingement of the respective spinal nerves, resulting in paresthesia, pain, and muscular weakness in the upper limb.

RADIOLOGIC MANIFESTATIONS

Some cranial thickening and increased density may be noticeable in infancy, and widespread changes are well advanced by age 5. Hyperostosis and sclerosis of the skull and tubular bones progress well into the third decade of life, when the disease tends to stabilize. The bones are enlarged in all dimensions (hyperostosis), which accounts for the progressive increases in body length and skeletal mass. Moreover, there is a moderate to marked increase in bony density (sclerosis). In addition, there is a disproportionate thickening of the cortices of many bones. Tubular bones so affected are massive, disproportionately long, and wide. They have less diaphyseal constriction than do normal bones and may have some alteration of the external contours. Flat bones that are involved with disease are abnormally thick. Narrowing of the medullary cavities may occur in some sites, but it is not a striking feature of the disease, and anemia is not a feature of sclerosteosis. Hyperostosis and sclerosis are most prominent in the skull and tubular bones.

In the skull, the changes are greatest in the base of the neurocranium and in the body of the mandible (Fig. 48.3). The base becomes increasingly sclerotic, and the cranial nerve foramina and vascular channels become progressively narrowed (Figs. 48.12–48.14, 48.18–48.25, and 48.27). The internal auditory and facial canals are constricted, and the optic foramina are deformed. The calvaria may be almost as severely affected. The head circumference can be increased, and the width of the vault may be enlarged as much as 3 cm. The overgrowth of the calvaria results in a diminution of cranial capacity. The hyperostosis results in the formation of a steep and elevated forehead, ocular hypertelorism, prominence of the supraorbital rims, and constriction of the orbits. The sella turcica may be enlarged. The mastoid air cells are obliterated, but the paranasal sinuses remain intact. Enlargement of the body of the mandible, which is often

severe, results in prognathism and malocclusion. The mandibular rami are less involved. The facial bones are the least affected, which explains the clinically noticeable relative midfacial hypoplasia.

The long bones are massive, with cortical hyperostosis and some alteration of their external appearance. One of the most prominent features of the disease is the change in the hands (Fig. 48.10). The metacarpals and proximal phalanges are the most severely involved; they lack the usual modeling and are usually gently curved. The middle and distal phalanges, since they are less involved, appear relatively small. They may be more deformed, however. The distal phalanges may show a bizarre radial kinking, most frequent in the index finger. Often the entire finger has a radial deviation. As mentioned above, about 90% of patients have some cutaneous syndactyly, and some also have osseous syndactyly (Fig. 48.10A). The changes involving the metatarsals and phalanges of the feet are similar, and bilateral partial cutaneous webbing of the second and third toes is not infrequent (11, 13, 16).

The clavicles and the ribs are widened and dense. The scapulae and the pelvis are sclerotic and somewhat thickened but are not expanded. The sclerosis in the pelvis tends to spare the iliac wings, which are somewhat narrow.

Case Reports

Case 1. *Sclerosteosis, craniotubular hyperostosis, and sclerosis. Characteristic facial deformity and appearance. Progressive constriction of neural and venous vascular foramina. Involvement of cranial nerves I, II, VII, VIII and X bilaterally; dysarthria and ataxia. Progressive elevation of intracranial pressure. Accelerated, excessive growth. Cutaneous syndactyly of left second, third, and fourth fingers. Hyperostosis and sclerosis of temporal bones with concentric narrowing of internal and external auditory canals, Fallopian canal, and middle ear cleft. Decompression of right transverse and sigmoid sinus for relief of total extrinsic jugular outflow obstruction.*

The patient was a black girl age 11 years 9 months with three distant relatives reported to have sclerosteosis (Witkop CJ, personal communication). She was born with cutaneous syndactyly involving the left second, third, and fourth fingers that required surgical correction (Fig. 48.10A). Onset of gradual loss of hearing was first suspected at age 3, when the patient received five aspiration myringotomies for recurrent serous otitis media. The audiogram at age 6 revealed a flat bilateral conductive hearing impairment with an average pure-tone loss of 35 dB in the speech frequency range. At age 10 years 9 months, the patient developed bifrontal headaches with progressive difficulties with vision and was found to have bilateral optic nerve atrophy with marked elevation of intracranial pressure.

On *admission* at age 11 years 9 months, the patient's height was 177 cm (Fig. 48.1), and her weight was 75 kg. Her face was ovoid, with a steep and high forehead. She had ocular hypertelorism, slight exophthalmos, broadening of the nasal base, relative hypoplasia of the midfacial area, and a square, prognathic mandible. A bilateral facial nerve paresis added to the characteristic expressionless facial appearance (Fig. 48.2).

Neurologic examination revealed: (a) slight hyposmia, (b) bilateral optic nerve atrophy, (c) bilateral facial nerve paresis, (d) slight tenth nerve paresis, and (e) mild dysarthria and ataxia.

Radiologic examination of the skull showed a significant increase in the diameter and density of the calvaria, with apparent obliteration of the diploic space. Hyperostosis and sclerosis were most prominent in the base and temporal bones (Figs. 48.3, 48.12, and 48.13). The body of the mandible showed distinct hyperplasia. The foramina of

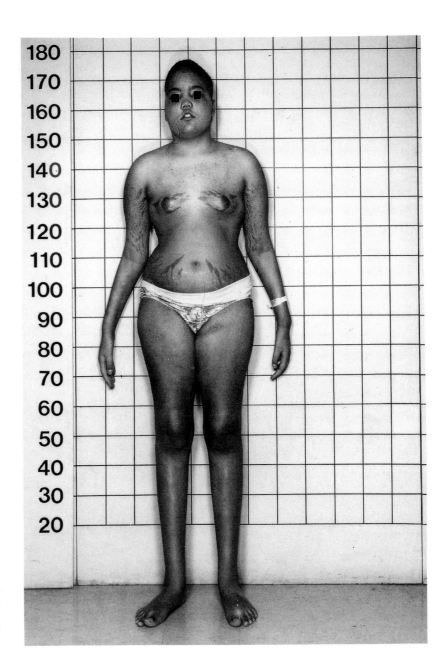

Figure 48.1. Girl age 11 years 9 months whose accelerated skeletal development began early in childhood, resulting in elongation of tubular bones with excessive height at 177 cm.

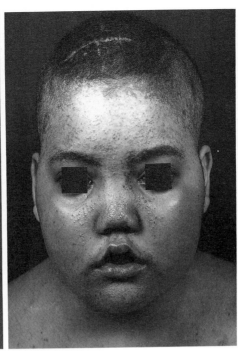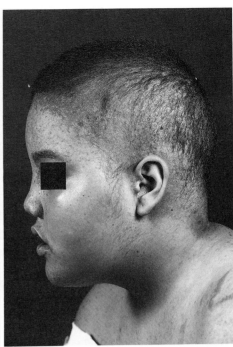

Figure 48.2. The high forehead, the ocular hypertelorism, the broad root of the nose, the relative midfacial hypoplasia, and the square and prognathic mandible associated with the bilateral facial paresis create the unmistakable facial expression.

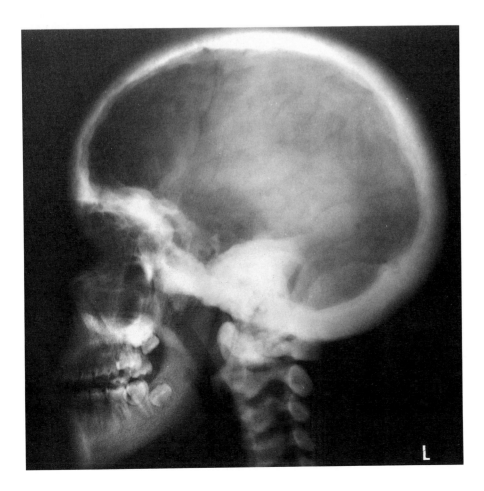

Figure 48.3. Lateral radiograph of skull. The striking increase in thickness and density of most bones is greatest in the base of the neurocranium, especially in the petrous portions of the temporal bones. The calvaria shows slight involvement; the hyperostosis and sclerosis of the inner and outer tables appear to have obliterated the diploë. The sella turcica is enlarged, and the inner cortex is lost along the floor and the dorsum. No mastoid air cells are visible, yet the paranasal sinuses are well pneumatized. The body of the mandible is greatly thickened.

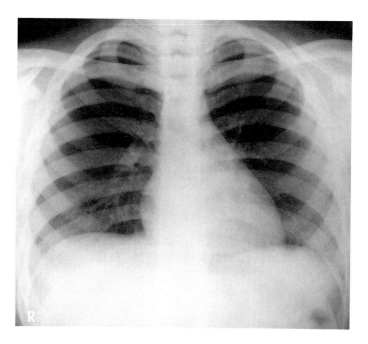

Figure 48.4. Anteroposterior (AP radiograph of chest. The increased diameter and the density of the clavicles and ribs are clearly visible.

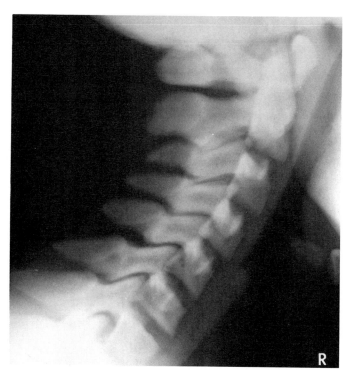

Figure 48.5. Lateral radiograph of cervical spine. There is diffuse sclerosis of all portions of the cervical vertebrae, but the third through sixth vertebral bodies are partially spared.

exit for cranial nerves II, V, and VII–XII displayed obvious concentric narrowing bilaterally.

The clavicles and ribs were wide and sclerotic (Fig. 48.4). Sclerosis was more striking in the spine than that seen in most reported cases, and only in the thoracic and midcervical regions was there some sparing of the vertebral bodies (Figs. 48.5 and 48.6). The pelvis showed a marked sclerosis but no hyperostosis (Fig. 48.7).

The long bones were enlarged, and the cortices were thick and sclerotic. The epiphyseal ossification centers were much less affected than other portions of the bones, so that many epiphyses appeared to be relatively flat (Figs. 48.8 and 48.9). In the hand, cutaneous syndactyly was still recognizable, even though the major portion had been surgically corrected on the left side. The metacarpal and phalangeal bones showed striking changes. The abnormalities in the feet were as severe as those in the hands (Fig. 48.10*A* and *B*).

Computed tomography of the skull and brain confirmed the calvarial thickening. It also showed a moderate, bilateral parietal lobe atrophy but no ventricular abnormality.

Otologic examination revealed a slight concentric narrowing of the osseous external auditory canals and a firm fixation of the malleus bilaterally. Cochlear function studies showed a bilateral asymmetrical conductive hearing loss with a speech reception threshold of 55 dB in the right ear and 35 dB in the left ear (Fig. 48.11). Discrimination was 100% bilaterally. Electronystagmographic studies displayed a vertical nystagmus, increasing on right and left lateral gaze. Caloric responses were markedly diminished. Eye tracking and refixation movements were severely disturbed. Radiographs of the temporal bones, including multidirectional tomograms, revealed a strikingly severe diffuse hyperostosis and sclerosis of all portions of the temporal bones. The middle ear clefts were markedly constricted (Figs. 48.12 and 48.13). The internal acoustic and facial canals displayed an almost thread-like lumen. The lower portion of the sigmoid groove and the jugular foramen were almost totally obliterated (Figs. 48.12 and 48.13). The venous phase of the carotid angiogram demonstrated marked narrowing of the left transverse sinus and sigmoid sinus, almost complete obstruction of the lower segment of the right sigmoid sinus, and near-total occlusion of the right jugular bulb (Fig. 48.14*A*). The right and left jugular venograms showed a min-

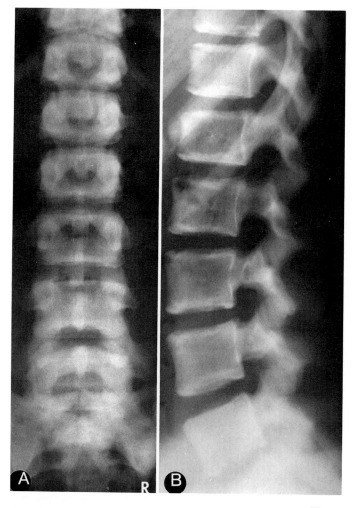

Figure 48.6. AP and right lateral radiographs of lumbar spine. There is moderately severe generalized sclerosis, without the sparing of the vertebral bodies reported in other cases.

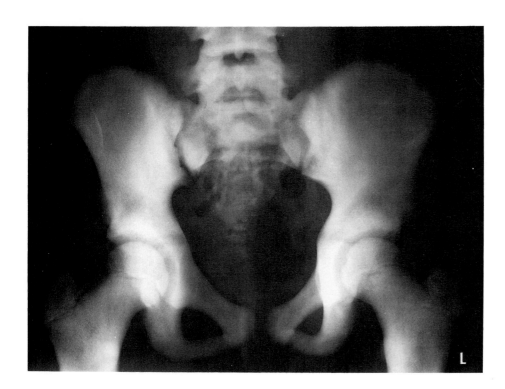

Figure 48.7. Posteroanterior (PA) radiograph of pelvis. The generalized sclerosis is quite striking, yet the bones do not appear disproportionately wide. Notice the normal proportion of the ischial and pubic rami. The sclerosis is greatest along the medial portions of the iliac bones and about the acetabular cavities.

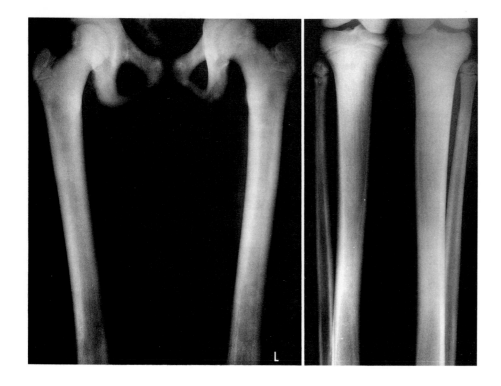

Figure 48.8. AP radiographs of upper and lower legs. The long bones are sclerotic and elongated, especially in the diaphyses. There is some cortical thickening but no widening of the medullary cavities.

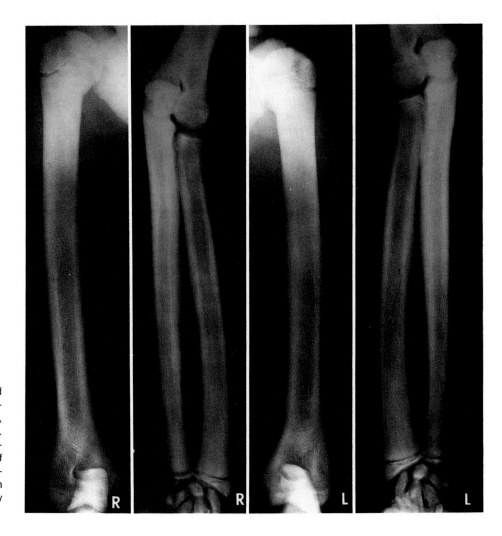

Figure 48.9. AP radiographs of arms and forearms. The bones are sclerotic and relatively widened, particularly in the diaphyses, which accounts for the decreased modeling. Although the cortices are thickened, the medullary cavities are only slightly expanded or of normal width in most areas. The epiphyseal ossification centers are much less affected than the rest of the bones and appear moderately flattened in the elbow and wrist.

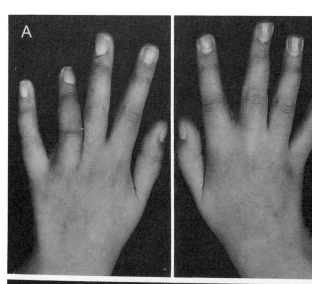

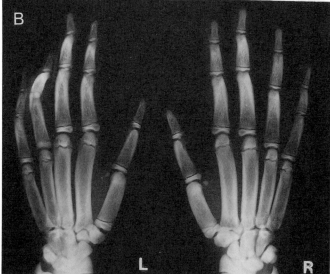

Figure 48.10. A. Slight cutaneous syndactyly involving the second, third, and fourth digits, moderate camptodactyly of left fourth digit and slight camptodactyly of other digits, slight onychodysplasia of left third digit, and tendency toward axial deviation of some digits.

Figure 48.10. B. PA radiographs of hands. The carpal bones and the epiphyseal ossification centers of the distal parts of the radius and ulna are of about normal size. The other bones are strikingly elongated and disproportionately wide. The changes are most marked in the second and third rays. Except in the thumbs, all of the metacarpals and phalanges show a slight radial bowing. The deformity of the left ring finger is the result of contracture of the proximal interphalangeal joint and moderate bowing of the middle phalanx.

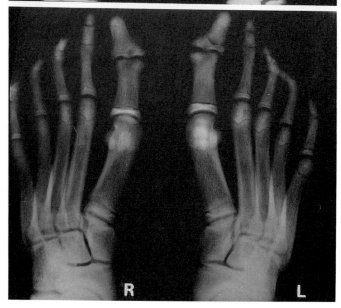

Figure 48.10. C. Dorsal-plantar radiographs of feet. The changes in the metatarsals and phalanges are similar to those in the hands except that the phalanges and medial metacarpals are less bowed. The middle and distal phalanges are relatively short, and there is hallux valgus.

imal remaining lumen of the left sigmoid sinus and jugular bulb and extreme constriction of the right jugular bulb (Fig. 48.14B).

At *operation*, because of the increased intracranial pressure associated with jugular outflow obstruction and bilateral facial paresis, the right sigmoid sinus, the right jugular bulb, and almost the entire right facial nerve were decompressed. Antrum, aditus, and attic were extremely constricted. The lumina of the lower portion of the sigmoid sinus and of the jugular bulb were maximally constricted. After the decompression, however, these venous channels reexpanded to their original normal sizes. Concentric new bone formation resulted in a very marked constriction of the entire middle ear cleft immobi-

lization of the ossicular chain, fracture of the stapedial arch at the base, and narrowing and distortion of the oval window niche. The posterior cranial fossa and the foramen magnum were decompressed in a second stage by the neurosurgeon. The patient made an uneventful recovery, her vision and mental functions improved remarkably, and intracranial pressure returned to normal and remained so for the next couple of years. Biopsy of the right mastoid process revealed conspicuous broadening of the bony trabeculae of the spongiosa, resulting in progressive obliteration of the marrow spaces and sclerosis (Fig. 48.15).

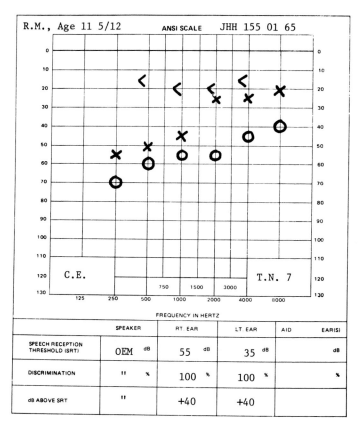

Figure 48.11. Audiogram of patient in Case 1.

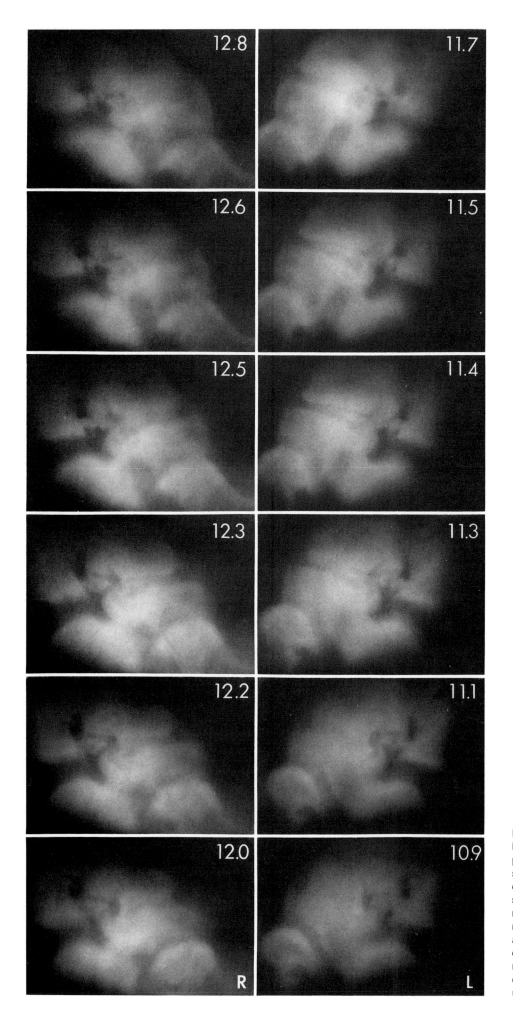

Figure 48.12. AP polytomograms of right and left temporal bones at corresponding levels. All portions of the temporal bone are massive in size and sclerotic. The hyperostosis resulted in complete obliteration of air cells and marrow spaces and in severe constriction of the internal auditory canal, middle ear cleft, and external auditory meatus (*Sects. 12.5* and *12.3* (right), and *11.5* and *11.4* (left)). These structural changes eventually led to compression of cranial nerves, immobilization of middle ear ossicles, and distortion of the cochlear and vestibular fenestrae.

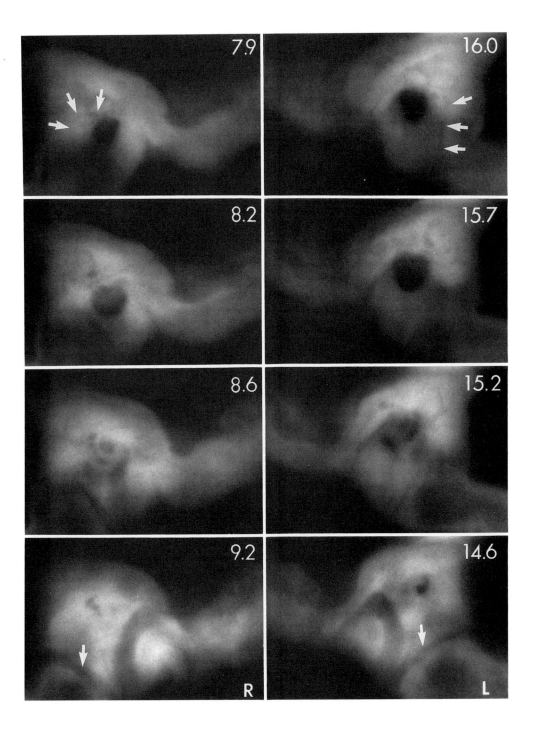

Figure 48.13. Lateral polytomograms of right and left temporal bones. The narrowing of the epitympanic recess, the enlargement of the outer middle ear ossicles, and the distortion and constriction of the tympanic and mastoid segments of the Fallopian canal *(arrows)* are recognizable in *Sections 7.9* (right) and *16.0* (left). The carotid canal appears normal, but the inferior portion of the sigmoid groove and the jugular foramen *(arrows)* are almost totally obliterated (*Sects. 9.2* (right) and *14.6* (left)).

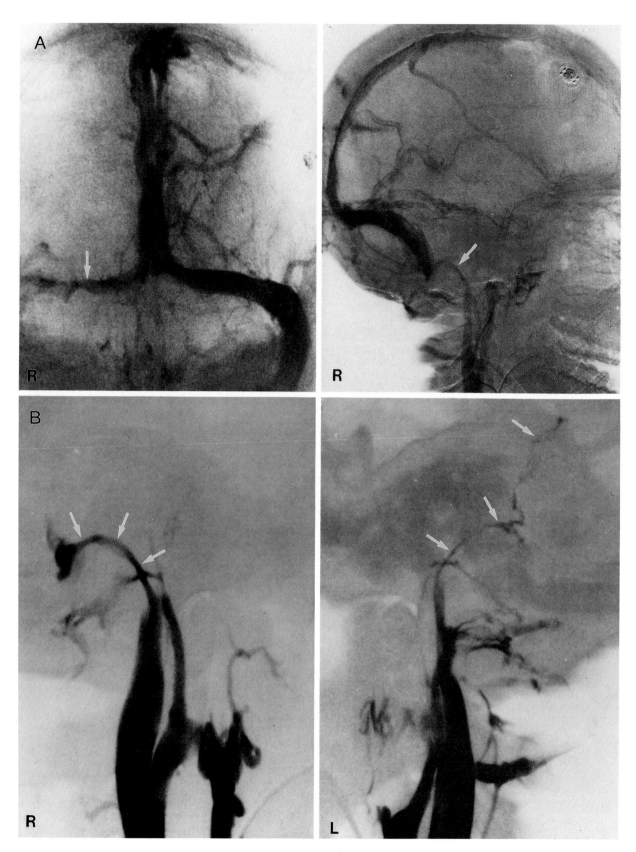

Figure 48.14. **A.** *Left:* Venous phase of carotid angiogram, AP subtraction study. The severe constriction of the left transverse sinus *(arrow)* with total occlusion at its junction with the left sigmoid sinus and the near-total obliteration of the caudad end of the right sigmoid sinus are well shown. *Right:* Venous phase of carotid angiogram, right lateral subtraction study. The near-total occlusion of the right jugular bulb and the adjacent sigmoid sinus are clearly evident *(arrow)*. The diploë, which appears to be obliterated on the standard radiographs (Fig. 48.2), is clearly shown to be preserved and relatively thick on this and the other subtraction studies. **B.** Right and left retrograde jugular venograms confirm the thread-like lumen of the left jugular bulb and sigmoid sinus *(arrows)* and the extreme narrowing of the right jugular bulb *(arrows)*.

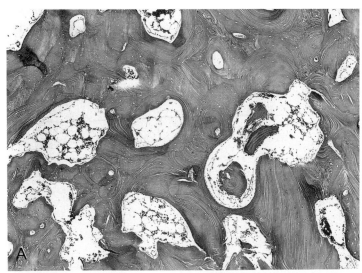

Figure 48.15. **A.** Biopsy from right mastoid process. Progressive obliteration of the marrow spaces caused by widening of the bony trabeculae and minimal bone remodeling have led to advanced sclerosis of the spongiosa in the tip of the mastoid. (Hematoxylin and eosin, ×65.)

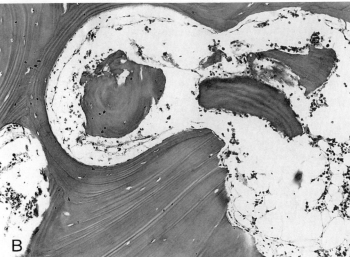

Figure 48.15. **B.** The osseous lamellae are arranged in parallel and concentric patterns. (×175.)

Case 2. *Sclerosteosis, craniotubular hyperostosis, and sclerosis with typical facial deformity and features. Excessive growth. Involvement of cranial nerves II, VII, and VIII. History of recurrent episodes of alternating facial palsy and subsequent progressive bilateral facial paresis since age 18 months. Decompression of mastoid segment of right facial nerve at age 11. Long-standing history of progressive headaches. History of decompression of right anterior cranial fossa and unroofing of right orbit for acute loss of vision in right eye. Hyperostosis and sclerosis of temporal bones with extreme narrowing of internal acoustic and Fallopian canal and middle ear cleft. Total obliteration of tympanic segment of Fallopian canal with expulsion of facial nerve into severely constricted and distorted round window niche. Compression fixation of stapes. Complete obliteration of round window niche. Progressive headaches during past 7 years. Sudden death presumably from acute compression of medulla oblongata.*

The patient was a 31-year-old Afrikaner man with no family history of sclerosteosis. His clinical features were previously discussed by Klintworth (16) and Hamersma (25). At age 18 months, the patient developed recurrent episodes of facial palsy, which initially were unilateral, affecting each side alternately, lasting about 3 months and subsequently becoming bilateral. The recoveries were incomplete and left the patient with synkinesis and muscle contractions.

At *operation,* at age 11 years, he underwent a surgical decompression of the vertical segment of the right facial nerve. The stapes was found to be fixed in a narrow oval window niche. By age 18 years, the bilateral facial palsy had become complete with no detectable muscle contraction on either side, and a reconstructive procedure was performed to correct the drooping of his lower lip (Fig. 48.16). Progressive bilateral hearing loss had been noticed before age 10 years, requiring him to wear a hearing aid in the left ear. He had had a long history of headaches.

On *physical examination,* at age 23 years, the patient's height was 199.4 cm, and his weight was 90.7 kg. His head was large with a circumference of 65 cm (Fig. 48.16). The forehead was high and steep. There was a marked ocular hypertelorism, exophthalmos, and proptosis. The root of the nose was flat and broad, and the mandible was square and prognathic. The midfacial area appeared hypoplastic. Complete bilateral facial palsy prevented closure of the mouth and both eyes and created an unmistakable facial expression (Fig. 48.16).

Radiologic examination of the skull revealed marked hyperostosis and sclerosis of the calvaria and base. At age 24 years, he suffered an acute loss of vision in the right eye and consequently underwent an anterior fossa decompression and an unroofing of the right orbit. The right optic nerve appeared unremarkable at that time, but the orbital cavity had become quite constricted.

Otologic examination revealed a severe bilateral conductive hearing loss with some loss of bone conduction up to 2000 Hz, with a sharp high-frequency loss, an average pure-tone loss of 60 dB, and a discrimination score of 100% in both ears (Fig. 48.17). During the subsequent 7 years the patient continued to have severe headaches. He later died suddenly in his office, presumably from an acute compression of the medulla oblongata.

Examination of the temporal bones reveals immediately apparent histologic features of sclerosteosis involving the temporal bone: *(a)* the overall increase in size or hyperostosis, *(b)* the increased bony density or sclerosis, and *(c)* their effect on the structures within the petrous pyramid. Hyperostosis and sclerosis are the result of *(a)* an increase in apposition of lamellar bone laid down by the periosteum covering the petrous pyramid (Figs. 48.18 and 48.19) and lining the major vascular and neural channels traversing it (Figs. 48.18–48.23, 48.26, and 48.27) and *(b)* deposition of lamellar bone in the spongiosa of the petrous pyramid (Figs. 48.22–48.26). Since the abnormal modeling is restricted to the lamellar bone, the endochondral and endosteal bone of the cochlear and vestibular capsules are un-

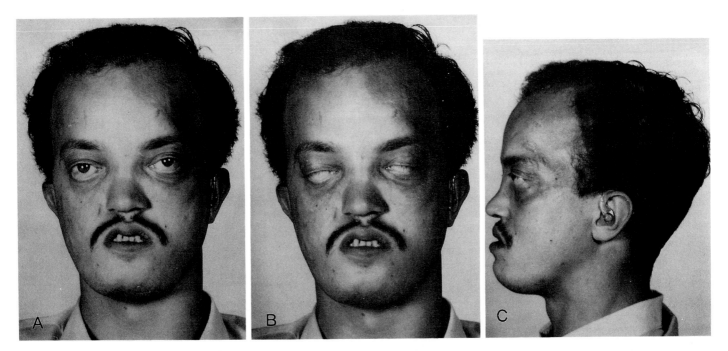

Figure 48.16. Patient at 23 years of age. **A.** and **C.** Enlargement of the head, high and steep forehead, ocular hypertelorism, exophthalmos and proptosis, the flat and broad root of the nose, and the square and progna- thic mandible are readily recognizable. **B.** Bilateral facial palsy prevented closure of the eyes and mouth and created, with the midfacial hypoplasia, unmistakable facial expression.

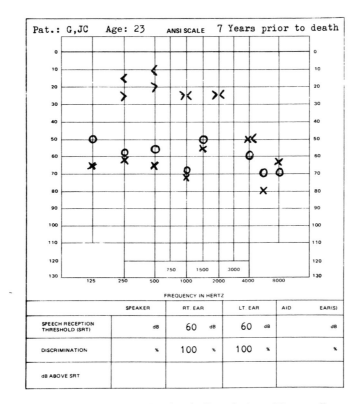

Figure 48.17. Audiogram of patient in Case 2 at age 23 years, 7 years before death.

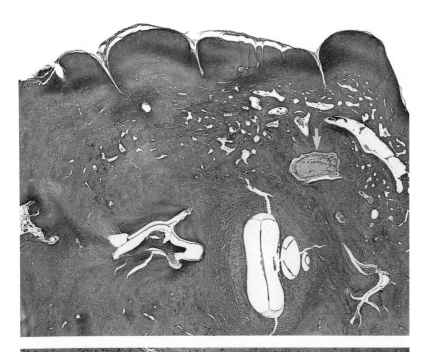

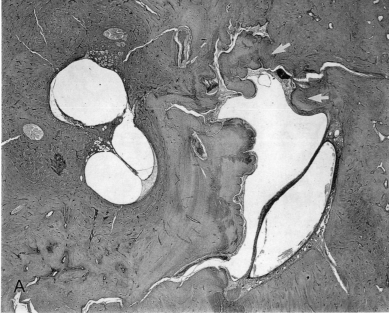

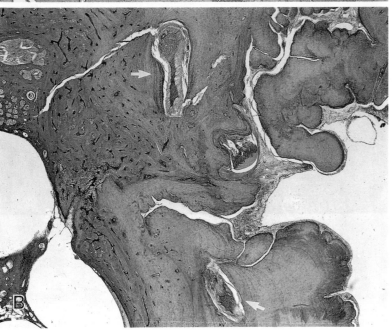

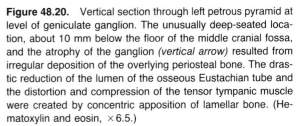

Figure 48.20. Vertical section through left petrous pyramid at level of geniculate ganglion. The unusually deep-seated location, about 10 mm below the floor of the middle cranial fossa, and the atrophy of the ganglion *(vertical arrow)* resulted from irregular deposition of the overlying periosteal bone. The drastic reduction of the lumen of the osseous Eustachian tube and the distortion and compression of the tensor tympanic muscle were created by concentric apposition of lamellar bone. (Hematoxylin and eosin, ×6.5.)

Figure 48.21. **A** and **B.** Vertical section through right petrous pyramid anterior to oval window. The anterior tympanic segment of the Fallopian canal is deeply embedded (**B,** *arrow*) and severely constricted, and the epitympanic space is almost totally obliterated by the new lamellar bone formation (**A,** *arrow*). (Hematoxylin and eosin, ×10.3 and 32.5, respectively.)

affected, and their configuration and the architecture of the cochlear modiolus remain unaltered (Fig. 48.19). The disease, however, does affect all structures made of lamellar bone, such as the cortex of the temporal bone, the boundaries of the middle ear cleft, the architecture of the oval and round windows, and the ossicular chain. It also affects the Fallopian canal, the canals for the carotid artery, sigmoid sinus, and jugular bulb, the passages for the ninth, tenth, and eleventh cranial nerves, and the internal and external auditory canals. It slightly alters the configuration of the cochlear and vestibular aqueducts and the intraosseous portion of the endolymphatic sac. In addition, it results in an obliteration of the majority of marrow spaces and possibly of previously existing air cells. Periosteal new bone formations are compromising the lumen of the external auditory canals and, by entrapment of squamous epithelium, have given rise to a large external cholesteatoma in the left outer ear canal (Fig. 48.27A). The internal auditory canals have become constricted to a thread-like lumen, causing a severe pressure atrophy of the cochlear, vestibular, and facial nerves and their branches (Figs. 48.18, 48.20, 48.21, and 48.27) and a slight reduction of the cell population of the spiral and vestibular ganglia. The lumen of the Fallopian canal rapidly decreases along the course of the tympanic segment of the facial canal (Figs. 48.20 and 48.21) to become totally obliterated above the oval window after the facial nerve has been forcibly extruded into the oval window niche (Figs. 48.22 and 48.23). The severely atrophic nerve continues its course thereafter to the stylomastoid foramen in a very small canal (Fig. 48.25A). The Eustachian tube is severely affected in its cartilaginous portion by extrinsic compression. New bone formations almost completely obliterate its lumen along its osseous portion (Fig. 48.26). Extensive proliferations of periosteal bone arising from the walls of the middle ear cavity have obliterated the greater portion of the middle ear space (Fig. 48.23), almost occluded the oval and round windows, and immobilized the stapedial arch by compression (Fig. 48.23). In a similar fashion, malleus and incus

have become totally immobilized in the attic and aditus by a concentric compression of new bone formations and even by bony ankylosis (Figs. 48.24 and 48.25). The communication from the aditus to the antrum has become reduced to a small cleft (Figs. 48.21, 48.25, and 48.27). Continuous proliferation of lamellar bone has led to thickening of the bony trabeculae and progressive obliteration of once-existing air cells and marrow spaces and therefore to massive sclerosis of the entire temporal bone. The bony canal of the internal carotid artery has become reduced in diameter, and the caliber of the internal carotid artery has accordingly become considerably smaller (Figs. 48.18 and 48.26). The lumen of the sigmoid sinuses is markedly reduced. Both jugular bulbs are narrow. The right one displays a severe stenosis as a result of a localized proliferation of periosteal bone (Fig. 48.27B). The foramina of exit for cranial nerves IX, X and XI are somewhat reduced in diameter but not to the extent of compressing the nerves (Fig. 48.27A and C). On the right a localized proliferation of periosteal bone severely compromises the passage of the glossopharyngeal nerve within the neural compartment of the jugular foramen (Fig. 48.27A). Both cochlear aqueducts are completely obliterated near their junction with the lower basal turn of the cochlea. The vestibular aqueducts, however, are patent.

The structural changes found can fully explain the mechanisms involved in the malfunction of the Eustachian tube, in the interference with sound conduction, and in the impairment of cochlear, vestibular, and facial nerve function. They demonstrate how the proliferation of bone in the external auditory meatus can give rise to external canal cholesteatomas with their local and other potential secondary complications. Most important, perhaps, they clearly delineate the principles involved in the reduction of the arterial blood supply to the brain and in the spectacular interference with the venous drainage from the brain that may well represent one of the main reasons ultimately responsible for the lethal complications of the disease.

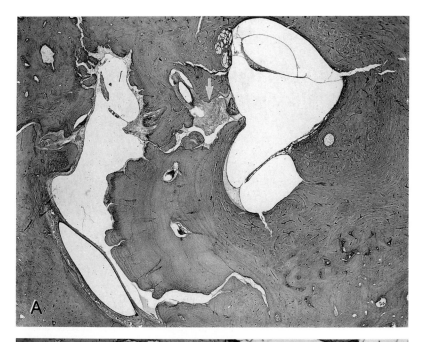

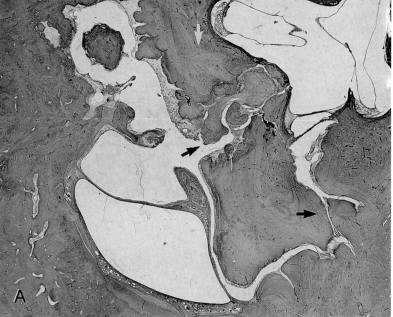

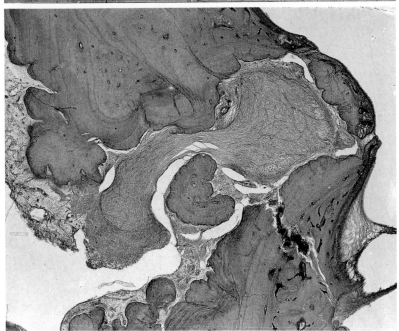

Figure 48.22. Vertical sections through right **(A)** and left **(B, opposite page)** temporal bone level of anterior portion of stapes footplate. The facial nerve is being squeezed out of the Fallopian canal into the oval window niche by concentric apposition of the lamellar bone *(vertical arrows)*. The proliferation of periosteal bone resulted in an almost complete obliteration of the window niches *(oblique arrow)*. The enormous hyperostosis of the promontory nearly reaches the undersurface of the tympanic membranes *(horizontal arrow)*. (Hematoxylin and eosin, ×10.3.)

Figure 48.23. Vertical sections through right **(A)** and left **(B, opposite page)** temporal bones at level of oval and round windows. The Fallopian canal has become totally obliterated by bone *(vertical arrows)*. The extruded facial nerve occupies all of the available space in the constricted oval window niche within and around the stapedial arch. The increase in thickness and irregularity of the middle ear portion of the stapedial footplate and the anterior stapedial crus reflects the participation of these structures in the proliferation of lamellar bone. Concentric apposition of bone from the lower promontory and the floor of the hypotympanum created an almost complete occlusion of the round window niches *(horizontal arrows)*. The greater portion of the tympanic cavities is occupied by bone. (Hematoxylin and eosin, ×10.3 and 32.2, respectively.)

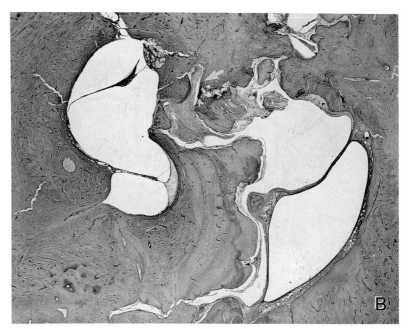

Figure 48.22.   B.

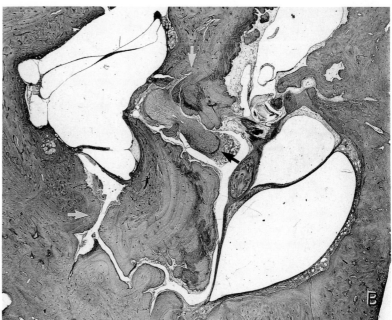

Figure 48.23.   B.

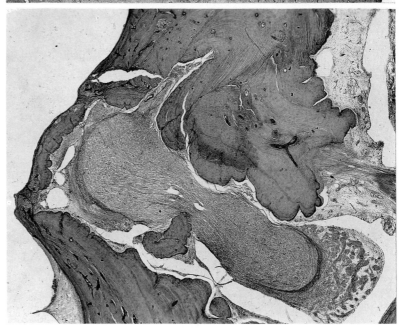

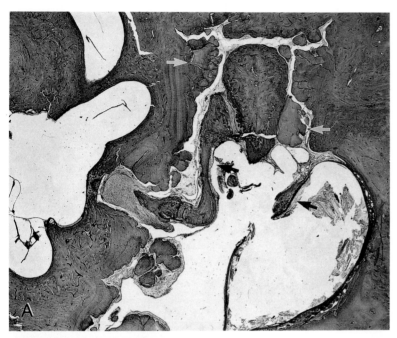

Figure 48.24. A and B (opposite page). Vertical sections through left temporal bone at level of ossicular chain. Massive concentric proliferations of lamellar bone from the walls of the attic produced jamming and osseous ankylosis in several locations *(horizontal arrows)*. The malleus and incus show evidence of increased replacement of endochondral bone and obliteration of marrow spaces by lamellar bone. A large external canal cholesteatoma extends through a central tympanic membrane perforation into the middle ear cavity and has begun to erode the long process of the incus *(oblique arrows)*. (Hematoxylin and eosin, ×10.3 and ×28.4, respectively.)

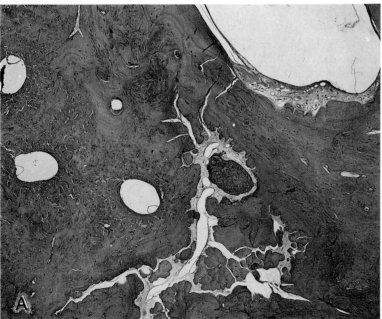

Figure 48.25. Vertical sections through right **(A)** and left **(B, opposite page)** temporal bones at level of short process of incus. Mushroom-like proliferations of lamellar bone arising from the walls of the aditus jam the incus and form solid bony ankyloses in several locations *(horizontal arrows)*. Only a small cleft of an air space remains as a communication with the antrum *(vertical arrow)*. Atrophy of the left facial nerve within the obviously constricted mastoid segment of the Fallopian canal is easily recognizable *(oblique arrow)*. Irregular sphere-like bony formations compromise the lumen of the left external auditory canal *(oblique arrow)*. (Hematoxylin and eosin, ×10.3.)

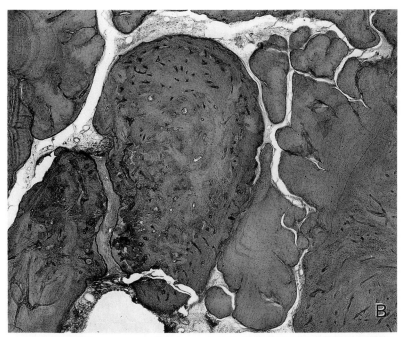

Figure 48.24.   B.

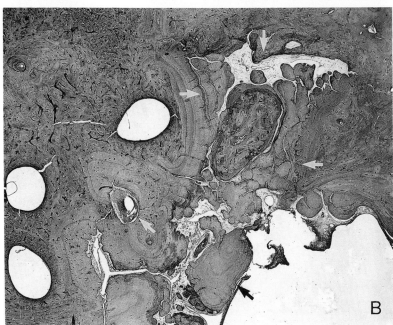

Figure 48.25.   B.

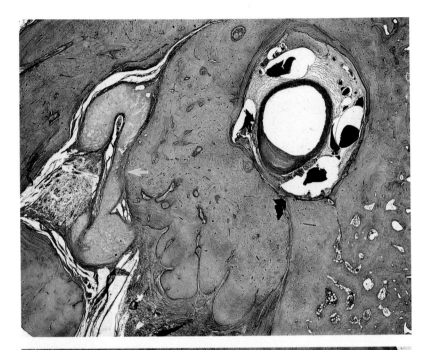

Figure 48.26. Vertical section through right petrous apex, demonstrating narrowing of bony canal of internal carotid artery and vessel lumen. Proliferation of lamellar bone lateral to the carotid canal produced an extrinsic compression of the cartilaginous portion of the Eustachian tube *(arrow)*. (Hematoxylin and eosin, ×10.3.)

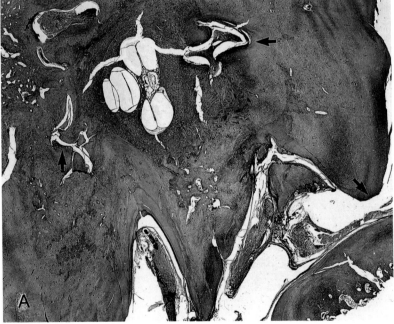

Figure 48.27.   A. Vertical section through right petrous pyramid at level of neural compartment of jugular foramen. The thread-like internal acoustic meatus contains the extremely atrophic seventh and eighth cranial nerves *(horizontal arrow)*. A star-like cleft *(vertical arrow)* represents the collapsed osseous portion of the Eustachian tube. Intrinsic and extrinsic new bone formation resulted in narrowing of the bony canals of the ninth and tenth cranial nerves and almost total obliteration of their intracranial apertures *(oblique arrows)*. (Hematoxylin and eosin, ×5.3.)

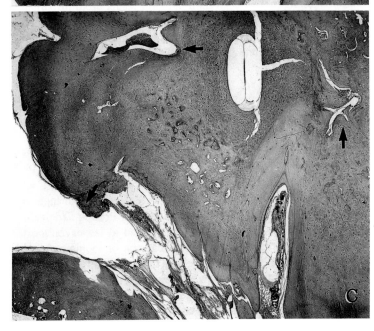

Figure 48.27.   B. Vertical section through right temporal bone at level of jugular bulb. A broad-based hemispherical proliferation of periosteal bone almost completely obliterates the already severely reduced vascular lumen *(arrow).* (×5.2.)

Figure 48.27.   C. Vertical section through left petrous pyramid at level of neural compartment of jugular foramen. As on the opposite side, the internal acoustic meatus and its containing nerves, the osseous canals of the glossopharyngeal and vagus nerve, and their respective nerves, and the Eustachian tube display the same degree of constriction and atrophy *(arrows).* (×5.3.)

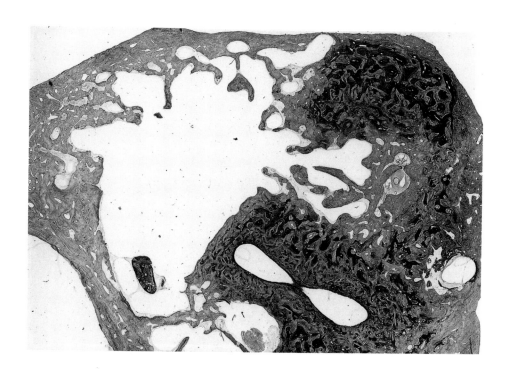

Figure 50.7. Vertical section through right temporal bone near posterior tangent of lateral semicircular canal. Cross-section through non-ampullated end of posterior semicircular canal reveals extensive destruction of its bony wall with creation of a fistula. (Hematoxylin and eosin, ×7.)

Case 2.

A 41-year-old man was admitted to the Francis Scott Key Medical Center (formerly Baltimore City Hospital) in July 1929 with cough for 5 months, chest pain, and weight loss. The clinical diagnosis was advanced bronchogenic carcinoma involving the left recurrent laryngeal nerve and secondary pneumonitis documented by history, physical findings, and radiographs. The serologic test for syphilis was negative and sputum tests for acid-fast bacilli were negative. Four months after admission death occurred after a progressive febrile course.

Otologic examination was made 4 months prior to death. The patient denied any difficulties with hearing and control of balance. The external canals, tympanic membranes, and middle ears appeared normal. The 512 steel fork did not refer, air conduction was better than bone conduction, and bone conduction was normal bilaterally. The audiogram showed an abrupt, bilateral loss of acuity for all frequencies above 1024 Hz by air conduction.

Postmortem examination showed: *(a)* squamous cell carcinoma of the left bronchus with metastases to the right lung, pericardium, hilar lymph nodes, liver, kidneys, suprarenals, and spleen; *(b)* tumor involvement of the left recurrent laryngeal nerve; *(c)* dilatation of the heart and chronic passive congestion of the lungs and viscera; *(d)* generalized arteriosclerosis; *(e)* no abnormalities in the brain and meninges; and *(f)* no macroscopic or microscopic evidence of syphilis. The locations of osseous lesions and temporal bone sections are shown in Figures 50.1 and 50.8–50.21.

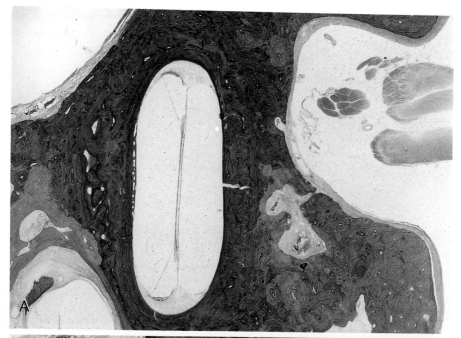

Figure 50.17. **A.** Vertical sections through right temporal bone near center of basal turn of cochlea with two osseous lesions adjacent to anterolateral wall of internal auditory canal. (Hematoxylin and eosin, ×11.5.)

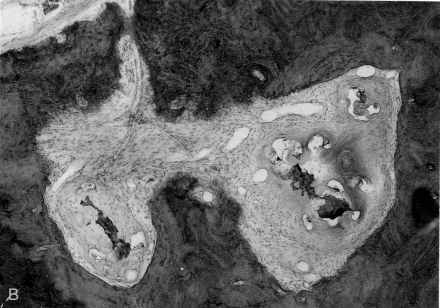

Figure 50.17. **B.** In two adjacent lesions, bony sequestra are embedded in partially necrotic fibrous tissue surrounded by granulation tissue including mostly empty calcified irregular cystic spaces. (×110.)

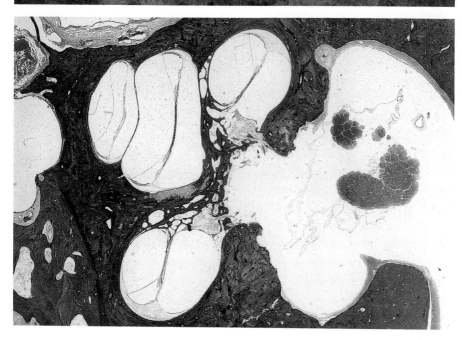

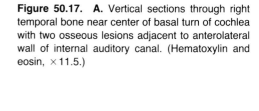

Figure 50.18. Vertical, anterior, paramodiolar section through right cochlea with small osseous lesion in superolateral wall of internal auditory canal adjacent to dura. (Hematoxylin and eosin, ×11.5.)

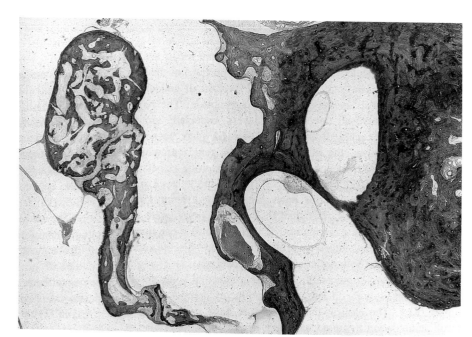

Figure 50.19. Vertical section of right temporal bone at level of ossicular chain. Multiple osseous lesions with bony sequestra are disseminated throughout the malleus and incus, resulting in localized synostosis of the incudomalleolar articulation. (Hematoxylin and eosin, ×11.)

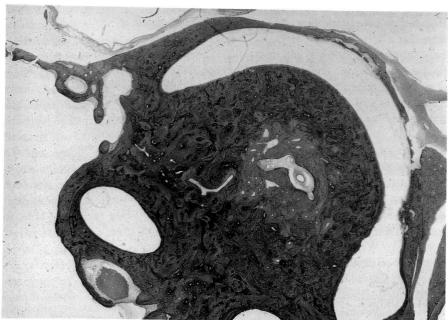

Figure 50.20. Vertical section through right temporal bone at level of superior semicircular canal. An extensive osseous lesion involves the outer bony canal wall. The dura is over the necrotic bone. Underlying the sequestrated bone is an almost acellular, reactive connective tissue that protrudes in several places into the canal lumen. (Hematoxylin and eosin, ×11.)

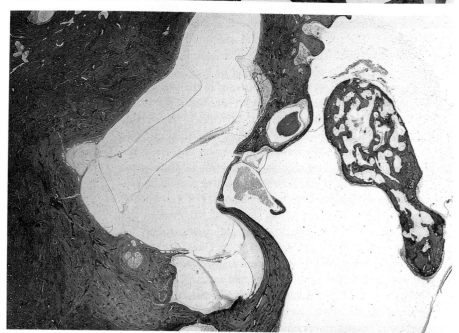

Figure 50.21. Vertical section through left temporal bone at level of oval window. The extent of osseous lesions involving the left malleus, with the formation of bony sequestra, is identical with that found in the right malleus. (Hematoxylin and eosin, ×11.5.)

51/ Craniotubular Scleroses

Part 1
Osteopathia Striata

Linear striations in the tubular bones and pelvis were first observed in several members of a family in 1921 (1), but it was only after 1950 that its association with cranial sclerosis was recognized (2) and that impairment of hearing was considered part of this syndrome (3). Its autosomal dominant inheritance was established in 1972 (2).

The clinical expression of osteopathia striata is considerably varied, with some affected individuals being essentially asymptomatic. Craniomegaly, a square configuration of the face, frontal bossing, impairment of hearing, and radiodense vertical striations in the predominantly long tubular bones represent the most prominent clinical features (2).

RADIOGRAPHIC MANIFESTATIONS

The head is frequently enlarged. The calvaria, skull base, and temporal bones are sclerotic and frequently display hyperostosis. The paranasal sinuses may be totally or partially obliterated. The frontal sinuses can be aplastic. The ribs and pelvis may exhibit patchy sclerosis, and the iliac bones occasionally demonstrate fan-shaped linear striations. In general, delicate but occasionally more coarse radiodense vertical striations are characteristic findings predominantly in the long tubular bones. The femoral neck, the distal femur, and the proximal tibia are their predilective locations. Patchy sclerosis may be found in the carpus and torus as well as in the diaphyses of the long bones (2).

The hearing loss associated with this disease results from progressive narrowing of the middle ear cleft with impingement on and immobilization of the ossicular chain and distortion of the vestibular fenestra with jamming of the stapes footplate.

Case Reports

Case 1. *Osteopathia striata with extensive sclerosis and hyperostosis of calvaria, skull base, and facial and temporal bones. Smallness and constriction of orbits with narrowing of optic foramina. Complete obliteration of frontal and sphenoid sinuses, partial occlusion of ethmoid and maxillary sinuses. Upward slanting and narrowing of external and internal auditory canals. Severe constriction of middle ear clefts with immobilization of ossicular chain on right side. History of progressive hearing loss since age 4, requiring a hearing aid at age 9, and ear troubles associated with Eustachian tube dysfunction and recurrent malodorous otor-*

rhea. Maximal conductive hearing loss of right ear and mild mixed hearing impairment of left ear. Incipient cortical cataracts. Striking vertical radiodense striations in head, neck, and distal ends of femora and proximal ends of tibiae. Diabetes mellitus. Family history of diabetes in grandmothers and great grandmothers on both sides and one aunt with similar abnormal head configuration.

A 46-year-old white woman with a long history of difficulties with her ears and hearing loss whose bony abnormality of the skull was first noted in early childhood was seen. The onset of a progressive hearing loss was first detected at age 4, requiring the use of amplification at 9 years of age. She has had repeated episodes of serous and perforative purulent otitis media since an early age, suggesting dysfunction of the Eustachian tubes. The family history was positive for diabetes on both sides. One aunt had a similar abnormal head configuration.

Physical examination at age 20 revealed normal body proportions and sexual development. The head was large and square with an elevated steep forehead, prominent bony ridges, and a broad and flattened nasal bridge with a hypertelorism (Fig. 51.1.1).

Otologic examination revealed irregular, concentrically narrowed, upward-slanting external auditory canals exposing only the central portion of the tympanic membranes. The malleus was fixed on the right side but could not be visualized on the left side. The right ear showed a 55-dB conductive hearing loss, while the left ear showed a 16-dB mixed loss. Discrimination was excellent bilaterally (100%).

Ophthalmoscopic examination (slit-lamp) demonstrated an incipient posterior cortical cataract bilaterally.

Radiologic examination disclosed a dense osteosclerosis of the calvaria, skull base, and facial and temporal bones with smallness and narrowing of the orbits and optic foramina (Fig. 51.1.2). The frontal and sphenoid sinuses were totally obliterated, and the ethmoid and maxillary sinuses were subtotally obliterated (Fig. 51.1.3). The mastoid and petrous bones exhibited extensive sclerosis and hyperostosis with severe constriction of the middle ear clefts and impingement on the malleus and incus on the right side. The external and internal acoustic meati were concentrically narrowed and slanted upward (Fig. 51.1.4). The medial portions of the iliac bones revealed a broad vertical band of sclerosis involving the full width of the acetabulum and ischial bones on each side of the pelvis (Fig. 51.1.5). Obvious radiodense vertical striations were noted in the heads, necks, and distal ends of the femora and proximal ends of the tibiae (Fig. 51.1.6).

At *operation*, the right external canal was reconstructed to improve the use of amplification, and the middle ear was explored. The concentric narrowing of the middle ear cleft had resulted in impingement on and immobilization of the ossicular chain. The oval and round window niches were concentrically narrowed and distorted, resulting in jamming of the stapedial footplate. No stapedotomy was considered for obvious reasons. (The skeletal manifestations of this patient were discussed in an earlier publication (4).)

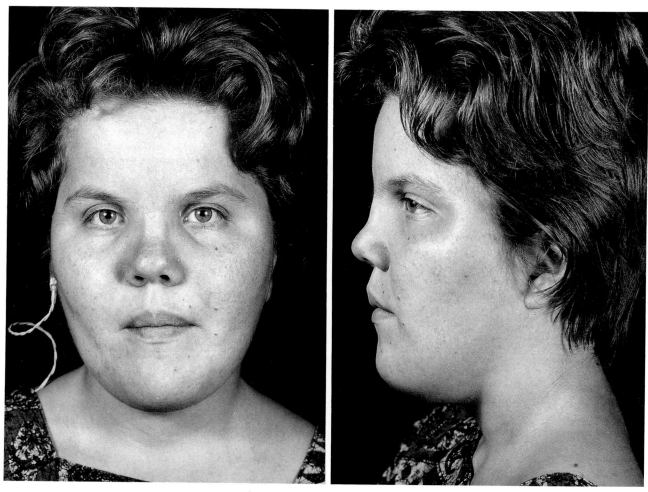

Figure 51.1.1. The patient's face is somewhat large and square. It displays prominent bony ridges, a broad and flattened nasal bridge with an unusual distance between the eyes, and fullness in the malar areas. The jaw is square and tilted slightly to the left.

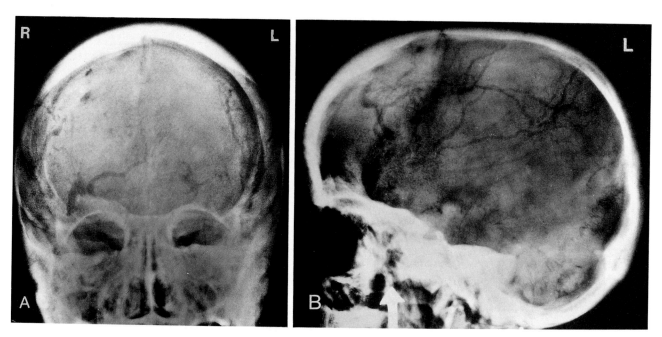

Figure 51.1.2. Frontal **(A)** and later **(B)** projections of the skull demonstrate the dense sclerosis involving the calvaria, skull base, orbital roofs, and mastoid portions of the temporal bones. The orbits are small and constricted. The frontal and sphenoid sinuses are totally obliterated.

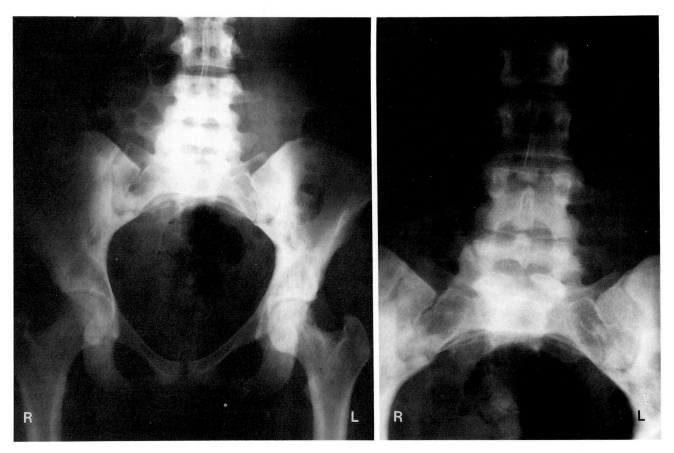

Figure 51.1.5. A broad vertical band of sclerosis involves the medial portion of the iliac bones, the acetabulum, and the ischial bones bilaterally. Faint vertical striations are recognized in the femoral heads and necks.

The lumbar spine displays a mild scoliosis. The portions of the iliac bone adjacent to the sacroiliac articulations display marked sclerosis. (Courtesy of Dr. V. A. McKusick.)

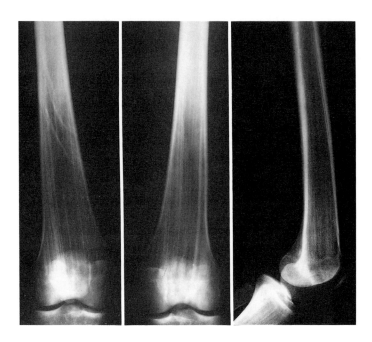

Figure 51.1.6. The lower femora and upper tibiae show the characteristic coarse vertical striations confirming the diagnosis of osteopathia striata. (Courtesy of Dr. V. A. McKusick.)

Case 2. *Osteopathia striata with diffuse sclerosis and hyperostosis involving the calvaria, skull base, and temporal bones. Vertical striations in short and long tubular bones. Constriction of middle ear cleft with impingement on ossicular chain. Concentric narrowing and upward slanting of external and internal auditory canals. Bilateral mixed hearing loss. Bilateral progressive hearing impairment since childhood, requiring amplification bilaterally by age 20. Recurrent serous and perforative otitis media since infancy, necessitating aspiration myringotomies and placement of middle ear ventilation tubes. Family history of short stature and macrocephaly in both parents and one sister.*

A 26-year-old white woman with a history of repeated episodes of serous and purulent perforative middle ear infections and progressive bilateral loss of hearing since early childhood that required repeated placement of ventilating tubes was seen. Both parents and one sister were of short stature and macrocephalic.

On *physical examination* at age 10 years 8 months, her height was short and her head was large with a circumference of 57 cm. The forehead was steep and elevated. The root of her nose was broad and flat, there was an ocular hypertelorism, the midface was flat, and the broad and square mandible created an unmistakable facial expression. Except for a foreshortening of the fifth digits and big toes, the hands and feet appeared normal. The oral examination re-vealed a high palatal arch, a submucosal palatal cleft, a bifid uvula, and an upper and lower overcrowding of the teeth resulting from retention of multiple deciduous teeth.

On *otologic examination,* the bony external canals were slanted upward and were tortuous and narrow, limiting visualization of the tympanic membranes to the posterior third. Cochlear function studies disclosed a bilateral mixed hearing loss.

Radiologic examination revealed a marked diffuse sclerosis and hyperostosis of the calvaria, skull base, and facial and temporal bones (Fig. 51.1.7A and B). The lumbar spine, pelvis, and femoral heads exhibited a markedly increased bony density (Fig. 51.1.7C). The femoral heads and necks, the distal end of the femora, and the proximal and distal ends of the tibiae demonstrated noticeable vertical striations (Fig. 51.1.7B–E). Sequential axial and coronal computed tomography (CT) scans of the temporal bones demonstrated a severe general sclerosis and hyperostosis with constriction of the middle ear clefts, localized impingement on the ossicular chain, and upward slanting and narrowing of the external and internal auditory canals (Fig. 51.1.8A and B).

During the past several years, the patient had noticed a gradual decrease in her sense of smell. There was no evidence of optic nerve atrophy, papilledema, or facial weakness, but there was extensive calcification of the choroid plexus in the occipital horns of the lateral ventricles (Fig. 51.1.7A and B).

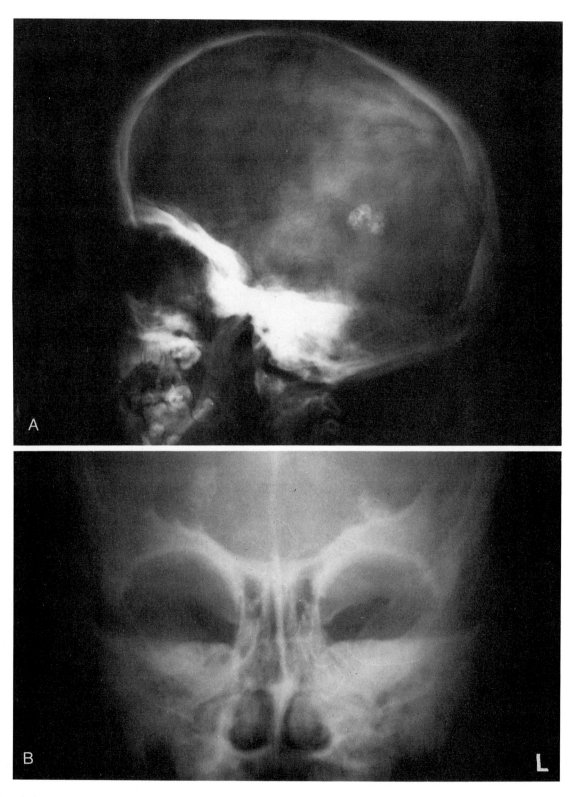

Figure 51.1.7. **A.** Lateral projection of the skull demonstrates marked sclerosis involving the base and temporal bones and calcification of the choroid plexus in the lateral ventricles. **B.** PA view of the skull shows absence of the frontal sinuses and partial obliteration of the maxillary sinuses.

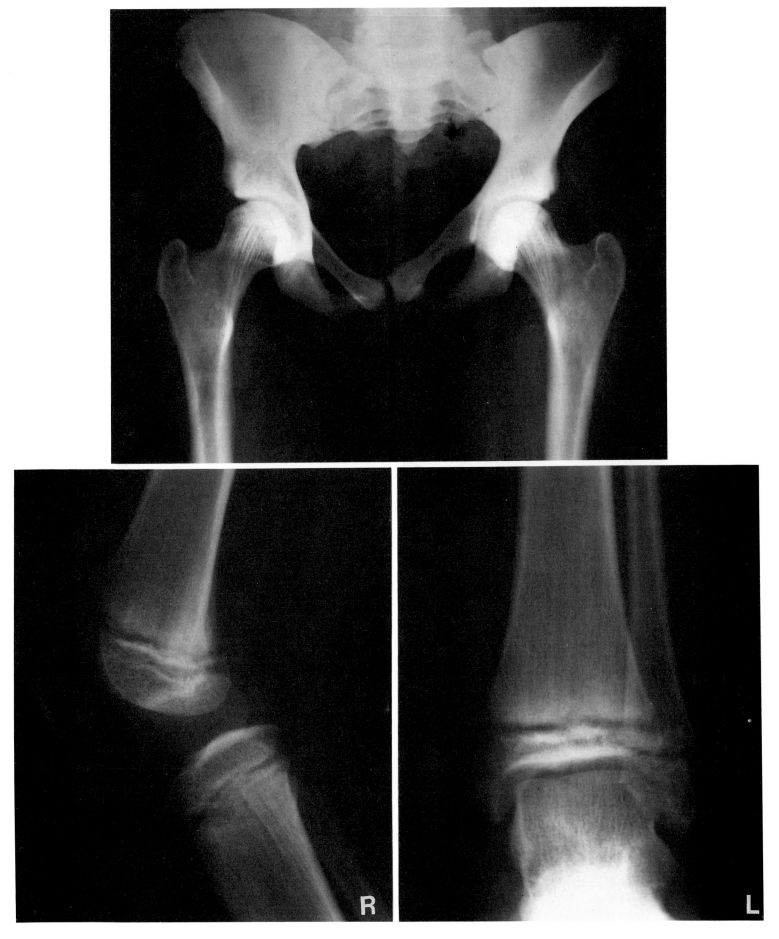

Figure 51.1.7. **C.** Extensive sclerosis involves the sacrum, iliac bones, acetabula and femoral heads. The striations in the femoral necks are clearly visible. **D** and **E.** Radiodense vertical striations are recognized in right distal femora and in right proximal and left distal tibiae.

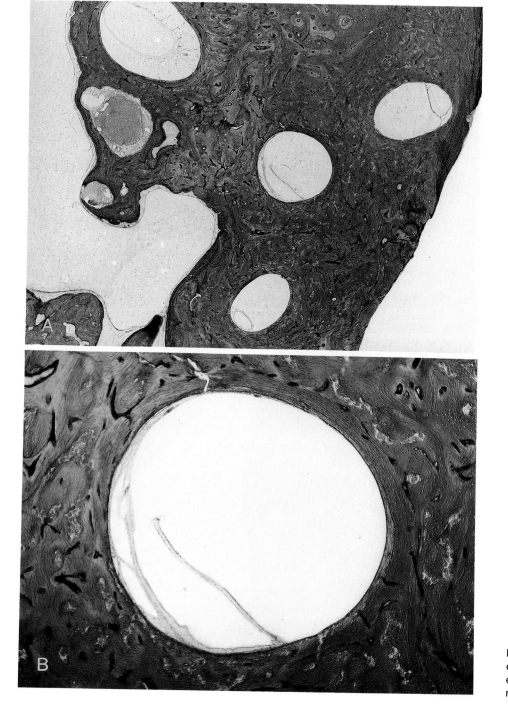

Figure 52.7. **A.** Vertical section through right temporal bone at level of sinus tympani with cross-sections through lateral and posterior semicircular canals. (Hematoxylin and eosin, ×15.)

Figure 52.7. **B.** Cross-section through the lateral semicircular canal, near its nonampullated end, demonstrates a rupture of the membranous canal. (×65.)

Case Report

Case 1.

The patient was a 65-year-old white man with a 10-year history of progressive hearing loss, intermittent high-pitched tinnitus in the right ear, and numerous characteristic episodes of rotatory vertigo with nausea and vomiting, resistant to any form of medical therapy. The audiogram revealed a marked, slightly trough-shaped impairment in all frequencies for air and bone conduction on the right side, with a maximal loss of 75 dB at 500 and 1000 cycles. The left ear disclosed a mild, gradually sloping sensorineural high-tone loss with a speech reception threshold of 25 dB. The vestibular examination showed no spontaneous nystagmus but did reveal paresis of the right lateral semicircular canal with diminished responses to caloric stimulation.

Microscopic examination of the right temporal bone reveals extreme ectasia of the cochlear duct in all turns except the lower region of the lower basal turn (Figs. 52.1A, 52.2A, 52.3, and 52.4). The marked distension of Reissner's membrane resulted in occlusion of the helicotrema (Fig. 52.2A). Reissner's membrane displays an existing rupture in the lower basal turn as well as evidence of several, probably old, healed tears in the first and second cochlear turns (Figs. 52.3 and 52.4). The organ of Corti is peculiarly collapsed throughout all turns (Fig. 52.4C). This collapse differs distinctly from the one usually observed with postmortem changes, and it is in marked contrast to the normal appearance of the organ of Corti in the opposite ear. Some hair cells are recognizable, but the distorted architecture precludes reliable evaluation. The external sulcus cells, stria vascularis, and spiral ligament show no gross abnormalities. The spiral ganglion cells exhibit some patchy partial atrophy in the upper basal and apical turns. For the most part, the cochlear nerve fibers appear unremarkable. The saccule displays a slight dilatation of the utricular recess. Its macula and peripheral nerve fibers appear within normal limits. The canalis reuniens is not dilated. The utricle displays a uniform distension that obliterates the posterior third of the perilymphatic cistern (Fig. 52.5A). A large protrusion of its wall extends into the common crus of the superior and posterior semicircular canals (Fig. 52.6). In addition, the utricular wall has many smaller saccular herniations at its junction with the semicircular canals (Fig. 52.6A). The sensorineural epithelium and nerve fibers are unremarkable. The membranous lateral semicircular canal reveals a rupture near the junction with the utricle (Fig. 52.7). The cristae of all semicircular canals, their sensorineural epithelium, and nerve fibers are unremarkable.

Of particular interest is the presence of several cystic lesions located within the sensorineural epithelium of the superior and posterior cristae and in the submacular region of the utricle (Figs. 52.8–52.11). In the region beneath the sensorineural epithelium of the utricular macula, there are two large and several small interstitial spaces that are lined by a single endothelial layer and contain a homogeneous eosinophilic fluid with a few peripheral vacuoles (Fig. 52.8). Similar cystic spaces are found in the cristae of the ampullae of the superior and posterior semicircular canals (Figs. 52.9–52.11). Their location is on the sloping side of the crista at the periphery of the sensorineural epithelium and transition to the planum semilunatum. They are situated within the epithelium and contain a finely granular, almost amorphous, eosinophilic colloidal liquid. There are no accumulations of mononuclear cells in the surrounding tissue or around adjacent capillaries. They do not look like viral lesions. It is presently unclear whether they represent an incidental finding, could possibly be related to a viral infection, or have any relation to the etiology to this patient's Ménière's disease.

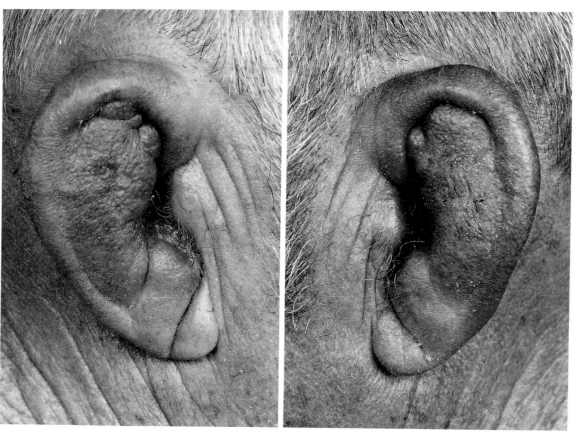

Figure 53.1. The auricles display the characteristic features of relapsing polychondritis: diffuse inflammatory swelling, thickening, loss of land- marks, and concentric narrowing with partial collapse of the entrance to the external auditory canals.

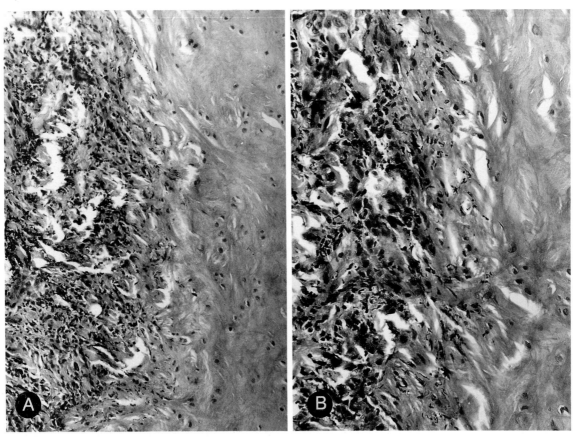

Figure 53.2.   A and **B.** The histopathology of this biopsy from the aural cartilage reflects the typical changes found in relapsing polychondritis: disintegration with fragmentation of the cartilage and replacement by a chronic inflammatory granulation tissue. (Hematoxylin and eosin, x140 and x260, respectively.)

Case 2. *Relapsing polychondritis with involvement of both external ears, nasal pyramid and septum, and Eustachian tubal, laryngeal, and tracheal cartilages. Deformity of auricles with partial collapse of membranous external auditory canals. Saddle nose deformity with collapse of columella. Partial collapse of upper trachea with subglottic stenosis, requiring tracheostomy. Chondrosternal cartilage involvement. Past history of multiple allergies, extrinsic asthma, and recurrent dermatitis.*

The patient was a 49-year-old woman who at age 29 presented with a 3-month history of itching, erythematous swelling, pain, and tenderness of both auricles and external auditory canals. This condition had progressed in spite of oral and systemic penicillin over several weeks but had temporarily improved after a 3-week course of prednisone. She subsequently developed hoarseness. Since childhood she had suffered from extrinsic asthma and recurrent dermatitis, and she was allergic to a number of air-borne allergens.

On *otologic examination,* both auricles were hyperemic, swollen, greatly thickened, and somewhat tender. The external auditory canals were concentrically narrowed, filled with exudate, and involved in a diffuse dermatitis that also affected the outer layer of the drums. Both arytenoid cartilages were hyperemic and edematous and slightly limited in mobility, but the vocal cords appeared anatomically and functionally normal. There was no tenderness or impairment of cochlear and vestibular function. The nose and nasopharynx were unremarkable.

Five years later, the patient developed redness and tenderness of her lower nasal pyramid and nasal congestion. The cartilaginous portion of her septum became very swollen, hyperemic, and tender. She began to have intermittent mild epistaxis and had noticed increasing tenderness of her tracheal and chondrosternal cartilages and episcleritis. Over the next 12 years, the patient had numerous exacerbations and remissions, resulting in complete resorption of her auricular and nasal cartilages, leaving her with distorted floppy ears and a saddle nose deformity (Fig. 53.3). Progressive destruction of her laryngeal and tracheal cartilages resulted in a partial collapse of the upper trachea and a subglottic stenosis requiring a tracheostomy. At operation, the cricoid cartilage and upper tracheal rings were very soft, and the tracheal mucosa was very hyperemic and edematous.

All along she had been on prednisone varying in dose between 20 and 60 mg daily. After 10 years she finally reached a satisfactory control of her symptoms on 10 mg of prednisone and 200 mg of dapsone a day. A tracheoscopy at age 47, 18 years after the onset of her illness, disclosed a generalized narrowing of the tracheal lumen to about 9–10 mm, and a segmental loss of landmarks of the tracheal rings for a distance of about 1 inch.

Histologic examination, done earlier, had shown a widespread superficial disintegration and destruction of the left auricular cartilage associated with extensive subacute and chronic inflammation and vasculitis (Fig. 53.4).

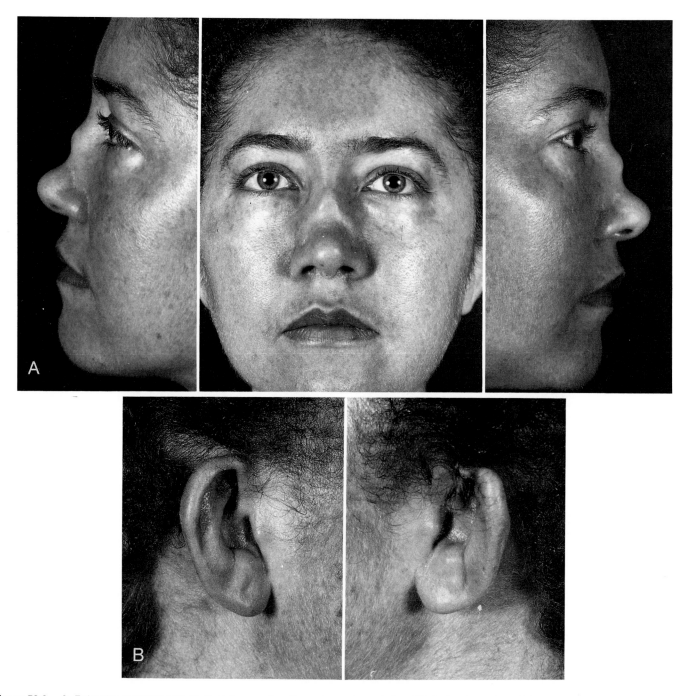

Figure 53.3. **A.** Relapsing polychondritis involves the nasal cartilages in about 63% of patients. Recurrent episodes may result in complete destruction of these cartilages and the development of the characteristic saddle nose deformity. **B.** The most prominent clinical manifestation in relapsing polychondritis is the destruction of the aural cartilage. This manifestation results in loss of structural support with floppiness, drooping, and destruction of the auricle and collapse of the cartilaginous outer ear canal.

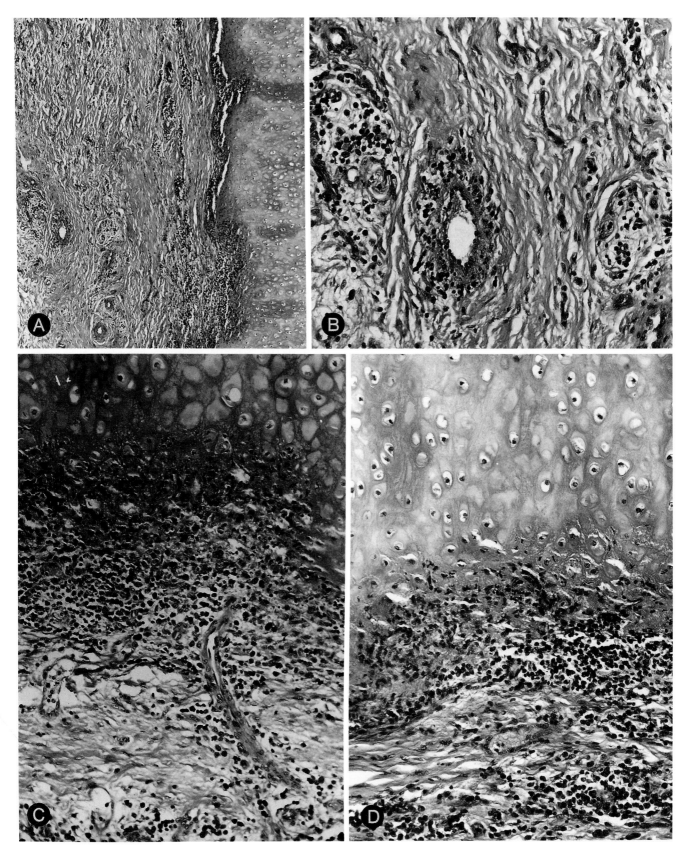

Figure 53.4. Biopsies from left auricle. **A.** In an earlier stage a narrow rim of infiltrating inflammatory cells, primarily lymphocytes, plasma cells, and macrophages, is seen along the chondrodermal junction in association with localized proteoglycan depletion of the cartilage. **B.** Several of the smaller vessels seen in *A* show evidence of vasculitis. **C.** In a subse- quent stage, granulation tissue invades and replaces the disintegrating cartilage. **D.** As lymphocytes infiltrate the cartilage, it loses its basophilic staining ability. Numerous chondrocytes disappear from their capsule, and the matrix becomes fragmented and disintegrates. (Hematoxylin and eosin, x65, x250, x250, and 380, respectively.)

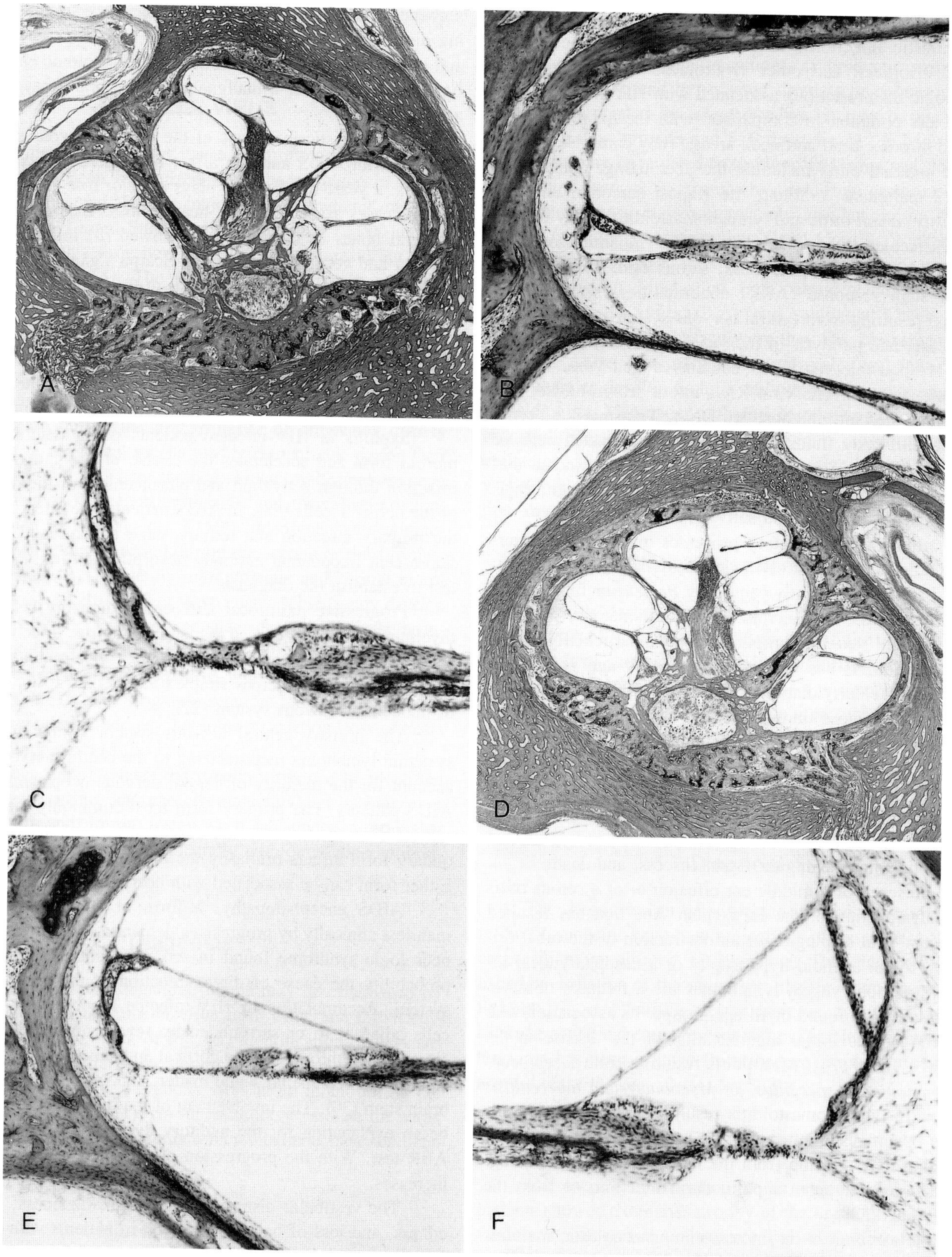

Figure 54.1. **A.** Vertical midmodiolar section of right cochlea, showing the flattening of the cochlea often found in rubella embryopathy, collapse of Reissner's membrane, and atrophy of the stria vascularis. **B.** Cross-section of scala media of lower third turn of cochlea, showing the severe atrophy of the stria, detachment of its upper end from the underlying spiral ligament, and dystrophy and medial displacement of the tectorial membrane into the internal sulcus and under Reissner's membrane. **C.** Cross-section of scala media in lower basal turn of cochlea. The tectorial membrane is "rolled-up" in the internal sulcus, covered by a single layer of endothelial cells. The stria vascularis is atrophic, and Reissner's membrane is collapsed. **D.** Vertical midmodiolar section of left cochlea. The configuration of the cochlear capsule is identical with the one on the opposite side *(A),* but the morphologic changes involving the scala media are less pronounced. **E.** Cross-section of scala media of upper middle turn of cochlea, revealing the detachment of the upper portion of the dystrophic stria vascularis from the spiral ligament and condensation and displacement of the tectorial membrane. **F.** Cross-section through scala media of lower basal turn of cochlea. The detachment of the dystrophic stria vascularis has much the same appearance as a cyst. (Hematoxylin and eosin, ×10, ×75, ×100, ×10, ×75, and ×100, respectively.)

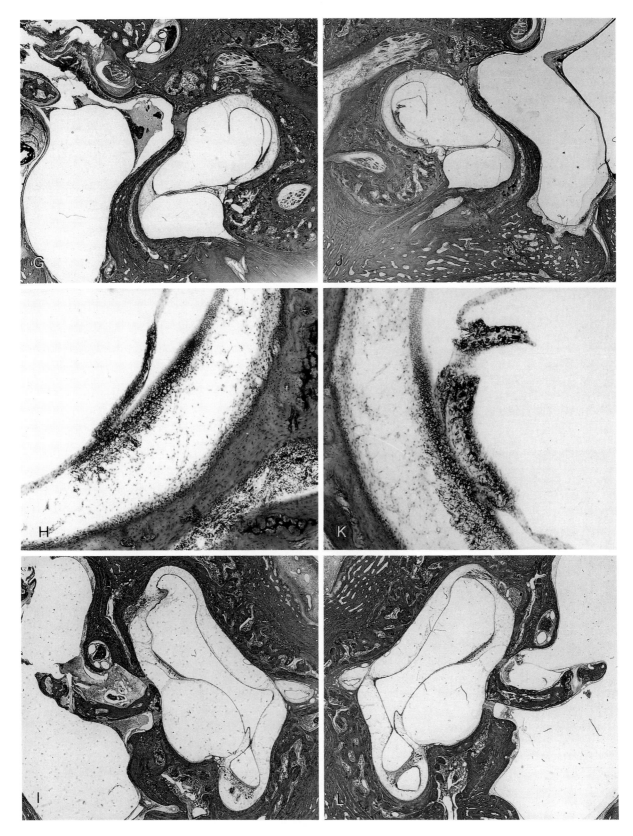

Figure 54.1. **G.** Vertical section through right temporal bone at anterior end of oval window. The saccule is collapsed, and its lateral wall is adherent to the macula sacculi. **H.** Higher power showing adherence of lateral wall of saccule to macula. **I.** Vertical section of right temporal bone at level of oval window, demonstrating a mild dysplasia of the stapedial arch but an essentially normal utricle. **J.** Vertical section through left temporal bone near anterior end of oval window, exhibiting the collapse of the saccule with adherence to the macula. **K.** Higher power showing distortion and adherence of lateral wall of saccule to macula. **L.** Vertical section through left temporal bone at level of vestibular fenestra with minor dysplasia of stapedial arch. (Hematoxylin and eosin, ×10, ×75, ×9, ×10, ×75, and ×9, respectively.)

ysis of the facial nerve is a decrease in the number of the T4 lymphocytes (22, 31). The facial nerve function generally returns over a period of 3 weeks to 3 months (31).

Magnetic resonance imaging of the brain with gadolinium enhancement may be of help in the differentiation between the central nervous system and peripheral nerve involvement (22).

Case Reports

Case 1. *Congenital rubella syndrome. Atresia of pulmonary valve and main pulmonary artery. Ventricular septal defect. Overriding aorta. Patent ductus arteriosus. Intimal proliferation of renal, mesenteric, prostatic, and iliac arteries with aneurysmal dilatation of right iliac artery. Microphthalmos and nuclear cataracts. Malformation of tentorium and ventricular pseudocysts. Severe hemolytic anemia, purpura, and jaundice. Centrolobular scarring and severe bilestasis. Retardation of intrauterine growth. Premature birth (week 28). Documented maternal rubella during first trimester of pregnancy. Scheibe-type cochlear malformation with flattening of bony capsule and anomalies involving the membranous cochlea and saccule.*

The patient was a 31-day-old premature infant boy (43 cm, 1790 g) born to a 19-year-old primigravida who had had documented rubella in the first trimester of pregnancy. At birth, the infant was found to have microphthalmia and hypospadias. Shortly thereafter, he developed petechial-like rash, progressive hepatosplenomegaly, hemolytic anemia, jaundice, congenital hepatitis, cardiomegaly, and respiratory distress and died of cardiorespiratory arrest on the 31st day. Although no definite assessment of his hearing was obtained, he failed to show response to sound stimuli.

Microscopic examination of the temporal bones reveals that both ears display a Scheibe-type malformation involving the cochlear duct and saccule, which is somewhat more marked on the right (Fig. 54.1A and D). Reissner's membrane is collapsed, to a great extent adherent to the stria vascularis, and plastered against the organ of Corti (Fig. 54.1B, C, E, and F). The stria is shorter, smaller, and less differentiated, often detached from the spiral ligament near the upper end, and pulled down and medially by Reissner's membrane (Fig. 54.1B, C, E, and F). In many places the tectorial membrane is rolled up and lying in the internal sulcus, encased in a sheath of flattened endothelial cells (Fig. 54.2C). Nowhere is it found in a normal position covering the organ of Corti. In some places there is what appears to be a single-layered membrane covering the internal sulcus and extending under Reissner's membrane. The organ of Corti is essentially normal in appearance. The hair cells are plentiful, and the pillar cells are unremarkable. In some regions, some pink homogeneous material is found in the internal sulcus. A single layer of undifferentiated endothelial cells is present where normally the Claudius, Hensen, and Böttcher cells are found. The first cochlear neuron is unremarkable. The saccule is partially collapsed, with a portion of the membrane being adherent to the macula (Fig. 54.1G, H, K, and L). A number of large endothelial cells are lying along this membrane near the point of adhesion. The utricle, all three semicircular canals, and the endolymphatic sac are normal in appearance. In the left ear, Reissner's membrane in much of its length is pulled away from the bony wall at its external attachment, rolling up the upper portion of the stria vascularis. In some places the detachment of the stria vascularis has much the same appearance as a cyst (Fig. 54.1F).

Case 2. *Congenital rubella syndrome. Documented maternal rubella during tenth week of pregnancy. Premature birth at 7 months. Death 18 hours after delivery. Positive viral cultures from newborn infant at birth.*

Microscopic examination of the temporal bones reveals that the morphologic changes are minimal and limited to the right ear. Reissner's membrane is adherent throughout its entire length to the organ of Corti (Fig. 54.2). The tectorial membrane is somewhat distorted under Reissner's membrane. The stria vascularis is unremarkable, and the organ of Corti appears normal. Utricle, saccule, semicircular canals, and endolymphatic sac as well as the first cochlear neuron are normal in appearance.

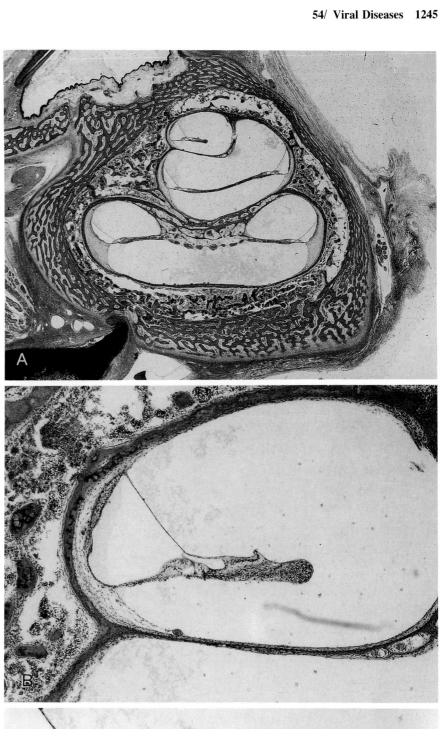

Figure 54.2. A. Vertical midmodiolar section of right cochlea with normal configuration of cochlear capsule. (Hematoxylin and eosin, ×10.)

Figure 54.2. B and **C.** Cross-sections of lower third turn of cochlea, displaying the collapse of Reissner's membrane, dysplasia of the tectorial membrane, and cystic dysplasia of the stria vascularis. (×50 and ×100, respectively.)

References

1. Davies LE, Johnson LG. Viral infections of the inner ear: clinical, virologic, and pathologic studies in humans and animals. Am J Otolaryngol 1983;4(5):347–362.

2. Davies LE, James CG, Fiber F, et al. Cytomegalovirus isolation from a human inner ear. Ann Otol Rhinol Laryngol 1979;88:424–426.

3. Westmore GA, Pickard BH, Stern H. Isolation of mumps virus from the inner ear after sudden deafness. Br Med 1979;1:14–15.

4. Lindsay JR, Hemenway WG. Inner ear pathology due to measles. Ann Otol Rhinol Laryngol 1954;63:754–771.

5. Stagno S, Reynolds DW, Amos CS, et al. Auditory and visual defects resulting from symptomatic and subclinical congential cytomegaloviral and *Toxoplasma* infections. Pediatrics 1977;59:669–678.

6. Reynolds DW, Stagno S, Subbs G, et al. Inapparent congenital cytomegalovirus infection with elevated cord IgM levels: causal relationship with auditory and mental deficiency. N Engl J Med 1974;290:291–296.

7. Hanshaw JB. Cytomegalovirus. In: Remington JS, Klein JO, eds. Infectious diseases of the foetus and newborn infant. Philadelphia: WB Saunders, 1976:107–155.

8. Mitschke H. Der Höhrsturz, eine mögliche zentrale Manifestation der Zytomegalie-Infektion Erwachsener. Laryngol Rhinol Otol 1978;57:876–881.

9. Stagno S, Reynolds DW, Huang ES, et al. Congenital cytomegalovirus infection: occurrence in an immune population. N Engl J Med 1977;296:1254–1258.

10. Congenital and perinatal cytomegalovirus infection. In: Berkow R, ed. Merck manual of diagnosis and therapy. 16th ed. Rahwah, New Jersey: Merck & Co, 1992:2039–2044.

11. Stagno S, Pass RF, Reynolds DW. Comparative study of diagnostic procedures for congenital cytomegalovirus infection. Pediatrics 1980;65:251–257.

12. Davies LE, Johnson LG, Kornfeld M. Cytomegalovirus labyrinthitis in an infant: morphological, virological and immunofluorescent studies. J Neuropathol Exp Neurol 1981;40:9–19.

13. Kimura RS. Distribution, structure and function of dark cells in the vestibular labyrinth. Ann Otol Rhinol Laryngol 1969;72:542–561.

14. Trybus RI, Karschner MA, Kerstetter PP, et al. The demographics of deafness resulting from maternal rubella. Am Ann Deaf 1980;125:977–984.

15. Katz SL. Rubella (German measles). In: Wyngaarden JB, Smith LH, eds. Cecil textbook of medicine. 18th ed. Philadelphia: WB Saunders, Chap 337, 1988;2:1776–1777.

16. Karmody CS. Subclinical maternal rubella and congenital deafness. N Engl J Med 1968;278:809–814.

17. Mesner MA, Forrest JM. Rubella—high incidence of defects in children considered normal at birth. Med J Aust 1974;1:123–126.

18. Bordley JE, Brookhauser PE, Hardy J. Prenatal rubella. Acta Otolaryngol (Stockh) 1968;66:1–9.

19. Everberg G. Deafness following mumps. Acta Otolaryngol (Stockh) 1957;48:397–403.

20. Lindsay JR, Davey PR, Ward PH. Inner ear pathology in deafness due to mumps. Ann Otol Rhinol Laryngol 1960;69:918–935.

21. Smith CA, Gussen R. Inner ear pathologic features following mumps infection: report of a case in an adult. Arch Otolaryngol 1976;102:108–111.

22. Lalwani AK, Sooy CD. Otologic and neurologic manifestations of the acquired immunodeficiency syndrome. Otolaryngol Clin North Am 1992;25(6):1183–1197.

23. Church J. Human immunodeficiency virus (HIV) infection at Childrens Hospital of Los Angeles: recurrent otitis media or chronic sinusitis as the presenting process in pediatric AIDS. Immunol Allergy 1987;9:25–32.

24. Marcusen DC, Sooy CD. Otolaryngologic and head and neck manifestations of acquired immunodeficiency syndrome (AIDS). Laryngoscope 1985;95:401–405.

25. Sooy CD. Impact of AIDS on otolaryngology–head and neck surgery. In: Meyers EN, ed. Advances in otolaryngology–head and neck surgery. Chicago: Year Book Medical Publishers, 1987;1:1–27.

26. Petito CK, Navia BA, Cho ES, et al. Vacuolar myelopathy pathologically resembling subacute combined degeneration in patients with the acquired immunodeficiency syndrome. N Engl J Med 1985;312:874–879.

27. McGill T. Mycotic infections of the temporal bone. Arch Otolaryngol 1978;104:140–144.

28. Phillips TJ, Dover JS. Medical progress: recent advances in dermatology. N Engl J Med 1992;326:167–178.

29. Smith ME, Canalis RF. Otologic manifestations of AIDS: the otosyphilis connection. Laryngoscope 1989;99:365–372.

30. Levy RM, Bredesen DE, Rosenblum ML. Neurological manifestations of the acquired immunodeficiency syndrome (AIDS) experience at UCSF and a review of the literature. J Neurosurg 1985;62:475–495.

31. Schielke E, Pfister HW, et al. Peripheral facial nerve palsy associated with HIV infection. Lancet 1989;1:553–554.

55/ Temporal Bone Fractures

MECHANISMS OF CRANIAL FRACTURES

Three factors determine the nature of a cranial fracture: *(a)* the location and form of the injury, *(b)* the velocity and mass of the object inflicting the injury, and *(c)* the direction in which the force has been applied.

Not all areas of the calvaria are equally resistant to a fracture. The resistance is greatest in the frontal bone. It decreases to one-half in the parietal bone and to one-fourth in the zygomatic region. The cranial vault has a certain amount of elasticity. An impact on a broad surface produces a local indentation. Because of the elasticity and configuration of the skull, the force generated over the surface of the impact results in the creation of one or more linear fractures (Fig. 55.1). These linear fractures generally run in and parallel to the direction of the impact but often deviate as they follow recognized lines of stress within the skull. In many instances, linear fractures continue from the calvaria into the base, and most basal skull fractures arise in this manner. Any attempt to identify a basal skull fracture radiographically should, therefore, begin with the search for a linear fracture in the calvaria from where it may be followed down into the base (1).

Fractures involving the base of the skull may be limited to that area. The majority, however, occur in combination with fractures of the calvaria. Depending on the location, course, and characteristics, several forms may be distinguished: *(a)* frontobasal fractures, *(b)* laterobasal fractures, *(c)* posterobasal fractures, *(d)* combined frontobasal, laterobasal, or posterobasal fractures, and *(e)* impression or ring fractures (Fig. 55.1).

Fractures of the petrous bone are estimated to occur in about 75% of all forms of basal skull fractures and, as a rule, all middle cranial fossa fractures, with the exception of a few unusual fractures involving the clivus and posterior clinoid process (1, 2).

Fractures of the temporal bone represent a form of laterobasal or posterobasal skull fracture. They result from a bursting mechanism caused by deformation of the entire skull following an impact on a broad surface of the lateral or posterior aspect of the calvaria. Their greatest damage does not occur at the site of impact but rather at some distance away from it, in an area of maximal tension and minimal elasticity. The base of the skull, because of its irregular architectural structure, becomes the predilective site for these fractures commonly referred to as indirect or bursting fractures.

Fractures of the base of the skull that involve the temporal bone have in the past conventionally been classified as *(a)* longitudinal fractures, *(b)* transverse fractures, or *(c)* combined longitudinal and transverse fractures of the petrous pyramid (3–5). This classification was based on the course and plane of the principal fracture in relation to the long axis of the petrous pyramid. Such a classification, however, represented an obvious oversimplication. There is abundant histologic evidence that many of these hitherto considered "typical" fractures have ramifications in several different planes and directions that escape radiologic detection and that there are documented combinations and variations of fractures that no longer fall into any one of these "typical" categories (6–8). A certain number of fractures, because of their pattern, actually represent compound fractures of the petrous pyramid. In spite of this well-recognized shortcoming, for the time being it may be convenient for diagnostic and didactic purposes to adhere in principle to the long-established, conventional classification but to add the additional category of compound fractures.

Longitudinal fractures of the petrous pyramid are basically middle fossa fractures, whereas transverse fractures represent a combination of posterior and middle fossa fractures. Longitudinal fractures of the petrous pyramid are far more frequently observed than transverse, combined, or compound fractures (9).

LONGITUDINAL FRACTURES OF THE PETROUS PYRAMID

Longitudinal fractures of the petrous pyramid may account for up to 85% of all temporal bone fractures (7). This fracture is usually the result of an impact to the temporal or parietal area rather than to the frontal or occipital region (4, 5, 10, 11). Occasionally, it may occur bilaterally, and it can represent a bursting fracture caused by bilateral compression of the skull (12, 13). In one series, the temporal bones were involved bilaterally in 34 (23%) of 146 longitudinal fractures (12).

In general, the fracture originates in the squamous portion of the temporal bone or in the parietal bone and descends downward into the external auditory canal (Fig. 55.2). Less frequently, it begins in the occipital bone from where it courses forward horizontally across the mastoid to enter the outer ear canal (Fig. 55.2). In this instance the fracture may be associated with a separation of the lambdoidal or parietomastoid suture. On entering the external auditory canal, it usually follows the posterosuperior canal wall, traverses the tympanic annulus at about 11 o'clock on the right and 1 o'clock on the left, generally lacerating the posterosuperior quadrant of the tympanic membrane, and continues in the tegmen tympani in an anterior and medial direction along the anterior border of the petrous pyramid, parallel to its long axis (Fig. 55.3A and B). As a rule, it avoids the inner ear capsule, continues toward the geniculate ganglion, and follows the semi canal of the tensor tympani muscle or the carotid canal toward the region of the Gasserian ganglion, the foramen lacerum, or the foramina of the middle cranial fossa (Fig. 55.3B). A longitudinal fracture may exceptionally course along the posterior aspect of the pyramid (Fig. 55.3D) (7). One-fourth of the longitudinal fractures may extend to the opposite side along the sphenobasilar suture (Fig. 55.3D and E). In a rare instance the fracture may cause a separation of the lambdoidal or parie-

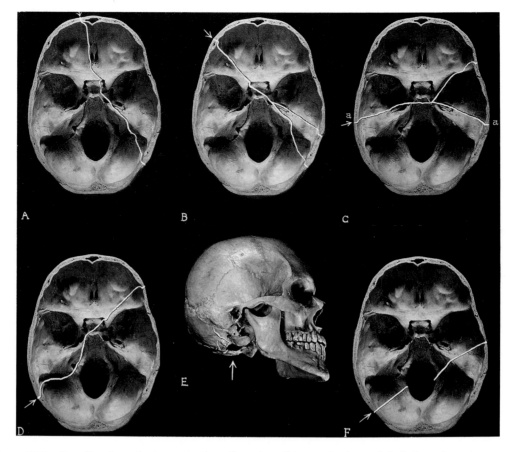

Figure 55.1. Prevailing linear fracture or fractures through section or entire base of skull after a force *(arrows)* has been applied to a broader surface in different areas of the calvaria and skull base.

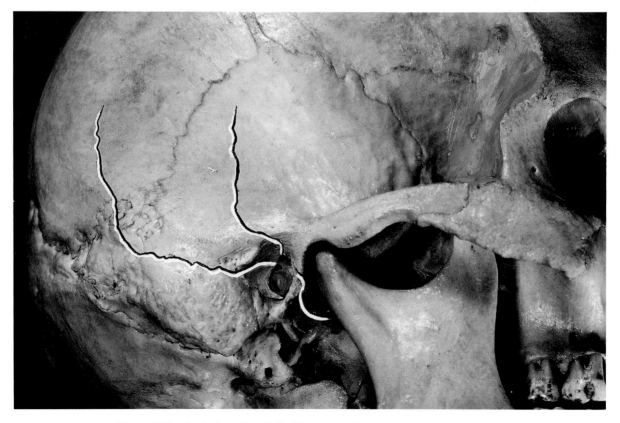

Figure 55.2. Beginning of longitudinal fracture as it involves the right temporal bone.

rous
celle
temp
and
stape
loca
infor
resis
appr

reco

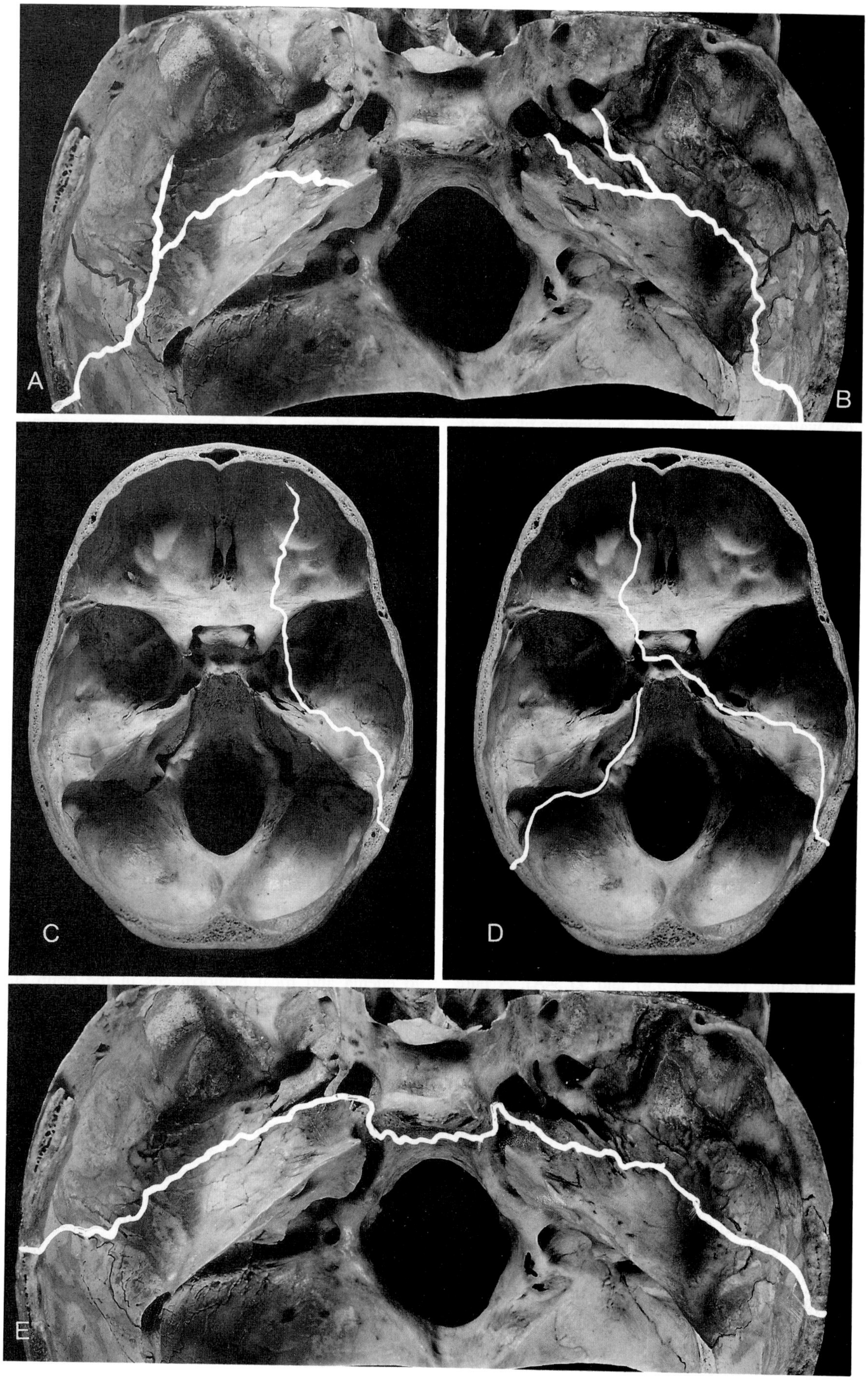

Figure 55.3.   A–E. Continuation of longitudinal fracture as it courses through the middle cranial fossa and beyond and its relation to the long axis of the petrous pyramid.

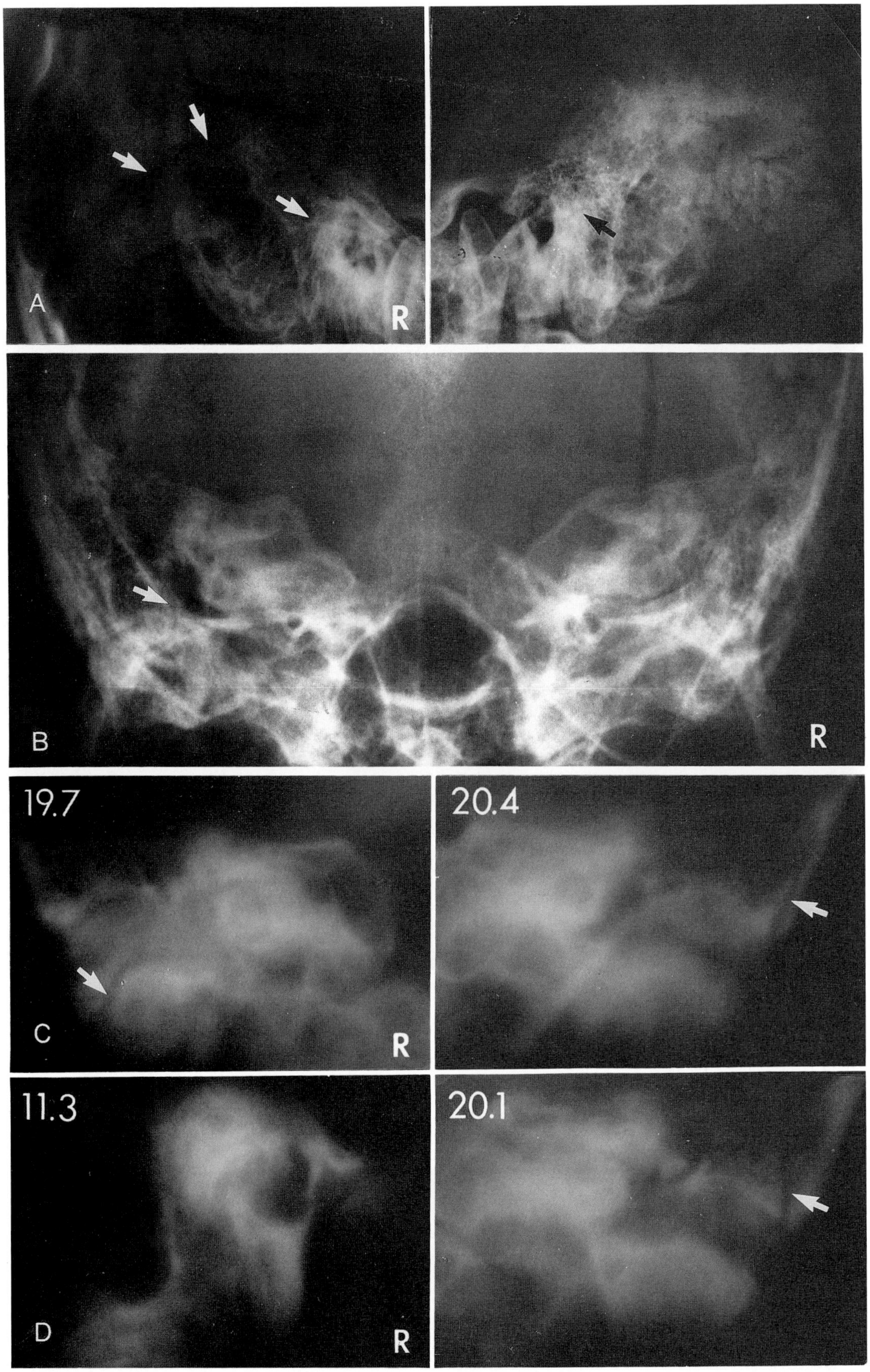

Figure 55.12. Lateral (Schüller) projection of temporal bone **(A)**, AP view of skull **(B)**, and complex motion AP **(C,** *Sects. 19.7, 20.4,* and *20.1*) and lateral **(D)** tomograms of petrous pyramids of a 36-year-old man who sustained bilateral laterobasal skull and bilateral, predominantly longitudinal pyramidal fractures in a motorcycle accident. There were narrowing of the right ear canal and leakage of CSF and blood from both ears. Additional fractures involving both outer ear canals are readily visible *(arrows).*

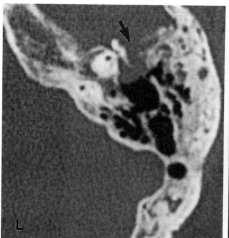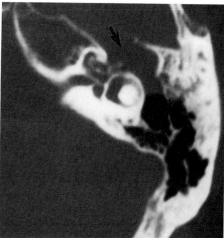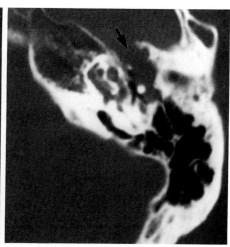

Figure 55.13. Axial CT scans through left temporal bone of a 35-year-old American Indian man who at age 20 had been struck by a car and suffered a longitudinal fracture of the petrous pyramid. He presented with a history of progressive hearing loss in the left ear. On examination, a soft tissue mass, covered by meatal skin, was protruding downward from the medial roof of the external auditory canal, and a whitish mass was noted behind the eardrum, hanging down from the attic. The CT scan revealed a large tegmental defect *(arrows),* and magnetic resonance imaging showed a herniation from the temporal lobe into the middle ear. At operation, the tegmental defect, which extended from the superior petrosal sinus laterally into the roof of the external meatus, measured 1.5 × 1.6 cm. It was closed from above after reposition of the cerebral hernia with a temporalis fascia and muscle flap supporting a plate of cortical bone.

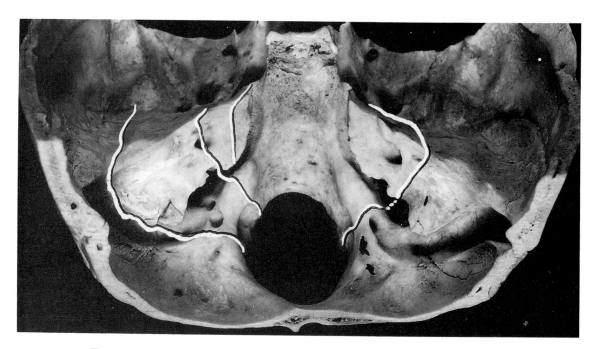

Figure 55.14. Course and direction of transverse fractures involving the petrous pyramid.

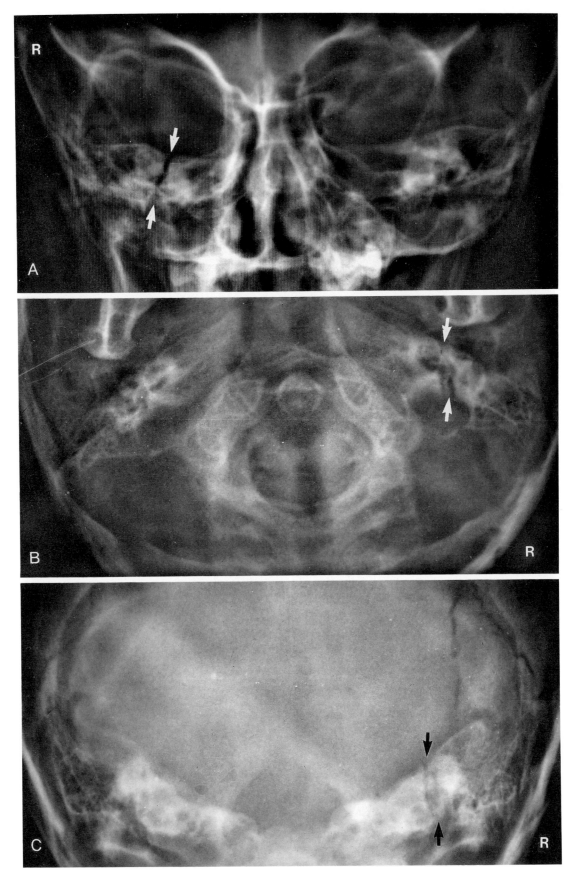

Figure 55.16. PA (transorbital) projection of petrous pyramids **(A)** and submentovertical **(B)** and AP **(C)** projections of skull of an 8-year-old boy who suffered a right posterobasal skull fracture with a transverse fracture of the right petrous pyramid *(arrows)*.

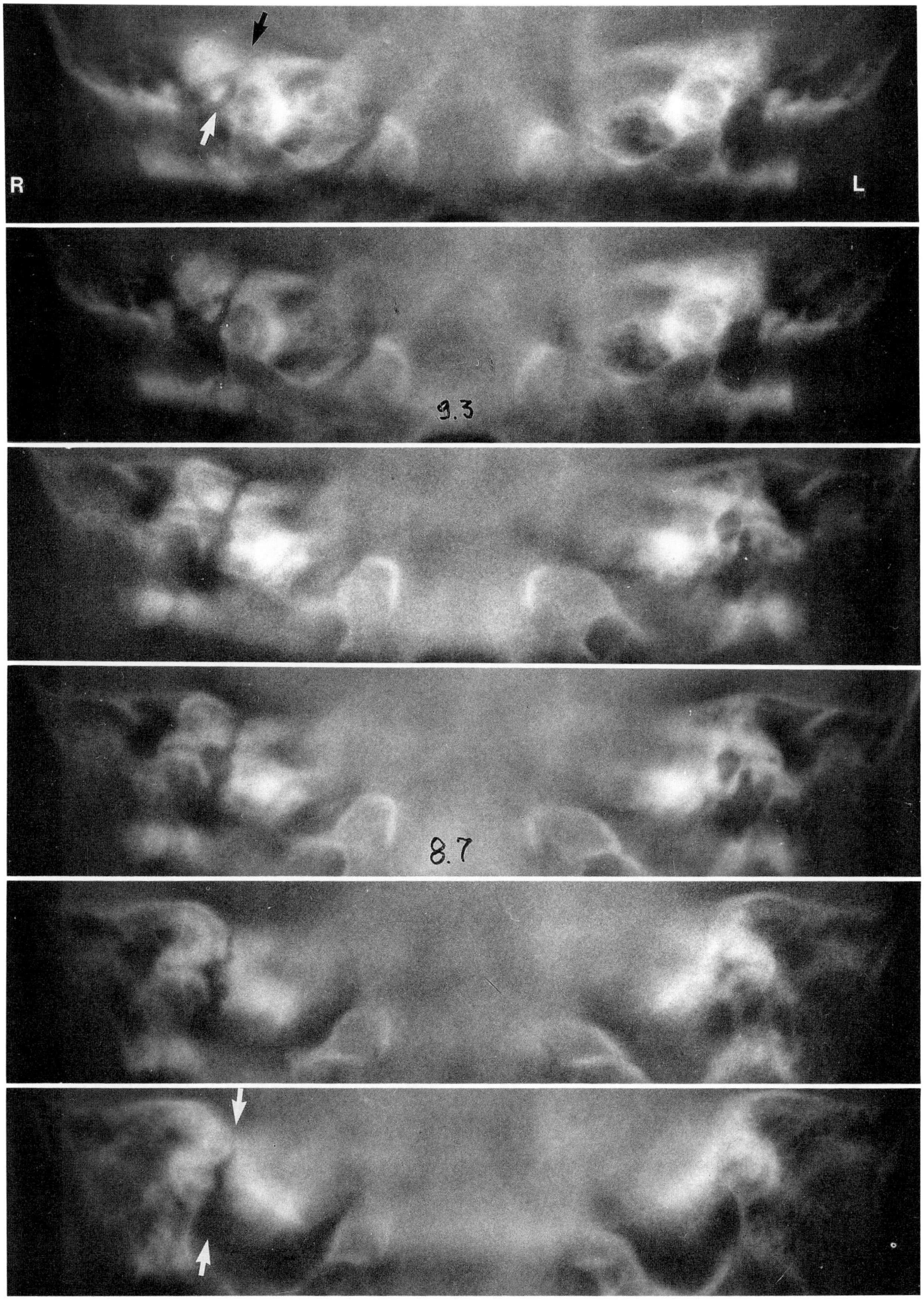

Figure 55.17. Complex motion AP tomograms of temporal bones of a 36-year-old man who had sustained an oblique transverse fracture of the right petrous pyramid from a backward fall on an icy street with impact on the right occipital area. The fracture involves the roof of the jugular bulb, vestibular labyrinth, and cochlea and resulted in total loss of cochlear and vestibular function with a noticeable separation of the bony fragments *(arrows).*

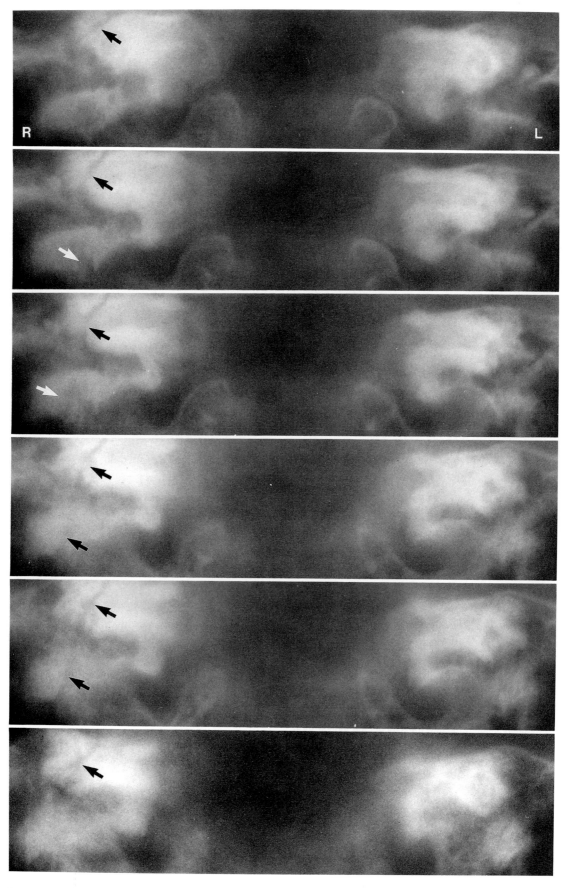

Figure 55.20. Complex motion AP tomograms of temporal bones of an adult man with a transverse fracture across the right petrous pyramid, tra- versing the vestibular labyrinth *(arrows)*, destroying its function but sparing the cochlea with preservation of hearing.

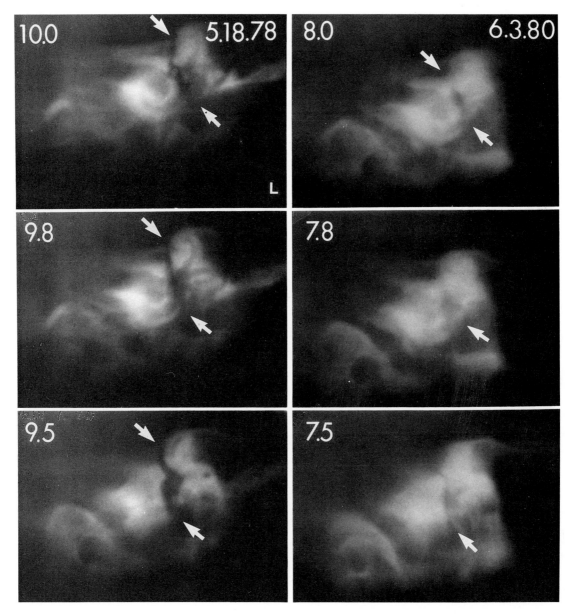

Figure 55.21. Complex motion AP tomograms of left temporal bone of an 8-year-old boy who was hit by a truck and sustained an oblique transverse fracture of the pyramid with total loss of hearing and vestibular function, subsequently resulting in development of an otogenic meningitis. Repeat tomograms 2 years later showed only a partial osseous union of the originally wide-open fracture cleft and an incomplete bony obliteration of the cochlea and vestibular labyrinth.

external auditory canal unless the transverse fracture is combined with a longitudinal fracture of the petrous pyramid.

The transverse fracture may establish a communication along its cleft between the subarachnoid space of the posterior fossa and the middle ear or the Eustachian tube. As the cerebral spinal fluid drains through the Eustachian tube into the nose, it may be mistaken for a CSF leak from the cribriform plate or one of the paranasal sinuses. Because of its communication with the middle ear cleft, the transverse fracture becomes an open skull fracture.

The immediate, large-amplitude, third-degree nystagmus beating toward the undamaged ear, accompanied by vertigo, nausea, and vomiting, gradually subsides over 2–3 weeks. During walking, a tendency to sway to the side of the involved labyrinth may exist for months. A mild spontaneous or a positional nystagmus may persist for months or years or indefinitely.

Isolated partial or total loss of either cochlear or vestibular function has been recognized as the result of limited microfractures. These fractures more frequently involve the cochlear capsule than the labyrinthine capsule (28–30).

The immediate facial palsy is most often permanent, unless timely surgical repair is instituted.

The transverse fracture of the petrous pyramid may be recognized radiographically in the conventional Stenvers, transorbital, and submentovertical projections and in multidirectional and axial and coronal (Figs. 55.15–55.23) CT tomograms. Fractures of the inner ear capsule often remain visible for the rest of the patient's life because of their tendency to heal only with a fibrous rather than an osseous union in the endochondral capsule layer (Fig. 55.21) (3). For any fracture to be recognized, it has to be close to the film, the cleft has to have a certain width, the fractured bone must have a sufficient density, the central x-ray beam must coincide with the fracture plane, and the plane has to be perpendicular to the x-ray film.

COMBINED LONGITUDINAL AND TRANSVERSE FRACTURES OF THE PETROUS PYRAMID

Combined longitudinal and transverse fractures probably account for less than 5–7% of fractures of the petrous pyramid. The mechanisms are identical with the ones involved in either of these fractures.

The transverse fracture branches off the longitudinal fracture at either a right or an oblique angle (Fig. 55.22). It usually traverses the cochlear and vestibular capsule and follows the internal acoustic meatus toward the foramen magnum (Figs. 55.22 and 55.23).

This fracture combines the anatomical and clinical features of both the longitudinal and the transverse fracture. By establishing a direct communication between the posterior cranial fossa, the middle ear cleft, and the external auditory canal, it becomes an open skull fracture in more than one way.

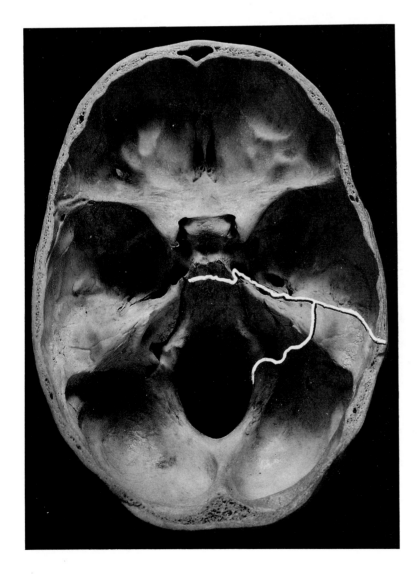

Figure 55.22. Course and direction of combined longitudinal and transverse fracture involving the right petrous pyramid.

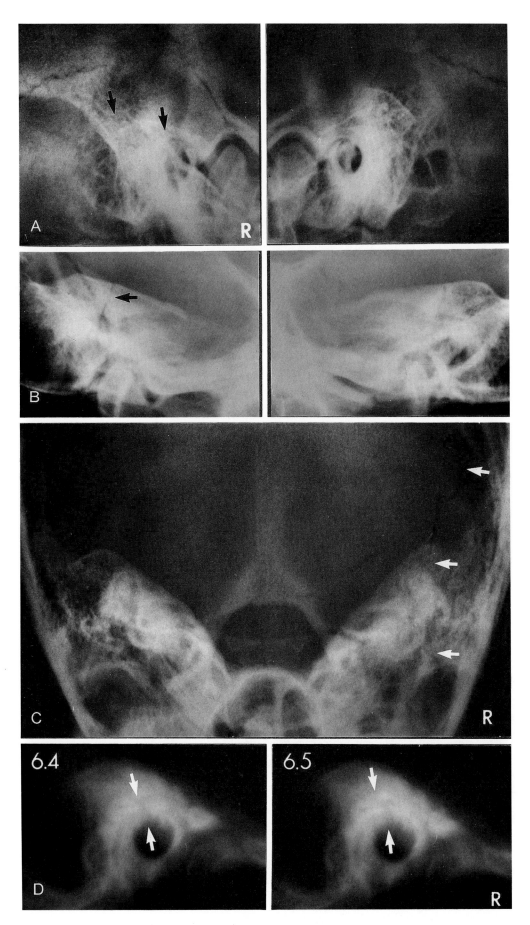

Figure 55.23. Lateral (Schüller) **(A),** longitudinal (Stenvers) **(B),** and sagittal AP **(C)** projections of temporal bones and complex motion lateral tomograms **(D)** of right temporal bone of a 20-year-old woman who sustained a combined longitudinal and transverse fracture of the right petrous pyramid in an automobile accident. There was bleeding from the right middle ear and a laceration of the canal skin, a paralytic nystagmus and anacusis, absence of tearing of the right eye, and progressive facial paresis. One of the fracture lines is seen in the tomograms, bisecting the lateral semicircular canal and the Fallopian canal at the geniculate ganglion *(arrows).*

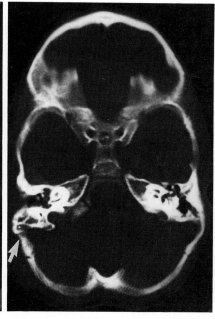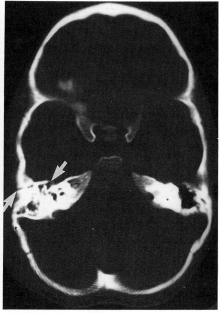

Figure 55.24. Axial CT scans of skull base with comminuted fracture through right temporal bone of a 31-year-old man. The fractures involved the squamous, mastoid, and posterior portions of the petrous pyramid but spared (protected) the entire inner ear capsule.

The combined fracture, like the transverse fracture, is characterized in most instances by total loss of cochlear and vestibular function and in about 50% of occurrences by an immediate loss of facial nerve function. It is associated with active bleeding and often with drainage of CSF from the middle ear and the external auditory canal. The CSF may leak into the middle ear from the subarachnoid space of both cranial fossae either directly or across the inner ear capsule. Cranial nerves IX, X, and XI are rarely injured, and this situation arises only when the fracture involves their neural compartments. These nerves are more likely traumatized by a ring fracture around the foramen magnum.

Recognition of a transverse pyramidal fracture is clinically important. The regularly associated loss of cochlear and vestibular function is usually total and permanent. The frequently accompanying facial nerve palsy, if improperly attended, may result in incomplete or altered return of seventh nerve function. As mentioned earlier, a transverse fracture may occasionally involve exclusively the cochlea or the labyrinth, in which instance function in the unaffected portion of the inner ear remains intact. In a rare situation, particularly when a transverse fracture is locally limited and affects only a portion of an inner ear capsule, cochlear and vestibular function may not immediately be totally destroyed. Eventually, however, most of the patients will lose all of their eighth nerve function as a result of associated secondary inner ear changes.

Of greater importance is the well-documented observation that the transverse fracture does not heal with an adequate bony union. Whereas the periosteal and endosteal layers of the otic and vestibular capsules are able to form new lamellar bone, the endochondral layer shows no evidence of participating in the repair. Consequently, in areas where the covering periosteal layer is very thin, no osseous unification is taking place, and the fracture cleft is being filled in with sparse fibrous tissue. This provides an open pathway for the spread of infection from the middle to the inner ear and hence to the subarachnoid space (Fig. 55.35) Thus there have been a number of well-documented instances of recurrent and delayed otogenic meningitis, often lethal, occurring weeks, months, and even many years after a transverse fracture of the pyramid. The clinical signs that should arise singly or in combination with the suspicion of a transverse fracture after a head trauma include: *(a)* partial or total loss of cochlear and vestibular function, *(b)* paralysis of the facial nerve, and *(c)* leakage of CSF from the middle ear. Once the clinical diagnosis has been established, a potentially lethal complicating meningitis can be treated or prevented.

COMMINUTED FRACTURES

Comminuted fractures no longer exhibit a predominant longitudinal or transverse fracture plane, although they may include components of each. Instead, the petrous pyramid is traversed by numerous fractures coursing at different levels, in different planes, and in various directions. This results in a considerable fragmentation of the entire pyramid (Figs. 55.24, 55.25, and 55.36). They actually occur far more frequently than hitherto suspected. One reason is that there are obvious transitional patterns from the hitherto-considered "classical" fracture to those complex fractures. By definition, they include all the features of the "standard" fractures as well as their disposition to complications. In fact, they have the highest incidence of meningeal complications. They may be recognized by their clinical manifestations, by their radiologic appearance, and above all by the histologic examination of the temporal bone.

OTHER FORMS OF TEMPORAL BONE FRACTURES

In addition to the longitudinal, transverse, combined, and compound fractures, there remains a small group of rare temporal bone fractures that should be mentioned merely for completeness. It includes: *(a)* an isolated fracture through the lower mastoid process that spares the middle ear but involves the external ear canal and the Fallopian canal (Figs. 55.26A and 55.28),

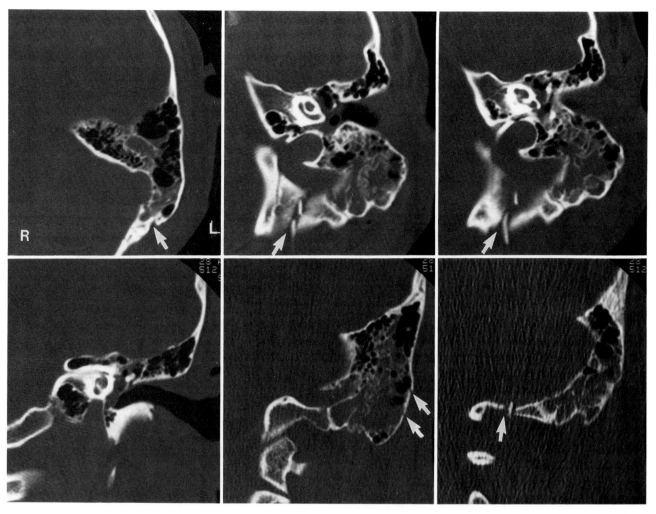

Figure 55.25. Serial axial CT scans of skull base with compound fracture of left temporal bone in a 22-year-old woman. The various fractures involved the medial and lateral cortex of the mastoid process, caused localized hemorrhages into the middle ear cleft and mastoid process, but did not affect cochlear, vestibular, and facial nerve function.

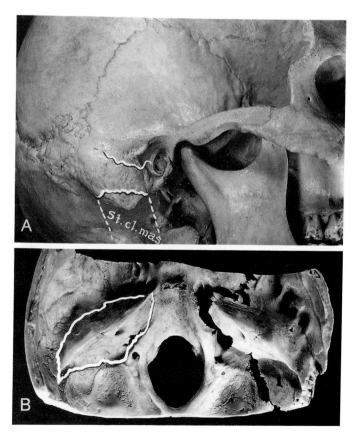

Figure 55.26. Pathways and directions of other temporal bone fractures. **A.** The fracture that transverses the mastoid process enters the external canal, may injure the lower mastoid segment of the facial nerve, but does not involve the middle ear. The fracture across the lower part of the mastoid process merely evulses the mastoid tip from the mastoid process. **B.** On the left, the fracture separates the petrous pyramid from the remaining portions of the left temporal bone. On the right, the fracture evulses the entire temporal bone from the surrounding skull base and calvaria.

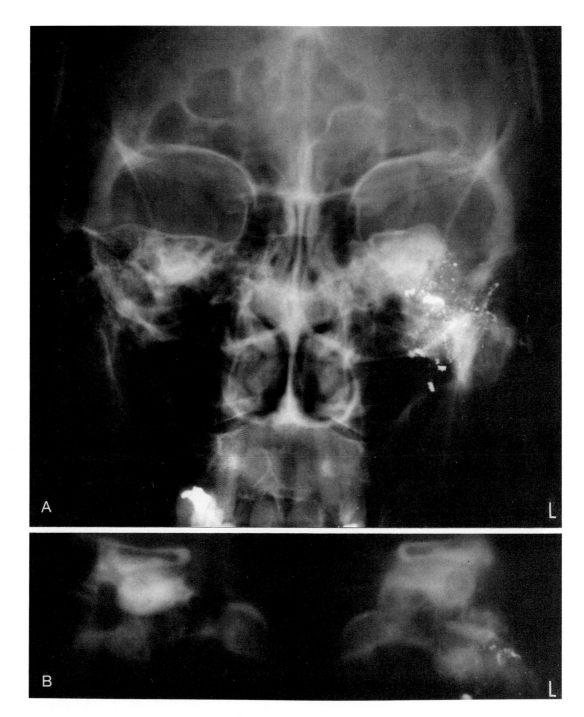

Figure 55.28. PA view of skull **(A)** and AP complex motion tomogram **(B)** of temporal bone bullet wound that resulted in shattering of the tympanic bone and inferior displacement of the mastoid process.

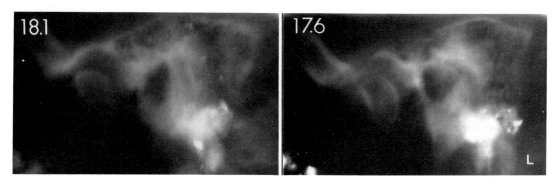

Figure 55.29. Lateral complex motion tomograms of left temporal bone in a young adult man with a gunshot wound that resulted in shattering of the lower mastoid process with injury to the facial nerve at the stylomastoid foramen.

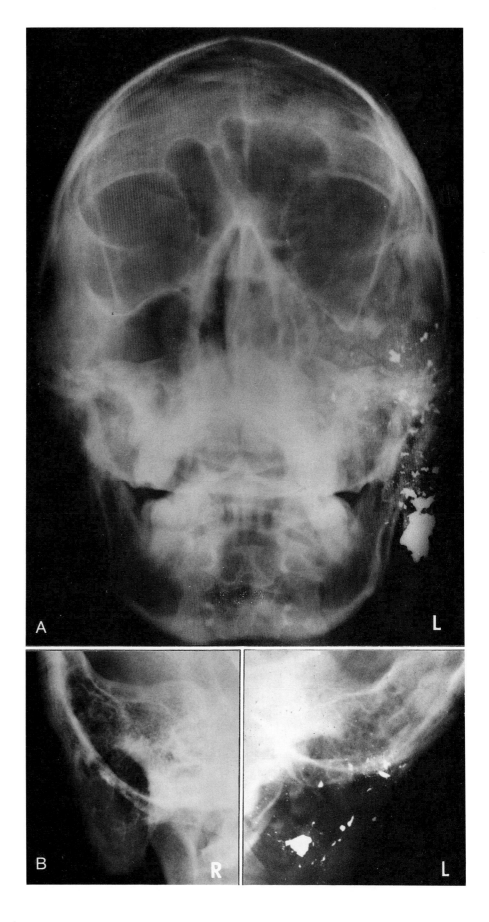

Figure 55.30.   PA view of skull **(A)** and tangential projections of mastoids **(B)** in an adult man with a gunshot wound of the left temporal bone. The gunshot resulted in a shattering of the mastoid process and involvement of the left maxillary sinus and inferior lateral wall of the orbit.

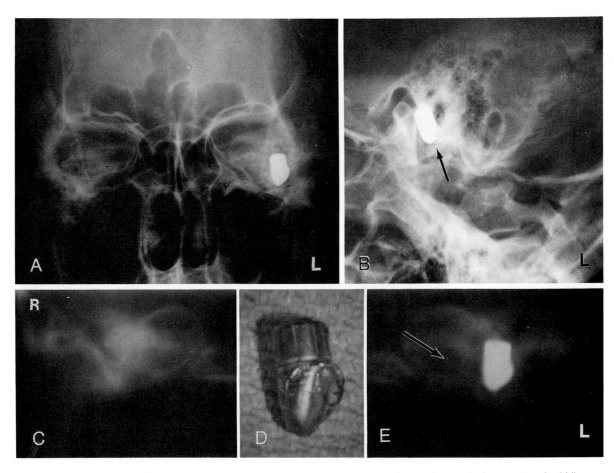

Figure 55.31   PA view of skull with transorbital projection of petrous pyramids **(A)**, lateral (Schüller) view of left temporal bone **(B)**, and AP complex motion tomograms of both petrous pyramids **(C)**, with a bullet **(D)** lodged in the left anterior external meatus and middle ear cavity of an adolescent man. Cochlear, vestibular, and facial nerve function were unimpaired.

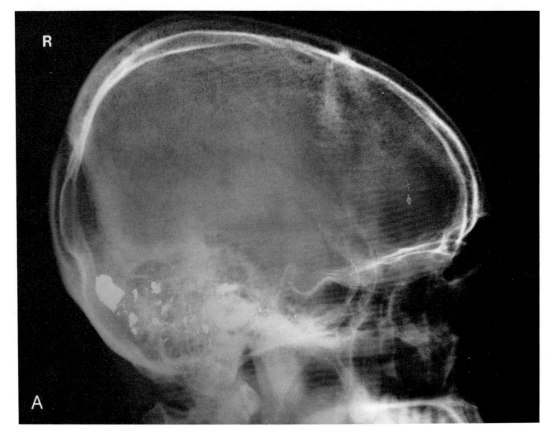

Figure 55.32.   Right lateral **(A)** and PA **(B)** views of skull and AP complex motion tomograms of right temporal bone **(C)** in an adult man with a gunshot injury to the right ear. The bullet has shattered the squamous, tympanic, and part of the petrous portion of the right temporal bone. Parts of the bullet are lodged in the attic, aditus, and mastoid antrum.

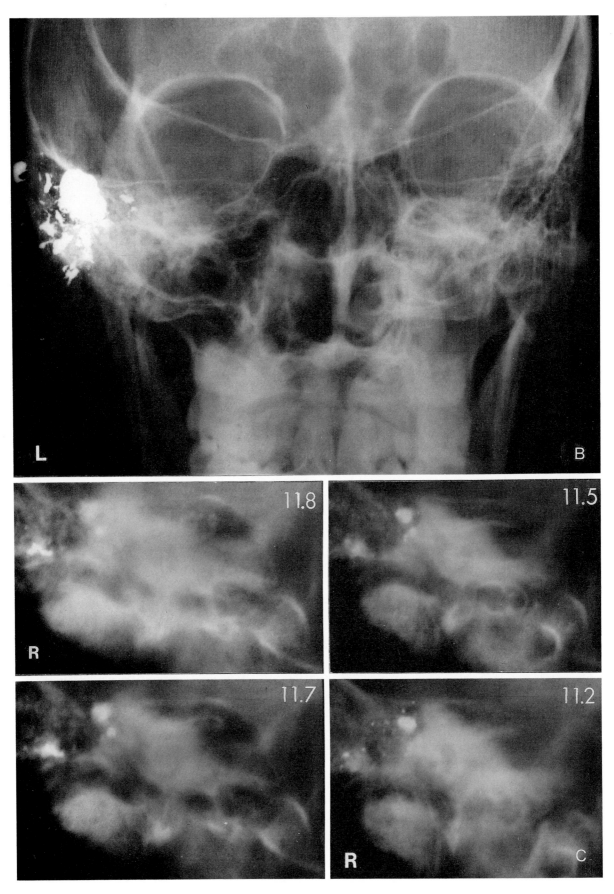

Figure 55.32.   B and **C.**

COMPLICATIONS

The most serious complications of a temporal bone fracture—extension of an infection in the middle ear cleft to the inner ear and subarachnoid space, injuries to the seventh and eighth cranial nerves and their end organs, and occasional involvement of cranial nerves IX, X, and XI—are discussed earlier. The laceration of the sigmoid sinus in a fracture of the mastoid process and the disruption of the carotid artery in an evulsive fracture of the petrous pyramid are also mentioned. In a rare instance a cranial pneumatocele may develop under the skin over the mastoid process, and occasionally a herniation of the arachnoid through a defect in the dura and the tegmental bone may give rise to a meningocele presenting in the antrum or epitympanic recess (Fig. 55.13). Displacement of brain tissue into the middle ear is a rare and grave complication. It is not uncommon for a fragment of meatal skin to become entrapped in a fracture involving the external auditory canal wall, a situation that subsequently results in a traumatic epidermoid inclusion cyst or cholesteatoma. Complications that require surgical intervention include: *(a)* recurrent or delayed meningitis, *(b)* persistent CSF leak, *(c)* persistent bleeding from a lacerated lateral sinus, *(d)* perilymph leak, *(e)* injury to the facial nerve with evidence of over 90% degeneration of its motor nerve fibers, and *(f)* traumatic cholesteatoma. Reconstruction of the ossicular chain is usually performed as an elective procedure at a later time.

In summary, more recent radiologic evidence and histopathologic observations necessitated a modification of the original classification of temporal bone fractures. For instance, longitudinal fractures, in addition to their most frequent vertical plane, may assume others, e.g., a horizontal plane. A transverse fracture may traverse the pyramid more often in an oblique than a perpendicular plane in relation to the long axis of the petrous bone, and the plane of that fracture may or may not be perpendicular to the floor of the posterior cranial fossa. The longitudinal, transverse, and combined pyramidal fractures frequently display a number of smaller or larger ramifications, departing in various directions. The fracture that shatters the pyramid must be regarded as a complex or compound fracture. This form of fracture has been seen more frequently. Case 4 is an example of such a fracture. It demonstrates the complexity of the anatomy and pathophysiology as well as the lethal endocranial complications of a compound pyramidal fracture. Bullet injuries are also typical examples of compound fractures.

Management of fractures of the temporal bone belong in the domain of the otologist and neuro-otologist who are familiar with the regional anatomy and possess the required surgical expertise.

Case Reports

Cases 1–5 illustrate the pertinent histopathologic changes found in the various temporal bone fractures and their effects on the middle ear, inner ear capsule, membranous labyrinth and cochlea, and seventh and eighth cranial nerves.

Case 1. *Extensive skull fracture involving the calvaria and base. Longitudinal fracture of left petrous pyramid. Microfractures involving the right cochlear and vestibular capsule.*

The patient had been an 18-year-old man who 18 hours before death had fallen 40 feet from a roof and sustained a fracture of the calvaria extending from the orbital plate of the right frontal bone posteriorly into the left basioccipital region, separating the sagittal suture. There were contusions involving the frontal, parietal, and temporal lobes and a massive subarachnoid hematoma.

Microscopic examination of the temporal bones reveals a longitudinal fracture involving the left petrous pyramid, shattering the tegmen, fracturing the Fallopian canal tangentially at the geniculate ganglion, producing an intraneural hematoma, and causing a massive hemorrhage into the middle ear air cell system and the cochlea (Fig. 55.33G and H). The right temporal bone exhibits scattered microfractures involving the floor of the internal auditory canal, the vestibular capsule, and the oval window area (Fig. 55.33A, E, and F). A widespread hemorrhage into the subarachnoid space of the right internal acoustic meatus can be seen (Fig. 55.33A and B). The right cochlear, vestibular, and facial nerves show extensive tears and intraneural hemorrhages (Fig. 55.33A–D).

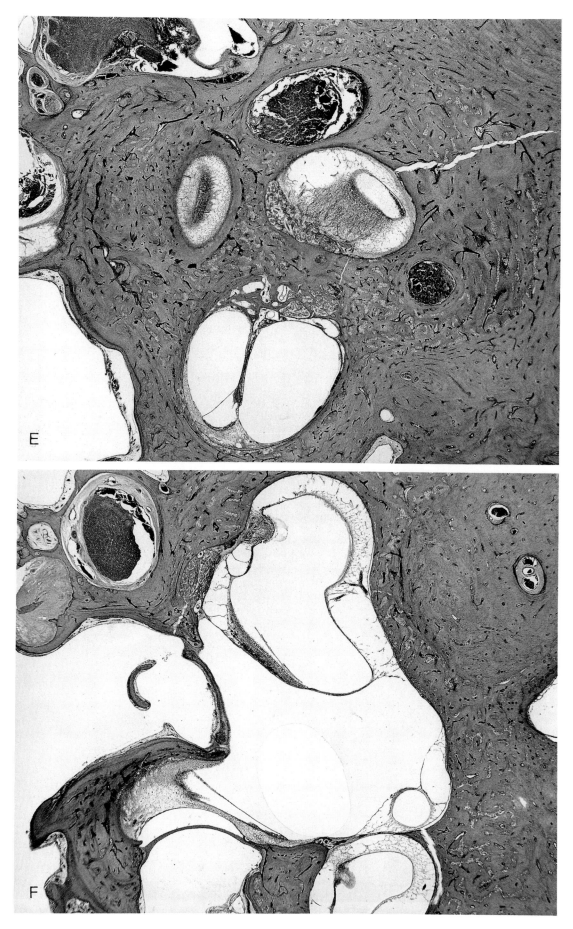

Figure 55.33.   E–H. Vertical sections through right **(E** and **F)** and left **(G** and **H)** temporal bones of the same patient as in **A–D.** Several microfractures involve the vestibular capsule **(E** and **F).**

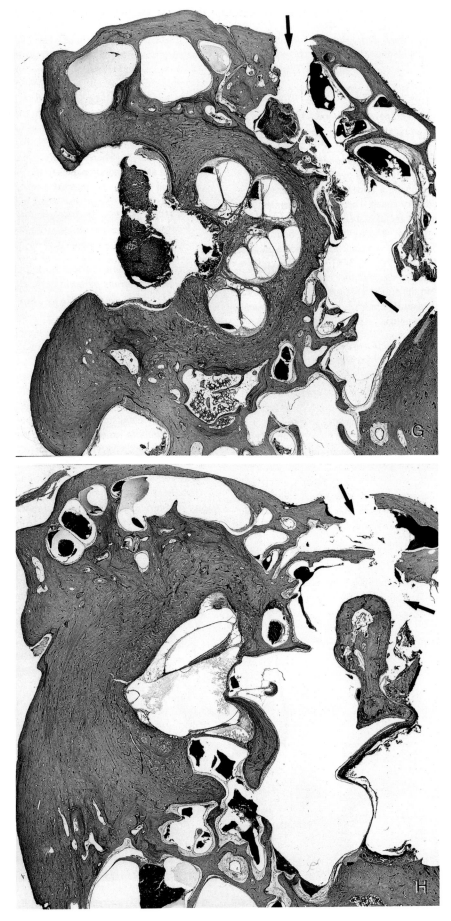

Figure 55.33.   G and **H.**

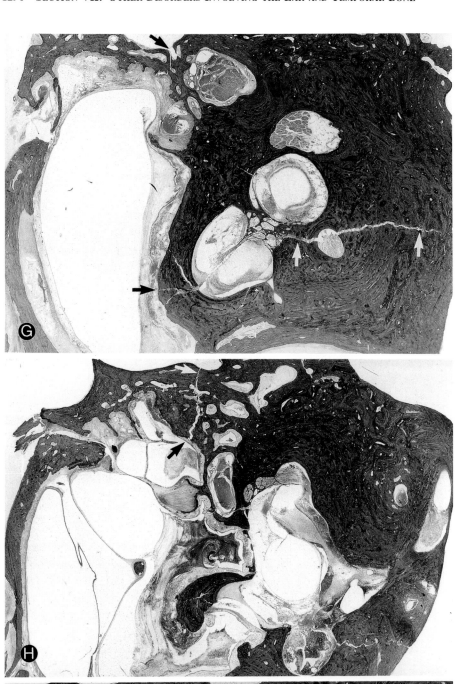

Figure 55.36. G. The horizontal longitudinal fracture continues posteriorly in a plane parallel to the skull base. Hairline fractures are recognized in the tegmen tympani, anterior vestibular capsule, and bone of the lower basal turn of the cochlea *(arrows)*. (Hematoxylin and eosin, ×9.)

Figure 55.36. H. A vertical fracture involves the tegmen tympani *(arrows)*. (×9.)

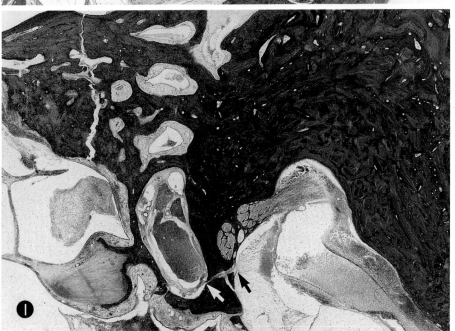

Figure 55.36. I. Another fracture connects the tympanic segment of the Fallopian canal with the perilymph compartment of the vestibule *(arrows)*. (×18.)

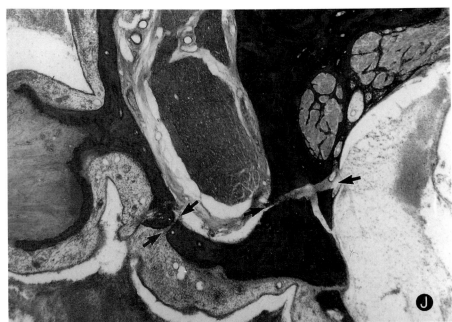

Figure 55.36. J. This fracture actually connects the middle ear mucosa with the vestibule *(arrows)*. (×40.)

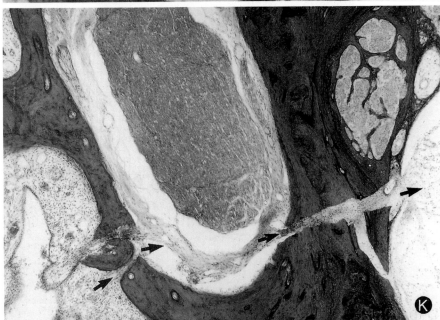

Figure 55.36. K. This fracture allowed the middle ear infection to extend to the perilymphatic space of the vestibule *(arrows)*. (×30.)

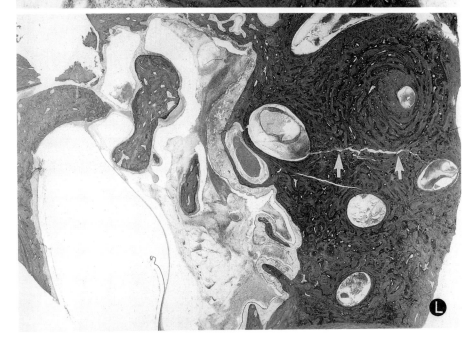

Figure 55.36. L. Inflammatory edema involving the middle ear mucosa and the purulent exudate in the tympanic cavity characterize the acute otitis media. The horizontal, longitudinal fracture connects the ampullated end of the lateral semicircular canal with the nonampullated end of the posterior semicircular canal *(arrows)*. (×9.)

References

1. DeGrood MPAM. Skull fractures. In: Vinken PJ, Bruyn GW, eds. Handbook of clinical neurology. Amsterdam: North Holland Publishing, Chap 17, 1975;17:387–402.

2. Schinz HR. Frakturen des Felsenbeines. In: Lehrbuch der Röntgendiagnostik. Stuttgart: Georg Thieme, 1966;3:493–494.

3. Ulrich K. Verletzungen des Gehöhrorgans bei Schädelbasisfrakturen. Acta Otolaryngol (Stockh) 1926;Suppl 6:1–150.

4. Skoog T. Studies of material of head injuries from the surgical clinic in Lund. Acta Chir Scand 1936;77:383–454.

5. Grove WE. Skull fractures involving the ear: clinical study of 211 cases. Laryngoscope 1933;49:678 and 833.

6. Kelemen G. Fractures of the temporal bone. Arch Otolaryngol 1944;40:333–373.

7. Kley W. Die Unfallchirurgie der Schadelbasis und der pneumatischen Raume. Arch Klin Exp Ohren-Nasen-Kehlkopfheilkd 1968;191:1–216.

8. Nager GT. Fractures of the temporal bone. Louis Clerf Lecture, June 23, 1982, Jefferson University School of Medicine, Philadelphia, Pennsylvania.

9. Brock W. Längsfraktur durch die Schläfenbeinpyramide mit Verletzung des inneren Ohres. Z Hals-Nasen-Ohrenheilkd 1933;34:349–377.

10. Durrer J. Mechanism of the laterobasal fractures. Acta Otolaryngol (Stockh) 1962;66:25–32.

11. Gurdjian ES, Lissner HR. Deformations of the skull in head injury studied by "stresscoat" technique quantitative determinations. Surg Gynecol Obstet 1946;83:219–233.

12. Grove WE. Military symposium. Management of injuries to middle and internal ear including fracture. Laryngoscope 1941;511:957–963.

13. Griffin JE, Altenau MM, Schaefer SD. Bilateral longitudinal temporal bone fractures: a retrospective view of seventeen cases. Laryngoscope 1979;89:1432–1435.

14. Hough JVD. Otologic trauma. In: Paparella MM, Shumrick DA, eds. Otolaryngology. Philadelphia: WB Saunders, Chap 27, 1980;II:1656–1679.

15. Guerrier Y. Ossicle lesions in closed skull injuries. Acta Otolaryngol Belg 1971;25(4):607–614.

16. Boenninghaus HG. Ohrverletzungen. In: Berendes J, Link R, Zöllner F, eds. Hals-Nasen-Ohrenheilkunde, Ohr I. Stuttgart: Georg Thieme, Chap 20, 1979:5.

17. Nassulphis P. Die Schädigung des Innenohres und seiner Nerven mach Schädeltrauma. Monatsschr Ohrenheilkd 1946;79:68–86 (part 1) and 1946;80:222–252 (part 2).

18. Schuknecht HF, Neff W, Perlman H. An experimental study of auditory damage following blows to the head. Ann Otol Rhinol Laryngol 1951;60:274–289.

19. Schuknecht HF. Mechanisms of inner ear injury from blows to the head. Ann Otol Rhinol Laryngol 1969;78:253–262.

20. Schuknecht HF, Davidson RC. Deafness and vertigo from head injury. Arch Otolaryngol 1956;63:513–528.

21. Ward PH. The histopathology of auditory and vestibular disorders in head trauma. Ann Otol Rhinol Laryngol 1969;78:227–238.

22. Makishima K, Snow JB. Pathogenesis of hearing loss in head injury. Arch Otolaryngol 1975;101:426–432.

23. Barber H. Positional nystagmus especially after head injury. Laryngoscope 1964;74:891–944.

24. Pfisterer H. Über den doppelseitigen Felsenbeinquerbruch. Monatsschr Unfallheilkd 1957;60(8):229–239.

25. Grove WE. Transverse fracture of the petrous pyramid. Arch Otolaryngol 1939;30:314.

26. McHugh HE. Facial paralysis in birth injury and skull fractures. Arch Otolaryngol 1963;78:443–455.

27. Proctor B, Gurdjian ES, Webster JE. The ear in head trauma. Laryngoscope 1959;66:16–59.

28. Nager FR. Zur Histologie der isolierten Schneckenfraktur. Pract Oto-Rhino-Laryngol (Basel) 1949;XI:134–141.

29. Klingenberg A. Die isolierte Schneckenfraktur bein Schädelbasisbrüchen. Z Hals-Nasen-Ohrenheilkd 1929;22:5–16.

30. Escher F. Die Otologische Beurteilung des Schädeltraumatikers. Pract Oto-Rhino-Laryngol (Basel) 1948;X(Suppl I):247.

31. Lange G, Kornhuber HH. Zur Bedeutung peripher- und zentral-vestibulärer Störungen nach Korftraumen. Arch Ohren-Nasen-Kehlkofpheilkd 1962;179:366.

32. Barber HO. Head injury: audiological and vestibular findings. Ann Otol 1969;78:239.

33. Harker LA, McCabe BF. Temporal bone fractures and facial nerve injury. Otolaryngol Clin North Am 1974;7:425.

34. Tos M. Course and sequelae of 248 petrosal fractures. Acta Otolaryngol (Stockh) 1973;75:353.

35. Pearson BW, Frederickson JM. Trauma of the temporal bone. In: English GM, ed. Otolaryngology. Philadelphia: Harper & Row, Chap 13, 1982;4:1–23.

56/ Various Aspects of Normal and Pathologic Anatomy

ANATOMY

Corpuscles of Vater-Pacini

The corpuscles of Vater-Pacini represent one of several forms of sensory nerve endings found in connective tissue. They have a predominantly oval shape measuring $1-4 \times 2$ mm in diameter, and when dissected from fresh tissue, they may be visible to the naked eye as a white bulb. Their characteristic structure reveals a thick capsule and a number of concentric lamellae in an onionskin-like (layered) arrangement. Each corpuscle is supplied by one or more thick myelinated nerve fibers that lose their myelin sheath first and then their neurolemma among the specialized layers in its elongated central core. The concentric capsule layers are separated from each other by a single flat layer of connective tissue. Each layer contains a fluid and longitudinally and transversely oriented connective tissue fibers. The capsule and concentric lamellae arise from the connective tissue sheath surrounding the penetrating nerve fibers. Within the cellular inner bulb the axon branches out and gives rise to an elongated dense convolution of fine branches that almost totally occupy its inner space, and it is surrounded by the ramifications of a second thin axon. A small artery enters the corpuscle together with the nerve fibers and gives rise to a capillary network between the lamellae (1–3).

The corpuscles of Vater-Pacini register and convey sensations of touch. They are found in the deep layers of the skin, under mucous membranes, in loose connective tissue, in the mesentery, pancreas, heart, conjunctiva, and cornea, and in different locations in the temporal bone (Fig. 56.1). In the temporal bone they may be observed in the jugular bulb (Fig. 56.1F and G), in the mucoperiosteum of the middle ear cleft, and in the bone accompanying small nerves and vessels. Figure 56.1 demonstrates their form and some of their locations in the temporal bone.

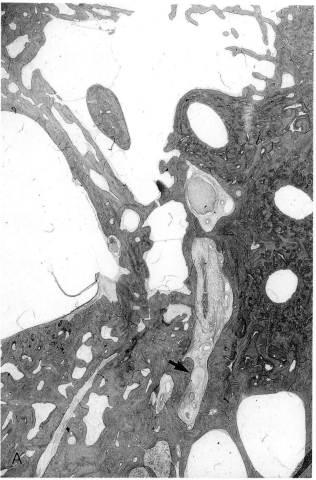

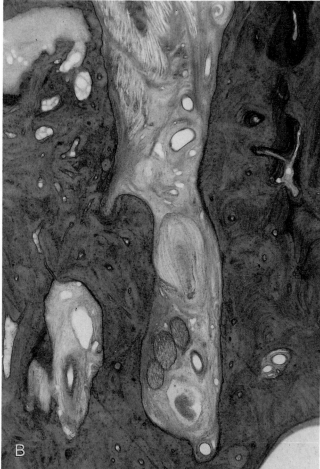

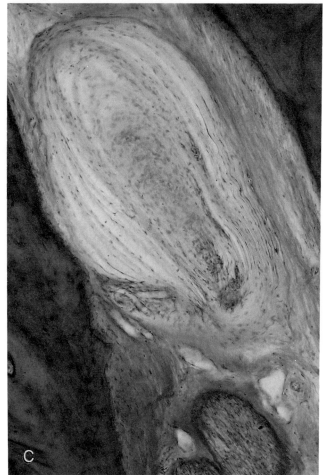

Figure 56.1. Corpuscles of Vater-Pacini. A. Vertical section through right temporal bone near mastoid segment of facial canal of a 37-year-old white man. It shows the location of a single corpuscle of Vater-Pacini 1 cm beneath the lower end of the stapedius muscle *(arrow)*. **B.** The corpuscle is near three fascicles of the auricular branch of the vagus nerve (nerve of Arnold). **C.** The corpuscle has an ovoid form and consists of a capsule and concentric lamellae in an onionskin-like arrangement. (Hematoxylin and eosin, ×10, ×30, and ×110, respectively.)

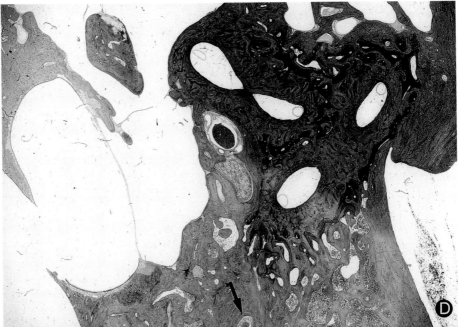

Figure 56.1 D. Vertical section through right temporal bone near upper end of vertical segment of Fallopian canal in a 16-year-old white woman. It shows a cross-section through the facial nerve and stapedius muscle and the location of a single corpuscle of Vater-Pacini above the jugular bulb *(arrow)*. (×10.)

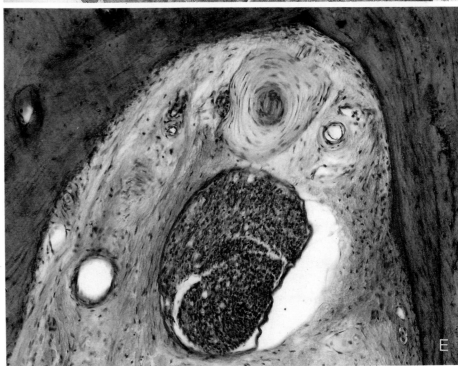

Figure 56.1 E. The corpuscle is located near the auricular branch of the vagus in its osseous canal, accompanied by blood vessels. (×150.)

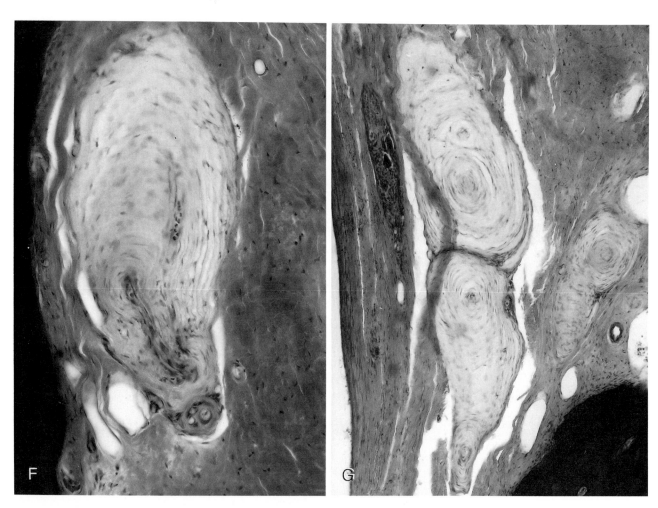

Figure 56.1. **F.** Single corpuscle of Vater-Pacini in vertical section of right temporal bone in a 40-year-old white woman. The ovoid corpuscle displays a capsule, a system of numerous concentric lamellae in an onion-skin-like arrangement, and a central cavity in which the axon or axons branch out and give rise to an elongated dense convolution of fine ramifi-cations. A small artery enters the corpuscle at the lower pole together with three thick myelinated fibers and supplies a capillary network between the lamellae. **G.** Corpuscles of Vater-Pacini are sometimes found in clusters, as seen here. (Hematoxylin and eosin, ×200 and ×100, respectively.)

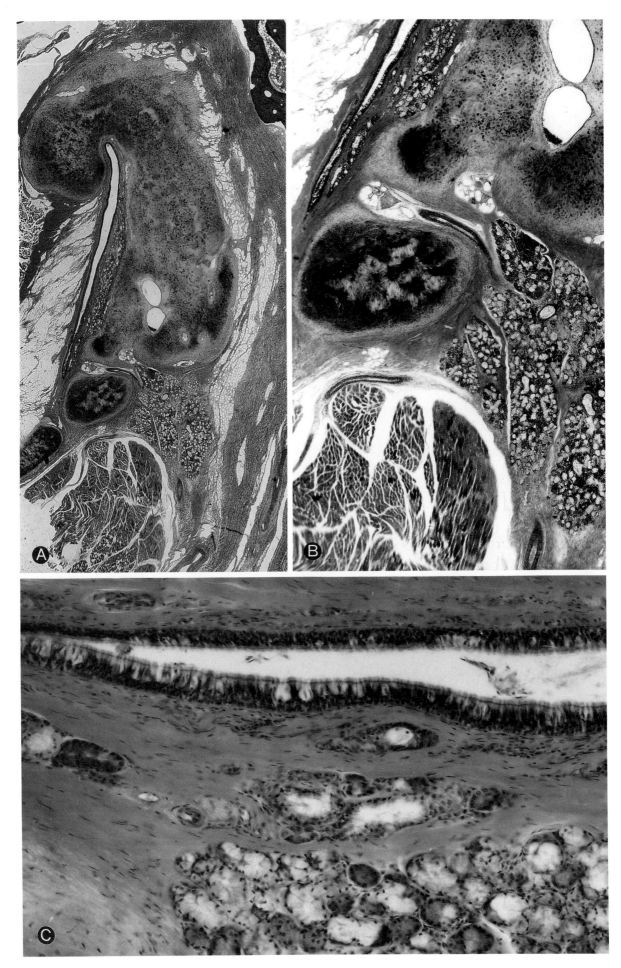

Figure 56.2. Eustachian tube. A. Vertical section through cartilaginous portion of right Eustachian tube and its adjacent muscles, tensor veli palatini muscle (near the left margin) and levator veli palatini muscle (near the lower margin). The cartilage is elastic. **B.** Compound tubuloalveolar glands secrete mucus via ducts opening into the tubal lumen, and blood vessels supply the mucosa. **C.** The epithelium is pseudostratified and composed of tall columnar ciliated cells with many goblet cells interspersed between them. Throughout the lamina propria a great many lymphocytes and collections of lymphoid tissue are recognized. (Hematoxylin and eosin, ×8, ×40, and ×200, respectively.)

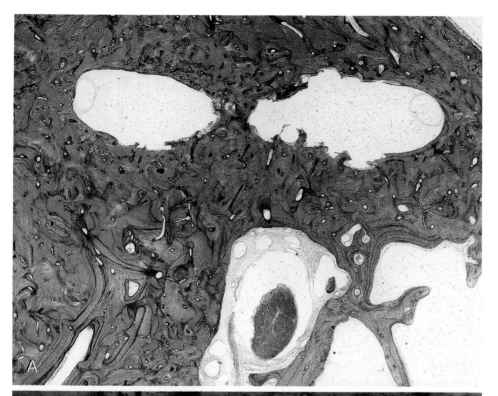

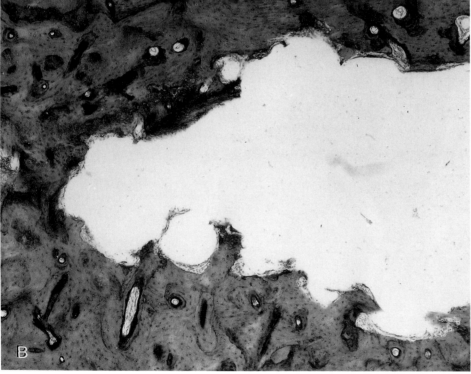

Figure 56.5. Irregular endosteal bone resorption involving the semicircular canals. A. Vertical section through left temporal bone near posterior tangent of lateral semicircular canal, displaying the areas of irregular resorption of endosteal and adjacent endochondral capsule layers. (Hematoxylin and eosin, ×25.)

Figure 56.5. B. The mechanism of this bone resorption is not fully understood. These occasional observations, however, are of no clinical significance. (×60.)

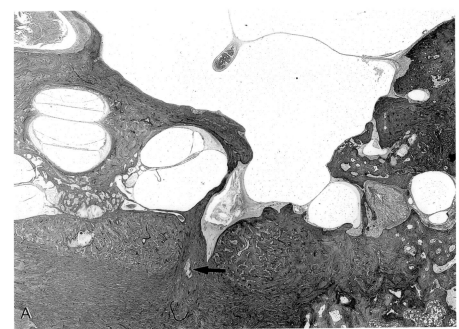

Figure 56.6. Cochlear aperture of cochlear aqueduct. A. Horizontal section through right temporal bone near level of round window in an adult. The cochlear aqueduct *(arrow)* is about to join the scala tympani of the lower basal turn of the cochlea. (Hematoxylin and eosin, ×10.)

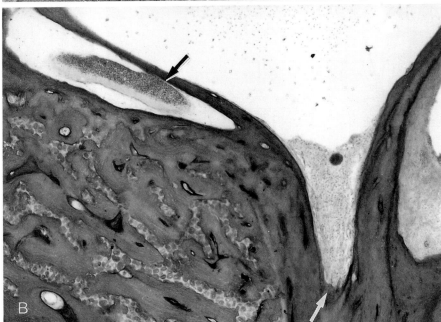

Figure 56.6. B. The cochlear aqueduct is opening into the scala tympani *(white arrow)*. To its left is a longitudinal section through its accompanying vein *(black arrow)*. (×40.)

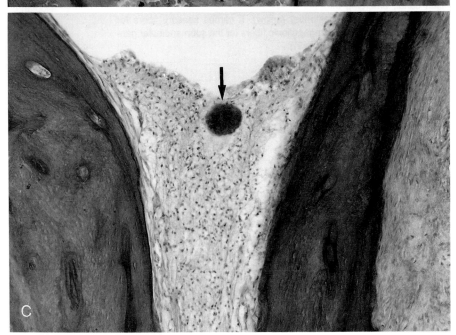

Figure 56.6. C. The cochlear aqueduct contains a loose meshwork of arachnoid tissue with a single psammoma body *(arrow)*. (×85.)

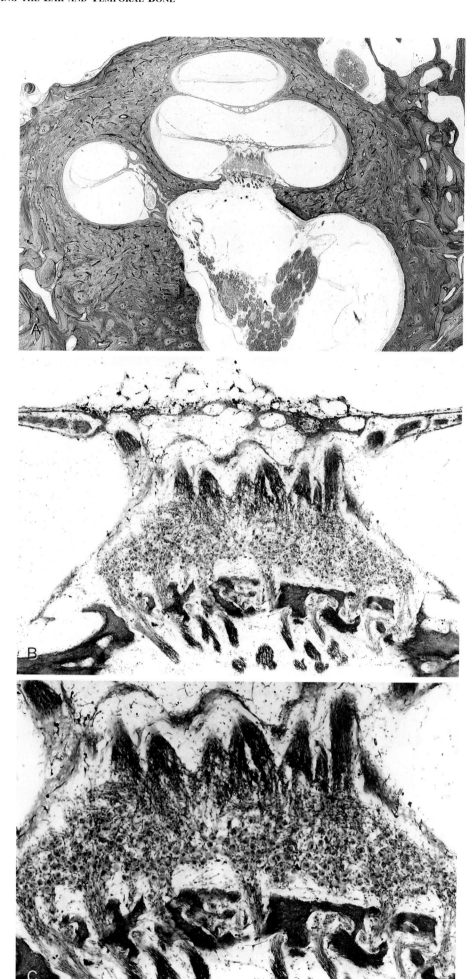

Figure 56.10.   Morphology of cochlear nerve at entrance into cochlear modiolus. A. Vertical, anterior paramodiolar section through right temporal bone in an adult with a cross-section through the spiral foraminal tract. (Hematoxylin and eosin, ×7.)

Figure 56.10.   B and **C.** As the cochlear nerve enters the cochlear modiolus, it divides into small fascicles that transverse the bone in individual canaliculi to form the spiral ganglion. From the spinal ganglion the peripheral nerve fibers leave in bundles to enter the osseous spiral lamina in a segmental, ascending spiral arrangement. (×70 and ×100, respectively.)

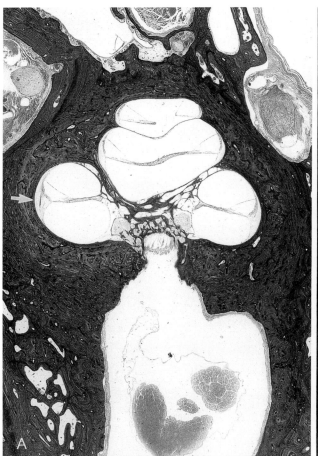

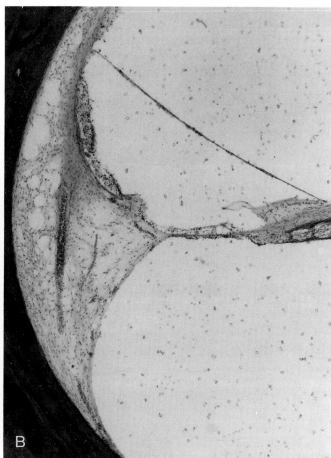

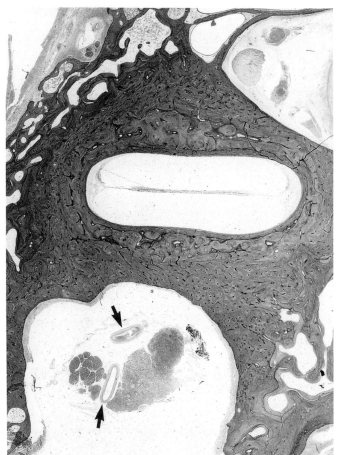

Figure 56.11 (above). Venous system of spiral ligament. A. Vertical, anterior paramodiolar section of right temporal bone in an adult with a longitudinal section through a "straight" vessel in the spiral ligament of the lower basal turn of the cochlea. **B.** The "straight" vessels in the spiral ligament follow a more-or-less direct course between the scalae connecting the radiating arterioles with the collecting venules. They vary in size and may well represent arteriovenous anastomoses that can bypass the spiral capillary network (see Chapter 4). (Hematoxylin and eosin, ×10 and ×90, respectively.)

Figure 56.12 (left). Anterior inferior cerebellar artery (AICA) inside internal auditory canal (IAC). Vertical section through left temporal bone in an adult. Occasionally, a loop of the AICA, of which two cross-sections are recognized *(arrows),* is found within the IAC. (Hematoxylin and eosin, ×12.)

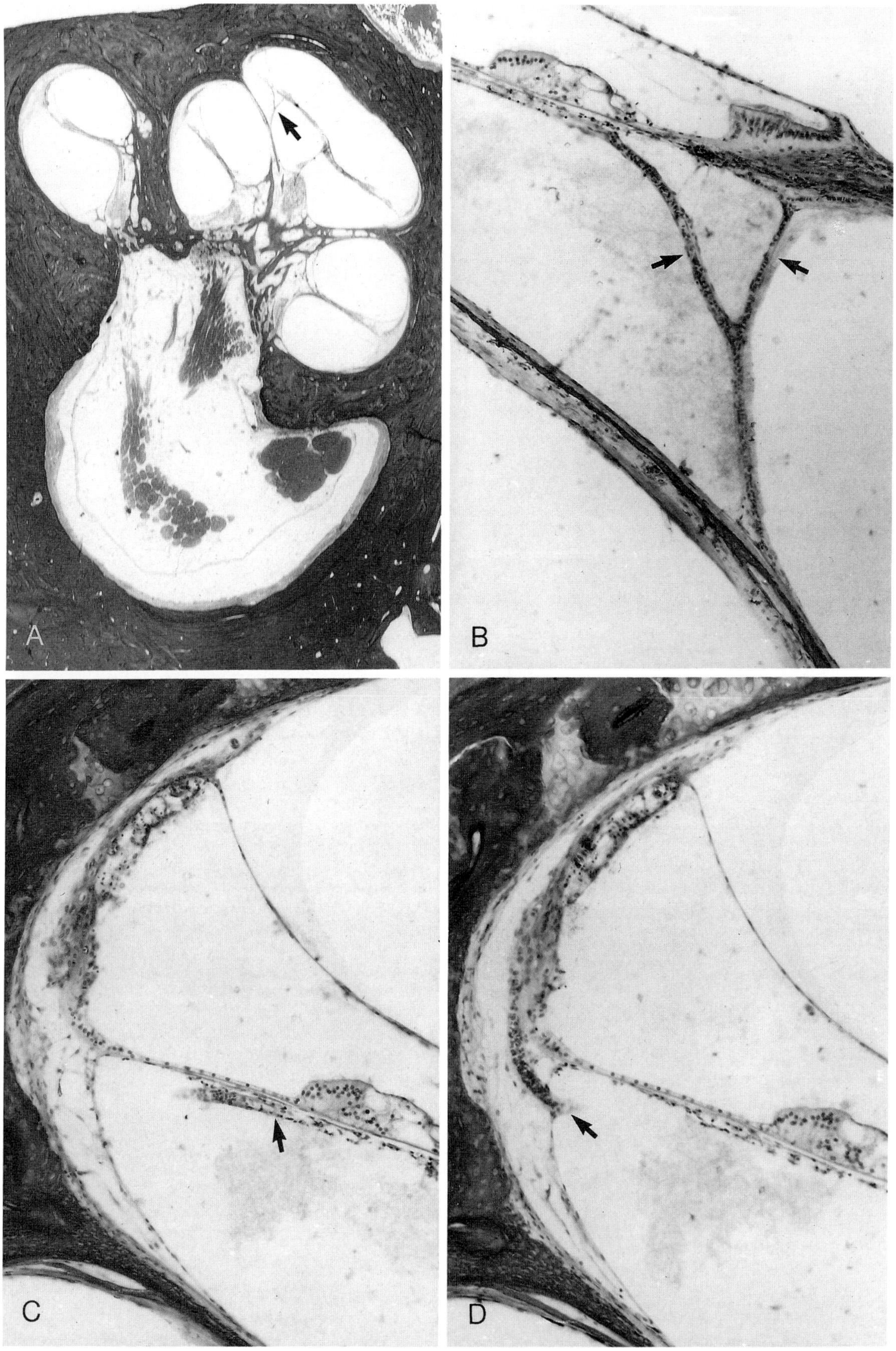

Figure 56.13. Abnormal blood vessel in scala tympani. A. Vertical, anterior paramodiolar section through right temporal bone of an adult with an abnormal blood vessel transversing the scala tympani of the lower apical turn of the cochlea *(arrow)*. **B.** This arteriole is a branch of an external radiating arteriole of the lower middle turn of the cochlea. It divides within the scale tympani into a medial and a lateral branch *(arrows)*. The medial branch anastomoses on the undersurface of the osseous spiral lamina with the arcading vessels of the tympanic lip and basilar membrane *(arrow)*. **C** and **D.** The lateral branch continues laterally beneath the membranous portion of the basal membrane *(arrow, C)*, enters the lower half of the spiral ligament **(D)**, and anastomoses with the capillary networks of that ligament **(D)**. (See Chapter 4.) (Hematoxylin and eosin, ×8, ×130, ×130, and ×130, respectively.)

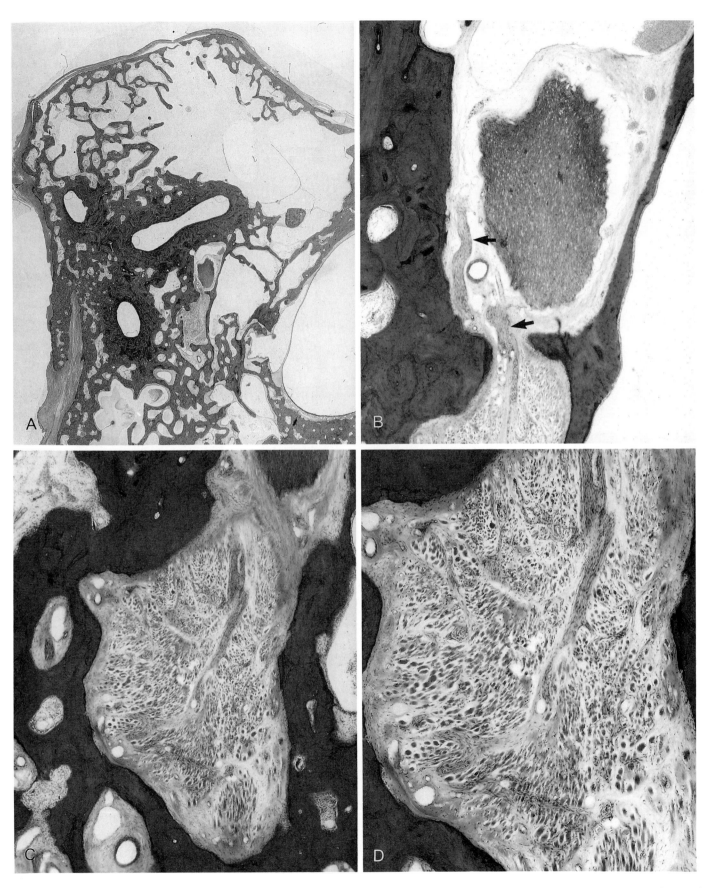

Figure 56.14. Innervation of stapedius muscle. A. Vertical section through left temporal bone at level of stapedius muscle and Fallopian canal. **B.** The nerve to the stapedius muscle arises from the facial nerve in the upper mastoid segment of the Fallopian canal. It is seen here as it leaves the parent nerve, next to the stylomastoid artery, as it enters the muscle *(arrows).* **C** and **D.** The complex innervation pattern of the stapedius muscle is demonstrated. (Hematoxylin and eosin, ×6, ×45, ×45, and ×65, respectively.)

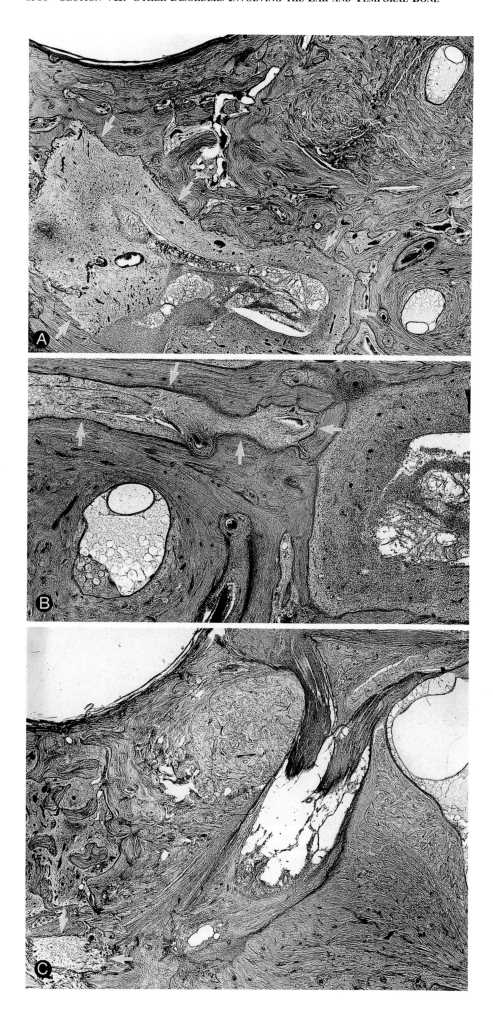

Figure 56.18. Coalescent petrous apicitis. A. Horizontal section through right petrous pyramid in a 10-year-old girl with subacute coalescent mastoiditis and petrous apicitis. The large osteolytic cavity in the apex is situated just anterior to (to the left of) the cross-section of the nonampullated end of the superior semicircular canal *(arrows)*. (Hematoxylin and eosin, ×22.)

Figure 56.18. B. The large abscess cavity occupying the mastoid process, recognized to the right of the ampullated end of the superior semicircular canal, is extending to the petrous apex along two recognized avenues: the lateral perilabyrinthine cell tract above the ampullated end of the superior canal *(arrows);* and the subarcuate fossa seen to the right and below that segment of the canal. (×22.)

Figure 56.18. C. The level of this section is just below the roof of the IAC. It demonstrates a longitudinal section of the intracanalicular, labyrinthine, and tympanic segments of the facial nerve and of the superior division of the vestibular nerve. In the left lower corner, there is a tangential section through the abscess in the petrous apex *(arrows)*. (See Chapter 12 for petrocitis.)

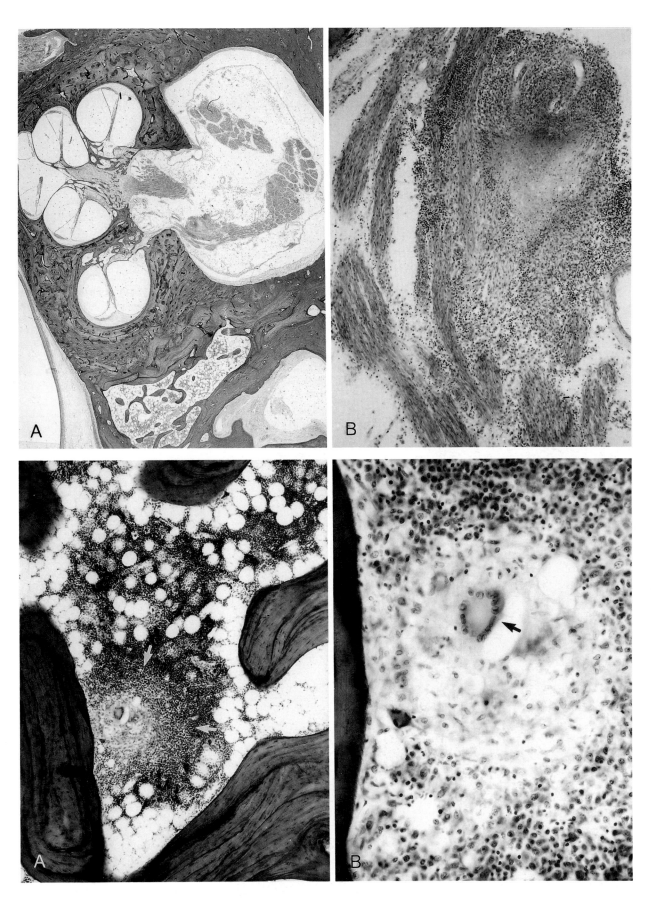

Figure 56.19 (upper). **Tuberculosis. A.** Vertical section through right temporal bone in an adult who died from tuberculous meningitis. **B.** The subarachnoid space within the IAC contains a purulent exudate and a conglomerate of tubercles with a caseous center surrounded by epithelioid histiocytes. A mantle of lymphocytes, plasma cells, and monocytes surrounds the epithelioid cell zone. (Hematoxylin and eosin, ×7 and ×75, respectively.)

Figure 56.20 (lower). **A.** Miliary tubercle in marrow space of right petrous apex of a young adult who died from exudative pulmonary tuberculosis with hematogenous dissemination *(arrows).* **B.** A striking feature of the tuberculous granuloma is the presence of multinucleate giant cells *(arrow).* In this Langhans' giant cell, formed by fusion of several epithelioid cells, the nuclei are arranged in a ring surrounding an eosinophilic cytocenter. (Hematoxylin and eosin, ×160 and ×40, respectively.)

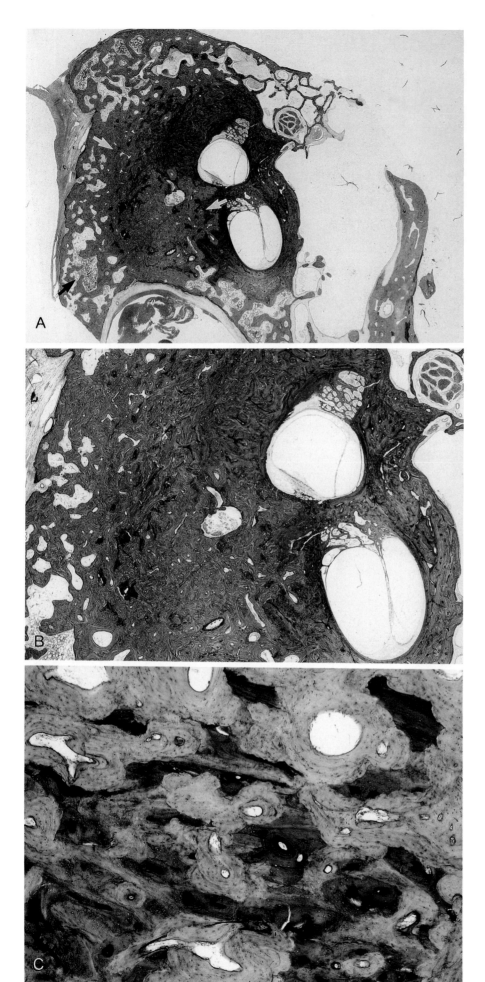

Figure 56.21. Osteitis deformans (Paget). A. Vertical section through left temporal bone just anterior to oval window margin in an elderly man with a moderate-sized, somewhat ill-defined, asymptomatic area of pagetoid bone remodeling *(arrows).* (Hematoxylin and eosin, ×6.)

Figure 56.21. B. It is situated between the medial cortex of the pyramid and the anterior vestibule and lower basal turn of the cochlea. (×13.)

Figure 56.21. C. The mosaic pattern created by the irregularly oriented and ill-assorted units representing several generations of bone, joined by cement lines, is characteristic for and identifies the arrested final phase of pagetoid bone remodeling. (×55.)

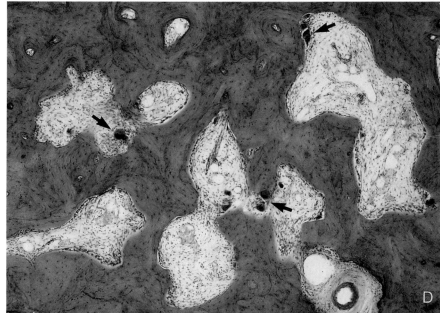

Figure 56.21. D. Destruction of the original and subsequent generations of bone begins in adjacent marrow spaces with erosion along the surface by mononucleated osteoclasts and with lacunar erosion by mononucleated and multinucleated osteoclasts *(arrows).* (×55.)

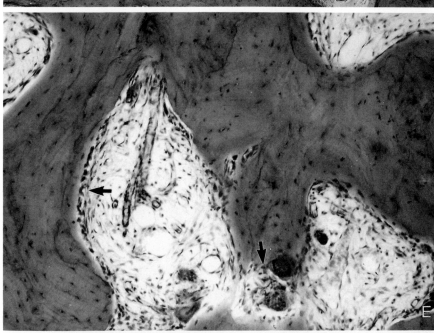

Figure 56.21. E. In areas of active bone transformation, osteoclastic bone absorption and osteoblastic rimming with deposition of osteoid can be seen side by side, occasionally lining the same trabecula *(arrows).* (×145.)

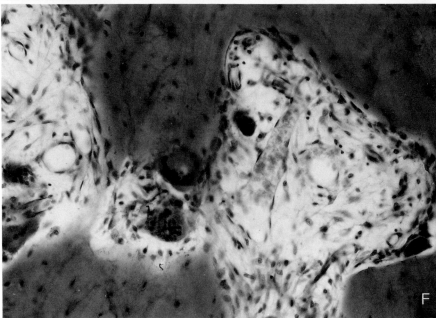

Figure 56.21. F. The marrow is replaced by a vascular, cellular, fibrous tissue. (×240.)

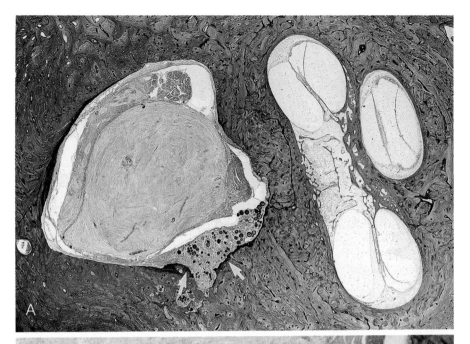

Figure 56.22. Meningioma. A. Vertical, anterior paramodiolar section through left temporal bone of a 54-year-old man with multiple intracranial meningiomas and multiple bilateral schwannomas of the seventh and eighth cranial nerves, associated with an intracanalicular meningioma *(arrows)* (neurofibromatosis type 2). (Hematoxylin and eosin, ×11.)

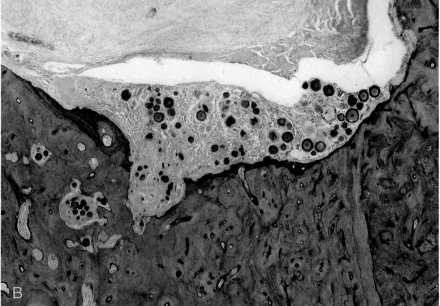

Figure 56.22. B. The meningioma within the IAC is of the psammomatous subgroup that includes numerous concentric calcifications. (×35.)

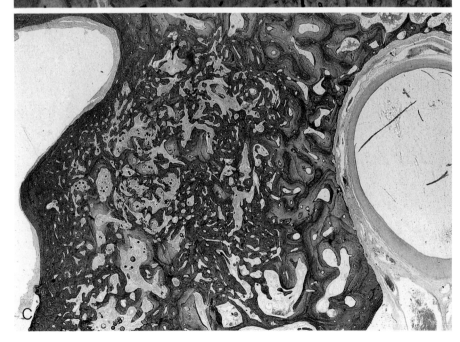

Figure 56.22. C. The psammoma extensively invaded the underlying bone, giving rise to a reactive sclerosis of the endochondral bone. (×20.)

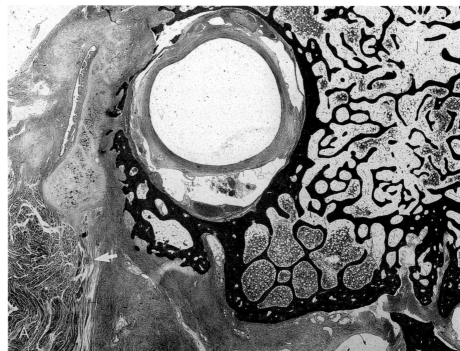

Figure 56.23. Trichiniasis. A. Vertical section through right petrous apex of an adult, demonstrating the location of a larva of *Trichinella spiralis* encysted in the striated voluntary levator veli palatini muscle *(arrow).* The infection, now less common than in the past, is still found in approximately 5% of autopsies performed in the United States. (Hematoxylin and eosin, ×7.5.)

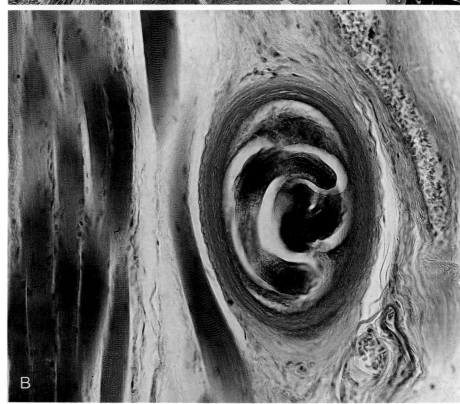

Figure 56.23. B. Once the larva penetrates the muscle fibers, it grows in size, coils in a corkscrew fashion, and proceeds to encyst. The infected muscle fiber is destroyed by the inflammatory process, and a fibrous wall or capsule develops around the larva, producing a cyst averaging 1 mm or less in diameter. Ultimately, the wall of the cyst and larva may calcify. (×270.)

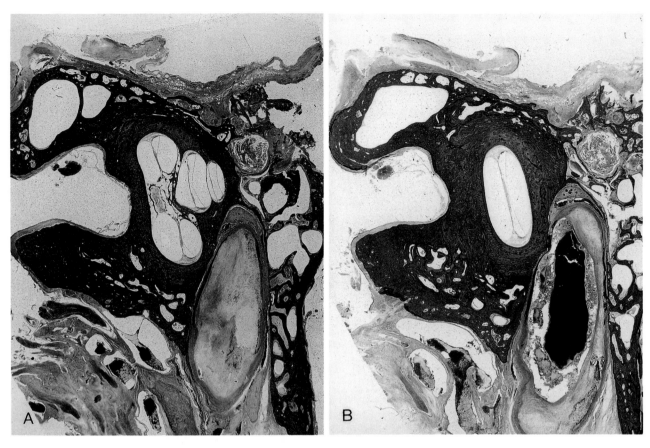

Figure 56.24. Thrombosis of internal carotid artery. A. Vertical para-modiolar section through left temporal bone in an adult who died shortly after thrombosis of left intratemporal carotid artery. **B.** The arteriosclerotic thrombosis is in the process of being organized. (Hematoxylin and eosin, ×6 for both.)

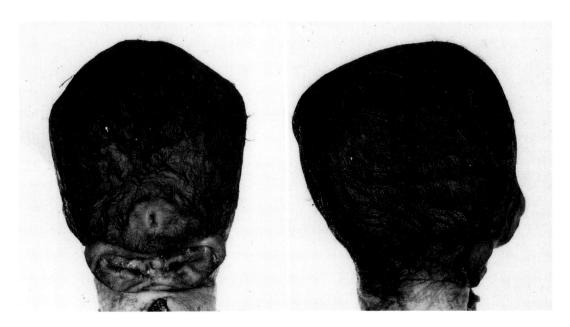

Figure 56.25. Development anomalies. Extreme displacement of malformed auricles (melotus) to anterior neck in association with other severe developmental anomalies of head.

References

1. Von Möllendorff W. Peripheres nerven System. In: Von Möllendorff W, ed. Lehrbuch der Histologie. 24th ed. Jena: G Fischer, 1940:257–272.
2. Goss MC. History of the nervous system. In: Goss MC, ed. Anatomy of the human body by H Gray. 28th ed. Philadelphia: Lea & Febiger, Chap 11, 1966:895–896.
3. Bloom W, Fawcett DW. Encapsulated terminal sensory endings. In: Bloom W, Fawcett DW, eds. A textbook of histology. 10th ed. Philadelphia: WB Saunders, 1975:363–364.

Figure and Table Credits

The following figures and tables have been reproduced with permission from the sources listed below.

Figures	*Sources*
1.2, 1.3, 1.4	Brödel M. Three unpublished drawings of the anatomy of the human ear. Philadelphia: WB Saunders, 1946.
1.5, 1.6	Anson BJ, Donaldson JA. Surgical anatomy of the temporal bone. 3rd ed. Philadelphia: WB Saunders, 1981.
1.8	Hawkins JE Jr. Hearing anatomy and acoustics. In: Best CH, Taylor NE eds. The physiological basis of medical practice. 8th ed. Baltimore: Williams & Wilkins, 1965.
1.9	Blum W, Fawcett DW. A textbook of histology. 9th ed. Philadelphia: WB Saunders, 1968.
1.10	Hawkins JE Jr. Hearing anatomy and acoustics. In: Best CH, Taylor NE eds. The physiological basis of medical practice. 8th ed. Baltimore: Williams & Wilkins, 1965.
1.13, 1.14, 1.15	Beck CHL. Anatomie und Histologie des Ohres. In: Berendes J, Link R, Zöllner F, eds. Hals-Nasen-Ohrenheilkunde in Praxis und Klinik, 2: Aufl, Ohr I. Stuttgart: Georg Thieme, Chap 2, 1979;5:1–60.
1.20	Brödel M. Three unpublished drawings of the anatomy of the human ear. Philadelphia: WB Saunders, 1946.
1.21	Anson BJ, Donaldson JA. Surgical anatomy of the temporal bone. 3rd ed. Philadelphia: WB Saunders, 1981.
1.22	Wersall J, Lundquist PG. Morphological polarization of the mechanoreceptors of the vestibular and acoustic system. In: Graybiel A, ed. Second symposium on the role of the vestibular organs in space exploration. NASA publication no. Sp-115. Washington, DC: National Aeronautics and Space Administration, 1966.
1.23	Spoendlin A. The innervation of the organ of Corti. J Laryngol 1967;81:717.
1.27, 1.28A&B	Hardy M. Observations on the innervation of the macula sacculi in man. Anat Rec 1934; 59(4):403–418.
1.29	deBurlet HM. Zur Innervation der Macula Sacculi bei Säugetieren. Anat Anz 1924;84:26–32.
1.30	Lorenté de No R. Etudes su l'anatomie et la physiologie du labyrinthe de l'oreille et du VIII 'nerv. Trav Lab Rech Biol Madrid 1926;24:53–153.
4.3, 4.4, 4.5, 4.6, 4.7, 4.8, 4.9A&B	Nager GT, Nager M. The arteries of the human middle ear, with particular regard to the blood supply of the auditory ossicles. Ann Otol Rhinol Laryngol 1953;62:923–950.
4.10	Axelsson A. The vascular anatomy of the cochlea in the guinea pig and in man. Acta Otolaryngol Suppl (Stockh) 1968;243:1–134.
4.11	Schuknecht HF, Gulya AJ. Anatomy of the temporal bone with surgical implications. Philadelphia: Lea & Febiger, 1986.
4.12	Axelsson A. The vascular anatomy of the cochlea in the guinea pig and in man. Acta Otolaryngol Suppl (Stockh) 1968;243:1–134.
4.13	Smith CA. Capillary area of the membranous labyrinth. Ann Otol Rhinol Laryngol 1954;63:435–447.
4.14, 4.15	Axelsson A. The vascular anatomy of the cochlea in the guinea pig and in man. Acta Otolaryngol Suppl (Stockh) 1968;243:1–134.
5.1	Paparella MM, Shumrick DA, Gluckman JL, Meyerhoff WI, eds. Otolaryngology, Vol II: Otology and neuro-otology. 3rd ed. Philadelphia: WB Saunders, Chap 20, 1991;II:1191–1226.
5.2	Anson BD. Morris' human anatomy. 12th ed. New York: McGraw-Hill, Sect X, Part II, 1966.
5.3, 5.4A–F, 5.5, 5.6, 5.7A–P, 5.8, 5.9	Paparella MM, Shumrick DA, Gluckman JL, Meyerhoff WI, eds. Otolaryngology, Vol II: Otology and neuro-otology. 3rd ed Philadelphia: WB Saunders, Chap 20, 1991;II:1191–1226.
5.10A, 5.11A	Lowry RB. The Nager syndrome (acrofacial dysotosis): evidence for autosomal dominant inheritance. Birth Defects 1977;13(3C):195–200.
5.12, 5.13, 5.14, 5.15A&B, 5.17, 5.18, 5.19A–C, 5.20A&B	Paparella MM, Shumrick DA, Gluckman JL, Meyerhoff WI, eds. Otolaryngology, Vol II: Otology and neuro-otology. 3rd ed. Philadelphia: WB Saunders, Chap 20, 1991;II:1191–1226.
5.21, 5.22, 5.23, 5.24, 5.25	Nager GT, Chen SCA, Hussels IE. A new syndrome in two females: Klippel-Feil deformity, conductive deafness and absent vagina. Birth Defects 1971;VII(6):311–317.
6.1	Mündnich K, Terrahe K. Missbildungen des Ohres. In: Berendes J, Link R, Zöllner F, eds. Hals-

Nasen-Ohrenheilkunde in Praxis und Klinik, Ohr I. Stuttgart: Georg Thieme, Chap 18, 1979;5:1–49.

7.1, 7.2, 7.3A&B, 7.4A&B, 7.5, 7.6A&B, 7.7A&B, 7.8A–F, 7.9A–Y, 7.10A&B, 7.11A&B	Proctor B, Nager GT. The facial canal: normal anatomy, variations and anomalies. Ann Otol Rhinol Laryngol 1982;91(5):33–61.
8.1A–F	Kennedy DN, El Sirsi HH, Nager GT. The jugular bulb in otologic surgery: anatomic, clinical and surgical considerations. Otolaryngol Head Neck Surg 1986;94(1):6–15.
8.3, 8.4	Nager GT. Paget's disease of the temporal bone. Ann Otol Rhinol Laryngol 1975;Suppl 22(3):1–32.
8.5A&B, 8.6A&B	Kennedy DN, El Sirsi HH, Nager GT. The jugular bulb in otologic surgery: anatomic, clinical and surgical considerations. Otolaryngol Head Neck Surg 1986;94(1):6–15.
8.7A–C, 8.8A&B, 8.9A–E	Nager GT. Paget's disease of the temporal bone. Ann Otol Rhinol Laryngol 1975;Suppl 22 (3):1–32.
8.10A–D	Nager GT, Stein SA, Dorst JP, et al. Sclerosteosis involving the temporal bone: clinical and radiologic aspects. Am J Otolaryngol 1983;4(1):1–17.
10.5.3A&B	Glorig A, Gerwin KS. Otitis media: pathology of acute and chronic otitis media and their complications. In: Proceedings of the national conference, Callier Hearing and Speech Center, Dallas, Texas. Springfield, Illinois: Charles C Thomas, 1972.
10.5.4A–D	Nager GT. Meningiomas involving the temporal bone: clinical and pathological aspects. Springfield, Illinois: Charles C Thomas, 1964.
12.1A–D	Nager GT. Mastoid and paranasal sinus infections and their relation to the central nervous system. Clin Neurosurg 1967;14:288–313.
12.2A, 12.3A&B, 12.4A&B, 12.6A&B, 12.8A&B, 12.10, 12.12A–G, 12.17, 12.18, 12.21C, 12.27A–D, 12.29B	Glorig A, Gerwin KS. Otitis media: pathology of acute and chronic otitis media and their complications. In: Proceedings of the national conference, Callier Hearing and Speech Center, Dallas, Texas. Springfield, Illinois: Charles C Thomas, 1972.
12.31	Proctor B, Nager GT. The facial canal: normal anatomy, variations and anomalies. Ann Otol Rhinol Laryngol 1982;91(5):33–61.
12.33, 12.34A–D, 12.35A–D, 12.36, 12.37A–D, 12.38, 12.39, 12.52, 12.53, 12.54A&B, 12.66	Nager GT. Mastoid and paranasal sinus infections and their relation to the central nervous system. Clin Neurosurg 1967;14:288–313.
13.5A–C	Nager GT. Meningiomas involving the temporal bone: clinical and pathological aspects. Springfield, Illinois: Charles C Thomas, 1964.
13.11A–D	Nager GT. Cholesteatomas of the middle ear: pathogenesis and surgical indication. In: McCabe BF, Sade G, Abramson M, eds. Cholesteatoma. First International Conference. Birmingham, Alabama: Aesculapius Publishing, 1977:193–203
13.12A&B, 13.13, 13.14A&B, 13.15, 13.16, 13.17, 13.18, 13.21	Nager GT. Theories on the origin of attic retraction cholesteatomas. In: Shambaugh GE Jr, ed. Fifth International Workshop on Middle Ear Microsurgery and Fluctuant Hearing Loss. Northwestern University Medical School, Chicago, Illinois, February 29–March 5, 1976. Huntsville, Alabama: Strode Publications, 1976.
13.19, 13.20	Nager GT. Cholesteatomas of the middle ear: pathogenesis and surgical indication. In: McCabe BF, Sade G, Abramson M, eds. Cholesteatoma. First International Conference. Birmingham, Alabama: Aesculapius Publishing, 1977:193–203
13.23A–C	Glorig A, Gerwin KS. Otitis media: pathology of acute and chronic otitis media and their complications. In: Proceedings of the national conference, Callier Hearing and Speech Center, Dallas, Texas. Springfield, Illinois: Charles C Thomas, 1972.
13.26A&B	Nager GT. Cholesteatomas of the middle ear: pathogenesis and surgical indication. In: McCabe BF, Sade G, Abramson M, eds. Cholesteatoma. First International Conference. Birmingham, Alabama: Aesculapius Publishing, 1977:193–203
13.27	Nager GT. Theories on the origin of attic retraction cholesteatomas. In: Shambaugh GE Jr, ed. Fifth International Workshop on Middle Ear Microsurgery and Fluctuant Hearing Loss. Northwestern University Medical School, Chicago, Illinois, February 29–March 5, 1976. Huntsville, Alabama: Strode Publications, 1976.
14.1.9	Glorig A, Gerwin KS. Otitis media: pathology of acute and chronic otitis media and their complications. In: Proceedings of the national conference, Callier Hearing and Speech Center, Dallas, Texas. Springfield, Illinois: Charles C Thomas, 1972.
14.4.1	Avery ME, McAfee JG, Guild HG. The course and prognosis of reticuloendotheliosis (eosinophilic granuloma. Schüller-Christian disease and Letterer-Siwe disease). Am J Med 1957;22:646–652.
15.3, 15.4, 15.14, 15.16, 15.18, 15.23, 15.33	Hyams VJ, Batsakis JG, Michaels L. Tumors of the upper respiratory tract and ear. Washington, DC: Armed Forces Institute of Pathology, 1988.
16.1, 16.6, 16.10	Hyams VJ, Batsakis JG, Michaels L. Tumors of the upper respiratory tract and ear. Washington, DC: Armed Forces Institute of Pathology, 1988.

17.7	Hyams VJ, Batsakis JG, Michaels L. Tumors of the upper respiratory tract and ear. Washington, DC: Armed Forces Institute of Pathology, 1988.
19.5	Hyams VJ, Batsakis JG, Michaels L. Tumors of the upper respiratory tract and ear. Washington, DC: Armed Forces Institute of Pathology, 1988.
20.2, 20.3, 20.5, 20.9	Hyams VJ, Batsakis JG, Michaels L. Tumors of the upper respiratory tract and ear. Washington, DC: Armed Forces Institute of Pathology, 1988.
21.8, 21.21,21.22,21.23, 21.24, 21.28, 21.29, 21.30, 21.31, 21.32, 21.35, 21.46, 21.49, 21.50, 21.52	Hyams VJ, Batsakis JG, Michaels L. Tumors of the upper respiratory tract and ear. Washington, DC: Armed Forces Institute of Pathology, 1988.
23.1, 23.3, 23.6, 23.7, 23.8A&B, 23.9, 23.10A–E	Nager GT. Acoustic neurionomas: pathology and differential diagnosis. Arch Otolaryngol 1969;89:68–95.
23.24	Nager GT. Association of bilateral VIIth nerve tumors with meningiomas in von Recklinghausen's disease. Laryngoscope 1964;74:1220–1261.
23.25, 23.26	Nager GT. Acoustic neurinomas: pathology and differential diagnosis. Arch Otolaryngol 1969;89:68–95.
23.27, 23.28, 23.29, 23.30, 23.31, 23.32, 23.33, 23.34, 23.35, 23.49, 23.50, 23.51	Nager GT. Association of bilateral VIIth nerve tumors with meningiomas in von Recklinghausen's disease. Laryngoscope 1964;74:1220–1261.
23.52	Nager GT. Meningiomas involving the temporal bone: clinical and pathological aspects. Springfield, Illiniois: Charles C Thomas, 1964.
24.1, 24.2, 24.3, 24.4, 24.5, 24.6, 24.7, 24.8, 24.9, 24.10, 24.11, 24.12, 24.13, 24.14, 24.15, 24.16, 24.17, 24.18, 24.19	Nager GT. Neurinomas of the trigeminal nerve. Am J Otolaryngol 1984;5:301–333
25.2	Proctor B, Nager GT. The facial canal: normal anatomy, variations and anomalies. Ann Otol Rhinol Laryngol 1982;91(5):33–61.
25.3, 25.4	Nager GT. Meningiomas involving the temporal bone: clinical and pathological aspects. Springfield, Illinois: Charles C Thomas, 1964.
25.5	Nager GT. Association of bilateral VIIth nerve tumors with meningiomas in von Recklinghausen's disease. Laryngoscope 1964;74:1220–1261.
27.1, 27.2, 27.3A&B, 27.4A–G, 27.5, 27.6A&B, 27.7, 27.8A–D, 27.9A&B	Nager GT. Meningiomas involving the temporal bone: clinical and pathological aspects. Springfield, Illinois: Charles C Thomas, 1964.
27.11A–D, 27.12, 27.13, 27.14A–C, 27.15A–C, 27.16A&B, 27.17, 27.18A&B, 27.19, 27.20A&B, 27.21, 27.22	Nager GT, Masica DN. Meningiomas of the cerebello-pontine angle and their relation to the temporal bone. Laryngoscope 1970;80:863–895.
27.25, 27.26, 27.27A–C, 27.28A–C, 27.29, 27.30, 27.31A–E	Nager GT. Meningiomas involving the temporal bone: clinical and pathological aspects. Springfield, Illinois: Charles C Thomas, 1964.
27.32, 27.33, 27.34A–C, 27.35A&B, 27.36A–C, 27.37, 27.38, 27.39, 27.40A&B	Nager GT, Heroy J, Hoeplinger M. Meningiomas invading the temporal bone with extension to the neck. Am J Otolaryngol 1983;4:297–324.
28.1, 28.2A&B, 28.3, 28.4A–E, 29.5A–E, 28.6, 28.7A&B, 28.8, 28.9A&B, 28.10A&B, 28.11A&B, 28.12, 28.13A–C, 28.14A–C, 28.15A–C, 28.16A&B, 28.17A&B, 28.18A&B, 28.19A–C, 28.20A&B, 28.21A&B	Nager GT. Gliomas involving the temporal bone: clinical and pathological aspects. Laryngoscope 1967;77:454–488.
30.1	Nager GT. Acoustic neurinomas: pathology and differential diagnosis. Arch Otolaryngol 1969;89:68–95.
30.2A&B, 30.3, 30.4A–D, 30.5A&B, 30.6A–D, 30.7A–C	Nager GT. Epidermoids involving the temporal bone: clinical, radiological and pathological aspects. Laryngoscope Suppl 2 1975;85(12):1–22.
30.7A–C, 30.8A–C, 30.9A–C, 30.10, 30.11A&B, 30.12, 30.13A&B	Nager GT. Epidermoids (congenital cholesteatomas) involving the temporal bone. Otolaryngology 1991;1:1–24.
30.14A&B, 30.15A–C	Nager GT. Epidermoids involving the temporal bone: clinical, radiological and pathological aspects. Laryngoscope Suppl 2 1975;85(12):1–22.
31.10A&B, 31.11A–C, 31.12A–C, 31.13A–E, 31.14	Kennedy DW, Nager GT. Glomus tumor and multiple endocrine neoplasia. Otolaryngol Head Neck Surg 1986;94:644–648.
36.1A–C, 36.2A–C, 36.3A–C	Nager GT. Meningiomas involving the temporal bone: clinical and pathological aspects. Springfield, Illinois: Charles C Thomas, 1964.
36.4	Hardy M, Crowe SJ. Early asymptomatic acoustic tumor. Report of six cases. Arch Surg 1936;32:292–301.
37.1	Nager GT. Acoustic neurinomas: pathology and differential diagnosis. Arch Otolaryngol 1969;89:68–95.
37.11A–F, 37.12A&B, 37.13	Taxy JB. Renal adenocarcinoma presenting as a solitary metastasis. Cancer 1981;48(9):2056–2062.

42.1A–C, 42.2A–C, 42.3, 42.4A–C, 42.5A–C, 42.6	Nager GT. Solitary (unicameral) cysts involving the temporal bone. Laryngoscope 1986;96:666–674.
43.1A&B	Glorig A, Gerwin KS. Otitis media: pathology of acute and chronic otitis media and their complications. In: Proceedings of the national conference, Callier Hearing and Speech Center, Dallas, Texas. Springfield, Illinois: Charles C Thomas, 1972.
43.7A–C, 43.8A–D, 43.9A&B, 43.10	Nager GT, Vanderveen, TS. Cholesterol granuloma involving the temporal bone. Ann Otol Rhinol Laryngol 1976;85:204–211.
44.1A–C, 44.2A–D, 44.3A–H, 44.7A–C, 44.9A–C	Nager GT. Histopathology of otosclerosis. Arch Otolaryngol 1969;89:157–179.
44.11	Nager GT. Clinical pathologic correlates of conductive deafness. Trans Am Acad Otolaryngol 1973;77:267–285.
44.12A–C, 44.14A&B	Nager GT. Histopathology of otosclerosis. Arch Otolaryngol 1969;89:157–179.
44.18, 44.19A–C, 44.20A&B, 44.21A&B, 44.22A&B, 44.23, 44.24, 44.25, 44.26A&B, 44.27A&B, 44.28, 44.29, 44.30, 44.31, 44.32, 44.33	Nager GT. Sensorineural deafness and otosclerosis. Ann Otol Rhinol Laryngol 1966:75:481–512.
44.34, 44.35, 44.36A–C, 44.37, 44.38, 44.39A–C, 44.40, 44.41, 44.42A&B, 44.43A-C, 44.44A–C, 44.45, 44.46, 44.47A–C	Nager GT, Jafek B. Histopathologic findings following surgical procedures for stapedial ankylosis. Ann Otol Rhinol Laryngol Suppl 15 1974;83(5):1–30.
44.48. 44.49	Nager GT. Ein Paar weiblicher eineiiger Zwillinge mit klinisch sowie anatomisch konkordanter Otosklerose und ahnlichem Horgewinn durch Fenestration. Acta Otolaryngol (Stockh) 1955;45:42–58.
45.3, 45.5, 45.13, 45.14, 45.19A&B, 45.20A&B, 45.21A–D, 45.22A&B, 45.23A&B, 45.24A&B, 45.25, 45.26A&B, 45.27, 45.28A&B, 45.29A&B, 45.30A&B, 45.31A–C, 45.32A&B, 45.33A&B, 45.34A&B, 45.35A&B, 45.36A&B, 45.37A&B, 45.38A&B	Nager GT. Paget's disease of the temporal bone. Ann Otol Rhinol Laryngol 1975;Suppl 22(3):1–32.
46.1, 46.2, 46.7A&B, 46.9, 46.25A&B, 46.27A&B, 46.29A, 46.34	Nager GT. Osteogenesis imperfecta of the temporal bone and its relation to otosclerosis. Ann Otol Rhinol Laryngol 1988;97(6):585–593.
47.1, 47.2	Uehlinger E. Fibröse Dysplasia (Jaffé-Lichtenstein): Osteofibrosis deformans juvenilis (Uehlinger); Albrightsches Syndrome. In: Schinz HR, Baensch WE, Frommhold W, Glauner R, Uehlinger E, Wellauer J, eds. Lehrbuch der Röntgendiagnostik. 6th ed. Band II/Teil I. Stuttgart: Georg Thieme, 1979;II:947–982.
47.3, 47.4A–C, 47.5A&B, 47.6, 47.7A–C, 47.8, 47.9A–C, 47.10, 47.11, 47.12, 47.13A&B, 47.14, 47.15A&B, 47.16, 47.17, 47.18A&B, 47.19, 47.20A&B, 47.21A–D, 47.22A&B, 47.23A&B, 47.24, 47.25, 47.26A&B, 47.27, 47.28, 47.29A&B, 47.30, 47.31A&B, 47.32, 47.33, 47.34, 47.35, 47.36, 47.37, 47.38, 47.39A&B, 47.40A&B, 47.41A–C, 47.42A–D	Nager GT, Kennedy DW, Lopstein E. Fibrous dysplasia: a review of the disease and its manifestations in the temporal bone. Ann Otol Rhinol Laryngol Suppl 92 1982;91(3):1–52.
47.43, 47.44, 47.45	Nager GT, Holliday MJ. Fibrous dysplasia of the temporal bone update with case reports. Ann Otol Rhinol Laryngol 1984;93:630–633.
48.3, 48.4, 48.5, 48.6, 48.7, 48.9, 48.10A–C, 48.11, 48.12, 48.13, 48.14, 48.15	Nager GT, Stein SA, Dorst JP, et al. Sclerosteosis involving the temporal bone: clinical and radiologic aspects. Am J Otolaryngol 1983;4(1):1–17.
48.16A&B, 48.17, 48.18B, 48.19A, 48.20, 48.21A&B, 48.22A&B, 48.23A&B, 48.24A&B, 48.25A&B, 48.26, 48.27A&B	Nager GT, Hamersma H. Sclerosteosis involving the temporal bone: histopathologic aspects. Am J Otolaryngol 1986;7:1–16.
50.1, 50.4B, 50.5B, 50.11A&B, 50.13B	Nager GT, Nager M. Multiple areas of necrosis and anaplerosis throughout the temporal bone. Ann Otol Rhinol Laryngol 1955;63:923–939.
50.15	Nager GT. Histopathology of otosclerosis. Arch Otolaryngol 1969;89:157–179.
50.16B, 50.19, 50.20	Nager GT, Nager M. Multiple areas of necrosis and anaplerosis throughout the temporal bone. Ann Otol Rhinol Laryngol 1955;63:923–939.
54.1A–F, 54.1G,H,J,K	Bordley JE, Brookhauser PE, Hardy J. Prenatal rubella. Acta Otolaryngol (Stockh) 1968;66:1–9.
47.1, 47.2, 47.3	Van Tilburg W. Fibrous dysplasia. In: Vinken PJ, Bruyn GW, eds. Handbook of clinical neurology. Amsterdam: North Holland Publishing, 1972;14:163–212.
54.1	Davies LE, Johnson LG. Viral infections of the inner ear: clinical, virologic, and pathologic studies in humans and animals. Am J Otolaryngol 1983;4(5):347–362.

Index

Numbers followed by *f* or *t* indicate page numbers for figures or tables, respectively.